Master the Boards
USMLE®

Step 2 CK

Sixth Edition

Other Titles by Conrad Fischer

Master the Boards USMLE® Step 3

Other Titles from Kaplan Medical

USMLE Step 2 CK Lecture Notes

Dr. Pestana's Surgery Notes

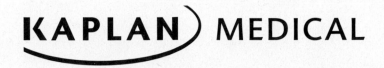

KAPLAN) MEDICAL

Master the Boards
USMLE®

Step 2 CK

Sixth Edition

Conrad Fischer, MD

© 2021, 2019, 2017, 2015, 2013, 2011 by Conrad Fischer, MD

The authors of the following sections have granted Conrad Fischer, MD, and Kaplan Publishing exclusive use of their work:

Victoria Hastings, DO, MPH, MS: Part 8, Obstetrics, and Part 9, Gynecology

Niket Sonpal, MD: Part 4, Surgery; Part 7, Pediatrics; and Part 16, Patient Safety

Alina Gonzales-Mayo, MD, Mena Mirhom, MD, and Niket Sonpal, MD: Part 12, Psychiatry

Philip J. Koehler III, DO, MS: Part 5, Sports Medicine

Published by Kaplan Publishing, a division of Kaplan, Inc.
1515 W. Cypress Creek Road
Fort Lauderdale, FL 33309

10 9 8 7 6 5 4 3 2
ISBN Retail: 978-1-5062-5458-6

10 9 8 7 6 5 4 3 2
ISBN Course: 978-1-5062-8038-7

Kaplan Publishing print books are available at special quantity discounts to use for sales promotions, employee premiums, or educational purposes. For more information or to purchase books, please call the Simon & Schuster special sales department at 866-506-1949.

Table of Contents

For Test Changes or Late-Breaking Developments

kaptest.com/retail-book-corrections-and-updates

The material in this book is up-to-date at the time of publication. However, the Federation of State Medical Boards (FSMB) and the National Board of Medical Examiners (NBME) may have instituted changes in the test after this book was published. Be sure to carefully read the materials you receive when you register for the test. If there are any important late-breaking developments—or any changes or corrections to the Kaplan test preparation materials in this book—we will post that information online at **kaptest.com/retail-book-corrections-and-updates.**

Conrad Fischer, MD, is program director of the Internal Medicine residency program at Brookdale University Hospital and Medical Center, as well as professor of medicine at Touro College of Osteopathic Medicine in New York City. He teaches USMLE Steps 1, 2, and 3; Internal Medicine Board Review and Attending Recertification; and USMLE Step 1 Physiology.

Section Authors

Niket Sonpal, MD, is assistant professor at Touro College of Osteopathic Medicine in New York City and a fellow of the American College of Physicians. He is a practicing gastroenterologist and hepatologist focusing on men's health and women's health and co-author of the best-selling books *Master the Boards: USMLE Step 2 CK* and *Master the Boards: USMLE Step 3.* Dr. Sonpal teaches USMLE, COMLEX, and American Board of Internal Medicine review.

Victoria Hastings, DO, MPH, MS, is a resident physician in obstetrics and gynecology at New York Presbyterian Brooklyn Methodist Hospital. She received her master of public health degree in biostatistics and epidemiology from Saint Louis University and her doctorate in osteopathic medicine with a master of science from NYIT College of Medicine. She is section editor of the obstetrics and gynecology chapters in *Master the Boards: USMLE Step 3.* She teaches obstetrics, gynecology, and biostatistics for USMLE Steps 1, 2, and 3.

Philip J. Koehler III, DO, MS, is a resident in physical medicine and rehabilitation. He completed an Osteopathic Manipulative Medicine (OMM) teaching fellowship at the Philadelphia College of Osteopathic Medicine.

Previous contributions by Elizabeth August, MD, Alina Gonzalez-Mayo, MD, and Mena Mirhom, MD.

Peer Reviewers/Section Editors

Pharmacology (throughout the book): Ed El Sayed

Cardiology: Yury Malyshev, Hal Chadow

Dermatology: Nikct Sonpal

Emergency Medicine: Sandra Scott

Endocrinology: Chris Paras

Fungal, Tropical, and Animal-Borne Diseases: Richard Cofsky

Gastroenterology: Niket Sonpal

Hematology: Hamza Minhas

Infectious Diseases: Richard Cofsky

Nephrology: Muhammad Bakhtyar Khan

Neurology: Alexander Andreev

Obstetrics/Gynecology: Victoria Hastings

Oncology: Hamza Minhas

Pediatrics: Conrad Fischer

Preventive Medicine: Herman Lebovitch

Psychiatry: Mena Mirhom, Peter You

Pulmonology: Seth Wenig, Sonu Shani

Radiology: Niket Sonpal

Rheumatology: Chris Paras

Sports Medicine: Philip Koehler

Surgery: Conrad Fischer

Acknowledgments

The authors wish to acknowledge the expert attention to detail of Dr. Ana Franceschi and Dr. Gabriel Vílchez Molina.

Niket Sonpal wishes to acknowledge Mr. Navin Sonpal, Mahendra Patel, Raj Patel, and Dr. Mukul Arya for their unwavering support, hope, and stance by me through thick and thin. Without them my path to becoming a physician would not have been possible.

Victoria Hastings wishes to acknowledge her husband, who lifts me up and pushes me to achieve great things.

Introduction

About the USMLE Step 2 CK Examination

The USMLE Step 2 CK (Clinical Knowledge) is typically taken as the second test in a series of 3 certifying examinations that are necessary to obtain a license to practice medicine in the United States. **Step 2 CK is usually taken in medical school between the end of years 3 and 4.**

- Step 2 CK is more clinically based than Step 1. Although there is no requirement to take Step 1 before Step 2 CK, that is the typical sequence for U.S. graduates. According to the test maker, the questions on Step 2 CK measure the ability to apply medical knowledge, skills, and understanding of clinical science as they pertain to patient care (under supervision), with emphasis on health promotion and disease prevention.

- Step 2 CS (Clinical Skills) is the second part of the USMLE Step 2 exam; it uses model patients to test the ability to perform in a real clinical setting.

> The most common mistake in preparation is doing the same single question bank over and over! Do **as many** different questions as you can.

Step 2 CK Examination Structure

USMLE Step 2 CK is a computer-based test that will not exceed 318 questions taken over a 9-hour period.

- Eight blocks, each one 60 minutes
- Once you have completed a block or 60 minutes has run out, you will not be able to go back to any questions in that block.
- The total break time throughout the day will be 45 minutes. The computer will keep track of your break time. Be sure not to exceed the 45 minutes or you will be penalized by having time deducted from your last block of the test.

USMLE Step 2 CK uses 2 types of questions: single best answer (most common type) and sequential.

> USMLE Step 2 CK questions have to be unequivocally clear. If an area is controversial, USMLE will avoid it, and ask only what is clear. The exam will not trick you.

Single Best Answer

The majority of Step 2 CK questions are multiple-choice questions that follow a clinical vignette. The basic structure is:

- History of present illness
- Physical examination
- Possibly laboratory and radiologic tests

There are 5 basic question types (and consequently, the very structure around which this book is created):

- What is the **most likely diagnosis?**
- What is the **best initial diagnostic test?**
- What is the **most accurate diagnostic test?**
- What **physical finding** is most likely to be associated with this patient?
- What is the **best initial therapy?**

> The phrase "most appropriate" can be very difficult to interpret. It is not always clear whether it means "first," "best," or "most accurate."

When the question reads: "**What is the most appropriate next step in management?**" this can refer to a test or a treatment. The phrase "most appropriate next step" can also be referred to as action, management, or simply what should you do next?

The most frequently asked question on Step 2 CK is "**What is the most likely diagnosis?**" As a result, many of the chapters in this book have a specific section labeled "What is the most likely diagnosis?" One of the many unique attributes of the *Master the Boards* format is that the diseases are presented with the specific goal of answering these questions.

Sequential

A smaller number of Step 2 CK questions are multiple questions that follow a single clinical story or vignette. Once you answer the first question, you will not be able to go back to the original question. That is because the second and third questions may give a clue to the answer to the first question.

Some of the questions in the sequence are *matching* questions, i.e., 4 and 26 separate answers are presented, and you must select the most appropriate one(s). Several cases may use the same answers. The answers can be used once, more than once, or not at all.

Score Reporting

You must answer 60–70% of questions correctly to get a passing score.

- Your correct answers are converted to a 3-digit score (as of publication, typically ranging from 190–280).
- Score reports and transcripts will show your 3-digit score and either "Pass" or "Fail." Score reports (but not transcripts) will also show your performance on certain topics, intended to help you assess your strengths and weaknesses.

As of publication, the 3-digit **passing score** was 209, but that score does (and will) increase over time. The reason is simple: Current medical students continue to improve their knowledge. The **average score** is currently 240, but that will also rise as students improve their knowledge.

There are always a number of new or experimental questions on each exam to test new questions for future exams. Every attempt is made to keep the exam fair and ensure it serves as an accurate measure of your knowledge level.

> USMLE Step 1 is moving to pass/fail. This raises the stakes for Step 2 CK enormously: it is the only chance you have to distinguish yourself from other candidates with a high score.

Registration

For the most accurate and up-to-date information about registration and Test Day procedures, go to usmle.org. At the time of publication, the registration fee is $645 for U.S. medical students and $965 for IMGs.

When to Take Step 2 CK

Frequently, medical students wonder when they should take Step 2 CK. The answer to that question depends on your background and level of knowledge.

- Remember, U.S. graduates do not have to take Step 2 CK in order to participate in the annual residency match. However, international graduates must take Step 2 CK to be ECFMG-certified, a requirement to participate in the match.
- The vast majority of U.S. graduates take Step 1 at the end of year 2 of medical school.
  - In fact, some schools require students to pass Step 1 in order to be allowed into year 3 and clinical rotations.
  - Some international schools—particularly those in the Caribbean in which virtually the entirety of the class is headed for residency in the United States—will soon follow this pattern as well.
  - Here is the bottom line: if there is no score on USMLE Step 1, it means the only chance you have to distinguish yourself from the other candidates is Step 2, making this test an enormously high-stakes exam.

Timing can be a factor for some U.S. graduates, too. For example, if you have a great Step 1 score and you are applying to a moderately competitive specialty, you may want to delay your Step 2 CK exam until after you have applied and interviewed for residency. The next section looks at some hypothetical scenarios.

Residency and the Exam

Another frequently asked question is, "How late can I take Step 2 CK and still be competitive in the match?" The Electronic Residency Application Service (ERAS) opens for applications in September.

- To be competitive, plan on having your application complete by the middle of September.
- You may think that program directors are sitting in their offices on opening day waiting for applications to come in over ERAS so they can give out interviews. That is not true.
- Many programs do not consider an application "complete" until they have received every single part of the application. Often, the Medical School Performance Evaluation (MSPE) does not go out from U.S. schools until October and, in some cases, November.

If you think it is better to fail than to pass with a low grade, you are wrong. **You cannot hide the grade on previous attempts at Step 2 CK.** It is better to delay your test than to risk a lower grade. Unfortunately, it is true that if you wait to take Step 2 CK until September or October, you will lose interview spots. However, if you take the test prematurely and fail or pass with a minimal score, that grade will follow you around through your entire application process. I would go so far as to say that **it would be better to sit out a year and fully prepare than take a chance on a failing or low grade**.

▶ **TIP**

Do not take the exam before you are ready. You cannot retake Step 2 CK if you pass with a poor grade. It is better to delay so that you can prepare more than to take the exam ill-prepared.

Students often wonder, "Is Step 1 or Step 2 CK more important to my future?" Step 1 may be perceived as a "harder" examination; however, the pass rate for first-time U.S. graduate test takers is about 93%. On the other hand, for many clinically oriented specialties, the perception may be that your performance on a clinically oriented examination such as Step 2 CK is more important than an examination more oriented to basic sciences. Step 2 CK is vastly more important than any other test because it is the *only* test that has a numeric score.

▶ **TIP**

Step 2 CK is the only exam with a score. Don't blow it! This is your main chance to shine.

> USMLE is the only worldwide, uniform measure across medical schools.

KAPLAN MEDICAL

What Do Program Directors Look For?

Program directors all agree on a few important criteria:

- Where you went to school
- USMLE Step 2 CK scores
- Transcript and MSPE (U.S. graduates)
- Visa status (international graduates)

Other criteria such as research, publications, recommendation letters, extra-curricular activities, and personal statement are much harder to define and are not universally valued.

- Some programs may highly prize research, while others may not even look at your publications until after you arrive for an interview.
- The personal statement often has no value because it says nothing personal or original about you at all.
- Letters of recommendation often all sound the same.

The reason that USMLE carries such importance is because it is the only world-wide, uniform measure across schools.

- If you are a U.S. medical student, how do you prove to a program director that you have greater value than a student applying from a school with a very highly prized and famous name? Your USMLE score may be the only thing that gives you an edge.
- If you are from a school with a highly prized and famous name, how do you prove that you are a better applicant than another candidate from a similarly highly prized and famous name school? The answer is your transcript and USMLE score.
- If you are an international graduate, how do you overcome the fact that you need a visa or perhaps you are applying as an older graduate? The answer is the same: your USMLE score.

Is this fair? Is it right? The system is generally fair. The test taken by U.S. and international graduates is the same. The test is not graded on a curve. That means that theoretically, everyone taking the test on a particular day could get a 270. Whether or not you think it's right, one thing we know for sure is that the USMLE is of colossal importance to your professional future.

How Do I Get Clinical Experience?

Nothing makes an international student more anxious than the programmatic requirement for "United States Clinical Experience." The truth is, unless you are at an international school that is specifically geared to return you to the United States, you are often simply not going to be able to get this U.S. experience. Do not worry!

An "observership" or "externship" is of extremely inconclusive value.

Many future doctors obtain residency each year as international graduates without U.S. clinical experience. A high score on Step 2 CK is also far more valuable than some "fake" experience where you "hang around" an office.

How is "observing" measurable? What did you do there? I know you will get anxious about this. If you can get meaningful U.S. experience, that's great; however, a higher score on Step 2 CK is always valuable.

After separating applicants into groups based on where they went to school and for international graduates based on their visa status, the program director often has no readily quantifiable way to assess the applicant. There is enormous pressure to make sure that the pool she selects into the residency is highly qualified. Research, observerships, and clinical grades are hard to measure.

- Is one school a harder grader than another?
- Does one school practice grade inflation so that all the transcripts show high grades?
- Does another school fail many students to prove they are serious?

These are all factors that may be considered. Take time to understand how your credentials stack up.

What If I Failed?

The best way to show that your failure on Step 2 CK is not an accurate measure of your ability, knowledge, or intelligence is to pass with a very high score when you DO pass.

If you failed Step 1, there is a lot riding on your Step 2 CK grade. This book is constructed to help you pass.

Take your time. Study day and night. If you need more practice, use question banks to prepare and assess your knowledge base. If necessary, delay the exam until you are ready.

Several years ago, the size of incoming classes in U.S. medical schools started to increase after more than 30 years with the same class size. In addition, many new schools are opening.

U.S. medical students pass Step 2 CK at a rate of ~93%, doctors of osteopathic medicine (DO) pass at a rate of ~92%, and international graduates pass at a rate of ~71%.

This has an enormous impact on both U.S. and international graduates. In prior years, simply being a U.S. graduate automatically put you in the top half of the applicant pool in many specialties. That is no longer true. The incoming class size for U.S. schools will be increasing by several hundred every year for the next several years. This will increase the competition for everyone trying to get a good residency position.

Author's Note

You have worked very hard to get into medical school and to do well there. This is your last step. A great score on Step 2 CK will mean that all of your professional dreams in medicine are about to come true.

Now is the time to learn everything in this book. You can rest later. Practice hard and remember that everything you are learning here is medicine. It will help people.

A high grade on Step 2 CK is not a phony numerical statistic. What you are learning here will, with 100% certainty, help someone. You will save lives. You will relieve suffering. You will do good for humanity. It is with this emotional power that you should go forth to work hard and to test the limits of your endurance.

What you learn here, through your heart and mind and the power of your hands, will protect those who suffer in their hour of need.

I wish you well in your quest. If you see what you are learning here as "a bunch of stuff to cram in that you will forget," you will not get as good a grade and the information will quickly fade. If you can study knowing that a sick person that you have not yet met is depending on you, their very life is depending on you, then you will absorb this energy and make the studying you must do an act of devotion.

We—you and I—commit ourselves at this moment to our sacred calling. To offer humanity the best of our art, and to put the needs of others above our own needs, now and always.

Dr. Conrad Fischer

PART 1

Internal Medicine

Esophageal Disorders

Dysphagia (difficulty swallowing) is the essential feature of most esophageal disorders. Alarm symptoms include blood in stool, anemia, and weight loss. If any of these symptoms are present, perform an endoscopy to exclude cancer.

Hiatal Hernia

Hiatal hernia is a protrusion of the upper part of the stomach into the chest, generally caused by obesity weakening the diaphragm. It is associated with heartburn, chest pain, and dysphagia; symptoms can be indistinguishable from GERD.

Diagnosis is made by endoscopy or barium study.

> Weight loss has limited value when diagnosing an esophageal disorder, since it is seen in both dysphagia and odynophagia (pain while swallowing).

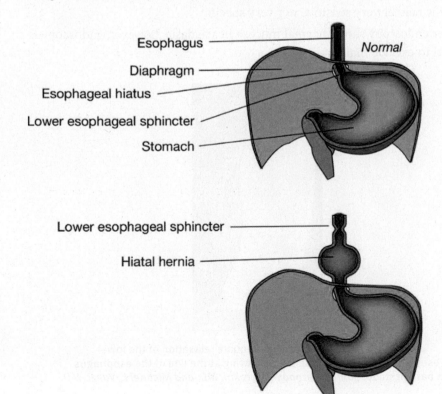

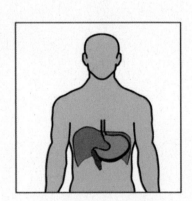

Figure 1.1 Sliding Hiatal Hernia. © Kaplan

The **best initial treatment** is weight loss and PPIs. If symptoms persist, proceed with surgical correction, e.g., Nissen fundoplication. Paraesophageal hernia is more likely to need surgery than gastric volvulus, obstruction, strangulation, and perforation.

Achalasia

Achalasia is the inability of the lower esophageal sphincter (LES) to relax due to a loss of the nerve plexus within the lower esophagus. The etiology is not clear. There is aperistalsis of the esophageal body.

"What Is the Most Likely Diagnosis?"

Look for:

- Young patient (age <50)
- Progressive dysphagia to both solids and liquids at the same time
- No association with alcohol or tobacco use

Diagnostic testing includes:

- Barium esophagram shows a "bird's beak" as the esophagus comes down to a point.
- Manometry ("**most accurate test**") will show a failure of the lower esophageal sphincter to relax.
- Chest x-ray may show some abnormal widening of the esophagus, but chest x-ray is neither very sensitive nor very specific.
- Upper endoscopy shows normal mucosa in achalasia; however, endoscopy is useful to exclude malignancy.

> In the esophagus, barium studies are acceptable to do first in most patients, although radiologic tests **always** lack the specificity of endoscopic procedures.

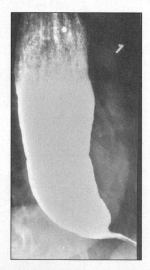

Figure 1.2 Achalasia, from inadequate relaxation of the lower esophageal sphincter; note the narrowing at the end of the esophagus on barium study. *Source: Farnoosh Farrokhi, MD, and Michael F. Vaezi, MD*

Treatment is simple mechanical dilation of the esophagus. There is no real "cure," i.e., nothing can restore the normal function of the missing neurological control of the esophagus.

- Pneumatic dilation (**highly effective**): placement of an endoscope that will allow a device to be inflated which will enlarge the esophagus
  - In <3% of patients, this treatment will cause perforation
  - Safer than surgery but slightly less effective; choosing between the two procedures may be difficult
- Surgical sectioning or myotomy to alleviate symptoms
- Botulinum toxin injection to relax the lower esophageal sphincter; however, the effects wear off in 3–6 months, requiring reinjection

> In the esophagus, only cancer and Barrett esophagus are diagnosed by biopsy.

Esophageal Cancer

"What Is the Most Likely Diagnosis?"

Look for:

- Age ≥50
- Dysphagia first for solids, followed later (progressing) to dysphagia for liquids
- Association with prolonged alcohol and tobacco use
- >5–10 years of GERD symptoms

> The single word *progressive* (or "from solids to liquids") is the **most important clue** to the diagnosis of esophageal cancer.

Diagnostic testing is as follows:

- Endoscopy is indispensable, since only a biopsy can diagnose cancer.
- Barium might be the **best initial test**, but no radiologic test can diagnose cancer.
- CT and MRI to determine the extent of spread into the surrounding tissues; they are not enough to diagnose esophageal cancer
- PET scan to determine the contents of anatomic lesions if uncertain whether they contain cancer; often used to determine whether a cancer is resectable

> For cancer, the radiologic test is **never** the "most accurate test."

> Local disease is resectable (removable), but widely metastatic disease is not.

Treatment is surgical resection. **No resection = no cure**. In addition, chemotherapy and radiation are used. For lesions that cannot be resected, stent placement can keep the esophagus open for palliation and to improve dysphagia.

Esophageal Spasm

The 2 forms of spastic disorders—diffuse esophageal spasm (DES) and nutcracker esophagus—are clinically indistinguishable. Both present with the sudden onset of chest pain unrelated to exertion. Initially, it is impossible to distinguish them from an atypical coronary artery spasm or unstable angina.

Symptoms include:

- Precipitated by drinking cold liquids
- Sudden, severe chest pain
- Normal EKG and stress test
- Normal esophagram and endoscopy

Diagnosis of DES and nutcracker esophagus (and distinguishing them) is done with manometry (**most accurate test**), which shows a different pattern of abnormal contraction in each.

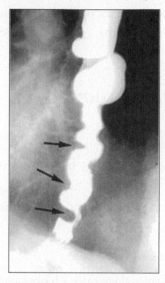

Figure 1.3 Esophageal spasm, as revealed by barium study, which shows a corkscrew appearance at the time of the spasm.
Source: Conrad Fischer, MD

Treatment of esophageal spastic disorders is as follows:

- CCBs (tricyclic antidepressants are an alternative); if those fail, sildenafil
- Nitrates (similar to treatment of Prinzmetal angina)
- PPIs in some cases

Eosinophilic Esophagitis

Patients with eosinophilic esophagitis have swallowing difficulty, food impaction, and heartburn. Look for a history of asthma and allergic diseases.

Endoscopy shows multiple concentric rings. The **most accurate test** is a biopsy finding eosinophils.

The **best initial treatment** is PPIs and the elimination of allergenic foods. If no response, swallowing steroid inhalers will allow for the topical use of steroids.

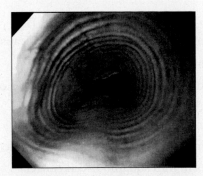

Figure 1.4 Eosinophilic Esophagitis. *Source: WikiCommons*

Infectious Esophagitis

A 43-year-old man recently diagnosed with AIDS comes to the ED with pain on swallowing that has become progressively worse over recent weeks. There is pain only when swallowing. CD4 count is 43 mm³. The patient is not currently taking any medications. What is the most appropriate next step in management?

a. Esophagram
b. Upper endoscopy
c. Oral nystatin swish and swallow
d. Intravenous amphotericin
e. Oral fluconazole

> The following pills cause esophagitis if in prolonged contact:
> - Doxycycline
> - Alendronate
> - Potassium chloride

Answer: E. The most commonly asked infectious esophagitis question is about esophageal candidiasis in a person with AIDS. Oral candidiasis (thrush) need not be present in esophageal candidiasis; one does not automatically follow from the other. Although other infections such as CMV and herpes can also cause esophageal infection, >90% of esophageal infections in patients with AIDS are caused by *Candida*. Empiric therapy with fluconazole is the best course of action; if that doesn't help, perform an endoscopy. Nystatin treats oral candidiasis; the oral "swish and swallow" form is not sufficient to control esophageal candidiasis. IV amphotericin is used for confirmed candidiasis that has not responded to fluconazole.

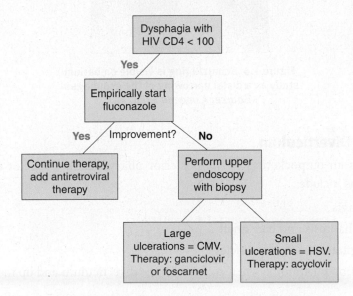

Figure 1.5 Management of Infectious Esophagitis

Rings and Webs

Schatzki ring and Plummer-Vinson syndrome both cause dysphagia.

- Schatzki ring is often caused by acid reflux
  - Associated with hiatal hernia, a type of scarring or tightening ("peptic stricture") of the distal esophagus
  - Associated with intermittent dysphagia
- Plummer-Vinson syndrome is associated with iron deficiency anemia
  - Can rarely transform into squamous cell cancer
  - Iron deficiency not caused by blood loss
  - More proximal than Schatzki
  - Rings are easily detected on barium studies of esophagus

Treatment is as follows:

- Schatzki ring: pneumatic dilation in an endoscopic procedure
- Plummer-Vinson syndrome: iron replacement at first, which may lead to resolution of the lesion

> "Steakhouse syndrome" is dysphagia from solid food, associated with Schatzki ring.

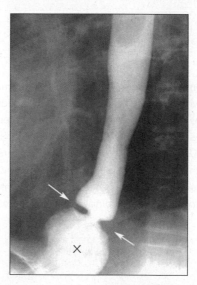

Figure 1.6 Schatzki ring is visible on barium study as a distal narrowing of the esophagus.
Source: Azmeena Laila, MD

Zenker Diverticulum

Zenker is an outpocketing of the posterior pharyngeal constrictor muscles. Symptoms include:

- Dysphagia
- Severe halitosis and bad smell
- Regurgitation of food particles
- Aspiration pneumonia when contents of the diverticulum end up in the lung

Diagnostic testing is barium study. Repair is made with surgery. There is no medical treatment.

▶ **TIP**

Do **not** answer nasogastric tube placement or upper endoscopy. These are dangerous to people with Zenker diverticulum and may cause perforation.

Scleroderma

Scleroderma patients present with symptoms of reflux and have a clear history of scleroderma or progressive systemic sclerosis. Manometry shows decreased lower esophageal sphincter pressure from an inability to close the LES.

Treatment is PPIs. The disorder is simply one of mechanical immobility of the esophagus.

▶ **TIP**

Manometry is the answer for achalasia, spasm, and scleroderma.

Mallory-Weiss Tear

Mallory-Weiss tear presents with upper GI bleeding after prolonged or severe vomiting or retching. Repeated retching is followed by hematemesis of bright red blood, or by black stool. There is no dysphagia.

There is no specific treatment, and it will resolve spontaneously. For severe cases with persistent bleeding, epinephrine injection or electrocautery can stop the bleeding.

Boerhaave syndrome is full penetration of the esophagus.

> Mallory-Weiss is a **nonpenetrating** tear of only the mucosa.

Epigastric Pain

The epigastric area is the part of the abdominal surface located just beneath the xiphoid process and between the 2 sets of ribs. It is above the umbilicus.

Pain in the epigastric area is common (up to 25% of the population at some point in their lives). Tenderness—increased pain on palpation or pressure in the epigastric area—is far less common.

> **Pain,** which is a complaint or sensation that is stated by the patient, is not the same thing as tenderness. **Tenderness** is a physical finding on examination.

A 44-year-old woman comes in reporting pain in the epigastric area for several months. She denies nausea, vomiting, weight loss, and blood in the stool. On physical examination no abnormalities are found. What is the most likely diagnosis?

a. Duodenal ulcer disease
b. Gastric ulcer disease
c. Gastritis
d. Pancreatitis
e. Functional dyspepsia
f. Pancreatic cancer

Answer: **E.** In the hospital, you will see far more patients with ulcer disease, pancreatic disorders, or cancer because those are the ones who are admitted. However, functional (non-ulcer) dyspepsia is by far the most common cause of epigastric pain (50–90% of all cases, especially age <60). Functional dyspepsia is virtually never a reason to be admitted to hospital.

How to Answer "What Is the Most Likely Diagnosis?" about Epigastric Pain	
If this is in the history:	**The most likely diagnosis is:**
Pain **worse** with food (70%)	Gastric ulcer
Pain **better** with food (70%)	Duodenal ulcer
Weight loss	Cancer, gastric ulcer
Tenderness	Pancreatitis
Bad taste, cough, hoarse	Gastroesophageal reflux
Diabetes, bloating	Gastroparesis
Nothing	Non-ulcer dyspepsia

> Patients hospitalized with epigastric pain are far more likely to have ulcers, biliary disease, pancreatic disease, cancer, and gastritis with bleeding.

Diagnostic Tests

Endoscopy is the only way to truly understand the etiology of epigastric pain from ulcer disease. Radiologic and barium testing are modest in accuracy at best. You cannot biopsy with radiologic testing.

> Only **endoscopy** can give a precise diagnosis.

▶ TIP

In the esophagus, barium study is a good place to start with testing, but in the stomach, barium is very poor.

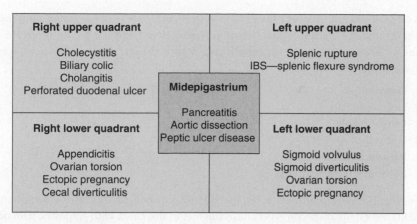

Right upper quadrant	Left upper quadrant
Cholecystitis Biliary colic Cholangitis Perforated duodenal ulcer	Splenic rupture IBS—splenic flexure syndrome

Midepigastrium

Pancreatitis
Aortic dissection
Peptic ulcer disease

Right lower quadrant	Left lower quadrant
Appendicitis Ovarian torsion Ectopic pregnancy Cecal diverticulitis	Sigmoid volvulus Sigmoid diverticulitis Ovarian torsion Ectopic pregnancy

Figure 1.7 Causes of Abdominal Pain by Location

Treatment of epigastric pains starts with PPIs. The various medications all have equal efficacy. Additionally:

- H2 blockers (nizatidine, cimetidine, famotidine) are less effective (but work in about 70% of patients)
- Liquid antacids (same efficacy as H2 blockers)

Gastroesophageal Reflux Disease

Gastroesophageal reflux disease (GERD) is the inappropriate relaxation of the lower esophageal sphincter, causing the acid contents of the stomach to come up into the esophagus. Symptoms of GERD are worsened by nicotine, alcohol, caffeine, chocolate, peppermint, late-night meals, and obesity.

There are no unique physical findings in GERD. It is a symptom complex most often diagnosed based on patient history. When the diagnosis is not clear, 24-hour pH monitoring may be considered to confirm the etiology.

Symptoms include sore throat, bad taste in the mouth (metallic), hoarseness, or cough. GERD may also show redness, erosions, ulcerations, strictures, or Barrett esophagus.

"What Is the Most Likely Diagnosis?"

GERD is the answer when you see "epigastric burning pain radiating up into the chest."

▶ TIP

You do not have to have **all** of these extra symptoms present in order to answer "GERD" as the most likely diagnosis.

> Misoprostol is always a wrong answer. Misoprostol, an artificial prostaglandin analogue, was designed to prevent NSAID-induced gastric damage. When PPIs arrived, misoprostol became obsolete—and a wrong answer on the test.

> USMLE Step 2 CK does **not** test dosing.

A 42-year-old man comes to the office with several weeks of epigastric pain radiating up under his chest which becomes worse after lying flat for an hour. He also has a "brackish" taste in his mouth and a sore throat. What is the next step in management?

a. Cimetidine
b. Liquid antacid
c. Lansoprazole
d. Endoscopy
e. Barium swallow
f. 24-hour pH monitoring

Answer: **C.** Lansoprazole is a PPI that should be used to control the symptoms of GERD. When the diagnosis is very clear (such as in this case), with epigastric pain going under the sternum, bad taste, and sore throat, confirmatory testing is not necessary. H2 blockers are effective in ~70% of patients but are clearly inferior to PPIs. Endoscopy does not diagnose GERD and is certainly not necessary when the diagnosis is so clear. Barium swallow shows major anatomic abnormalities of the esophagus and is worthless in GERD.

> Endoscopy will show nothing when there is only pyrosis (heartburn).

Endoscopy is indicated when there is:

- Signs of obstruction such as dysphagia or odynophagia
- Weight loss
- Anemia or heme-positive stools

Treatment starts with lifestyle management.

- Lose weight if obese
- Avoid alcohol, nicotine, caffeine, chocolate, mint
- Avoid eating within 3 hours of bedtime
- Elevate head of bed 6–8 inches

Additionally:

- **Mild or intermittent symptoms**: liquid antacids or H2 blockers
- **Persistent symptoms or erosive esophagitis**: PPIs (all equally effective)
- **Symptoms unresponsive to treatment** (5% of cases): surgical or anatomic correction to tighten the lower esophageal sphincter
  - Nissen fundoplication: wrapping the stomach around the lower esophageal sphincter
  - Endocinch: using a scope to place a suture around the LES to tighten it
  - Local heat or radiation of LES (causes scarring)

Barrett Esophagus

> Only endoscopy can determine the presence of Barrett esophagus.

Long-standing GERD leads to histologic changes in the lower esophagus with columnar metaplasia. Columnar metaplasia usually needs at least 5 years of reflux to develop. There are no unique physical findings or lab tests.

Biopsy is the only way to be certain of the presence of Barrett esophagus and/or dysplasia. This is indispensable because the biopsy drives treatment. Columnar metaplasia with intestinal features has the greatest risk of transforming into esophageal cancer.

> Each year, about 0.5% of people with **Barrett** esophagus progress to esophageal **cancer**.

Findings and Management	
Finding	**Management**
Barrett alone (metaplasia)	PPIs and rescope every 3–5 years
Low-grade dysplasia	PPIs and rescope every 6–12 months
High-grade dysplasia	Ablation with endoscopy: photodynamic therapy, radiofrequency ablation, endoscopic mucosal resection

Gastritis

Gastritis (sometimes called *gastropathy*) is inflammation or erosion of the gastric lining. Causes include:

- Alcohol
- NSAIDs
- *Helicobacter pylori*
- Portal hypertension
- Stress such as burns, trauma, sepsis, and multiorgan failure (e.g., uremia)

Atrophic gastritis is associated with vitamin B12 deficiency.

"What Is the Most Likely Diagnosis?"

Gastritis often presents with GI bleeding without pain. Severe, erosive gastritis can present with epigastric pain. NSAIDs or alcoholism in the history is a clue.

The GI bleeding can range from a mild "coffee-ground" emesis, to a large-volume vomiting of red blood, to a black stool (melena).

▶TIP

For gastritis, you cannot answer the "most likely diagnosis" question from the history and physical alone. There are no unique physical findings for gastritis.

Correlation of Manifestations with Volume of Bleeding	
Manifestation	**Volume of bleeding**
Coffee-ground emesis	5–10 mL
Heme (guaiac) positive stool	5–10 mL
Melena	50–100 mL

Diagnostic Tests

Only upper endoscopy can definitively diagnose erosive gastritis. Capsule endoscopy is not appropriate for upper GI bleeding if endoscopy is one of the choices.

Testing for *Helicobacter pylori* should also be performed because it would require treatment.

Although anemia may occur, there are no specific blood tests. Radiologic studies such as an upper GI series will not be specific enough.

Testing for *Helicobacter pylori*		
The test	**What is good about this test?**	**What is bad about this test?**
Endoscopic biopsy	The most accurate of all the tests	Requires an invasive procedure such as endoscopy
Serology	Inexpensive, easily excludes infection if it is negative	Lacks specificity; a positive test does not easily tell the difference between current and previous infection (rarely right)
Urea C^{13} or C^{14} breath testing	Positive only in active infection; 95% sensitive and specific	Requires expensive equipment in office
***H. pylori* stool antigen**	Positive only in active infection; 95% sensitive and specific	Requires stool sample

Treatment is PPIs. H2 blockers, sucralfate, and liquid antacids are not as effective.

> MALToma causes a false-negative *H. pylori* stool antigen.

Sucralfate is an inert substance (aluminum hydroxide complex) that coats the stomach. If sucralfate is presented as an answer choice on the exam, it is nearly always the wrong answer.

> **Stress ulcer prophylaxis is indicated in:**
> - Mechanical ventilation
> - Burns
> - Head trauma
> - Coagulopathy

Peptic Ulcer Disease

Peptic ulcer disease (PUD) includes duodenal ulcer (DU) and gastric ulcer (GU) disease. Causes of PUD include:

> The name "peptic ulcer disease" is a misnomer, based on the mistaken belief that the conditions were caused by the protein-digesting enzyme *pepsin*.

- *Helicobacter pylori* (**most common**)
- NSAIDs (**second most common**), due to their effect in inhibiting the production of the protective mucus barrier in the stomach
  - NSAIDs inhibit prostaglandins, and prostaglandins produce the mucus
  - NSAIDs produce more bleeding than pain
- Burns, head trauma, Crohn disease, gastric cancer, and gastrinoma (Zollinger-Ellison) (all less common)

▶ **TIP**

Alcohol and tobacco do **not** cause ulcers. They delay the healing of ulcers.

"What Is the Most Likely Diagnosis?"

PUD presents with recurrent episodes of epigastric pain that is described as dull, sore, and gnawing. Although the most common cause of upper GI bleeding is PUD, the majority of those with ulcers do not bleed. Tenderness and vomiting are unusual.

You cannot answer PUD as the "most likely diagnosis" based on symptoms alone.

Testing includes:

- Upper endoscopy (**most accurate test**) to distinguish DU and GU.
  - In those who are to undergo endoscopy, there is no point in doing noninvasive testing such as serology, breath testing, or stool antigen detection.
  - Endoscopy is the only method for detecting gastric cancer; cancer is present in 4% of those with GU but in none of those with DU.
- Radiologic testing, e.g., upper GI series, to detect ulcers (but cannot detect cancer or *H. pylori*)
- *H. pylori* testing: biopsy (**most accurate test**)

> - There is no way to diagnose PUD without endoscopy or barium studies.
> - There is no way to distinguish DU, GU, gastritis, and nonulcer dyspepsia without endoscopy.

> Changes in pain with eating are not specific enough to make a diagnosis of DU vs. GU.

Treatment is as follows:

- For PUD: PPIs (effective in far majority of cases) but will recur unless *H. pylori* is eradicated
  - DU is associated with *H. pylori* in >80–90% of cases
  - GU is associated with *H. pylori* in 50–70% of cases
- For *H. pylori*: PPIs + 2 antibiotics
  - Clarithromycin and amoxicillin is preferred
  - If no response, metronidazole, levofloxacin, or tetracycline are alternatives (**note this is the only use of tetracycline**)
  - Adding bismuth to a change of antibiotics may help to resolve treatment-resistant ulcers
  - Retest with stool antigen or breath test to confirm eradication of *Helicobacter*
  - Repeat endoscopy (for those with GU) to exclude cancer as a reason for not getting better

> Previous clarithromycin use for other reasons gives 30% failure in its use to treat *H. pylori*.

> Don't treat asymptomatic *Helicobacter*.

The only way to exclude cancer is with biopsy. You can test for *H. pylori* with noninvasive methods and treat it, but you cannot exclude gastric cancer noninvasively.

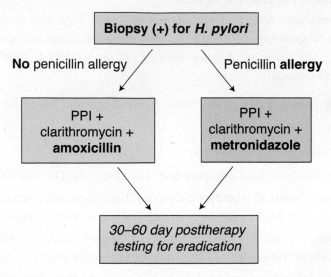

Figure 1.8 *Helicobacter pylori* Treatment in PUD

A 56-year-old woman comes to the clinic because her symptoms of epigastric pain from an endoscopically confirmed duodenal ulcer have not responded to several weeks of a PPI, clarithromycin, and amoxicillin. What is the most appropriate next step in management?

a. Refer for surgery
b. Switch the PPI to H2 blocker
c. Abdominal CT scan
d. Capsule endoscopy
e. Urea breath testing
f. Vagotomy
g. Add sucralfate

Answer: **E.** If there is no response to DU therapy with PPIs, clarithromycin, and amoxicillin, the first thought should be antibiotic resistance of the organism. Persistent *H. pylori* infection can be detected with urea breath testing, stool antigen detection, or a repeat endoscopy for biopsy. It would be very hard to choose between these, and that is why they are not all given as choices in this question. Capsule endoscopy cannot detect *H. pylori*. H2 blockers and sucralfate add nothing to a PPI and have less efficacy, not more.

> Stress ulcer prophylaxis *only* with:
> - Head trauma
> - Burns
> - Intubated patient
> - Sepsis **with** coagulopathy

> **Treatment failure most often stems from:**
> - Bacterial resistance
> - Nonadherence to medications
> - Alcohol
> - Tobacco
> - NSAIDs

Functional (Non-Ulcer) Dyspepsia

Functional (non-ulcer) dyspepsia (NUD) is epigastric pain that has no identified etiology. It can only be diagnosed after endoscopy. The pain of NUD can be identical to gastritis, PUD, gastric cancer, or reflux disease.

NUD is the most common cause of epigastric pain.

Treatment is as follows:

- **Age <60**: treat empirically with antisecretory therapy such as PPIs and scope only if symptoms do not resolve.
- **Age >60**: endoscopy is definitely indicated to exclude cancer.

NUD is not definitely associated with *H. pylori*; however, if symptoms do not resolve with initial therapy and *H. pylori* is present, you should try to treat it.

Symptoms persist + *H. pylori* present = Treat for *H. pylori*

> **Scope for dyspepsia** if patient is age >60, "alarm" symptoms are present (dysphagia, weight loss, anemia), or PPIs fail to control symptoms.

Functional dyspepsia is epigastric pain with a normal endoscopy.

Gastrinoma (Zollinger-Ellison Syndrome)

Less than 1% of those with ulcer disease have a gastrinoma.

"What Is the Most Likely Diagnosis?"

Look for a patient with ulcers that are:

- **Large** (>1–2 cm)
- **Recurrent** after *Helicobacter* eradication
- **Distal** in the duodenum
- **Multiple**

Once endoscopy confirms the presence of an ulcer, the most accurate diagnostic tests include:

- Lab testing (any of the following will confirm diagnosis)
  - High gastrin level off antisecretory therapy (PPIs or H2 blockers)
  - High gastrin level despite a high gastric acid output
  - Persistent high gastrin level despite injecting secretin
- Imaging (once diagnosis has been confirmed) to exclude metastatic disease
  - Abdominal CT/MRI is done first but has poor sensitivity, i.e., a negative test does not exclude metastases.
  - If CT/MRI is normal, somatostatin receptor scintigraphy (nuclear octreotide scan) is combined with endoscopic U/S to exclude metastatic disease.

Gastrinoma is often associated with **diarrhea** because **acid inactivates lipase**.

Hypercalcemia is the clue for multiple endocrine neoplasia from hyperparathyroidism.

> Gastrinoma is associated with a massive increase in the number of somatostatin receptors in the abdomen.

The **most accurate test** is always a functional test, such as looking at the response to secretin.

Local disease is removed surgically. Metastatic disease is unresectable and is treated with lifelong PPIs to block acid production.

Diabetic Gastroparesis

Longstanding diabetes leads to gastric dysmotility. Distention of the stomach and intestines is normally the most important stimulant to motility.

Gastroparesis is an autonomic neuropathy leading to dysmotility, caused by an inability to sense stretch in the GI tract.

"What Is the Most Likely Diagnosis?"

Look for a diabetic patient with chronic abdominal discomfort, "bloating," and constipation. There is also anorexia, nausea, vomiting, and early satiety.

> A 64-year-old patient with diabetes for 20 years comes to the office with several months of abdominal fullness, intermittent nausea, constipation, and a sense of "bloating." On physical examination, a "splash" is heard over the stomach on auscultation of the stomach when moving the patient. What is the most appropriate next step in management?
>
> a. Abdominal CT scan
> b. Colonoscopy
> c. Erythromycin
> d. Upper endoscopy
> e. Nuclear gastric emptying study
>
> Answer: **C.** When the diagnosis of diabetic gastroparesis seems clear, there is no need to do diagnostic testing unless there is a failure of therapy. Erythromycin or metoclopramide increases gastrointestinal motility. The most accurate test for diabetic gastroparesis is the nuclear gastric emptying study, although it is rarely needed.

Since diabetes can also be associated with GERD and diarrhea, confirmatory testing may be needed.

- **Best initial test**: upper endoscopy or abdominal CT to exclude a luminal gastric mass or an abdominal mass compressing the stomach
- **Most accurate test**: bolus of food tagged with technetium, a nuclear isotope; a delay in the emptying of food indicates gastroparesis

Treatment starts with dietary modification: blenderized foods, restored fluids, and corrected potassium and glucose levels.

- If no response to dietary modification, start metoclopramide. This will induce tardive dyskinesia, dystonia, and movement disorder in 1% of patients; other adverse effects are long QT and hyperprolactinemia.
- If metoclopramide is ineffective, answer erythromycin and antiemetics.
- If all medical treatment fails, do gastric electrical stimulation (gastric pacemaker).

> Metoclopramide *cannot* be used permanently: Dystonia and hyperprolactinemia will develop.

Gastrointestinal Bleeding

Upper and lower GI bleeds arise from 2 general groups of etiologies.

Etiology of Gastrointestinal Bleeding		
Location	**Upper**	**Lower**
Most common cause	Ulcer disease	Diverticulosis
Other causes	Esophagitis Gastritis Cancer Duodenitis Varices	Angiodysplasia Polyps IBD Cancer Upper GI bleeding Hemorrhoids

A 69-year-old woman comes to the ED with multiple red/black stools over the last day. Her medical history is significant for aortic stenosis. Her pulse is 115/min and blood pressure is 94/62 mm Hg. Physical examination is otherwise normal. What is the most appropriate next step in management?

a. Colonoscopy
b. Nasogastric tube placement
c. Upper endoscopy
d. Bolus of normal saline
e. CBC
f. Bolus of 5% dextrose in water
g. Consult gastroenterology
h. Check for orthostasis

Answer: **D.** Identifying the etiology of severe GI bleed is not as important as giving fluid resuscitation. There is no point in checking for orthostasis with the patient's systolic BP <100 mm Hg or when there is a tachycardia at rest. Endoscopy should be performed, but not as a first step. When BP is low, normal saline (NS) or Ringer lactate are better fluids to give than 5% dextrose in water (D5W). D5W does not stay in the vascular space to raise BP as well as NS.

> Assessing BP is the most important initial management for GI bleed.

Ischemic Colitis

Older patients with a history of DM, hypertension, and vascular disease are susceptible to ischemic colitis. It presents with left lower quadrant pain, mucosal friability on scope, and a clear demarcation between ischemic and normal tissue. It spares the rectum.

The condition is not life-threatening, and bleeding resolves without specific treatment.

Physical symptoms include:

- Orthostasis (>10-point rise in pulse when going from lying down to sitting/standing or ≥20 point drop in systolic BP when sitting up)
- Variceal bleeding (only form of GI bleed in which physical examination helps determine etiology)
  - The presence of the signs of liver disease helps establish the diagnosis.
  - Suspect variceal bleed when symptoms include vomiting blood +/□ black stool, spider angiomata and caput medusa, splenomegaly, palmar erythema, and/or asterixis

> - Initial management of GI bleeding is not based on the etiology; it is based on the severity.
> - For acute bleeding—especially when severe—it is far more important to replace fluids, check the hematocrit, platelets, and run coagulation tests such as PT or INR than it is to do an endoscopy.

Severity of Blood Loss Based on Hemodynamics	
Physical finding	**Percentage of blood loss**
Orthostasis	15–20%
Pulse >100 per minute	30%
Systolic BP <100 mm Hg	30%

Diagnostic testing is with nasogastric (NG) tube, but this has limited benefit. There is no treatment to be delivered through the NG tube, but it can guide where to start with endoscopy. If upper endoscopy will be done anyway, NG tube has a limited role.

- About 10% of those with red blood from the rectum have high-volume upper GI bleeding with "rapid transit time."
- The sensitivity of the NG tube is 70%. If you see bile in the aspirate, however, then you know the NG tube aspirate really is >95% sensitive.
- If the stool is black in a person with cirrhosis but there is no hematemesis, an NG tube showing red blood may tell you to use octreotide for varices and arrange urgent endoscopy for possible "banding" of varices.

> **80% of GI bleeding will stop spontaneously if the fluid resuscitation is adequate.** Most patients die of inadequate fluid replacement.

Additional Diagnostic Tests for GI Bleeding	
Test	**Indication**
Nuclear bleeding scan	Endoscopy unrevealing in a massive acute hemorrhage; lacks accuracy
Angiography	Specific vessel or site of bleeding needs to be identified prior to surgery or embolization of the vessel; used only in massive, nonresponsive bleeding
Capsule endoscopy	Small bowel bleeding; upper and lower endoscopy do not show the etiology
CT or MRI of abdomen	Not useful in GI bleeding
EKG, lactate level	Shows ischemia in severe bleeding

Treatment is as follows:

- **Fluid replacement** with high volumes (1–2 liters per hour) of saline or Ringer lactate in those with acute, severe bleeding
- **Packed red blood cells** if hematocrit <30 if patient is older or suffers from coronary artery disease; if patient is young, transfusion may not be needed until the hematocrit is very low (<20–25)
- **Fresh frozen plasma** if the PT or INR is elevated and active bleeding is occurring
- **Platelets** if <50,000 and there is bleeding
- **Reversal of anticoagulants**: andexanet alfa reverses Xa inhibitors (rivaroxaban, apixaban, edoxaban): idarucizumab reverses dabigatran; and prothrombin complex concentrate (PCC) reverses warfarin
- Endoscopy to determine the diagnosis and administer some treatment (band varices, cauterize ulcers, inject epinephrine into bleeding gastric vessels)
- IV PPI for upper GI bleeding
- Surgery to remove the site of bleeding if fluids, blood, platelets, and plasma will not control the bleeding

▶ TIP

Platelets are transfused when count is <50,000/μL and there is active bleeding. You would not transfuse platelets to prevent a spontaneous bleed unless the count was much lower (<10,000–20,000).

Esophageal and Gastric Varices

What do you do in addition to administering fluids, blood, platelets, and plasma?

- Octreotide (somatostatin) decreases portal pressure.
- Banding performed by endoscopy obliterates esophageal varices.
- Transjugular intrahepatic portosystemic shunting (TIPS) is used to decrease portal pressure in those who are not controlled by octreotide and banding.
- Propranolol or nadolol is used to prevent subsequent episodes of bleeding. Beta blockers such as propranolol will not do anything for the current episode of bleeding.
- Antibiotics to prevent spontaneous bacterial peritonitis (SBP) if ascites is present.
- Blakemore tube or balloon tamponade is rarely used as a temporary measure before TIPS procedure.

> Sclerotherapy is never the right answer if banding is technically possible.

Diarrhea

Antibiotic-Associated Diarrhea

Although clindamycin may be associated with the highest incidence of antibiotic-associated diarrhea and *Clostridioides difficile* (*C. diff*), any antibiotic can potentially cause diarrhea. Blood and white blood cells may be present in the stool. It usually presents several days or weeks after the start of antibiotics.

> For a patient with positive *C. diff* stool toxin but no symptoms, there is no treatment needed.

The best initial test is a stool *C. diff* toxin test. The most accurate test is PCR or NAAT.

Treatment is oral vancomycin (**most effective initial therapy**). If there is no response, switch to fidaxomicin.

> A 75-year-old man is admitted to the hospital with pneumonia. Several days after the start of antibiotics, he begins to have diarrhea. The stool *C. diff* toxin is positive, and he is started on vancomycin, which resolves the diarrhea after a few days. Two weeks later the diarrhea recurs and the *C. diff* toxin is again positive. What is the most appropriate next step in management?
>
> a. Treat with metronidazole orally.
> b. Retreat with vancomycin.
> c. Perform sigmoidoscopy, and treat only if pseudomembranes are found.
> d. Treat with metronidazole intravenously.
> e. Wait for stool culture.
> f. Treat with vancomycin intravenously.
>
> Answer: **B**. Recurrent episodes of *C. diff*-associated diarrhea are best treated with another course of vancomycin. Intravenous metronidazole is used only if oral therapy cannot be used, such as in a patient with an adynamic ileus. Stool is never cultured for *C. diff* because it simply will not grow in culture. Endoscopy looking for pseudomembranes will diagnose antibiotic-associated diarrhea but is not a necessary step given the availability of stool toxin assay.

> **Intravenous vancomycin** is always wrong for antibiotic-associated diarrhea since it will not pass the bowel wall.

Several considerations come to play in the treatment of *C. diff*:

- Both vancomycin (preferred) and fidaxomicin have better efficacy than metronidazole.
- Vancomycin is less expensive than fidaxomicin.
- If vancomycin is preferred but cannot be given orally, it can be given by enema.
- If there is a recurrence after vancomycin, give a tapered dose of vancomycin or fidaxomicin.
- After multiple recurrences, use bezlotoxumab or do fecal transplantation. Bezlotoxumab is an antibody against *C. diff* toxin.
- For fulminant, life-threatening infection, use vancomycin plus metronidazole.

> What is fulminant *C. diff*?
> - High WBC (>15,000)
> - Metabolic acidosis
> - High lactate
> - High creatinine (1.5× baseline)

▶ **TIP**

Switching to fidaxomicin is the answer when the case does not respond to vancomycin.

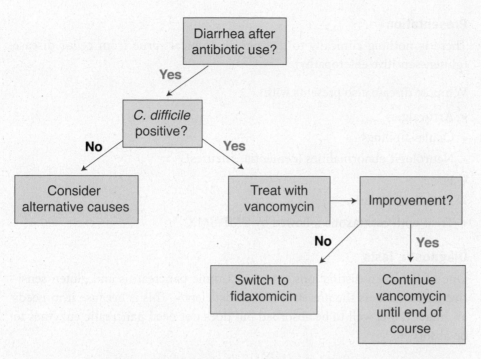

Figure 1.9 Antibiotic-Associated Diarrhea Algorithm

Malabsorption

Celiac disease is one of the most common types of malabsorption and can present as an adult. Chronic pancreatitis has a very similar presentation with fat malabsorption. Rare causes of fat malabsorption are tropical sprue and Whipple disease. All of these present with steatorrhea, defined as stool that is oily, greasy, floating, and foul-smelling.

All forms of fat malabsorption present with deficiency of fat-soluble vitamins such as vitamins A, D, E, and K. Hence, they can all present with the following:

Deficiencies and Manifestations	
Deficiency	**Manifestation**
Vitamin D	Hypocalcemia, osteoporosis
Vitamin K	Bleeding, easy bruising
Vitamin B12	Anemia, hypersegmented neutrophils, neuropathy

▶ **TIP**

Fat malabsorption frequently presents with **weight loss.**

Celiac disease is associated with:

- Thyroiditis
- Vitiligo
- Pernicious anemia
- Type I diabetes

Vitamin B12 needs an intact bowel wall **and** pancreatic enzymes to be absorbed.

Presentation

There is nothing clinically to distinguish tropical sprue from celiac disease (gluten-sensitive enteropathy).

Whipple disease also presents with:

- Arthralgias
- Ocular findings
- Neurologic abnormalities (dementia, seizures)
- Fever
- Lymphadenopathy
- Treat with ceftriaxone followed by TMP/SMX

Diagnostic Tests

One of the main distinctions between chronic pancreatitis and gluten sensitive enteropathy is the presence of iron deficiency. This is because iron needs an intact bowel wall to be absorbed but does not need pancreatic enzymes to be absorbed.

Unique tests for celiac disease:

- Anti-tissue transglutaminase (TTG) is the first test (can be falsely negative in IgA deficiency).
- Antiendomysial antibody
- IgA antigliadin antibody

The **most accurate diagnostic test** for celiac disease is a small bowel biopsy that shows flattening of the villi. Whipple disease and tropical sprue are also most accurately diagnosed with a bowel wall biopsy showing the specific organism.

Chronic Pancreatitis

Diagnostic testing includes:

- Abdominal x-ray: 50–60% sensitive for calcification of the pancreas
- Abdominal CT: 80–90% sensitive for pancreatic calcification
- MRCP or EUS with secretin enhancement is more accurate than CT scan
- Secretin stimulation test (**most accurate test**)
  - Place a nasogastric tube
  - Administer an IV injection of secretin
  - A normal pancreas will release a large volume of bicarbonate-rich fluids

---

> Celiac disease gives dermatitis herpetiformis in 10% of cases.

> Rice and wine are safe in celiac disease.

> Bowel biopsy is essential in celiac disease to exclude lymphoma.

> The abdominal x-ray is very specific for chronic pancreatitis when the test is abnormal.

> The angiotensin receptor blocker olmesartan gives a sprue-like illness.

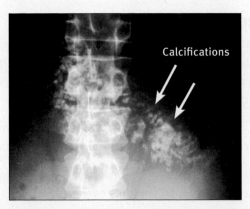

Figure 1.10 Chronic pancreatitis leads to calcification of the pancreas, visible on x-ray in 50–60% of patients. *Source: Conrad Fischer, MD.*

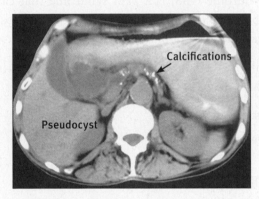

Figure 1.11 Abdominal CT scan has greater sensitivity and specificity in the detection of calcifications of the pancreas. *Source: Conrad Fischer, MD*

Treatment	
Disease	**Specific treatment**
Chronic pancreatitis	Enzyme replacement
Celiac disease	Avoid gluten-containing foods such as wheat, oats, rye, or barley
Whipple disease	Ceftriaxone, trimethoprim/sulfamethoxazole
Tropical sprue	Trimethoprim/sulfamethoxazole, doxycycline

> The D-xylose test is an old test that distinguished pancreatitis from bowel wall abnormalities. D-xylose test results are normal in pancreatic disorders.

Carcinoid Syndrome

Carcinoid syndrome presents with intermittent diarrhea in association with:

- Flushing
- Wheezing
- Cardiac abnormalities of the right side of the heart

The best initial diagnostic test is the urinary 5-hydroxyindoleacetic acid (5 HIAA) test. Treatment is octreotide, a synthetic version of somatostatin, to control the diarrhea.

Lactose Intolerance

No weight loss is associated with lactose intolerance because lactose is only one of several sugars to absorb. Lactose intolerance does not alter the absorption of any other nutrient such as fat, so there is no deficiency in calories. Vitamins are absorbed normally. Stool osmolality is increased.

Diagnosis is typically made by removing all milk-containing products from the diet and waiting a single day for resolution of symptoms.

Treatment is the avoidance of milk products, except yogurt. Oral lactase replacement is also effective and available over the counter.

Irritable Bowel Syndrome

Irritable bowel syndrome (IBS) is a pain syndrome that can have diarrhea, constipation, or both. IBS is not associated with weight loss. Pain does not automatically mean malabsorption.

There is no specific diagnostic test for IBS. It is a diagnosis of exclusion in association with a complex of symptoms.

The pain of IBS is:

- Relieved by a bowel movement
- Less at night
- Relieved by a change in bowel habit such as diarrhea

IBS is not associated with blood or WBCs in the stool.

Treatment is as follows:

- Fiber in the diet
- Antispasmodic agents such as hyoscyamine, dicyclomine, peppermint oil
- Tricyclic antidepressants (e.g., amitriptyline or SSRIs)

Additional treatment for **diarrhea-predominant IBS**:

- Rifaximin: nonabsorbed antibiotic with modest effect in diarrhea-predominant IBS
- Alosetron: inhibitor of serotonin with modest effect in IBS; needs special permissions to use
- Eluxadoline: mu-opioid receptor agonist for diarrhea IBS; relieves pain/slows bowel
- Probiotics: unclear (on the exam, do not choose)

Additional treatment **constipation-predominant IBS**:

- Fiber
- Polyethylene glycol (PEG): nonabsorbed bowel lubricant
- Lubiprostone (chloride channel activator): use if PEG doesn't work
- Linaclotide (guanylate cyclase agonist): use if PEG doesn't work

Inflammatory Bowel Disease

Inflammatory bowel disease (IBD) is an idiopathic disorder that presents with diarrhea, blood in the stool, weight loss, and fever. Both Crohn disease (CD) and ulcerative colitis (UC) have extraintestinal manifestations that can be identical in both diseases. These are:

- Arthralgias
- Uveitis, iritis
- Skin manifestation (erythema nodosum, pyoderma gangrenosum)
- Sclerosing cholangitis (more frequent in UC)

Both forms of IBD can lead to colon cancer. The risk of colon cancer is related to the duration of involvement of the colon. CD that involves the colon has the same risk of colon cancer as UC.

> Erythema nodosum is an indicator of disease activity.

> Pyoderma and primary sclerosing cholangitis do not change with the disease activity of IBD.

CD versus UC	
Crohn disease	**Ulcerative colitis**
Skip lesions	Curable by surgery
Transmural granulomas	Entirely mucosal
Fistulas and abscesses	No fistulas, no abscesses
Masses and obstruction	No obstruction
Perianal disease	No perianal disease

When should screening occur?

- After 8–10 years of colonic involvement, with colonoscopy every 1–2 years

Diagnostic testing includes:

- Endoscopy (**most accurate test** when disease can be reached by a scope)
- Radiologic testing (e.g., barium study) for CD that is mainly in the small bowel to detect any lesions
- Serologic testing when the diagnosis is still unclear

All IBD is associated with anemia.

ANCA and ASCA Results in IBD		
Test	**Crohn disease**	**Ulcerative colitis**
Antineutrophil cytoplasmic antibody (ANCA)	Negative	Positive
Anti-Saccharomyces cerevisiae antibody (ASCA)	Positive	Negative

Treatment is as follows:

- Steroids for acute exacerbations (both UC and CD)
- 5-ASA derivatives such as mesalamine for chronic maintenance of remission
- UC: Asacol (mesalamine) or Rowasa (mesalamine) if limited to the rectum
- CD: Pentasa (mesalamine) or ciprofloxacin + metronidazole for perianal CD
- Steroids: prednisone, budesonide
- Azathioprine and 6-mercaptopurine to wean patients off steroids
- Calcium and vitamin D for all
- Anti-TNF agents for fistulae and severe disease unresponsive to other agents
    - If it is not effective, check drug level.
    - If drug level is adequate, check for antibodies to the TNF inhibitor.
    - If antibodies are present, switch to another anti-TNF drug; if not, switch to another class of biological agent.
    - If there is no response, surgery is done.

> **IBD treatments**
> - Anti-TNF: adalimumab, infliximab, certolizumab, golimumab, etanercept
> - Anti-IL 12/23: ustekinumab

> Budesonide is a steroid specific to IBD. First pass effect is good for IBD treatment.

Neither form of IBD is routinely treated with surgery.

- UC can be cured, however, with colectomy.
- In CD, surgery is used exclusively for bowel obstruction. CD will tend to recur at the site of the surgery.

If the disease is refractory to all other treatments, give vedolizumab (alpha-integrin inhibitor).

Short Bowel Syndrome

Short bowel syndrome is seen in patients who have had least half of the small bowel removed, most often as a result of multiple surgeries to relieve obstruction in Crohn disease.

Symptoms include diarrhea, dehydration, and malnutrition and weight loss from steatorrhea. The key finding is deficiency in vitamins A, D, E, K, B12, calcium, magnesium, iron, and zinc—making it look like celiac disease.

Treatment starts with a diet that avoids high-fat foods.

- IV hyperalimentation may be needed long term
- Loperamide to slow the bowel; teduglutide is a GLP agonist that slows the bowel and increases surface area
- Vitamin supplementation

Small Intestine Bacterial Overgrowth

Small intestine bacterial overgrowth (SIBO) results from progressive dilation of the small bowel as the body's adaptation to resection. Normally the small bowel is sterile, but in SIBO the loss of the ileocecal valve lets bacteria in.

- Patients present with flatulence, bloating, diarrhea, and steatorrhea.
- Diagnose with small bowel aspirate with quantitative cultures.
- Treat with antibiotics (rifaximin first).

Microscopic Colitis

Microscopic colitis is caused by chronic, nonbloody, watery diarrhea. Tissue appears normal at the time of colonoscopy, but pathology of a biopsy reveals inflammation. In other words, there is colitis, but you can only see the cause under a microscope.

A clue to diagnosis is autoimmune disease in the patient history.

Varieties of microscopic colitis include lymphocytic, collagenous, and mastocytic. All may respond to steroids.

Diverticular Disorders

Diverticulosis

Diverticulosis (outpocketings of the colon) is so common on a standard meat-filled diet as to be routinely expected in those age >65. It is rarely seen in vegetarians.

Most patients are asymptomatic, but they may present with left lower quadrant abdominal pain, constipation, bleeding, and possible infection (diverticulitis).

Diverticulosis can occur anywhere in the colon, but in elderly patients, the sigmoid region is most involved, making it the most likely location for inflammation.

The **most accurate test** is colonoscopy. Barium studies are acceptable but less accurate. Bran, psyllium, methylcellulose, and increased dietary fiber are used to decrease the rate of progression and complications.

Diverticulitis

The "most likely diagnosis" question is easily answered when presented with an older patient with:

- Left lower quadrant pain and tenderness
- Fever
- Leukocytosis
- Possible palpable mass

Colonoscopy and barium enema are **dangerous** in acute diverticulitis because of increased risk of perforation. Infection weakens the colonic wall.

Patients with acute diverticulitis should not be fed.

Nausea, constipation, and bleeding may also be present, but they are too non-specific for diagnosis.

CT scan is the **best initial test**.

Treatment for the first bout of diverticulitis is medical if there are no complications warranting surgery. Treatment is antibiotics that cover the *E. coli* and anaerobes present in the bowel. Possible combinations include:

- Ciprofloxacin + metronidazole or ceftriaxone + metronidazole
- Beta-lactam/beta-lactamase combinations
  - Amoxicillin/clavulanate
  - Ticarcillin/clavulanate or piperacillin/tazobactam
  - Ertapenem (carbapenems)

Diverticulitis that is recurrent or not responsive to medical treatment will require resection of the affected loop of bowel. Surgery is also the answer for cases that involve perforation, fistula formation, abscess, stricture, or obstruction.

- Younger patients should have the colon resected more often than older patients because of the greater total number of recurrent episodes that will occur.
- Diverticular disease does not disappear despite treating episodes of diverticulitis or the use of fiber in the diet.

The most common complication after diverticulitis is abscess formation.

Colon Cancer Screening

The far majority of colon cancer deaths are preventable with screening.

Which of the following is the most effective method of screening for colon cancer?

a. Colonoscopy
b. Sigmoidoscopy
c. Fecal occult blood testing (FOBT)
d. Barium enema
e. Virtual colonoscopy with CT scanning
f. Capsule endoscopy

Answer: **A.** Since 40% of colon cancer occurs proximal to the rectum and sigmoid colon, colonoscopy is far more sensitive than sigmoidoscopy in detecting lesions. FOBT has more false-positives and false-negatives than colonoscopy; in addition, a positive FOBT must be followed up with colonoscopy. Barium study, virtual colonoscopy with CT, and capsule endoscopy do not allow for biopsy.

Virtual colonoscopy is never the correct answer for anything.

Capsule endoscopy is used to detect sources of bleeding in the small bowel not reachable by endoscopy.

The recommended frequency of screening is as follows:

- **Routine testing (2021 guidelines)**: beginning at age 45, do a colonoscopy every 10 years
- **If previous adenomatous polyp**: screen with colonoscopy every 3–5 years
- **If previous history of colon cancer**: screen with colonoscopy at 1 year after resection, then at 3 years, then every 5 years
- **If family history of colon cancer**:
  - **Single family member**: start screening 10 years earlier than the age at which the family member developed cancer or age 40 (whichever is younger); repeat the scope every 5 years if the family member was age <60
  - **3 family members, 2 generations, 1 premature (age <50)**, i.e., hereditary nonpolyposis colon cancer syndrome (HNPCC): start screening at age 25 with colonoscopy every 1–2 years
  - **Familial adenomatous polyposis** (FAP): beginning at age 12, do a sigmoidoscopy every year; FAP (the presence of thousands of polyps) is identified with an abnormal genetic test known as the adenomatous polyposis coli (APC) test

Anticoagulation in Colonoscopy

- Stop NOACs one day before colonoscopy, restart them the day after colonoscopy. (If colonoscopy is on Tuesday, skip Monday's dose and restart on Wednesday.)
- Stop warfarin 3–5 days before colonoscopy.
- Use the shortest period of time off warfarin in patients with metal heart valves.

Other Polyposis Syndromes

Peutz-Jeghers Syndrome

Peutz-Jeghers syndrome is characterized by multiple hamartomatous polyps in association with:

- Melanotic spots on the lips and skin
- Increased frequency of breast cancer
- Increased gonadal and pancreatic cancer

The frequency of colonoscopy screening is increased to every 3 years, starting at age 8.

Gardner Syndrome

Gardner syndrome is colon cancer in association with:

- Osteomas
- Desmoid tumors
- Other soft tissue tumors

> - Screen **age 8**: Peutz-Jeghers
> - Screen **age 12**: FAP, juvenile polyposis

Put Gardner syndrome in the same place in your brain as FAP regarding cancers outside the colon: It is similar to FAP in its long-term risk of colon cancer and has greater incidence of cancer of the thyroid, pancreas, and small bowel than FAP. Screen Gardner syndrome from the same starting age of 12 with sigmoidoscopy.

Turcot Syndrome

Turcot syndrome is colon cancer in association with:

- CNS malignancy

Juvenile Polyposis

Juvenile polyposis is colon cancer in association with:

- Multiple hamartomatous polyps
- Screen both upper and lower GI tracts at same intervals as FAP.

Pancreatic Disorders

Acute Pancreatitis

Acute pancreatitis is an acute inflammation of the pancreas. Causes include:

- Alcoholism and cholelithiasis (most common)
- Trauma
- Hypertriglyceridemia
- Hypercalcemia
- Infection
- Drug toxicity (pentamidine, didanosine, azathioprine, estrogens) or drug allergy (sulfa drugs such as furosemide, hydrochlorothiazide)
- Ductal obstruction, endoscopic retrograde cholangiopancreatography (ERCP), cystic fibrosis
- Scorpion sting

> Pancreatitis: a **stone**, a **stricture**, a **tumor**, or an **obstruction**

> ERCP-induced pancreatitis is preventable with rectal NSAIDs such as indomethacin.

"What Is the Most Likely Diagnosis?"

Suspect pancreatitis when the patient presents with acute epigastric pain, tenderness, and nausea/vomiting. Pain intensity is subjective and does not correlate with the degree of organ damage.

In severe cases there is hypotension and fever.

▶ **TIP**

The pain of pancreatitis goes **straight through** to the back "like a spear" stabbed into the abdomen. Cholecystitis pain goes **around the side** to the back.

Which of the following is associated with the worst prognosis in pancreatitis?

a. Elevated amylase

b. Elevated lipase

c. Intensity of the pain

d. Low calcium

e. C-reactive protein (CRP) rising

Answer: D. Severe pancreatic damage decreases lipase production and release, leading to fat malabsorption in the gut. Calcium binds with fat (saponifies) in the bowel, leading to calcium malabsorption. Although amylase and lipase are elevated in pancreatitis, there is no correlation between the height of these enzyme levels and disease severity.

Diagnostic testing includes:

- Amylase and lipase are elevated (**best initial tests**)
- CT scan or MRI (**most specific test**) (also detects pseudocysts)
  - Disease severity strongly correlates with the degree of necrosis seen on CT scanning.
  - Needle biopsy is indispensable for determining the presence of infection in those who have extensive necrosis (i.e., >30% necrosis).
- MRCP to determine etiology of the disease (e.g., stones, stricture, tumor)
- Plain x-ray shows a sentinel loop of bowel (air-filled piece of small bowel in left upper quadrant)
- CBC: leukocytosis, drop in hematocrit over time with rehydration
- Elevated LDH and AST
- Hypoxia, hypocalcemia

U/S has very poor accuracy; the overlying bowel blocks any precise imaging.

Treatment is as follows:

- NPO
- IV hydration at very high volume
- Analgesia
- PPIs decrease pancreatic stimulation from acid entering the duodenum
- If CT/MRI shows >30% necrosis, adding an antibiotic such as imipenem or meropenem may decrease mortality by limiting the development of infected, necrotic pancreatitis
  - Severe necrosis is an indication for needle biopsy to determine the presence of infection.
  - The only way to confirm an infection is with biopsy.

Infected, necrotic pancreatitis should be resected with surgical debridement to prevent ARDS and death.

Pseudocysts are drained with a needle if they are enlarging or painful.

Autoimmune (IgG4-Related) Pancreatitis

This is pancreatitis without the usual causes but with the unique feature of ANA and rheumatoid factor.

> High triglycerides can falsely decrease amylase levels.

> Abdominal CT scan is always performed with IV and oral contrast to better define and outline abdominal structures.

> MRCP is diagnostic, while ERCP is for treatment (to place stents, remove obstructing stones, and dilate strictures).

Symptomatic IgG4-related pancreatitis presents as a patient with recurrent jaundice, weight loss, and abdominal pain. Abdominal CT shows an enlarged, "sausage-shaped" pancreas, and serum IgG4 level is elevated.

> Autoimmune pancreatitis is easily confused with pancreatic cancer.

The key to diagnosis is the absence of significant alcohol intake or stones. Biopsy, if done to exclude pancreatic cancer, shows lymphocytic and plasma cell infiltrates.

IgG4-related pancreatitis is associated with Sjögren syndrome, autoimmune thyroiditis, interstitial nephritis, and sclerosing cholangitis.

Steroids give a robust response. Surgery is a wrong answer.

Pancreatic Cancer

Look for a patient with painless jaundice, weight loss, and a generally nontender epigastric area. Amylase and lipase are mostly normal, while bilirubin, alkaline phosphatase, and gamma-glutamyltranspeptidase (GGTP) are elevated.

> Depression + weight loss + jaundice = pancreatic cancer

CT scan reveals a pancreatic mass (90% of patients).

- If CT is negative, the next step is an endoscopic ultrasound with biopsy of the pancreatic lesions.
- If CT shows a clear lesion in the pancreas, the next step is surgical biopsy/ removal at same time.

> CA 19-9 follows response to treatment of pancreatic cancer.

Cystic neoplasms of the pancreas are cysts that have a small chance of turning into pancreatic cancer over time. Mucinous cystadenoma and intraductal papillary mucinous neoplasms are associated with elevated CEA and CA 19-9. Like cervical dysplasia, these neoplasms must be removed before the growth becomes invasive cancer. Also like cervical dysplasia, the invasive malignant potential of cystic neoplasms of the pancreas ranges from 0–70%.

There is no treatment for pancreatic cancer. Chemotherapy and radiation have little benefit. The 5-year survival rate is just 5%.

Liver Disease

All forms of chronic liver disease can produce:

- Ascites
- Coagulopathy (all clotting factors except VIII are made in liver)
- Asterixis and encephalopathy
- Hypoalbuminemia and edema
- Spider angiomata and palmar erythema
- Portal hypertension leading to varices
- Thrombocytopenia from splenic sequestration
- Renal insufficiency (hepatorenal syndrome)
- Hepatopulmonary syndrome

Everyone with cirrhosis should get an U/S every 6 months to screen for cancer. U/S is 95% sensitive at detecting cancer.

Ascites

Paracentesis should be performed if there is new-onset ascites, abdominal pain and tenderness, or fever.

Portal hypertension from cirrhosis is the etiology of the ascitic fluid if there is a low albumin level in the fluid.

Serum ascites albumin gradient (SAAG) is the difference or "gradient" between the serum and ascites. SAAG >1.1 is highly suggestive of portal hypertension.

SAAG: Correlating Level with Disease	
<1.1 g/dL	**>1.1 g/dL**
• Infections (except SBP) • Cancer • Nephrotic syndrome	• Portal hypertension • CHF • Hepatic vein thrombosis • Constrictive pericarditis

Spontaneous Bacterial Peritonitis

Spontaneous bacterial peritonitis (SBP) is infection without a perforation of the bowel. How the bacteria gets there isn't known. Causes include:

- *E. coli* (most common)
- Anaerobes (rare)
- Pneumococcus, a respiratory pathogen (reasons unknown)

Diagnostic testing includes:

- Cell count with >250 neutrophils (**best initial test**) is the basis upon which we start treatment.
- Gram stain (almost always negative)
- LDH level (too nonspecific)
- Fluid culture (**most accurate test**) but results are never available in time for treatment decisions

Treatment of SBP is with cefotaxime or ceftriaxone.

SBP frequently recurs. When the ascites fluid albumin level is quite low, prophylactic ciprofloxacin or trimethoprim/sulfamethoxazole is used to prevent SBP. If the ascitic fluid albumin is <1, prophylaxis against SBP is also needed. This is why everyone with new ascites needs a paracentesis even if there are no symptoms.

> All variceal bleeding with ascites needs SBP prophylaxis.

> Anyone with SBP needs lifelong prophylaxis against recurrence.

| Treatment of Specific Features of Cirrhosis ||
Feature	**Treatment**
Ascites and edema	Spironolactone and other diuretics. Serial paracenteses for large-volume ascites.
Coagulopathy and thrombocytopenia	FFP and/or platelets only if bleeding occurs
Encephalopathy	Lactulose and rifaximin
Hypoalbuminemia	No specific therapy
Spider angiomata and palmar erythema	No specific therapy
Varices	Propranolol and banding via endoscopy
Hepatorenal syndrome	Somatostatin (octreotide), midodrine
Hepatopulmonary syndrome	No specific therapy

Acute Alcoholic Hepatitis

Look for jaundice, anorexia, and weight loss over a few months with RUQ pain. Ascites, liver tenderness, and fever are often present.

Also look for:

- AST > ALT
- Elevated GGTP and bilirubin
- Elevated INR and prothrombin time (PT)

You must exclude viral and drug-induced hepatitis. If the discriminant factor is >32, treat with steroids.

$$\textbf{Discriminant factor} = \textbf{4.6} \times \textbf{(patient's PT} - \textbf{control PT)} + \textbf{bilirubin}$$

Severe alcoholic hepatitis has 50% mortality.

Hepatopulmonary Syndrome

This is lung disease and hypoxia entirely on the basis of liver failure. Look for orthodeoxia, which is hypoxia upon sitting upright. There is no specific therapy. If the liver's condition is this bad, the patient needs a transplant.

Causes of Cirrhosis

Alcoholic Liver Disease

This is a diagnosis of exclusion. The most accurate test—as with most causes of cirrhosis except sclerosing cholangitis—is a liver biopsy.

Alcohol, like all drugs causing liver disease, gives a greater elevation in AST compared to ALT. Viral hepatitis gives a higher ALT than AST. Binge drinking gives a sudden rise in GGTP.

There is no specific treatment.

Primary Biliary Cholangitis (PBC)

Answer primary biliary cirrhosis (PBC) as the "most likely diagnosis" when the question describes:

- Woman in 40s or 50s
- Fatigue and itching
- Normal bilirubin with an elevated alkaline phosphatase

The most characteristic features of PBC are xanthelasma/xanthoma (collection of cholesterol under the skin that is yellowish in color) and osteoporosis.

Diagnostic testing includes:

- Liver biopsy (**most accurate**)
- Antimitochondrial antibody (**most accurate blood test**)
- Bilirubin and IgM elevate in very advanced disease

> In PBC, obeticholic acid decreases fibrosis.

Treatment is ursodeoxycholic acid or obeticholic acid (decreases fibrosis).

Primary Sclerosing Cholangitis

Over 80% of primary sclerosing cholangitis (PSC) occurs in association with inflammatory bowel disease. Look for:

- Pruritus
- Elevated alkaline phosphatase and GGTP as well as elevated bilirubin level

Early PSC can look just like PBC. Bilirubin level can be normal in early disease.

Diagnostic testing includes:

- MRCP or ERCP (**most accurate test**) shows beading, narrowing, or strictures in the biliary system (MRCP is generally done because there is no therapeutic need for ERCP)
- Biopsy (only if done for other reasons, i.e., not essential for establishing a diagnosis)

> PSC is the **only** cause of cirrhosis for which a biopsy is **not** the most accurate test.

No treatment is effective for PSC. We try to dilate strictures, but nothing modifies the disease.

▶ TIP

PSC does not improve or resolve with resolution of the IBD. Even after a colectomy in ulcerative colitis, the patient may still progress to needing a liver transplantation.

Alpha 1-Antitrypsin Deficiency

Look for the combination of liver disease and emphysema (COPD) in a young patient (age <40) who is a nonsmoker. The question may throw in a family history of COPD at an early age. Treat by replacing the enzyme. The most frequently asked question is "What is the most likely diagnosis?"

> Inhaled aerosolized alpha 1-antitrypsin is used for lung disease.

> Hemochromatosis **may be found on routine testing** with mildly abnormal LFTs or iron levels.

> *Vibrio vulnificus, Yersinia,* and *Listeria* infections occur in hemochromatosis because these organisms feed on iron.

Hemochromatosis

This is a genetic disorder leading to overabsorption of iron in the duodenum. The mutation is the C282y gene.

Men present earlier than women because menstruation delays the onset of liver fibrosis and cirrhosis.

Look for a patient age 50s with mild increases in AST and alkaline phosphatase and:

- Fatigue and joint pain (pseudogout)
- Erectile dysfunction in men, and amenorrhea in women (from pituitary involvement)
- Skin darkening
- Diabetes
- Cardiomyopathy

Diagnostic testing includes:

- Iron study (**best initial test**) shows increased serum iron and ferritin, and decreased iron-binding capacity
- Liver biopsy for increased iron (**most accurate test**)
- EKG may show conduction defects
- Echocardiogram may show dilated or restrictive cardiomyopathy

A 54-year-old man is evaluated for fatigue, erectile dysfunction, and skin darkening. He is found to have transferrin saturation (iron divided by TIBC) >50%. His AST is 2 × the upper limit of normal. What is the next step to confirm the diagnosis?

a. Echocardiography
b. Glucose level
c. Abdominal MRI and HFE (C282y) gene testing
d. Liver biopsy
e. Prussian blue stain of the bone marrow
f. Deferoxamine
g. Deferasirox

Answer: **C.** MRI shows increased iron deposition in the liver. An abnormal MRI combined with an abnormal genetic test for hemochromatosis can spare the patient the need for a liver biopsy. Hemochromatosis has an association with diabetes, although glucose levels will not confirm a diagnosis of hemochromatosis. Prussian blue is the stain of blood cells for iron, used to diagnose sideroblastic anemia.

Treatment for those with an overabsorption of iron is phlebotomy. **Liver fibrosis can resolve** if phlebotomy is begun before cirrhosis develops.

If phlebotomy is contraindicated or if patient is anemic and has hemochromatosis from overtransfusion (e.g., thalassemia), use iron chelation therapy with deferasirox, deferiprone, or deferoxamine.

- Deferasirox and deferiprone are huge breakthrough medications because they are effective orally.
- Deferoxamine must be given lifelong by subcutaneous injection.

> Oral iron chelators:
> - Deferiprone
> - Deferasirox

Hepatitis

Hepatitis is an infection or inflammation of the liver.

- **Viral hepatitis A or B** (most cases of acute hepatitis)
- **Hepatitis C**: rarely presents with an acute infection; is found as "silent" infection on blood test or when patients present with cirrhosis
- **Hepatitis D**: seen exclusively in those who have active viral replication of hepatitis B
- **Hepatitis E** (worst in pregnancy, especially among patients from East Asia)

> Test all adults for hepatitis C regardless of risk factors.

> Sex, blood, perinatal (parenteral): **hepatitis B, C,** and **D**
> Food and water (enteric): **hepatitis A** and **E**
> - You **A**te hepatitis **A**; you **E**at hepatitis **E**.

There is no way to detect the etiology or specific type of hepatitis from the acute symptoms. All forms of acute hepatitis present with:

- Jaundice and dark urine
- Fever, weight loss, and fatigue
- Hepatosplenomegaly
- Nausea, vomiting, abdominal pain

Diagnostic testing includes:

- Increased direct bilirubin
- Increased ratio of alanine aminotransferase (ALT) to aspartate aminotransferase (AST)
- Increased alkaline phosphatase

Additionally, there are disease-specific tests:

- Hepatitis A, C, D, and E: IgM antibody for the acute infection and IgG antibody to detect resolution of infection (**best initial tests**)
- PCR for viral load (hepatitis B and C), which tells the amount of active viral replication; PCR is first thing to improve with treatment and is best correlate of treatment failure

> Older terms like "chronic active" or "chronic persistent" hepatitis are irrelevant. Answer "viral load by PCR."

> Aplastic anemia is a rare complication of acute hepatitis.

Serologic Patterns in Hepatitis B				
	Surface antigen	**e-Antigen**	**Core antibody**	**Surface antibody**
Acute or chronic infection	Positive	Positive	Positive IgM or IgG	Negative
Resolved, old, past infection	Negative	Negative	Positive IgG	Positive
Vaccination	Negative	Negative	Negative	Positive
"Window period"	Negative	Negative	Positive IgM, then IgG	Negative

Rituximab reactivates hepatitis B surface antigen carriers.

It is critical to test for the presence of hepatitis B surface antigen before initiating certain medications in a patient, because the medications will inhibit the part of the immune system that suppresses hepatitis B growth.

- Anti-CD20 medications (highest risk): rituximab, ofatumumab, obinutuzumab
- Anti-CD52: alemtuzumab
- HIV pre-exposure prophylaxis (PrEP): tenofovir and emtricitabine can reactivate hepatitis B when used in the short term and then stopped.

In diagnosing both hepatitis B and C, the level of viral particles should be tracked.

Hepatitis B DNA viral load is even more precise than e-antigen.

- PCR is used to measure the DNA of hepatitis B and the RNA of hepatitis C. Although PCR viral load level is not the right test for the initial diagnosis of these infections, it is the right test for determining if treatment has been successful.
- Elevated viral load also identifies the most accurate way to assess the degree of infectivity of the source patient. In other words, who is most likely to transmit the infection to a baby, to a sex partner, or via needle-stick?

Treatment

- **Hepatitis A and E** resolve spontaneously over a few weeks and are almost always benign conditions. Hepatitis E is also transmitted by the oral-fecal route and is more often seen in poor countries. Its most severe presentation is in pregnant women, in whom it can cause acute liver failure.
- **Hepatitis B** becomes chronic in 10% of patients and there is no treatment to prevent this (*chronicity* for hepatitis B is defined as persistence of surface antigen >6 months). If patients are positive for e-antigen with elevated DNA viral load, treatment is entecavir, adefovir, lamivudine, telbivudine, tenofovir, or interferon (note that interferon is an injection and has many side effects, including arthralgia/myalgia, leukopenia and thrombocytopenia, depression, and flu-like symptoms).
- **Acute hepatitis C**, in the few cases in which it is detected, should be treated. This decreases the likelihood of developing a chronic hepatitis C infection.

- **Chronic hepatitis C** is treated if PCR-RNA viral load is elevated. The goal of treatment is to reduce it to undetectable levels.
  - All treatment for hepatitis C is oral.
  - Treat with sofosbuvir plus ledipasvir or sofosbuvir plus velpatasvir.

> Acute hepatitis C is the only acute hepatitis that is treated.

The key points regarding treatment of hepatitis C are as follows:

- Acute hepatitis C *is treated*!
- Hepatitis C is the **only** form of **acute** hepatitis to be treated!
- All adults are tested for hepatitis C regardless of risk factors.
- Cure rates (i.e., rates of "sustained viral response") exceed 95–99%.
- This eliminates the need for liver transplant.

> Velpatasvir covers all genotypes of hepatitis C. On the test, if velpatasvir is one of the answer options, choose it!

What this means for Step 2 CK: If you *don't* see a hepatitis C question of some kind, we would be shocked!

Viral load testing has nearly eliminated the need for liver biopsy. Simeprevir, telaprevir, and boceprevir are always the wrong answer.

USMLE has to ask clear questions. The answer to the clear question is this: Hepatitis C can be effectively cured in the majority of cases. Be more concerned to know the following:

> Interferon is never used first-line in hepatitis C. However, for the exam you must know its side effects: arthralgia, myalgia, anemia, and depression.

- *Do not test* based only on risk factors (such as injection drug use).
- Anyone with detectable PCR RNA viral load needs treatment.
- **Genotype** predicts the response to therapy.
- **Viral load** assesses the effect of therapy. Viral load answers the question "Has there been an effect?"
- **Liver biopsy** determines how much damage there has been to the liver. If you are going to treat anyway because the viral load is elevated, there is no point in doing a liver biopsy.

Which of the following correlates best with an increased likelihood of mortality?

a. Bilirubin
b. Prothrombin time
c. ALT
d. AST
e. Alkaline phosphatase

Answer: B. All of these lab tests can be markedly elevated during acute hepatitis with little adverse significance except for prothrombin time (PT). If PT is elevated, there is a markedly increased risk of fulminant hepatic failure and death.

Which of the following is the best indicator that a pregnant woman will transmit infection to her child?

a. Bilirubin
b. e-Antigen
c. Surface antigen
d. Core IgM antibody
e. ALT
f. Anti-hepatitis B, e-antibody

Answer: **B.** The correct answer is e-antigen. The exam question may offer DNA polymerase or PCR for viral load as a choice instead of e-antigen. The only difference is that e-antigen is a **qualitative** test, meaning it is simply positive or negative. DNA viral load is a **quantitative** test, meaning it gives a level that is highly variable. It is like the gas tank in your car. Hepatitis B e-antigen tells you, "Gas present: yes or no." DNA viral load is like the gauge on your tank: It tells an amount. If a woman is positive for surface antigen, but the e-antigen is negative, only 10% of children will become infected with hepatitis B at birth. When both surface antigen and e-antigen are positive, 90% of children will be infected at birth. This is why **perinatal transmission is the most common method of transmission worldwide**.

Which of the following will become abnormal first after acquiring hepatitis B infection?

a. Bilirubin
b. e-Antigen
c. Surface antigen
d. Core IgM antibody
e. ALT
f. Anti-hepatitis B e-antibody

Answer: **C.** Surface antigen is a measure of actual viral particles. Bilirubin, ALT, and antibody production are a measure of the body's response to the infection.

Which of the following indicates that a patient is no longer a risk for transmitting infection to another person (active infection has resolved)?

a. Bilirubin normalizes
b. No e-antigen found
c. No surface antigen found
d. No core IgM antibody found
e. ALT normalizes
f. Anti-hepatitis B e-antibody

Answer: **C.** As long as surface antigen is present, there is still some viral replication potentially occurring. Even if surface antibody were one of the choices, the correct answer would still be surface antigen. Transmissibility ceases when DNA viral load or polymerase ceases, not when surface antibody appears. Jaundice (increased bilirubin) and elevated ALT will all normalize long before viral replication stops. You can definitely have viral replication, elevated DNA polymerase, and positive surface antigen with a normal ALT. Hepatitis B e-antibody will appear *prior to resolution* of all DNA polymerase activity. It is an indication that the acute infection is moving toward resolution, but it does not conclusively prove resolution has occurred.

ALT levels are not a good indication of the activity of chronic hepatitis. You can have significant infection with normal transaminase levels.

Which of the following best indicates the need for treatment with antiviral medication in chronic disease?

a. Bilirubin
b. e-Antigen
c. Surface antigen
d. Core IgM antibody
e. ALT
f. Anti-hepatitis B e-antibody

Answer: **B.** The person most likely to benefit from antiviral medication is the one with the greatest degree of active viral replication. Hepatitis B e-antigen is the strongest indicator of active viral replication. Although surface antigen means there is at least some active disease, it might be on the way to spontaneous resolution. Everyone with e-antigen also has surface antigen. The person with the worst disease (highest DNA polymerase) will benefit the most from treatment.

Adverse Effects of Hepatitis Medications	
Interferon	Arthralgias, thrombocytopenia, depression, leukopenia
Ribavirin	Anemia
Adefovir	Renal dysfunction
Lamivudine	None

Ribavirin causes anemia.

Wilson Disease

This is a disorder of abnormally decreased copper excretion from the body. Because of a decrease in ceruloplasmin, copper is not excreted and it builds up in the body in the liver, kidney, red blood cells, and nervous system.

"What Is the Most Likely Diagnosis?"

In addition to all the previously described features of cirrhosis and hepatic insufficiency, you will answer Wilson disease as the diagnosis if you see:

- Neurological symptoms: psychosis, tremor, dysarthria, ataxia, or seizures
- Coombs negative hemolytic anemia
- Renal tubular acidosis or nephrolithiasis

▶ TIP

Wilson disease gives psychosis and delusions—*not* the encephalopathic features or delirium that you would get with any form of liver failure.

Diagnostic testing includes:

- Slit-lamp examination for Kayser-Fleischer rings, a brownish ring around the eye from copper deposition (**best initial test**)
- Urine test shows abnormally increased amount of copper excretion after giving penicillamine (**most accurate test**)
- Ceruloplasmin is usually low
- Liver biopsy (most sensitive and specific) will detect abnormally increased hepatic copper

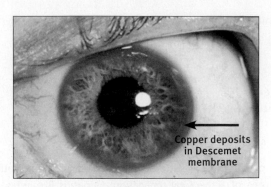

Figure 1.12 Copper deposits in Descemet membrane give a brownish ring around outer edge of the cornea.
Source: Herbert L. Fred, MD, and Hendrik A. van Dijk, MD

> Decreased ceruloplasmin level is not the most accurate test. This is the most common wrong answer. All plasma proteins can be decreased with liver dysfunction and cirrhosis.

> Penicillamine cannot be used with allergy to penicillin. Use zinc or trientine.

Treatment is penicillamine, which will chelate copper and remove it from the body (trientine is an alternative). Zinc is also used, which interferes with intestinal copper absorption.

Autoimmune Hepatitis

Look for young women with signs of liver inflammation with a positive ANA. More specific tests are liver-kidney microsomal antibodies, high gamma globulin (IgG), anti-smooth muscle antibodies, and anti-liver/kidney microsomal antibodies. The most accurate test is the liver biopsy. Treat with prednisone and or azathioprine.

Non-Alcoholic Fatty Liver Disease

Non-alcoholic fatty liver disease (NAFLD) is a common condition in which there is excess fat in the liver of those who don't consume alcohol. There are 2 types:

- **Non-alcoholic fatty liver (NAFL)** is relatively benign and is not associated with fibrosis or malignant potential.
- **Non-alcoholic steatohepatitis (NASH)** is associated with inflammation and fibrosis and the potential to progress to cirrhosis. NASH is potentially premalignant.

The disorder is associated with obesity, diabetes, hyperlipidemia, and corticosteroid use.

The most important diagnostic challenge is to exclude more serious liver disease.

- Liver function tests are often mildly abnormal.
- Biopsy (**most accurate test**) shows the microvesicular fatty deposits you would find in alcoholic liver disease, but without the history of alcohol use.

Treatment is correction of diabetes, obesity, and hyperlipidemia. There is no specific drug treatment to reverse NAFLD. Use vitamin E in everyone. NASH is treated with obeticholic acid. Obeticholic acid decreases progression, but it will not reverse severe fibrosis. If there is NASH and diabetes, the answer is pioglitazone.

Model for End-Stage Liver Disease (MELD) Score

MELD score predicts survival in cirrhosis and alcoholic hepatitis. It uses:

- Age
- Creatinine and the need for dialysis
- Bilirubin and INR

MELD score is critical in prioritizing who gets a donor liver first. High MELD means death sooner and, therefore, a higher priority for getting liver transplantation.

Benign Liver Lesions

Focal nodular hyperplasia (FNH) rarely grows or bleeds and never becomes malignant. The key fact for you is imaging shows "central stellate scarring," which is how you know it is benign. FNH is from hyperplastic hepatocellular growth around an abnormal blood vessel. No treatment is needed.

Hemangioma is mostly asymptomatic, found incidentally with a small number of patients experiencing RUQ pain. Ultrasound, CT, and MRI eliminate the need for biopsy in most cases. Lesions <5 cm get no treatment.

Unlike FNH, **hepatic adenoma** changes with hormone levels, and during pregnancy it may grow and even rupture. Adenomas can cause pain. Biopsy is the definitive diagnostic test. Because of adenomas have a small risk of malignancy, biopsy is more essential in adenoma than in the other lesions.

Focal nodular hyperplasia	Hemangioma	Hepatic adenoma
• Central scarring on imaging • No malignant potential	• Tuft of abnormal vessels • Imaging diagnostic • No malignant potential	• Grows with estrogen • Large ones may rupture • Small malignant potential

Pituitary Disorders

Pituitary Incidentaloma

By definition, an "incidentaloma" occurs in an asymptomatic patient. Tumor size determines the management.

Tumor size	Treatment
<1 cm	Prolactin level MRI (yearly)
>1 cm	Prolactin level MRI (yearly) 24-hour urine cortisol TSH, T4, LH, FSH, IGF Test visual fields for evidence of optic chiasm compression

Empty Sella Syndrome

Empty sella syndrome (ESS) is a disorder in which the pituitary is undersized, flattened, and not visible on MRI. ESS can be an incidental finding, and it is associated with surgery, obesity, and radiation therapy; however, 70% are idiopathic. When asked how to manage asymptomatic ESS, answer "Check thyroid and adrenal function."

Panhypopituitarism

Panhypopituitarism is caused by any condition that compresses or damages the pituitary gland.

- Tumor (e.g., metastatic cancer, adenoma, Rathke cleft cyst, meningioma)
- Trauma and radiation
- Hemochromatosis, sarcoidosis, and histiocytosis X
- Infection with fungi, TB, and parasites
- Autoimmune and lymphocytic infiltration

Anything that damages the brain—from tumor to stroke to infection to trauma—can cause panhypopituitarism.

Symptoms are based on the deficiencies of the specific hormone.

- **Deficiency of prolactin**: In men, there are never any symptoms of prolactin deficiency. In women, prolactin deficiency inhibits lactation after childbirth. *Pro*lactin literally means "in favor of" or "pro" lactation. If deficient, the patient cannot lactate normally.

- **Deficiency of growth hormone (GH)**: Children present with short stature and dwarfism. Adults have few symptoms because several other hormones—catecholamines, glucagon, cortisol—act as stress hormones; subtle findings include central obesity, elevated LDL/cholesterol, and reduced lean muscle mass.

- **Deficiency of luteinizing hormone (LH)** and **follicle-stimulating hormone (FSH)**: Men will not make testosterone or sperm; they will have erectile dysfunction and decreased muscle mass. Women will not be able to ovulate or menstruate normally and will become amenorrheic. Both will have decreased libido and decreased axillary, pubic, and body hair.

	Kallmann syndrome	Klinefelter syndrome
Etiology	KAL-1 mutation	47 XXY karyotype
Relation to FSH and LH	Decreased FSH and LH from decreased GnRH	Androgen deficiency through insensitivity to FSH and LH despite high FSH/LH
Other characteristics	Anosmia Renal agenesis (50% of patients)	Tall
Treatment	Replace testosterone	Replace testosterone

Symptoms of hypothyroidism and hypoadrenalism will be covered in the sections devoted to those glands.

Hyponatremia is common secondary to hypothyroidism and isolated glucocorticoid underproduction. Potassium level remains normal because aldosterone is not affected and aldosterone excretes potassium.

MRI detects compressing mass lesions on the pituitary.

Diagnostic testing:

- The initial tests for suspected panhypopituitarism are TSH, T4, IGF, estrogen, testosterone, LH, FSH, and prolactin.
- For suspected GH deficiency, the **best initial stimulatory test** is injecting growth hormone–releasing hormone (GHRH). The normal response to GHRH is a rise in GH level.

Specific Diagnostic Tests for Each Hormone	
Standard blood tests	**Abnormality confirmed with**
Low thyroid-stimulating hormone (TSH) and low thyroxine levels	Decreased TSH response to thyrotropin-releasing hormone (TRH)
Decreased adrenocorticotropic hormone (ACTH) and decreased cortisol level	Normal response to cosyntropin stimulation of the adrenal. Cortisol will rise (adrenal is normal) in recent disease, but abnormal in chronic disease because of adrenal atrophy. No response (rise) in ACTH level with corticotropin-releasing hormone (CRH). An elevated baseline cortisol level excludes pituitary insufficiency.
Decreased LH and FSH levels Decreased testosterone level	No confirmatory test
GH levels low, but this finding is not helpful since GH is pulsatile and maximum at night.	No response to GH-releasing hormone (GHRH) No response to arginine infusion
Prolactin level low, but not helpful	No response to TRH

Older, less useful tests are:

- **Metyrapone** inhibits 11-beta hydroxylase, which decreases the output of the adrenal gland. Metyrapone should normally cause ACTH levels to rise because cortisol goes down. Cortisol is the feedback inhibition on the pituitary.
- **Insulin stimulation:** The normal effect of insulin-inducing hypoglycemia is a rise in GH level. GH increases glucose levels because it is a stress hormone. "Insulin-induced hypoglycemia" as a test is always the wrong answer.

Replace deficient hormones with:

- Cortisone
- Thyroxine (only after cortisone has been replaced)
- Testosterone and estrogen
- Recombinant human growth hormone

> Do not answer dexamethasone for deficiency of adrenal steroid hormones. It has no mineralocorticoid activity.

Posterior Pituitary

The 2 products of the posterior pituitary are antidiuretic hormone (ADH) and oxytocin. There is no deficiency disease described for oxytocin. Oxytocin helps uterine contraction during delivery, but delivery still occurs even if it is absent. ADH deficiency is also known as central diabetes insipidus.

Acromegaly

Acromegaly is the overproduction of GH, leading to overgrowth of soft tissue throughout the body. Causes include:

- Pituitary adenoma (95% of cases)
- MEN syndrome when it is combined with a parathyroid/pancreatic disorder such as gastrinoma or insulinoma
- Ectopic GH or GHRH production from a lymphoma or bronchial carcinoid (rare)

"What Is the Most Likely Diagnosis?"

Acromegaly enlarges soft tissue like cartilage and bone, resulting in:

- Increased hat, ring, and shoe size
- Carpal tunnel syndrome and obstructive sleep apnea from soft tissues enlarging
- Body odor from sweat gland hypertrophy
- Coarsening facial features and teeth widening from jaw growth
- Deep voice and macroglossia (big tongue)
- Colonic polyps, skin tags, and colon cancer
- Arthralgias from joints growing out of alignment
- Hypertension resistant to treatment for unclear reasons (50% of cases)
- Cardiomegaly and CHF
- Erectile dysfunction from increased prolactin cosecreted with the pituitary adenoma
- Hyperglycemia

Lab tests will show glucose intolerance and hyperlipidemia, which contribute to the cardiac dysfunction.

- Insulin-like growth factor (IGF-1) level (**best initial test**)
- Glucose suppression test (**most accurate test**) (normally, glucose should suppress GH)
- MRI, only after the laboratory identification of acromegaly

Treatment is as follows:

- Transsphenoidal resection of the pituitary (70% success rate); larger adenomas are harder to cure
- Medications
  - Cabergoline: dopamine inhibits GH release
  - Octreotide or lanreotide: somatostatin inhibits GH release
  - Pegvisomant: GH receptor antagonist inhibits IGF release from the liver
- Radiation only when there is no response to surgery or medication

> Abuse of GH can give the same presentation as acromegaly.

> Prolactin levels are tested because of cosecretion with GH.

> If GH is an **anti**insulin, why does it make an **insulin-like** growth factor? Only the effect on proteins and amino acids is insulin-like.

Diabetes Insipidus

(See the Nephrology chapter for evaluation and management of diabetes insipidus.)

Hyperprolactinemia

High prolactin can seem confusing because so many causes have nothing to do with a pituitary adenoma. Causes of elevated prolactin include:

- Physiologic causes: pregnancy, intense exercise, renal insufficiency, and increased chest wall stimulation
- Hypothyroidism, because extremely high TRH levels will stimulate prolactin secretion

- Acromegaly, because prolactin can be cosecreted with GH
- Cutting the pituitary stalk, which eliminates dopamine delivery to the anterior pituitary (dopamine inhibits prolactin release)
- Certain drugs: antipsychotics, methyldopa, metoclopramide, opioids, tricyclic antidepressants, and verapamil

> Verapamil is the only calcium blocker to **raise prolactin level.**

Symptoms include:

- Women: galactorrhea, amenorrhea, infertility
- Men: erectile dysfunction, decreased libido
- While men may experience gynecomastia, men very rarely experience galactorrhea

After the prolactin level is found to be high, diagnostic tests include:

- Thyroid function tests
- Pregnancy test
- BUN/creatinine (kidney disease elevates prolactin)
- LFTs (cirrhosis elevates prolactin)

> Always **exclude pregnancy first** in any woman with a high prolactin level.

MRI is done after prolactin level is confirmed to be high, secondary causes like medications are excluded, and patient is confirmed to not be pregnant.

> With any endocrine disorder, MRI of the head should never be done first.

Treatment is as follows.

- Dopamine agonists: cabergoline is better tolerated than bromocriptine, whose side effects include orthostasis, lightheadedness, and nausea/vomiting
- Transsphenoidal surgery if no response to medications
- Radiation (rarely needed)

Asymptomatic hyperprolactinemia does not need treatment.

Gynecomastia

This is an increase in size of breast tissue arising from:

- Klinefelter syndrome
- Hyperprolactinemia
- Drugs (spironolactone, opiates, oral ketoconazole, estrogen)
- Liver and renal failure (which elevate prolactin levels)
- Testicular lesions (Sertoli cells make estrogen)

Testing should be done to exclude these disorders. Do mammography to exclude cancer.

Treatment is as follows:

- Tamoxifen
- Testosterone replacement if there is testosterone-deficiency
- Surgery for refractory and idiopathic cases

Thyroid Disorders

What to Look for in Hypothyroidism and Hyperthyroidism	
Hypothyroidism	**Hyperthyroidism**
Bradycardia	Tachycardia, palpitations, arrhythmia (atrial fibrillation)
Constipation	Diarrhea (hyperdefecation)
Weight gain	Weight loss
Fatigue, lethargy, coma	Anxiety, nervousness, restlessness
Decreased reflexes	Hyperreflexia
Cold intolerance	Heat intolerance
Hypothermia (hair loss, edema)	Fever

Hypothyroidism

Hypothyroidism is almost always has a single cause: failure of the thyroid gland due to burnt-out Hashimoto thyroiditis. The acute phase is rarely perceived. Occasionally hypothyroidism is caused by amiodarone or dietary deficiency of iodine.

"What Is the Most Likely Diagnosis?"

Hypothyroidism is characterized by almost all bodily processes being slowed down—except menstrual flow, which is increased.

> High TSH (double normal) + Normal T4 = Treatment

When TSH is very high (more than double the upper limit of normal) with normal T4, replace hormone. When TSH is less than double the normal, get antithyroid peroxidase/antithyroglobulin antibodies. If antibodies are positive, replace thyroid hormone.

> Antithyroid peroxidase antibodies tell who needs thyroid replacement when T4 is normal and TSH is high.

Diagnostic testing for hypothyroidism starts with TSH. If TSH is suppressed, measure free T4. If TSH is markedly elevated, the gland has failed.

Treatment is replacement of thyroid hormone with thyroxine.

Euthyroid sick syndrome is a condition in which clinically euthyroid patients with nonthyroidal systemic illness have low serum levels of thyroid hormones.

- T3 is low
- Reverse T3 (rT3) is high
- T4 can be low

> Real hypothyroidism has very high TSH. Euthyroid sick syndrome does not.

The mechanism of this abnormality is that T4 is converted to rT3, which is inactive, instead of T3, which is very active. The key is that TSH does not rise, so **it is not real hypothyroidism.** Euthyroid sick syndrome is not the same as subclinical hypothyroidism (i.e., elevated TSH with normal T4 and T3 and no symptoms), which is sometimes treated.

Treatment of euthyroid sick syndrome is directed toward the underlying illness. Thyroid hormone replacement is not indicated.

Hyperthyroidism

Etiology/"What Is the Most Likely Diagnosis?"	
Diagnosis	**Unique feature**
Graves disease	Eye (proptosis) (20%–40%) and skin (5%) findings, bruit
Subacute thyroiditis	Tender thyroid
Painless "silent" thyroiditis	Nontender, normal exam results
Exogenous thyroid hormone use	Involuted gland is not palpable
Pituitary adenoma	High TSH level

> Don't order thyroid function tests in patients with nonthyroid critical illness. The results will not be accurate.

Diagnostic testing includes:

- T4 (thyroxine): elevated in all forms of hyperthyroidism
- TSH: elevated in pituitary adenomas, but decreased in all others

> Only Graves disease has:
> - Eye and skin abnormalities
> - TSH receptor antibodies

Thyroid Antibodies	
Antibody name	**Significance**
Thyroglobulin	Detects recurrence of thyroid cancer
Thyroid-stimulating immunoglobulin (TSI)	• Confirms Graves disease • Not positive in toxic multinodular goiter
Thyroperoxidase antibody (TPO)	Confirms presence of Hashimoto thyroiditis

Lab Findings in Hyperthyroidism			
Diagnosis	**TSH**	**RAIU***	**Confirmatory**
Graves disease	Low	Elevated	Positive antibody testing
Subacute thyroiditis	Low	Decreased	Tenderness
Painless "silent" thyroiditis	Low	Decreased	None
Exogenous thyroid hormone use	Low	Decreased	History and involuted, nonpalpable gland
Pituitary adenoma	High	Not done	MRI of head
Toxic nodule	Low	Increased	Focal areas

*RAIU = radioactive iodine uptake

> TSH level is used to monitor hypothyroidism. In hyperthyroidism, however, free T4 levels are used to monitor the disease because TSH lags.

> Toxic nodule has focal uptake of radioactive iodine. Graves is diffuse.

Treatment is as follows:

- **Graves disease:** methimazole or propylthiouracil (PTU), then radioactive iodine
- **Subacute thyroiditis:** aspirin
- **Exogenous thyroid hormone use:** stop use
- **Pituitary adenoma:** surgery

- **Acute hyperthyroidism and "thyroid storm"**
  - Propranolol: blocks target organ effect, inhibits peripheral conversion of T4→T3
  - Thiourea drugs (methimazole [preferred] or PTU [preferred only in pregnancy]): block hormone production
  - Iodinated contrast material (iopanoic acid and ipodate): blocks the peripheral conversion of T4 to the more active T3; also blocks the release of existing hormone. Beta blockers must always be given before iodine replacement.
  - Steroids (hydrocortisone)
  - Radioactive iodine: ablates the gland for a permanent cure
- **Graves ophthalmopathy**: steroids (**best initial therapy**); if no response, radiation is used; severe cases may need decompressive surgery

Painless "silent" thyroiditis requires no treatment.

> Amiodarone always gives thyroid abnormalities, either high or low.

Thyroid Nodules

Thyroid nodules are very common and are palpable in as much as 5% of women and 1% of men. The vast majority of cases are benign (adenoma, colloid nodule, cyst).

There is rarely an association with clinically apparent hyperfunctioning or hypofunctioning.

> Papillary: most common
> Anaplastic: most lethal

A 46-year-old woman presents with a small mass she found on palpation of her own thyroid. A small nodule is found in the thyroid. There is no tenderness. She is otherwise asymptomatic and uses no medications. What is the most appropriate next step in management?

a. Fine-needle aspiration
b. Radionuclide iodine uptake scan
c. T4 and TSH levels
d. Thyroid ultrasound
e. Surgical removal (excisional biopsy)

Answer: **C.** If the patient has a hyperfunctioning gland (i.e., the T4 is elevated or the TSH is decreased), the patient does not need immediate biopsy. Malignancy is not hyperfunctioning. Ultrasound of thyroid is done to evaluate the size of the lesion but does not change the need for either thyroid function testing or needle aspiration.

Diagnostic testing includes:

- Biopsy with fine-needle aspiration for thyroid nodules >1.5 cm if patients have normal thyroid function (T4/TSH)
- U/S and radionuclide scans are not needed because they cannot exclude cancer

> Needle biopsy is the mainstay of thyroid nodule management.

When a patient has a nodule:

1. Perform thyroid function tests (TSH and T4).
2. If tests are normal, biopsy the gland.

A 46-year-old woman with a thyroid nodule is found to have normal thyroid function on testing. The fine-needle aspirate comes back as "indeterminant for follicular adenoma." What is the most appropriate next step in management?

a. Neck CT
b. Surgical removal (excisional biopsy)
c. Ultrasound
d. Calcitonin level

Answer: B. A follicular adenoma is a histologic reading that cannot exclude cancer. The only way to exclude thyroid malignancy is to remove the entire nodule. This is an indeterminant finding on fine-needle aspiration. A sonogram cannot exclude cancer. Calcitonin levels are useful if the biopsy shows medullary carcinoma.

Calcium Disorders

Hypercalcemia

Most patients are asymptomatic. Causes include:

- Primary hyperparathyroidism (PTH) (most common cause)
- Vitamin D intoxication
- Sarcoidosis and other granulomatous diseases
- Thiazide diuretics
- Hyperthyroidism
- Metastases to bone and multiple myeloma

Those who are symptomatic likely have cancer and hypercalcemia of malignancy (caused by a PTH-like particle) due to severe, acute symptomatic hypercalcemia. In those cases, symptoms include:

- Confusion, stupor, lethargy
- Constipation
- Cardiovascular: short QT and hypertension (mechanism not clear)
- Bone lesions: osteoporosis
- Renal: nephrolithiasis, DI, renal insufficiency

Treatment for acute hypercalcemia is as follows:

- Saline hydration at high volume
- Bisphosphonates: pamidronate, zoledronic acid
- Calcitonin (works faster than bisphosphonates)
- Prednisone when the cause is sarcoidosis or any granulomatous disease

> Primary hyperparathyroidism and cancer account for 90% of hypercalcemia patients.

A 75-year-old man with a history of malignancy is admitted with lethargy, confusion, and abdominal pain. His calcium is found to be markedly elevated. After 3 liters of normal saline and zoledronic acid, his calcium is still markedly elevated the next day. What is the most appropriate next step?

a. Calcitonin
b. Pamidronate
c. Plicamycin
d. Gallium
e. Dialysis
f. Cinacalcet

Answer: **A.** Calcitonin inhibits osteoclasts. The onset of action of calcitonin is very rapid, and it wears off rapidly. Bisphosphonates take several days to work. Plicamycin and gallium are older therapies for hypercalcemia that are no longer used (when given as answer choices for treatment, they are always wrong). Pamidronate is a bisphosphonate and does not add anything to the use of zoledronic acid. Dialysis would be used only for those in renal failure. Cinacalcet is an inhibitor of PTH release. If the hypercalcemia is from malignancy, PTH should already be maximally suppressed.

Furosemide is *not used* when urine output is adequate with hydration alone.

Hyperparathyroidism

Primary hyperparathyroidism is from:

- Solitary adenoma (80–85%)
- Hyperplasia of all 4 glands (15–20%)
- Parathyroid malignancy (1%)

Primary hyperparathyroidism often presents as an asymptomatic elevation in calcium levels found on routine blood testing. When there are symptoms, it can occasionally present with the signs of acute, severe hypercalcemia previously described. More often, there are slower manifestations such as:

- Osteoporosis
- Nephrolithiasis and renal insufficiency
- Muscle weakness, anorexia, nausea, vomiting, and abdominal pain
- Peptic ulcer disease (calcium stimulates gastrin)

Bone x-ray is not a good test for bone effects of high PTH. DEXA densitometry is better.

Besides high calcium and PTH levels, you will also find a low phosphate level, high chloride level, EKG with a short QT, and sometimes an elevated BUN and creatinine. Alkaline phosphatase may be elevated from the effect of PTH on bone.

▶ TIP

Preoperative imaging of the neck with sonography or nuclear scanning may be helpful in determining the surgical approach.

Treatment is surgical removal of the involved parathyroid glands (standard of care). Indications for removal of parathyroids:

- Bone disease (e.g., osteoporosis)
- Renal involvement including stones

- Age <50
- Calcium level consistently 1 point above normal

When surgery is not possible, give cinacalcet, which inhibits the release of PTH. Etelcalcetide is used for secondary hyperparathyroidism.

Hypocalcemia

Primary hypoparathyroidism is most often a complication of prior neck surgery, such as for thyroidectomy, in which the parathyroids have been removed. Other causes are:

- Hypomagnesemia: Magnesium is necessary for PTH to be released from the gland. Low magnesium will lead to increased urinary loss of calcium.
- Renal failure, which leads to hypocalcemia. The kidney converts 25 hydroxy-D to the more active 1,25 hydroxy-D.
- Vitamin D deficiency, which can be caused by inadequate sunlight exposure or insufficient intake. Unlike hypoparathyroidism, vitamin D deficiency has low phosphate and elevated alkaline phosphatase. PTH is elevated because calcium is low. Choose 25-hydroxyvitamin D as the best test of vitamin D levels. Deficiency causes:
  - Rickets: childhood disease of impaired long bone growth and craniotabes (soft skull bones)
  - Osteomalacia: adult disease of bone impairment (milder than rickets) and muscle pain
- Genetic disorders
- Fat malabsorption
- Low albumin states: for every 1 point decrease in albumin, calcium level decreases by 0.8; this is *not* symptomatic hypocalcemia, and no calcium replacement is needed

> Cow's milk has significant vitamin D only because **it is added**. The food with the highest naturally occurring level of vitamin D is **salmon**.

Signs of neural hyperexcitability in hypocalcemia:

- Chvostek sign (facial nerve hyperexcitability)
- Carpopedal spasm
- Perioral numbness
- Mental irritability
- Seizures
- Tetany (Trousseau sign)

> Low calcium = twitchy and hyperexcitable
>
> High calcium = lethargic and slow

Testing is EKG, which shows a prolonged QT that may eventually cause arrhythmia. Slit lamp exam shows early cataracts.

Treatment is calcium replacement and activated vitamin D. This is given orally if symptoms are mild/absent and intravenously if symptoms are severe.

Paget Disease of Bone

In Paget disease, osteoclasts and osteoblasts work out of sync, deforming the bone. Paget disease of bone can become osteosarcoma.

Most patients are asymptomatic. An elevation in alkaline phosphatase is found, accompanied by normal gamma-glutamyl transpeptidase (GGTP) and normal bilirubin. Abnormalities are found on skeletal survey.

In symptomatic disease, the most common symptom is bone pain.

Diagnostic testing includes nuclear (technetium) bone scan finding patchy areas of osteoblastic activity (**most accurate test**).

Treatment is as follows:

- For asymptomatic disease: no treatment needed
- When there is pain: bisphosphonates
- When there is bone pain and NSAIDs have failed: calcitonin

Adverse effects of therapy modalities for Paget disease of bone are as follows.

> Paget disease gives high-output CHF.

Adverse Effects			
Bisphosphonate	**PPIs**	**Octreotide, Lanreotide**	**Cabergoline**
• Jaw necrosis • Flulike symptoms • Esophagitis	• Low calcium • Low magnesium • Low iron • Low B12 • *C. difficile* • Pneumonia	• Gallstones • Cholecystitis	Heart valve disease

Adrenal Disorders

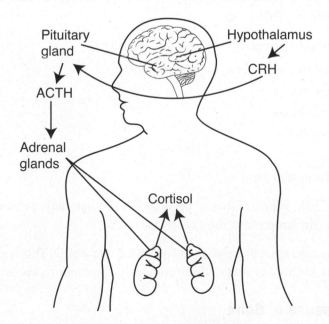

Figure 2.1 Pituitary-Adrenal Axis

Hypercortisolism

Cushing syndrome can be used interchangeably with the term *hypercortisolism*. **Cushing disease** is a term used for the pituitary overproduction of ACTH. Hypercortisolism can also be from the ectopic production of ACTH from carcinoid or cancer or from overproduction autonomously in the adrenal gland. Prednisone and other glucocorticoid use can cause the same manifestations.

Etiology of Hypercortisolism	
Cause of hypercortisolism	**Frequency**
Pituitary ACTH (Cushing disease)	70%
Adrenals	15%
Unknown source of ACTH	5%
Ectopic ACTH (cancer, carcinoid)	10%

Presentation includes:

- **Fat redistribution**: "moon face," truncal obesity, "buffalo hump," thin extremities, increased abdominal fat
- **Skin**: striae, easy bruising, decreased wound healing, and thinning of skin
- **Osteoporosis**
- **Hypertension** from increased sodium resorption in the kidney and increased vascular reactivity
- **Menstrual disorders** in women
- **Erectile dysfunction** in men
- **Cognitive disturbance** from decreased concentration to psychosis
- **Polyuria** from hyperglycemia and increased free water clearance

Diagnostic testing focuses on establishing the presence of hypercortisolism and then identifying the cause of the hypercortisolism.

1. Establish the Presence of Hypercortisolism

The 24-hour urine cortisol is the **best initial test to confirm the presence** of hypercortisolism. If elevation occurs, hypercortisolism is confirmed.

If urine cortisol is not among the answer choices, choose the 1-mg overnight dexamethasone suppression test, which should suppress morning cortisol.

- If suppression occurs, hypercortisolism can be excluded.
- Expect to see some false positives in the presence of depression, alcoholism, and obesity.

2. Establish the Cause of Hypercortisolism

ACTH testing is the **best initial test to determine the cause or location** of hypercortisolism.

- Decreased ACTH means there is an **adrenal source**.

> Low ACTH level = Adrenal source

- Elevated ACTH means one of two possible sources:
  - **Pituitary source** (suppresses with high-dose dexamethasone): Once ACTH is elevated and suppresses with high-dose dexamethasone, do an MRI to scan the brain. If no clear pituitary lesion is seen, sample the inferior petrosal sinus for ACTH, possibly after stimulating the patient with corticotropin-releasing hormone (CRH). Elevated ACTH from the venous drainage of the pituitary confirms the pituitary as the source. The petrosal venous sinus must be sampled because some pituitary lesions are too small to be detected on MRI.
  - **Ectopic production** (does not suppress with high-dose dexamethasone): If ACTH is elevated and you cannot find a defect in the pituitary either with MRI or petrosal sinus sampling, do a chest scan looking for an ectopic source of ACTH production (e.g., lung cancer, carcinoid tumor). You must **always confirm the source of hypercortisolism with biochemical tests** before you perform imaging studies.

> ACTH high? Do a high-dose dexamethasone test.
> - Suppression = pituitary
> - No suppression = ectopic or cancer

Cortisol is also a stress hormone that is an anti-insulin. It has an aldosterone-like effect on the kidney's distal tubule of excreting potassium and hydrogen ions. It causes the following:

- Hyperglycemia
- Hyperlipidemia
- Hypokalemia
- Metabolic alkalosis
- **Leukocytosis** from demargination of WBCs (At least 50% of WBCs in the blood are on the vessel wall waiting for an acute stress to come into circulation. They are like "parked police cars" waiting to be called.)

> A normal midnight salivary cortisol test excludes hypercortisolism.

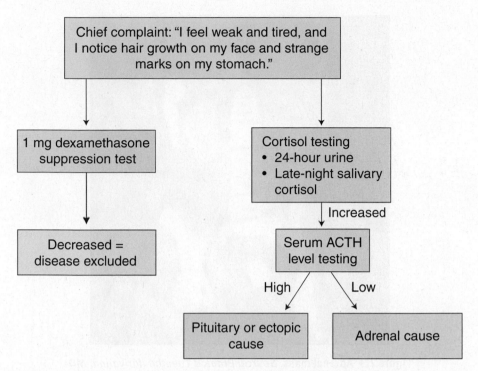

Figure 2.2 Hypercortisolism Diagnostic Evaluation, Part 1

▶ TIP

At least 10% of the population has an abnormality of the pituitary on MRI. If you start with a scan, you may remove the pituitary when the source is in the adrenals.

Treatment is surgical removal of the source of the hypercortisolism.

- Transsphenoidal surgery for pituitary sources
- Laparoscopic surgery for adrenal sources
- Pasireotide, a somatostatin analog, if surgery is not successful
- Mifepristone, which inhibits cortisol receptors throughout the body, if surgery is not possible
  - If adrenal cancer cannot be fully resected or there is metastatic disease that cannot be identified, give mitotane, an inhibitor of steroidogenesis that is also cytotoxic to adrenal tissue.

Pasireotide controls unresectable pituitary ACTH overproduction.

Mitotane cleans up adrenal cancer mets!

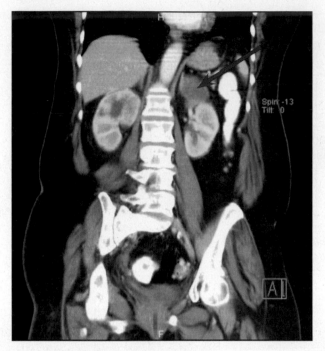

Figure 2.3 Adrenal mass. *Source: Pramod Theetha Kariyanna, MD*

How far should you go in the evaluation of an unexpected, asymptomatic adrenal lesion found on CT?

- Metanephrines of blood or urine to exclude pheochromocytoma
  - **Do these first**, because operating on a pheochromocytoma without proper premedication such as phenoxybenzamine (alpha blocker) is dangerous.
- Renin and aldosterone levels to exclude hyperaldosteronism
- 1 mg overnight dexamethasone suppression test

> 4% of the population has adrenal "incidentaloma." **Do not start with a scan or you will remove the wrong organ.**

Features of Incidental Adrenal Masses	
Favoring Benign Status	**Suspicious for Malignancy**
• Size <4 cm • Low density (<10 Hounsfield units) • High/rapid contrast washout	• Size >4 cm • High density (>10 Hounsfield units) • Low/slow contrast washout • Rapid rate of growth (>1 cm/year)

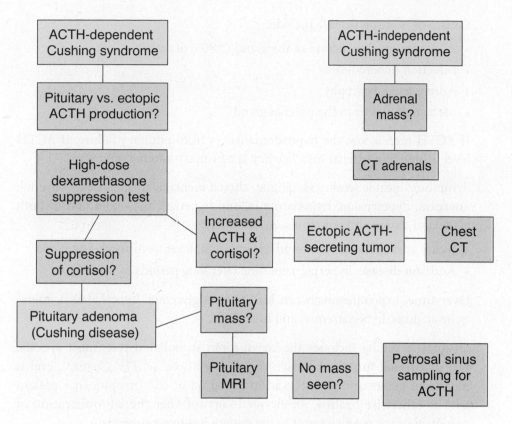

Figure 2.4 Hypercortisolism Diagnostic Evaluation, Part 2

Confirmatory Laboratory Findings in Adrenal Disorders			
	Adrenal	**Pituitary**	**Ectopic**
ACTH level	Low	High	High
Petrosal sinus	Not done	High ACTH	Low ACTH
High-dose dexamethasone	No suppression	Suppresses	No suppression

Hypoadrenalism

Acute adrenal insufficiency is an adrenal crisis, while chronic adrenal insufficiency (or *Addison disease*) is a progressive hypofunctioning of the adrenal cortex. These conditions are different severities of the same disorder.

Causes of acute adrenal crisis include:

- Hemorrhage, surgery, hypotension, or trauma that rapidly destroys the gland
- Sudden removal of chronic high-dose prednisone (steroid)
- Loss of the pituitary (rare, because aldosterone is not under the control of ACTH)

Causes of Addison disease include:

- Autoimmune destruction of the gland (>80% of cases)
- Infection (tuberculosis)
- Adrenoleukodystrophy
- Metastatic cancer to the adrenal gland

If ACTH level is low, the hypoadrenalism is from pituitary failure. If ACTH level is high, the adrenal insufficiency is a primary adrenal failure.

Symptoms include weakness, fatigue, altered mental status, nausea, vomiting, anorexia, hypotension, hyponatremia, and hyperkalemia—common in both acute and chronic presentations. Additionally:

- **Acute adrenal crisis**: profound hypotension, fever, confusion, and coma
- **Addison disease**: hyperpigmentation over long periods of time

Over time, hypoadrenalism can lead to hypoglycemia, hyperkalemia, metabolic acidosis, hyponatremia, and high BUN.

Eosinophilia is common in hypoadrenalism.

Diagnostic testing includes the cosyntropin stimulation test (**most specific test of adrenal function**). Cosyntropin is synthetic ACTH. Cortisol level is measured before and after the administration of cosyntropin. In a patient who is otherwise healthy, an elevated cortisol after the administration of cosyntropin is a positive test, i.e., the patient has hypoadrenalism.

▶ **TIP**

In acute adrenal crisis, treatment is more important than testing.

Treatment is as follows:

- Replace steroids with hydrocortisone. Dexamethasone cannot be used because it has no mineralocorticoid activity.
- If there is still evidence of postural instability, administer fludrocortisone, a steroid hormone that is very high in mineralocorticoid or aldosterone-like effect.

Increase the dose of steroids in stress.

- Use mineralocorticoid supplements in primary adrenal insufficiency if the patient is on oral steroids such as cortisone.

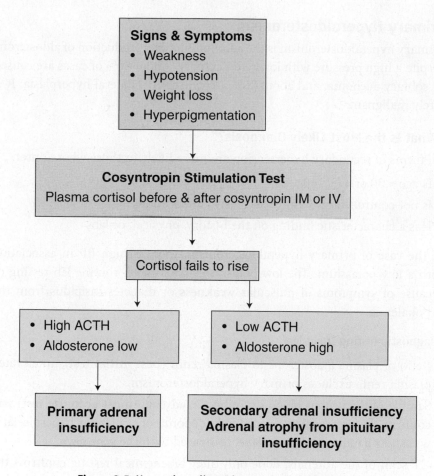

Figure 2.5 Hypoadrenalism Diagnostic Test Algorithm

A patient is brought to the ED after a car accident during which he sustains severe abdominal trauma. On hospital day 2, the patient becomes markedly hypotensive without evidence of bleeding. There is fever, a high eosinophil count, hyperkalemia, hyponatremia, and hypoglycemia. What is the most appropriate next step in management?

a. CT scan of the adrenals
b. Draw cortisol level and administer hydrocortisone
c. Cosyntropin stimulation testing
d. ACTH level
e. Dexamethasone suppression testing

Answer: **B.** In a patient with suspected acute adrenal insufficiency, it is critical to administer hydrocortisone. This is more important than diagnosing the etiology. Hydrocortisone possesses sufficient mineralocorticoid activity to be lifesaving. In addition, hydrocortisone will increase the BP because there is a permissive effect of glucocorticoids on the vascular reactivity effect of catecholamines. BP will come up fast with steroids because norepinephrine will be more effective on constricting blood vessels.

Primary Hyperaldosteronism

Primary hyperaldosteronism is the autonomous overproduction of aldosterone despite a high pressure with low renin activity. About 80% of cases are caused by solitary adenoma, and about 20% are caused by bilateral hyperplasia. It is rarely malignant.

"What Is the Most Likely Diagnosis?"

All forms of secondary hypertension are more likely in those whose onset:

- Is age <30 or age >60
- Is not controlled by 3 antihypertensive medications
- Has a characteristic finding on the history, physical, or labs

> High BP +
> Hypokalemia = Primary
> hyperaldosteronism

In the case of primary hyperaldosteronism, there is high BP in association with a low potassium. The low potassium is found on routine lab testing or because of symptoms of muscular weakness or diabetes insipidus from the hypokalemia.

Diagnostic testing includes:

- Ratio of plasma aldosterone to plasma renin (**best initial test**); an elevated plasma renin excludes primary hyperaldosteronism.
- Sample of the venous blood draining the adrenal (**most accurate test**) will confirm the presence of a unilateral adenoma or unilateral hyperplasia; it will show a high aldosterone level compared with the vena cava.
- CT scan of the adrenals, done only after biochemical testing confirms the following:
  - Low potassium
  - High aldosterone despite a high-salt diet
  - Low plasma renin
  - Aldosterone-to-plasma renin ratio >20:1 **and** aldosterone >15 = primary hyperaldosteronism

> Metabolic alkalosis
> is common in
> hyperaldosteronism.

▶ **TIP**

Never start with a scan in endocrinology. There are too many incidental lesions of the adrenal.

Treatment is as follows:

- Laparoscopy for unilateral adenoma
- Eplerenone or spironolactone for bilateral hyperplasia and patients who cannot have surgery (spironolactone causes gynecomastia and decreased libido because it is anti-androgenic)
- Amiloride (less effective)

Pheochromocytoma

Pheochromocytoma is a nonmalignant lesion of the adrenal medulla autonomously overproducing catecholamines despite a high BP.

"What Is the Most Likely Diagnosis?"

Pheochromocytoma is the answer when there is:

- Hypertension that is episodic in nature
- Headache
- Sweating
- Palpitations, tremor, and tachycardia

Diagnostic testing includes:

- Level of free metanephrines in plasma (**best initial test**)
- 24-hour urine collection for metanephrines will confirm diagnosis (more sensitive and more accurate than urine vanillylmandelic acid [VMA])
- Direct measurements of epinephrine and norepinephrine
- CT or MRI of the adrenal glands, done only after biochemical confirmation of pheochromocytoma
- If CT or MRI is negative, MIBG scan (a nuclear isotope scan) can detect the location of pheochromocytoma that originates outside the adrenal gland

Treatment is phenoxybenzamine, an alpha blocker (**best initial therapy**). Surgical removal of the lesion is done laparoscopically.

> Orthostatic hypotension occurs between hypertension episodes.

Pancreatic Islet Cell Tumors

Pancreatic islet cell tumors are rare tumors of the pancreas that begin in neuroendocrine islet cells.

Insulinoma

Insulinoma is diagnosed with the presence of hypoglycemia and elevated insulin. Most of these tumors are benign.

Testing includes:

- Low glucose + high C-peptide (**best initial test**)
- 72-hour fasting with high C-peptide + absence of ketosis (**most specific test**)
- CT of abdomen (pancreas)

Treatment is surgical removal, done laparoscopically.

Glucagonoma

Glucagonoma is diagnosed with hyperglycemia and weight loss that is 100% of pancreatic origin. Most of these tumors are malignant. Glucagonoma is associated with necrolytic migratory erythema, a characteristic skin lesion.

Treatment is octreotide (somatostatin) and surgical resection.

VIPoma

VIPoma is characterized by secretory, high-volume watery diarrhea; hypokalemia; and achlorhydria.

- Low osmotic gap for diarrhea, low iron/B12
- Testing includes high vasoactive intestinal peptide (VIP) + CT/MRI/ endoscopic U/S showing a lesion in the pancreas
- Somatostatin drugs: octreotide or lanreotide

Treatment is surgical resection.

Multiple Endocrine Neoplasia (MEN) Syndromes

MEN 1	MEN 2A	MEN 2B
• Parathyroid • Anterior pituitary • Pancreatic islet cells	• Parathyroid • Medullary thyroid • Pheochromocytoma	• Mucosal neuroma • Medullary thyroid • Pheochromocytoma • Marfanoid

Diabetes Mellitus

Diabetes mellitus (DM) is defined as persistently high fasting glucose levels >125 mg/dL on at least 2 separate occasions.

The most common symptoms are polyuria, polydipsia, and polyphagia. Decreased wound healing is common.

> Antibodies to glutamic acid decarboxylase (GAD) are present in type 1 diabetes.

- **Type 1 DM** (insulin deficiency)
  - Onset typically in childhood
  - Insulin dependent from an early age
  - Not related to obesity
- **Type 2 DM** (insulin resistance)
  - Onset typically in adulthood
  - Directly related to obesity
  - More resistant to diabetic ketoacidosis (DKA) than type 1

> Screen obese patients for diabetes.

A diagnosis of diabetes is made with one of the following:

- Two fasting blood glucose >125 mg/dL
- Single blood glucose >200 mg/dL with the preceding symptoms
- Increased glucose level on oral glucose tolerance testing

Hemoglobin A1c >6.5% is a diagnostic criterion and is the best test to follow treatment response over several months.

Treatment of DM focuses on a goal HbA1c <7%.

- Diet, exercise, and weight loss (controls up to 25% of type 2 DM cases without the need for medications)
  - Decreasing the amount of adipose tissue helps decrease insulin-resistance
  - Exercising muscle does not need insulin
- Oral hypoglycemic medication
  - Metformin (**best initial drug treatment**): works by blocking gluconeogenesis; does not cause weight gain (contraindicated in those with renal dysfunction because it can accumulate and cause metabolic acidosis)
  - Sulfonylureas are not used as first-line therapy because they increase insulin release from the pancreas, thereby driving the glucose intracellularly and increasing obesity.
- DPP-IV inhibitors (sitagliptin, saxagliptin, linagliptin, alogliptin) block the metabolism of the incretins (called glucose insulinotropic peptide [GIP] and glucagon-like peptide [GLP]).
- The incretins (GIP and GLP) increase insulin release and decrease glucagon release from the pancreas. They are secreted into the bloodstream when food (especially carbohydrates) enters the duodenum and is metabolized by dipeptidyl peptidase-IV (DPP-IV). The incretins normally have a half-life of only 1–2 minutes, but adding a DPP-IV inhibitor will markedly lengthen that. Semaglutide is the first oral GLP agonist.
- SGLT2 inhibitors (empagliflozin, dapagliflozin, canagliflozin, ertugliflozin) are added when 2 or 3 other oral hypoglycemic medications have not been effective. They inhibit the resorption of glucose in the proximal convoluted tubule after it has been filtered. The extra sugar in the urine increases the likelihood of urinary tract infections and fungal vaginitis. This is the most common question on SGLT2 inhibitors on Step 2 CK.
- Incretin mimetics (exenatide, liraglutide, albiglutide, dulaglutide) are a direct replacement of incretins. They are generally given after the DPP-IV inhibitors have been tried, because they must be administered by injection. Incretin agonists also markedly slow gastric motility and decrease weight. The management of incretins is confusing because they have several names.
- Thiazolidinediones (glitazones) provide no clear benefit over the other hypoglycemic medications. They are relatively contraindicated in CHF because they increase fluid overload.
- Nateglinide and repaglinide stimulate insulin release in a similar manner to sulfonylureas but do not contain sulfa. They do not add any therapeutic benefit to sulfonylureas.
- Alpha glucosidase inhibitors (acarbose, miglitol) are agents that block glucose absorption in the bowel. They add about half a point decrease in HgA1c. They cause flatus, diarrhea, and abdominal pain. They can be used with renal insufficiency.

> Hemoglobinopathies that can falsely decrease the HbA1c:
> - Sickle cell disease
> - G6PD
> - Thalassemia

> Semaglutide is the first oral GLP agonist.

> Metformin does not cause hypoglycemia. It is the safest drug to start in newly diagnosed diabetics.

> **Insulin pump:**
> - Standard of care for type 1 DM
> - Uses rapid insulin

- Pramlintide is an analog of a protein called amylin that is normally secreted with insulin. Amylin decreases gastric emptying, decreases glucagon levels, and decreases appetite.

If the patient is not controlled with oral hypoglycemic agents, **add insulin**. Again, the goal of treatment is HgA1c <7%. (Dosing is not tested on the exam.)

- Insulin glargine gives a steady state of insulin for the entire day.
- Glargine provides much steadier blood levels than NPH insulin, which is dosed 2×/day.
- Long-acting insulin is combined with a short-acting insulin such as lispro, aspart, or glulisine.
- Regular insulin is sometimes used as the short-acting insulin.

> The term "glucagon-like peptide" is confusing, because GLP actually inhibits/suppresses glucagon.

The incretins are glucose insulinotropic peptide (GIP) and glucagon-like peptide (GLP).

- DPP-IV inhibitors block their metabolism.
- All slow gastrointestinal motility.

Pharmacokinetics of Insulin Formulations			
Insulin formulation	**Onset**	**Peak action**	**Duration**
Lispro, aspart, and glulisine	5–15 minutes	1 hour	3–4 hours
Regular	30–60 minutes	2 hours	6–8 hours
NPH	2–4 hours	6–7 hours	10–20 hours
Glargine, detemir	1–2 hours	No peak	24 hours
Degludec	2–4 hours	No peak	36 hours

Diabetic Ketoacidosis

Although more common in those with type 1 diabetes, diabetic ketoacidosis (DKA) can definitely present in those with type 2 diabetes.

Patients present with:

- Hyperventilation
- Possibly altered mental status
- Metabolic acidosis with an increased anion gap
- Hyperkalemia in blood, but decreased total body potassium because of urinary spillage
- Increased anion gap on blood testing
- Serum is positive for ketones
- Nonspecific abdominal pain
- "Acetone" odor on breath
- Polydipsia, polyuria

Treat with large-volume saline and insulin replacement. Replace potassium when the potassium level comes down to a level approaching normal. Correct the underlying cause: noncompliance with medications, infection, pregnancy, or any serious illness.

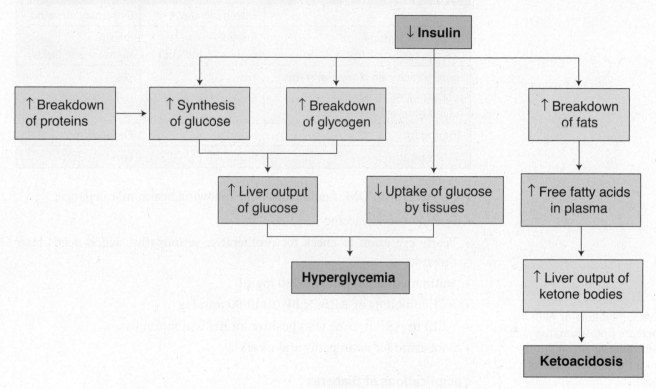

Figure 2.6 Action of Insulin Insufficiency in Diabetes Mellitus

A 57-year-old man is admitted to intensive care with altered mental status, hyperventilation, and a markedly elevated glucose. Which of the following is the most accurate measure of the severity of his condition?

a. Glucose level

b. Serum bicarbonate

c. Urine ketones

d. Blood ketones

e. pH level on blood gas

Answer: B. Serum bicarbonate level is a way of saying "anion gap." If bicarbonate is low, the anion gap is increased and the patient is at risk of death. If serum bicarbonate is high, it does not matter how high the glucose is, in terms of severity. Hyperglycemia is not the best measure of the severity of DKA. The glucose can be markedly elevated without the presence of ketoacidosis. Urine ketones mean very little. Although blood ketones are important, they are not all detected.

Nonketotic Hyperosmolar Syndrome (NKHS)

NKHS and DKA have important similarities and differences.

	NKHS	DKA
Glucose level	Extremely elevated	Extremely elevated
Best initial therapy	Insulin + high-volume fluids	Insulin + high-volume fluids
Hypertonicity alters mental status	Yes	Yes
Hypertonicity causes seizures and brain abnormalities	More common	Less common
Anion gap	Normal	Elevated
Serum bicarbonate	Normal	Low

All patients with DM should receive the following health maintenance:

- Pneumococcal vaccine
- Yearly eye exam to check for proliferative retinopathy, which needs laser therapy
- Statin medication if LDL >100 mg/dL
- ACE inhibitors or ARBs if BP **>140/90** mm Hg
- ACEI or ARB if urine tests positive for microalbuminuria
- Foot exam for neuropathy and ulcers

Complications of Diabetes

Mismanaged diabetes puts the patient at risk of developing dangerous complications.

- **Cardiovascular complications**: myocardial infarction, stroke, and CHF from premature atherosclerotic disease (all significant risk)
  - BP goal in those with diabetes is at least **<140/90 mm Hg**
  - Diabetes is considered an equivalent of coronary disease for treatment of LDL, and goal is <100 mg/dL when initiating treatment with statins
- **Diabetic nephropathy**
  - Early in the disease, microalbuminuria may develop (i.e., albumin 30–300 mg per 24 hrs)
  - Dipstick for urine becomes trace positive at 300 mg of protein per 24 hours.
  - Screening recommendation for those with diabetes is annual testing for microalbuminuria, plus an ACE inhibitor or ARB when it is present. These agents are proven to decrease the rate of progression of nephropathy by decreasing intraglomerular hypertension and decreasing damage to the kidney.

> If ACE inhibitors or ARBs increase potassium, use patiromer or zirconium to keep the potassium level normal.
>
> Do not stop the ACE inhibitor or ARB!

- **Gastroparesis** (an immobility of the bowels): After several years, DM decreases the ability of the gut to sense the stretch of the walls of the bowel. Stretch is the main stimulant to gastric motility. Symptoms include bloating, constipation, early satiety, vomiting, and abdominal discomfort. Treatment is metoclopramide or erythromycin, which increases gastric motility. If no response, choose a gastric pacemaker.

- **Retinopathy**: DM's effect on microvasculature is especially apparent in the eye. In the United States, nearly 25,000 people go blind from DM each year. The only treatment for nonproliferative retinopathy is tighter control of glucose. Aspirin does not help retinopathy. When neovascularization and vitreous hemorrhages are present, it is called proliferative retinopathy. This is treated with laser photocoagulation, which markedly retards the progression to blindness. VEGF inhibitors treat severe retinopathy.

> **Retinopathy:** Vascular endothelial growth factor (VEGF) inhibitors help.

- **Neuropathy**: Damage to microvasculature damages the vasa nervorum that surrounds large peripheral nerves. This leads to decreased sensation in the feet—the main cause of skin ulcers of the feet, which lead to osteomyelitis. When the neuropathy leads to pain, treatment is with pregabalin, gabapentin, or tricyclic antidepressants.

Hypoglycemia

The most common reason for hospital admission in diabetes is hypoglycemia—not DKA or new-onset diabetes. The most common cause is error in treatment, e.g., excess medication or inappropriate dose adjustment, particularly as renal insufficiency decreases insulin requirements. Treat by giving glucose and/or glucagon either intravenously or by inhalation.

Other causes of hypoglycemia are:

- **Insulinoma**: low glucose + high insulin/C-peptide; remove lesion surgically
- **Insulin autoimmune antibodies**: autoantibodies present
- **Sulfonylurea abuse**: urine metabolites of sulfonylureas found; elevated C-peptide and proinsulin
- **Surreptitious use of insulin/suicide**: low C-peptide, low pro-insulin

Hormone-Related Conditions

Hirsutism

Hirsutism is male-pattern hair growth in women. It can develop from any of several causes.

- Medications, such as minoxidil, valproic acid, phenytoin
- Emotional distress/depression
- Polycystic ovary syndrome (PCOS), Cushing syndrome, congenital adrenal hyperplasia, androgen medication use, androgen-secreting tumor, or carcinoma

Virilization is more severe than hirsutism. Symptoms include clitoromegaly, deepening of the voice, irregular menstrual periods, acne, and increased muscle mass.

Testing should be done when patients present with irregular menstrual periods and signs of virilization.

- Prolactin
- DHEA
- Testosterone
- FSH/LH
- 17-hydroxyprogesterone

Manage hirsutism with oral contraceptives, antiandrogens (spironolactone, finasteride), metformin (only in PCOS).

Polycystic Ovary Syndrome

Polycystic ovary syndrome (PCOS) is the most common cause of oligomenorrhea in the United States, with a dramatically high incidence that is rising. The following criteria are used to diagnose PCOS:

- Clinical hirsutism and/or high testosterone/DHEA
- Irregular menstruation
- 10 cysts on pelvic sonogram with enlarged ovary (>10 cm)

Diagnosis requires **only 2 of these criteria**. The idea that a pelvic sonogram is required to establish a diagnosis is a *common error*. If the patient meets the other 2 criteria, sonogram is *not* needed. Also note that LH/FSH ratio is not part of the diagnostic criteria.

Treatment of PCOS is a multisystem approach.

- PCOS is a "prediabetic" state—some of the same mechanisms that cause insulin resistance also interfere with aromatization of testosterone to estrogen, leading to higher androgen levels in these patients.
- LH/FSH alterations occur afterward.
- Metabolic health is very important in these patients, so BP, lipids, glucose, and weight must all be followed diligently and managed.
- Irregular menstruation is a problem in PCOS because a woman's uterine lining must be shed regularly; otherwise, there may be conversion to uterine hyperplasia (premalignant). Treatment is OCPs containing progesterone to regulate menstruation.
- Spironolactone (last-line) for patients with hirsutism, but only after lifestyle management, metformin, and OCPs have been tried.

Cardiology 3

Syncope

Syncope is loss of consciousness due to insufficient blood flow to the brain. Cardiovascular problems are one cause, but syncope can also arise from neurological causes or from toxins or metabolic problems.

The first step in the evaluation of loss of consciousness from syncope is to confirm that the patient has definitely lost consciousness. Just because a person falls to the floor or is less responsive does not mean there is syncope. Evaluate loss of consciousness as follows:

Was the loss of consciousness sudden or gradual?

- **Sudden loss** usually has a cardiac or neurologic etiology, such as arrhythmia or seizure.
- **Gradual loss** usually stems from toxins or metabolic problems, such as hypoglycemia, hypoxia, or drug intoxication.
- Vasovagal syncope can be sudden or gradual in onset.

Was the regaining of consciousness sudden or gradual?

- **Sudden regaining** usually has a cardiac etiology, such as arrhythmia, valve disease, or ischemia.
- **Gradual regaining** usually stems from tonic-clonic, generalized seizures (exception: absence seizure).

Note that people do not seize and wake up right away. They have a post-ictal state of confusion that can last up to 24 hours.

If the **loss and regaining are both sudden**, the next step is a cardiac exam as follows:

- **Exam normal**: arrhythmia, needs EKG, telemetry monitor, and troponin level
- **Exam abnormal**: needs echocardiogram; exclude AS, HOCM, MS

> Patients with true syncope are not able to hear people speaking. Urinary or bowel incontinence is too nonspecific to be useful.

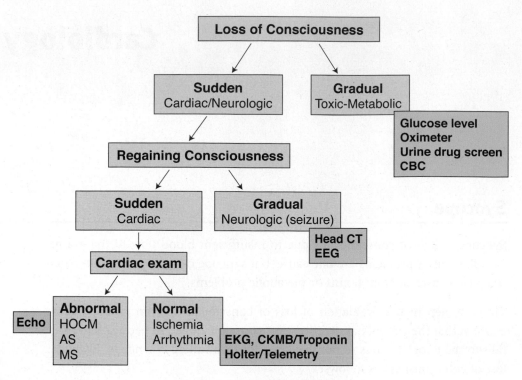

Figure 3.1 Syncope Evaluation

Treatment

Treatment of syncope is based on the history and physical examination. Routinely get a head CT, EKG, cardiac enzymes, and echocardiogram.

- Those inpatient are placed on cardiac telemetry to monitor for an arrhythmia.
- Those discharged home have a 24-hour Holter monitor placed for the same purpose.

> 90% of mortality from syncope is due to cardiac causes.

Coronary Artery Disease

Coronary artery disease (CAD) (also called atherosclerotic or ischemic heart disease) describes insufficient perfusion of the coronary arteries due to an abnormal narrowing of the vessels, resulting in insufficient oxygen delivery to the myocardial tissue.

When chest pain is equivocal or the history is uncertain, understanding the risk factors is critical for establishing a diagnosis of CAD. The most clearly agreed-upon risk factors for CAD are:

- DM (**most serious**)
- Hypertension (**most common**)
- Family history of premature CAD
- Hyperlipidemia

- Tobacco smoking
- Age >45 (men) and age >55 (women)
- Renal disease

The presence of CAD risk factors can help answer the question, "Which of the following is the most likely diagnosis?" when the patient is young or the presentation is equivocal.

Diabetes Mellitus

When followed over a long period of time (e.g., 10 years), it has been found that patients with DM have the highest rates of CAD.

Hypertension

Hypertension (BP >140/90 mm Hg) is more common than DM, with □20% of the total U.S. population (60 million people) suffering from hypertension. Nearly 50% of these people are unaware that they are hypertensive.

Family History of Premature CAD

Only **premature CAD in a first-degree relative** (sibling or parent) is a risk factor for CAD. "Premature CAD" is defined as male relative age <55 or female relative age <65.

In other words, if CAD developed in elderly relatives or if the relatives were grandparents, cousins, or aunts/uncles, there is no specific risk factor for CAD.

On the exam, the most common mistake about risk factor involves family history, i.e., students mistake CAD in elderly relatives (including their own parents) as a risk factor. The key is that the CAD in a relative must be premature.

> **Unproven risk factors** for CAD include elevated homocysteine, *Chlamydia* infection, and elevated C-reactive protein. There is no reason to measure, follow, or intervene therapeutically on these factors. They are wrong answers.

A 48-year-old woman is seen for chest pain that has been recurring for several weeks. The pain is not reliably related to exertion. She is comfortable now. The location of the pain is retrosternal. The pain is sometimes associated with nausea, it does not radiate beyond the chest, and there is no shortness of breath. She has no medical history. What is the most likely diagnosis?

a. Gastroesophageal reflux disease (GERD)
b. Unstable angina
c. Pericarditis
d. Pneumothorax
e. Prinzmetal angina

Answer: **A.** When a patient has chest pain and the etiology is not likely to be cardiac ischemia, a GI disorder such as GERD is the likely cause. Other common GI disorders associated with chest pain are ulcer disease, cholelithiasis, duodenitis, and gastritis. If a woman, age 48, has chest pain with no risk factors, ischemic heart disease is unlikely to be the cause. By age 55–60, however, the protective effect of menstruation and naturally-occurring estrogen has worn off, and the rates of CAD will at least equal the rates in men.

▶**TIP**

Menstruating women virtually never have myocardial infarction.

▶**TIP**

Overall, more women will die of heart disease than men.

Hyperlipidemia

Which of the following is the most dangerous to a patient in terms of risk for CAD?

a. Elevated triglycerides
b. Elevated total cholesterol
c. Decreased high density lipoprotein (HDL)
d. Elevated low-density lipoprotein (LDL)
e. Obesity

Answer: **D**. Marked elevation in LDL is by far the most dangerous portion of a lipid profile for a patient. Low HDL is also associated with a poor long-term prognosis but is not as dangerous as elevated LDL. Although elevated triglycerides are potentially dangerous, that is not as reproducible in terms of poor outcome as elevated LDL. Treatment of an isolated elevated triglyceride level is less clearly beneficial than treatment of an elevated LDL. Obesity, particularly that resulting in increasing abdominal girth, is associated with increased cardiac mortality. However, much of the danger of obesity is from its association with other abnormalities such as hyperlipidemia, diabetes, and hypertension.

> Measurement of lipid subtypes such as lipoprotein has no benefit.

Takotsubo Cardiomyopathy

A postmenopausal woman develops chest pain immediately on hearing the news of her son's unexpected death. She develops acute chest pain, dyspnea, and ST segment elevation in leads V2 to V4 on EKG. Elevated troponin confirms an acute myocardial infarction. Coronary angiography is normal including an absence of vasospasm on provocative testing. EKG reveals apical left ventricular "ballooning." What is the presumed mechanism of this disorder?

a. Absence of estrogen
b. Massive catecholamine discharge
c. Plaque rupture
d. Platelet activation
e. Emboli to the coronary arteries

Answer: **B**. Takotsubo cardiomyopathy is acute myocardial damage most often occurring in postmenopausal women immediately following an overwhelming, emotionally stressful event. Examples are divorce, financial issues, earthquake, lightning strike, and hypoglycemia. This leads to "ballooning" and left ventricular dyskinesis. As with ischemic disease, manage with beta blockers and ACE inhibitors. Revascularization will not help, since the coronary arteries are normal.

> Sudden, overwhelming emotional stress and anger can cause chest pain and sudden death.

Correcting which of the following risk factors for CAD will result in the most immediate benefit for the patient?

a. Diabetes mellitus
b. Tobacco smoking
c. Hypertension
d. Hyperlipidemia
e. Weight loss

Answer: **B.** Smoking cessation results in the greatest immediate improvement in patient outcomes for CAD. Within 1 year after stopping smoking, the risk of CAD decreases by 50%, and within 2 years after stopping smoking, risk is reduced by 90%.

Chest Pain Presentation

"What Is the Most Likely Diagnosis?"

For every 100 people presenting to the ED with chest pain:

- <10% end up having a myocardial infarction as the cause
- ≥50% have no cardiac disease at all

The heart is a muscle, and like any muscle, when it is starved for oxygen it will produce a sore-muscle type of pain when ischemic. Ischemic pain is described as:

- Dull or "sore"
- Squeezing or pressure-like

Qualities of the pain that go against ischemia are:

- Sharp ("knifelike") or pointlike
- Lasts for a few seconds

Three features of chest pain effectively rule out ischemia as the cause of the pain:

- Changes with respiration (pleuritic)
- Changes with position of the body
- Changes with touch of the chest wall (tenderness)

Ischemic pain is not tender, positional, or pleuritic, so any one of these features would exclude ischemia as a cause of the chest pain (□95% negative predictive value). On the USMLE exam, a 95% negative predictive value is generally enough to allow you to answer the question correctly. When the pain is described as changing with respiration, with bodily position, or upon touching the chest wall, do *not* answer ischemia or CAD as the cause of the chest pain.

> **GI disorder** is the most common *non-ischemic* cause of chest pain.

Characteristics of Ischemic Pain	
Duration	Stable angina: >2 to <10 min ACS: >10 to 30 min
Provoking factors	Physical activity, cold, emotional stress
Associated symptoms	SOB, nausea, diaphoresis, dizziness, lightheadedness, fatigue
Quality	Squeezing, tightness, heaviness, pressure, burning, aching **NOT**: *sharp, pins, stabbing, knifelike*
Location	Substernal
Alleviating factors	Rest
Radiation	Neck, lower jaw & teeth, arms, shoulders

Causes of Chest Pain		
If the case describes...	**Answer as "most likely diagnosis"**	**Answer as "most accurate test"**
Chest wall tenderness	Costochondritis	Physical examination
Radiation to back, unequal BP between arms	Aortic dissection	Chest x-ray with widened mediastinum, chest CT, MRI, or TEE confirms the disease
Pain worse with lying flat, better when sitting up, young (<40)	Pericarditis	Electrocardiogram with ST elevation everywhere, PR depression
Epigastric discomfort, pain better when eating	Duodenal ulcer disease	Endoscopy
Bad taste, cough, hoarseness	Gastroesophageal reflux	Response to PPIs; aluminum hydroxide and magnesium hydroxide; viscous lidocaine
Cough, sputum, hemoptysis	Pneumonia	Chest x-ray
Sudden-onset shortness of breath, tachycardia, hypoxia	Pulmonary embolus	Spiral CT, V/Q scan
Sharp, pleuritic pain, tracheal deviation	Pneumothorax	Chest x-ray

There are some nonspecific symptoms of chest pain that will not be helpful in determining a diagnosis.

- Nausea
- Fever (suggests PE or pneumonia as the cause)
- Sweating (diaphoresis)
- Anxiety

Diagnostic Tests

- Electrocardiogram (EKG) (**best initial test** for all forms of chest pain)
  - In the office-based, ambulatory setting, the EKG is normal most of the time.
- Enzymes (CK-MB/troponin)
  - In the office-based, ambulatory setting, cardiac enzymes are not the answer when evaluating chronic or stable chest pain.
  - In the ED when you are evaluating acute cases of chest pain, enzymes should be used, after the EKG.
- Stress (exercise-tolerance) testing
  - Exercise tolerance testing (ETT) is indispensable for evaluating chest pain when etiology is not clear and EKG is not diagnostic.
  - ETT is based on 2 factors
    - Factor 1: **You can read the EKG**; ischemia is detected by ST segment depression on the EKG (if EKG cannot be read due to a baseline abnormality, do nuclear isotope uptake [thallium or sestamibi] or echocardiographic detection of wall motion abnormalities to detect ischemia)
    - Factor 2: **Patient can exercise**, i.e., can increase heart rate >85% of maximum (maximum heart rate = 220 minus the patient's age)
- Alternate methods for increasing myocardial oxygen consumption if patient cannot exercise
  - Dipyridamole or adenosine plus a nuclear isotope such as thallium or sestamibi
  - Dobutamine plus echocardiogram
    - Dobutamine will increase myocardial oxygen consumption and provoke ischemia detected as wall motion abnormalities on echo (i.e., dyskinesia, hypokinesia)
    - Contraindications to dobutamine include ventricular arrhythmias, severe hypertension, LV outflow obstruction, beta blocker

▶ **TIP**

Baseline EKG abnormalities may be caused by left bundle branch block, left ventricular hypertrophy, pacemaker use, and the effect of digoxin.

- Normal myocardium will pick up nuclear isotopes such as thallium in the same way that potassium is picked up by the sodium/potassium ATPase. If the myocardium is alive and perfused, thallium or other nuclear isotopes will be picked up. Abnormalities will be detected by seeing decreased thallium uptake.
- Normal myocardium will move on contraction. Abnormalities on echocardiogram will be detected by seeing decreased wall motion. This is also referred to as dyskinesis, akinesis, or hypokinesis.

- In office/ambulatory clinic, when chest pain for days/weeks: **no enzymes**
- In ED, when chest pain for minutes/hours: **yes enzymes**

Stress testing is used when the etiology of chest pain is uncertain and the EKG is not diagnostic.

Dipyridamole may provoke bronchospasm. Avoid in asthmatics.

Ischemia gives **reversible** wall motion or thallium uptake between rest and exercise. Infarction is irreversible, or "fixed."

▶**TIP**

Ischemia versus infarction: Ischemia, or simply decreased perfusion, will be detected by seeing a **reversal** of the decrease in thallium uptake or wall motion that will **return to normal** after a period of rest.

Use of Exercise Tolerance Testing					
Test	**Exercise tolerance**	**Exercise thallium**	**Exercise echo**	**Dipyridamole thallium**	**Dobutamine echo**
Indication	Determine presence of ischemia	Inability to read the EKG, baseline ST segment abnormalities	Same as exercise thallium	Inability to exercise to target heart rate	Same as dipyridamole thallium
Ischemia detected	ST segment depression	Decreased uptake of nuclear isotope	Wall motion abnormalities	Decreased uptake of nuclear isotope	Wall motion abnormalities

A man with atypical chest pain is found to have normal nuclear isotope uptake in his myocardium at rest. On exercise, there is decreased uptake in the inferior wall. Two hours after exercise, the uptake of nuclear isotope returns to normal. What is the next step in management?

a. Coronary angiography
b. Bypass surgery
c. Percutaneous coronary intervention (e.g., angioplasty)
d. Dobutamine echocardiography
e. Nothing; it is an artifact

Answer: **A.** This patient has reversible ischemia on the stress test: exactly the person who needs angiography. If the presentation of anginal chest pain is 100% specific for coronary disease, there is not much point in doing a stress test. Even if it comes back negative, the patient likely has coronary disease. The stress test is precisely for when you are not sure of etiology. When isotope uptake is normal at rest and decreases on exercise, you have found the person who can benefit from revascularization. You cannot determine what type of revascularization until after you know the anatomy. If there is no reversibility in ischemia between rest and exercise, there is little to be gained from revascularization. Irreversible ("fixed") defects mean dead (infarcted) myocardium. There is not much point in revascularizing dead tissue; it is too late. There *is* a point in revascularizing reversible defects. The tissue can be saved, and you can prevent infarction. Reversible perfusion defects need catheterization. Catheterization indicates which patients get bypass versus angioplasty versus medications alone.

▶**TIP**

The 2 methods that can detect ischemia in terms of using nuclear isotopes or echo are essentially equal in terms of sensitivity and specificity.

- Exercise thallium = Exercise echo
- Dipyridamole thallium = Dobutamine echo

Before administering a dipyridamole stress test, **stop caffeine.**

Coronary Angiography

Angiography is used to detect the anatomic location of coronary artery disease. Angiography is predominantly a test to detect the presence of narrowing that is best managed with surgery, angioplasty, or other methods of revascularization. Sometimes angiography is used if noninvasive tests such as EKG or stress testing are equivocal. Angiography is the **most accurate method** of detecting coronary artery disease.

Stenosis (narrowing) <50% of the diameter is insignificant. Surgically correctable disease generally begins with ≥70% stenosis.

> Angiography determines bypass **surgery** vs. **angioplasty**.

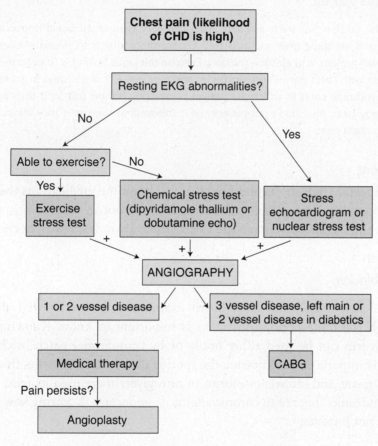

Figure 3.2 Chest Pain Diagnosis Algorithm

Holter Monitoring

The Holter monitor is a continuous ambulatory EKG monitor that records the rhythm; it is usually used for 24–48 hours but may be continued for months. Holter monitoring mainly detects rhythm disorders including atrial fibrillation (A-fib), flutter, ectopy such as premature beats, or ventricular tachycardia. Holter monitor does not detect ischemia and is not accurate for evaluating the ST segment.

> Holter monitoring is used mainly for **rhythm evaluation**.

A 48-year-old woman comes to the office with chest pain that has been occurring over the last several weeks. The pain is not reliably related to exertion. She is comfortable now. The location of the pain is retrosternal. She has no hypertension, and the EKG is normal. What is the most appropriate next step in management?

a. CK-MB
b. Troponin
c. Echocardiogram
d. Exercise tolerance testing
e. Angiography
f. CT angiography
g. Cardiac MRI
h. Holter monitor

Answer: **D.** Enzymes are to evaluate acute coronary syndromes. Serial troponin measurements are done prior to stress test. Echocardiography is to evaluate valve function, wall motion, and ejection fraction. Exercise tolerance testing is to evaluate stable patients with chest pain whose diagnoses are not clear. ETT is not used in acute coronary syndrome cases in which the patient is currently having pain and the diagnosis is already clear. Also, don't put patients on a treadmill to exercise if they are currently having chest pain.

Treatment

USMLE Step 2 CK is most concerned that you know the **medications that will lower mortality**. For a patient with chronic angina (not an acute coronary syndrome), the therapeutic options are easier. There are only a few right choices:

- Aspirin
- Beta blockers

USMLE Step 2 CK, like most board examinations, will not test dosing, although the route of administration is important to know. Knowing that nitroglycerin can be used either orally or by transdermal patch in chronic angina is important, but knowing the specific dose is not. Knowing that sublingual, paste, and intravenous forms of nitroglycerin are used in acute coronary syndromes, but not in chronic angina, is important. Knowing how much paste is not important.

Antiplatelet Therapy

> Ticagrelor is an antiplatelet medication added to aspirin. It is an alternative to prasugrel or clopidogrel.

Stable CAD patients and those without a stent only need aspirin.

ACE Inhibitors/Angiotensin Receptor Blockers

- Low ejection fraction/systolic dysfunction (best mortality benefit)
- Regurgitant valvular disease
- Cough is the most common adverse effect of ACE inhibitors, occurring in up to 7% of patients.

Beta Blockers

Beta blockers are the first-line therapy in patients with stable angina. They work by decreasing myocardial contractility, heart rate, and O_2 demand. Decreased heart rate prolongs diastole, which increases coronary perfusion. All beta blockers are equally effective in exertional angina; however, due to their side effects, nonselective beta blockers are rarely used.

Lipid Management

▶ TIP

Statins (HMG CoA reductase inhibitors)

- CAD with any LDL
- The goal is an LDL at least <70 mg/dL

Everyone will agree that with CAD, the goal of LDL should be at least **<70 mg/dL**. In primary prevention, start a statin if the 10-year risk of CAD is >7.5%. "High-intensity statin" means atorvastatin or rosuvastatin.

▶ TIP

CAD equivalents (statins should be used in all of these):

- Peripheral artery disease (PAD)
- Carotid disease
- Aortic disease (the aortic artery, not the valve)
- Stroke
- MI

What is clear on lipid management?

There is no cutoff point at which to start statin medications in those with coronary artery disease, stroke, or peripheral artery disease. *Everyone with this form of vascular disease* should be on a statin to lower LDL.

It is clear that *only* statins are associated with a definite mortality benefit in the management of hyperlipidemia in any circumstance.

> Which of the following is the most common adverse effect of statin medications?
>
> a. Rhabdomyolysis.
> b. Liver dysfunction.
> c. Renal failure.
> d. Encephalopathy.
> e. Hyperkalemia.
>
> Answer: **B.** At least 2–3% of patients taking statin medications will develop elevation of transaminases to the level where you will need to discontinue the medication. Myositis, elevation of CPK levels, or rhabdomyolysis will occur in less than 0.1% of patients. It is very rare to have to stop statins because of myositis. There is *no recommendation* to routinely test all patients for CPK levels in the absence of symptoms. On the other hand, all patients started on statins should have their AST and ALT tested as a matter of routine monitoring, even if no symptoms are present.

> Clear indications for the use of statins:
> - Acute coronary syndrome
> - MI or stenting
> - Any arterial disease
> - 10-year risk of CAD >7.5%

Other Lipid-Lowering Therapies

Niacin, gemfibrozil, and ezetimibe all have beneficial effects on lipid profiles. However, **none of them is the best initial therapy** because none of them has the clear mortality benefit in CAD that statins provide. **Statins have an antioxidant effect** on the endothelial lining of the coronary arteries that gives a benefit that transcends simply lowering the LDL number. When statin alone fails to achieve the LDL goal, add ezetimibe.

Ezetimibe: This agent definitely lowers LDL level. However, LDL levels are an imperfect marker of benefit with cholesterol-lowering therapies.

Niacin: Associated with glucose intolerance, elevation of uric acid level, and an uncomfortable "itchiness" from a transient release of prostaglandins. Although statins, exercise, and cessation of tobacco use will all raise the HDL level, niacin will raise HDL somewhat more.

Gemfibrozil: Fibric acid derivatives lower triglyceride levels somewhat more than statins; however, the benefit of lowering triglycerides alone has not proven to be as useful as the straightforward mortality benefit of statins. Use caution in combining fibrates with statins because of an increased risk of myositis. Routinely checking lipoprotein (Q) levels, apolipoprotein levels, or LDL particles provides no benefit.

PCSK9 Inhibitors

Evolocumab and alirocumab inhibit proprotein convertase subtilisin/kexin type 9 (PCSK9). PCSK9 inhibitors (injectable medications) do the following:

- Increase LDL clearance from the blood by blocking the breakdown of LDL receptors in the liver
- Decrease elevated LDL significantly in familial hypercholesterolemia
- Increase hepatic clearance of LDL massively, but do not lower mortality

With severe hyperlipidemia, if LDL is not controlled with a statin at maximum dose, try a PCSK9 inhibitor.

▶ **TIP**

Lipid-lowering therapy: What is clear?

- **Statins lower mortality the most.**
- **Adverse effects are well established.**

> Check AST and ALT when using statins.

Lipid-Lowering Medications and Their Adverse Effects	
Agent	**Adverse effect**
Statins	Elevations of transaminases (liver function tests), myositis
Niacin	Elevation in glucose and uric acid level, pruritus
Fibric acid derivatives	Increased risk of myositis when combined with statins
Cholestyramine	Flatus and abdominal cramping

Calcium Channel Blockers

Dihydropyridine calcium channel blockers (CCBs) such as nifedipine, nitrendipine, nicardipine, and nimodipine may actually increase mortality in patients with CAD because of their effect in raising heart rates. The best example of an increased heart rate is the "reflex tachycardia" developing from the use of nifedipine. This is probably the best explanation for the failure of the CCBs to decrease mortality.

Bottom line: Do *not* routinely use CCBs in CAD.

Use CCBs (verapamil/diltiazem) in CAD *only* with:

- **Severe asthma** precluding the use of beta blockers
- **Prinzmetal** variant angina
- **Cocaine-induced** chest pain (beta blockers are safe)
- Inability to control pain with maximum medical therapy

Adverse Effects of CCBs

- Edema
- Constipation
- Heart block (rare)

Ranolazine

Ranolazine is a sodium channel–blocking medication that treats angina. Ranolazine is added to those who still have pain despite aspirin, beta blockers, nitrates, and calcium blockers. It does not have a clear mortality benefit.

Revascularization

Angiography is indispensable in evaluating a patient for the possibility of revascularization, which is either coronary bypass surgery or angioplasty. Symptoms alone cannot tell the number of vessels involved, what vessels are involved, or the degree or percentage of stenosis.

Coronary artery bypass grafting (CABG) lowers mortality only in a few specific circumstances with very severe disease such as:

- Three vessels with at least 70% stenosis in each vessel
- Left main coronary artery occlusion
- Two-vessel disease in a patient with diabetes
- Persistent symptoms despite maximal medical therapy

None of the calcium channel blockers have been shown to lower mortality in CAD.

When studying medications, you must know **the clear adverse effects**. These USMLE Step 2 CK questions do not change over time.

Long-term mortality benefit from CABG is greater with the most severe disease such as left ventricular dysfunction. The immediate operative mortality may be greater in patients with an ejection fraction (EF) <35%, but in the long term, those with 3-vessel disease have improved survival with coronary bypass surgery if they survive the procedure.

Internal mammary **artery grafts last on average for 10 years** before they occlude, whereas saphenous **vein grafts remain patent reliably for only 5 years**. Half of vein grafts are patent at 10 years.

Percutaneous coronary intervention (PCI) is commonly referred to as angioplasty. The term *intervention* is more precise, because there are other interventions besides angioplasty. PCI is unquestionably the **best therapy in acute coronary syndromes**, particularly those with ST segment elevation. The mortality benefit of PCI has been much harder to demonstrate in chronic stable angina. Maximal medical therapy with aspirin, beta blockers, ACEIs/ARBs, and statins has proven to have equal or even superior benefit compared to PCI in stable CAD. PCI is more definitive in terms of decreasing dependence on medication and decreasing frequency of painful angina episodes.

> PCI is the best in **acute coronary syndromes**, particularly with ST segment elevation. PCI *does not* provide clear mortality benefit for stable patients.

Acute Coronary Syndromes

It is impossible to determine the precise etiology of acute coronary syndromes (ACS) from history and physical examination alone. The risk factors (e.g., hypertension, diabetes mellitus, tobacco) are the same as those described previously for CAD.

A 70-year-old woman comes to the ED with crushing substernal chest pain for the last hour. The pain radiates to her left arm and is associated with anxiety, diaphoresis, and nausea. She describes the pain as "sore" and "dull," and she clenches her fist in front of her chest. She has a history of hypertension. Which of the following is most likely to be found?

a. Decrease of >10 mm Hg in blood pressure on inhalation
b. Increase in jugular venous pressure on inhalation
c. Triphasic scratchy sound on auscultation
d. Continuous "machinery" murmur
e. S4 gallop
f. Point of maximal impulse displaced toward the axilla

Answer: **E.** Acute coronary syndromes are associated with an S4 gallop because of ischemia leading to noncompliance of the left ventricle. The S4 gallop is the sound of atrial systole as blood is ejected from the atrium into a stiff ventricle. A decrease of blood pressure is >10 mm Hg on inspiration is a pulsus paradoxus and is associated with cardiac tamponade.

An increase in jugulovenous pressure on inhalation is the **Kussmaul sign** and is most often associated with constrictive pericarditis or restrictive cardiomyopathy. A triphasic "scratchy" sound is a pericardial friction rub. Although pericarditis can occur as a complication of myocardial infarction (Dressler syndrome), this would not occur for several days after an MI and is much rarer than simple ventricular ischemia.

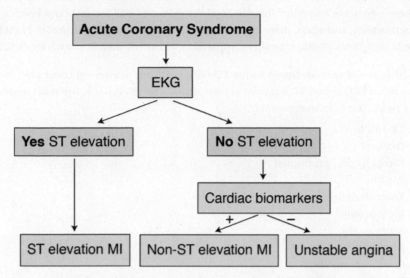

Figure 3.3 Acute Coronary Syndromes Diagnosis Algorithm

▶ **TIP**

A continuous "machinery" murmur is what would be found with a patent ductus arteriosus.

A displaced point of maximal impulse (PMI) is characteristic of left ventricular hypertrophy (LVH) as well as dilated cardiomyopathy. A displaced PMI is an anatomic abnormality that could not possibly occur with an acute coronary syndrome.

> There are **no specific physical findings** to allow you to answer a "most likely diagnosis" question in terms of ST elevation or depression without an EKG.

A 70-year-old woman comes to the ED with crushing substernal chest pain for the last hour. Which of the following EKG findings would be associated with the worst prognosis?

a. ST elevation in leads II, III, aVF
b. PR interval >200 milliseconds
c. ST elevation in leads V2–V4
d. Frequent premature ventricular complexes (PVCs)
e. ST depression in leads V1 and V2
f. Right bundle branch block (RBBB)

Answer: **C.** Leads V2 to V4 correspond to the anterior wall of the left ventricle. ST segment elevation most often signifies an acute myocardial infarction. ST elevation in leads II, III, and aVF is also consistent with an acute myocardial infarction, but of the inferior wall. Untreated, the mortality associated with an IWMI is <5% at 1 year after the event. With an AWMI, mortality untreated is closer to 30–40%. PR interval >200 milliseconds is first-degree atrioventricular (AV) block. **First-degree AV block has little pathologic potential** and, when isolated, requires no additional therapy. Ectopy such as PVCs and atrial premature complexes (APCs) are associated with the later development of more severe arrhythmias, but no additional therapy is needed for them if magnesium and potassium levels are normal. PVCs do not require any changes

> Do not walk into your USMLE Step 2 CK exam without knowing when you will expect each of the cardiac physical findings described here.

> **PVCs should not be treated**, even when associated with an acute infarction. Treatment of PVCs only worsens outcome.

in management. ST depressions in leads V1 and V2 are suggestive of a posterior wall myocardial infarction. These leads are read in the opposite direction of the rest of the leads. In other words, ST depression in leads V1 and V2 would be like ST elevation elsewhere—an acute infarction. Infarctions of the posterior wall are associated with a very low mortality, and again, there is no additional therapy to give because of it. Right bundle branch block (RBBB) is benign compared to a new left bundle branch block (LBBB).

A 70-year-old woman comes to the ED with crushing substernal chest pain for the last hour. EKG shows ST segment elevation in V2 to V4. What is the most appropriate next step in management?

a. CK-MB level
b. Oxygen
c. Nitroglycerin sublingual
d. Aspirin
e. Thrombolytics
f. Metoprolol
g. Atorvastatin
h. Angioplasty
i. Consult cardiology
j. Transfer patient to ICU
k. Troponin level
l. Morphine
m. Angiography
n. Clopidogrel

> All MIs get 2 antiplatelet drugs.

Answer: **D.** Aspirin lowers mortality with ACS, and it is critical to administer rapidly. With only 1 hour since the onset of pain, neither the CK-MB nor the troponin would yet be elevated. Morphine, oxygen, and nitroglycerin do not lower mortality, so are not as important as aspirin. Aspirin should be given simultaneously with activating the catheterization lab. Either clopidogrel, prasugrel, or ticagrelor is indicated in any patient with an acute MI. Transfer the patient to the ICU, but always initiate therapy and testing before doing so. Starting proper care first is critical. Thrombolytics or angioplasty should be done (and quickly), but aspirin should be given first. Aspirin and a second antiplatelet drug are then followed with another form of acute revascularization.

> Oxygen does *not* help nonhypoxic patients.

▶ **TIP**

On the USMLE Step 2 CK exam, consultation is almost **never** the correct choice. Do everything yourself.

> One of the most critical points of preparation is knowing the **order in which to do things**. It is not enough to know which tests and treatments must be done. You must be able to prioritize what is first.

A 70-year-old woman comes to the ED with crushing substernal chest pain for the last hour. An EKG shows ST segment elevation in V2 to V4. Aspirin and clopidogrel have been given to the patient to chew. What is the most appropriate next step in management?

a. CK-MB level
b. Oxygen
c. Nitroglycerin sublingual
d. Morphine
e. Thrombolytics
f. Metoprolol
g. Atorvastatin

h. Angioplasty

i. Troponin level

j. Lisinopril

Answer: H. Angioplasty is associated with the greatest mortality benefit of all the steps listed in this question. All of the answer choices are partially correct in that they should all be done for the patient. Nitrates should be given to the patient immediately, but they do not clearly lower mortality. Enzyme tests should be done, but within the first 4 hours of the onset of chest pain they will certainly be normal. Even if they are elevated, CK-MB and troponin levels would not alter the management. Beta blockers are associated with a decrease in mortality, but they are not critically dependent upon time. As long as the patient receives metoprolol sometime during the hospital stay and at discharge, she will derive benefit. The same is true of the use of statins and ACE inhibitors.

> CPR alone can raise cardiac enzymes.

Key issues in the management of ACS:

- Does the intervention/treatment lower mortality?
- Which intervention is most important to do first?

Diagnostic Tests		
Test	**Time to becoming abnormal**	**Duration of abnormality**
EKG	Immediately at onset of pain	ST elevation progresses to Q-waves over several days to a week
Myoglobin	1–4 hours	1–2 days
CK-MB	4–6 hours	1–2 days
Troponin	4–6 hours	10–14 days

The use of the troponin level has its limitations:

- Troponin cannot distinguish a reinfarction occurring several days after the first event.
- Renal insufficiency can result in false positive tests since troponin is excreted through the kidney.

Reinfarction

When a patient has a new episode of pain within a few days of the first cardiac event, the management is:

1. Perform an EKG to detect new ST segment abnormalities.
2. Check CK-MB levels.

After 2 days, the CK-MB level from the initial infarction should have returned to normal. A CK-MB level that is elevated several days after an initial myocardial infarction is indicative of a new ischemic event.

> CK-MB is better at detecting reinfarction. CK-MB should be gone in 24–48 hours.

Intensive Care Unit Monitoring

After the initial management is put in place, the patient should be monitored in an ICU. Continuous rhythm monitoring is essential to an improved survival:

- The most common cause of death in the first several days after a myocardial infarction is ventricular arrhythmia (ventricular tachycardia, ventricular fibrillation).
- Rapid performance of electrical cardioversion or defibrillation is available.

ST Segment Elevation Myocardial Infarction

All patients with ACS should receive 2 antiplatelet medications immediately upon arrival in the ED. Combine aspirin and a second agent (clopidogrel, prasugrel, or ticagrelor; all are inhibitors of the $P2Y_{12}$ receptor on the platelet).

- Two-drug therapy is specific to acute presentations, and especially to the use of coronary stenting.
- Two-drug antiplatelet drug therapy does not apply to chronic or stable coronary artery disease.

When angioplasty and stenting are planned, the answer is ticagrelor or prasugrel. Although all 3 $P2Y_{12}$ inhibitors are beneficial, the restenosis of stenting is best prevented by prasugrel or ticagrelor.

Clopidogrel

Best mortality benefit in **chronic** angina: aspirin and beta blockers.

- Used in:
    - Combination with aspirin on all acute coronary syndromes
    - Aspirin intolerance such as allergy
    - Recent angioplasty with stenting
- Rarely associated with thrombotic thrombocytopenic purpura

Prasugrel

- Indicated as antiplatelet medication
- **Best evidence for use**: angioplasty and stenting
- Dangerous in patients age ≥75: increased risk of hemorrhagic stroke
- Do not use if history of TIA or stroke

Ticlopidine

- Causes neutropenia and TTP

Angioplasty versus Thrombolytics

Angioplasty, or percutaneous coronary intervention (PCI), is superior to thrombolytics in terms of:

- Survival and mortality benefit
- Fewer hemorrhagic complications
- Reduced likelihood of developing complications of MI (less arrhythmia, less CHF, fewer ruptures of septum, free wall [tamponade] and papillary muscles [valve rupture])

The **standard of care** is that PCI is expected to be performed within 90 minutes of the patient arriving in the emergency department with chest pain.

> "Door to balloon time": **<90 minutes**

Complications of PCI

- **Rupture** of the coronary artery on inflation of the balloon
- **Restenosis** (thrombosis) of the vessel after the angioplasty
- **Hematoma** at the site of entry into the artery (e.g., femoral area hematoma)
- **Distal cholesterol embolization**; look for livedo reticularis, eosinophilia/eosinophiluria after catheterization, low complement, high ESR. There is no treatment.

Which of the following is most important in decreasing the risk of restenosis of the coronary artery after PCI?

a. Multistage procedure: i.e., doing 1 vessel at a time, with multiple procedures
b. Use of heparin for 3–6 months after the procedure
c. Warfarin use after the procedure
d. Placement of bare metal stent
e. Placement of drug-eluting stent (paclitaxel, sirolimus)

Answer: E. The placement of drug-eluting stents that inhibit the local T cell response has markedly reduced the rate of restenosis. Heparin is used at the time of the procedure but is not continued long term. Warfarin has no place in the management of coronary disease; it is useful for clots on the venous side of the circulation such as DVT or pulmonary embolus.

Rates of Restenosis within 6 Months of PCI

- No stenting: 30–40%
- Bare metal stent: 10–15%
- Drug-eluting stent: <5%

If there is a contraindication to the use of thrombolytics, the patient should be transferred to a facility that can perform PCI.

> Heme-positive brown stool is **not an absolute contraindication** to the use of thrombolytics.

Contraindications to Thrombolytics

- Major bleeding into the bowel (melena) or brain (any type of CNS bleeding)
- Recent surgery (within the last 2 weeks)
- Severe hypertension (>180/110 mm Hg)
- Nonhemorrhagic stroke within the last 6 months

> When it comes to administering thrombolytics, **lost time is lost heart muscle, and delay means death.** On the exam, you can answer "thrombolytics" in any patient with chest pain and ST segment elevation within 12 hours of the onset of chest pain.

A patient comes to a small rural hospital without a catheterization laboratory. The patient has chest pain and ST segment elevation. What is the most appropriate next step in management?

a. Angioplasty
b. Thrombolytics immediately
c. Cardiology consult

Answer: **B.** Immediate thrombolytics are far more beneficial than angioplasty delayed by several hours. The mortality benefit of thrombolytics extends to 12 hours from the onset of chest pain. The mortality benefit is as much as a 50% relative risk reduction within the first 2 hours of the onset of pain. This is why a patient with chest pain who arrives at the ED should receive thrombolytics within 30 min of coming through the door. A consult is almost never the right answer on USMLE Step 2 CK.

> "Door to needle time":
> **<30 minutes**

ACS Treatment Indications and Benefits	
Therapy	**In what cases is effect greatest?**
Aspirin	Everyone, as the best initial therapy
Clopidogrel or prasugrel or ticagrelor	• Those undergoing angioplasty or stenting, second antiplatelet drug with aspirin • 2 antiplatelet drugs in all MIs
Beta blockers	Everyone, effect is **not** dependent on time; started any time during admission
ACEI/ARB	Everyone, benefit best with ejection fraction <40%
Statins	Everyone, goal LDL <70 mg/dL
Nitrates	Everyone, no clear mortality benefit
Heparin	After thrombolytics/PCI to prevent restenosis, initial therapy with ST depression and other non-ST elevation events (unstable angina)
Calcium channel blockers	Can't use beta blockers, cocaine-induced pain, Prinzmetal or vasospastic variant angina

ST Segment Depression ACS

A man comes to the ED with chest pain for the last hour that is crushing in quality and does not change with respiration or the position of his body. An EKG shows ST segment depression in leads V2–V4. Aspirin and clopidogrel have been given. What is the most appropriate next step in management?

a. Low-molecular-weight heparin
b. Thrombolytics
c. Glycoprotein IIb/IIIa inhibitor (abciximab)
d. Nitroglycerin
e. Morphine
f. Angioplasty
g. Metoprolol

Answer: **A.** LMW heparin will prevent a clot from forming in the coronary arteries. Heparin does not dissolve clots that have already formed. When the patient has ACS and there is no ST segment elevation, thrombolytic therapy confers no benefit. Nitroglycerin, morphine, and oxygen are not associated with a reduction in mortality. ACE inhibitors and statins are used, but the mortality benefit is based on a low ejection fraction or increased LDL, respectively. Metoprolol should be used, but the timing of the beta blocker administration has not been proven, so it would not be considered urgent. There is tremendous urgency for heparin administration because we want to prevent the clot from growing further and closing off the coronary artery.

Glycoprotein IIb/IIIa Inhibitors (GPIIb/IIIa Inhibitors)

GPIIb/IIIa inhibitors (abciximab, tirofiban, eptifibatide) are used in patients with acute coronary syndromes who are to undergo angioplasty and stenting. These agents inhibit the aggregation of platelets.

Treatment Differences between Cardiac Events			
	Stable Angina	**Unstable Angina/Non-ST Elevation MI**	**ST Elevation MI**
Aspirin	Yes	Yes	Yes
Beta blockers	Yes	Yes	Yes
Nitrates	Yes	Yes	Yes
LMW heparin (enoxaparin)	No	Yes	Yes, but only after revascularization
GPIIb/IIIa meds	No	Yes	Yes
Thrombolytics	No	No	Yes, but not as good as PCI
CCBs	No	No	No
Warfarin	No	No	No
Antiplatelet drug	No	Yes	Yes

Absolute contraindications to thrombolytics:
- Major bleeding (bowel/brain)
- Recent surgery (≤2 weeks)
- Severe hypertension (>180/110 mm Hg)
- Nonhemorrhagic stroke (≤6 months)

Morphine is not useful in MI.

Bottom Line

a. tPA (thrombolytics) are beneficial **only with ST elevation MI or new LBBB**.

b. LMW heparin is best for **non-ST elevation MI**.

c. GP IIb/IIIa inhibitors are best for **non-ST elevation MI** in those undergoing PCI and stenting.

▶ **TIP**

Calcium channel blockers and warfarin have no mortality benefit in ACS.

GPIIb/IIIa inhibitors are used only with stenting.

▶ **TIP**

Low-molecular-weight heparin (enoxaparin) is superior to unfractionated heparin in terms of mortality benefit.

In non-ST elevation ACS, when all medications have been given and the patient is not better, urgent angiography and possibly angioplasty (PCI) should be done. **"Not better"** means:

- Persistent pain
- S3 gallop or CHF developing
- Worse EKG changes or sustained ventricular tachycardia
- Rising troponin levels

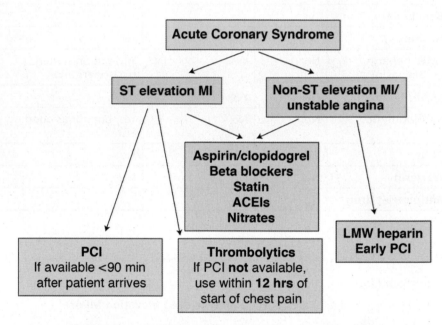

Figure 3.4 Acute Coronary Syndromes Treatment Algorithm

Complications of Acute Myocardial Infarction

▶ **TIP**

Complications of acute myocardial infarction are an excellent source of "What is the most likely diagnosis?" questions, the most common type of question on USMLE Step 2 CK.

All the complications of myocardial infarction can result in hypotension, so the presence of hypotension *will not help you* determine the diagnosis.

Bradycardia

Heart rate is key to establishing the diagnosis of post-MI complications.

Starving hearts have ventricular tachycardia— open it fast with PCI!

Sinus bradycardia is very common in association with MI because of vascular insufficiency of the sinoatrial (SA) node.

Third-degree (complete) AV block will have cannon A waves. They are the best way to distinguish third-degree AV block from sinus bradycardia before you obtain an EKG. Cannon A waves are produced by atrial systole against a closed tricuspid valve. The tricuspid valve is closed because the very essence of third-degree block is that the atria and ventricles are contracting separately and out of coordination with each other.

The cannon is the bounding jugulovenous wave bouncing up into the neck. Look for an association with right ventricular infarction and third-degree AV block. All symptomatic bradycardias are treated first with atropine and then (if the atropine is not effective) by placing a pacemaker.

Tachycardia

Right Ventricular Infarction

Look for the association with a new inferior wall MI and clear lungs on auscultation. You cannot get blood into the lungs if the blood cannot get into the heart. You can diagnose by flipping the EKG leads from the usual left side of the chest to the right side of the chest. ST elevation in RV4 is the most specific finding.

The right coronary artery supplies:

- Right ventricle (RV)
- AV node
- Inferior wall of the heart

> Right coronary supplies:
> SA node 60%
> AV node 90%

This is why up to 40% of those with an inferior wall myocardial infarction (IWMI) will have a right ventricular infarction. Treat RV infarctions with high-volume fluid replacement. Avoid nitroglycerin in RV infarctions; it markedly worsens cardiac filling.

Tamponade/Free Wall Rupture

It usually takes several days after an infarction for the wall to scar and weaken enough to rupture. Look for "sudden loss of pulse" in the case. Lungs are clear. It is a cause of pulseless electrical activity.

You can diagnose with emergency echocardiography. Emergency pericardiocentesis is done on the way into the operating room to repair it.

Ventricular Tachycardia/Ventricular Fibrillation

Both ventricular tachycardia and ventricular fibrillation can cause sudden death, and if they cause loss of pulse there is no way to distinguish them without an EKG. Both are treated with emergency electrical shock (cardioversion/defibrillation).

> These complications are the reason patients with acute MI are monitored in an ICU for the first several days after the infarction.

Valve or Septal Rupture

Both valve rupture and septal rupture present with new onset of a murmur and pulmonary congestion. Mitral regurgitation murmur is best heard at the apex with radiation to the axilla. Ventricular septal rupture is best heard at the lower left sternal border.

▶ **TIP**

Most accurate test: Echocardiogram for both valve rupture and septal rupture.

▶ **TIP**

You can't always depend on buzzwords like "step-up" for oxygenation. Often, the numbers are simply presented to you: "72% oxygen saturation is found on a sample of blood from the right atrium. 85% saturation is found on the right ventricular sample."

> Look for a **step-up in oxygen saturation** as you go from the right atrium to the right ventricle to hand you the diagnosis of **septal rupture**.

Intraaortic Balloon Pump

Intraaortic balloon pump (IABP) is the answer when there is acute pump failure from an anatomic problem that can be fixed in the operating room. IABP contracts and relaxes in sync with natural heartbeat. It helps give a "push" forward to the blood.

▶ **TIP**

IABP is **never** a permanent device. It serves as a bridge to surgery for valve replacement or transplant for 24–48 hours.

Extension of the Infarction/Reinfarction

When a patient presents with an inferior or anterior infarction, it is common for a second event to infarct a *second* geographic area of the heart.

Look for recurrence of pain, new rales on exam, a new bump up in CK-MBs, and even sudden onset of pulmonary edema.

Repeat the EKG and re-treat with angioplasty and sometimes thrombolytics in addition to the usual medications (aspirin, metoprolol, nitrates, ACE, statins).

Aneurysm/Mural Thrombus

Aneurysm or mural thrombus is detected with echocardiography. Most aneurysms do not need specific therapy. Mural thrombi, like all thrombi, are treated with anticoagulation.

"What Is the Most Likely Diagnosis?"	
Key feature	**Diagnosis**
Bradycardia, cannon A waves	Third-degree AV block
No cannon A waves	Sinus bradycardia
Sudden loss of pulse, jugulovenous distention	Tamponade/wall rupture
IWMI in history, clear lungs, tachycardia, hypotension with nitroglycerin	RV infarction
New murmur, rales/congestion	Valve rupture
New murmur, increase in oxygen saturation on entering the right ventricle	Septal rupture
Loss of pulse, need EKG to answer question	Ventricular fibrillation

Preparation for Discharge from Hospital

▶ TIP

Do not do a stress test if the patient remains symptomatic. These people clearly need angiography.

Do not do angiography if reversible signs of myocardial ischemia are absent on stress test. There is no point in revascularizing to myocardium that is dead (infarcted).

ACE inhibitors are **best for anterior wall infarctions** because of the high likelihood of developing systolic dysfunction. For patients who experience cough with an ACE inhibitor, give ARBs. The table summarizes discharge medications for patients post-MI.

Dipyridamole is **never** the right choice for coronary artery disease.

Discharge Medications Post-MI	
Therapy	**Comment**
Aspirin + P2Y$_{12}$ inhibitor	• Continue aspirin indefinitely. • Give P2Y$_{12}$ inhibitor ≥12 months
Beta blocker	• Start within 24 hours. • Reduces mortality as long as given before discharge.
Statin	All on high intensity statin after ACS. Goal LDL <70
ACEi/ARB	Anterior MI, heart failure, EF <40%
Spironolactone	EF <40% post MI

Prophylactic antiarrhythmic medications:

Do not use amiodarone, flecainide, or any rhythm-controlling medication to prevent the development of ventricular tachycardia or fibrillation. Do not be fooled by the question describing "frequent PVCs and ectopy." **Prophylactic antiarrhythmics increase mortality.**

Sexual Issues Postinfarction

This is a very frequently tested subject. The most commonly tested facts are:

1. Do not combine nitrates with sildenafil; hypotension can result because they are both vasodilators.

2. Erectile dysfunction postinfarction is most commonly from anxiety; however, of all the medications that cause erectile dysfunction, the most common is beta blockers.

3. The patient should wait until after an MI to reengage in sexual activity. If the patient is symptom-free, sexual activity may begin in 2–4 weeks. A small (inferior) MI requires a shorter wait before sex resumes than an anterior wall MI.

4. If the post-MI stress test is described as normal, the patient can reengage in any form of exercise program as tolerated, including sex.

Congestive Heart Failure

Congestive heart failure (CHF) is a dysfunction of the heart as a pump of blood, causing insufficient oxygen delivery to tissues and fluid accumulation in the lungs. There are 2 causes:

- **Systolic dysfunction**: decreased ejection fraction and dilation of the heart
- **Diastolic dysfunction** (inability of the heart to "relax" and receive blood): normal ejection fraction

The essential feature of CHF is shortness of breath (dyspnea).

Systolic Dysfunction

The most common cause of CHF is hypertension resulting in a cardiomyopathy or abnormality of the myocardial muscle. Initially, when caused by hypertension, ejection fraction is preserved. Over time, the heart dilates and causes systolic dysfunction and decreased ejection fraction. Valvular heart disease of all types results in CHF.

Myocardial infarction (MI) is a very common cause of dilated cardiomyopathy and decreased ejection fraction. When the heart is "dead" or infarcted, it will not pump. In the United States, CHF is the most common cause of hospital admission in adults. Those with CHF are admitted repeatedly for exacerbations.

▶ **TIP**

Infarction → Dilation → Regurgitation → CHF

Infarction, cardiomyopathy, and valve disease account for the vast majority of cases. Less common causes are:

- Alcohol
- Postviral (idiopathic) myocarditis
- Radiation
- Adriamycin (doxorubicin) use
- Chagas disease and other infections
- Hemochromatosis (also causes restrictive cardiomyopathy)
- Thyroid disease
- Peripartum cardiomyopathy
- Thiamine deficiency

Presentation

Even in its worst form (pulmonary edema), CHF is a clinical diagnosis. That means you should be able to identify the most likely diagnosis from the history and physical exam, without needing to use lab tests.

Dyspnea (shortness of breath) on exertion is the indispensable clue to diagnosis. In addition, look for:

- Orthopnea (shortness of breath that is worse when lying flat, relieved when sitting up/standing)
- Peripheral edema
- Rales on lung examination
- Jugulovenous distention (JVD)
- Paroxysmal nocturnal dyspnea (PND) (sudden worsening at night, during sleep)
- S_3 gallop rhythm (on the Step 2 exam, be prepared to identify the sound that may be played)

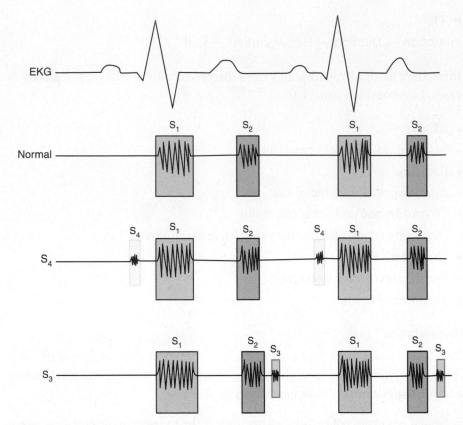

Figure 3.5 Timing of S_3 and S_4 Gallops in the Cardiac Cycle. *Source: Andrew Peredo, MD*

"What Is the Most Likely Diagnosis?" for Dyspnea	
Key feature	**Most likely diagnosis is...**
Sudden onset, clear lungs	Pulmonary embolus
Sudden onset, wheezing, increased expiratory phase	Asthma
Slower, fever, sputum, unilateral rales/rhonchi	Pneumonia
Decreased breath sounds unilaterally, tracheal deviation	Pneumothorax
Circumoral numbness, caffeine use, history of anxiety	Panic attack
Pallor, gradual over days to weeks	Anemia
Pulsus paradoxus, decreased heart sounds, JVD	Tamponade
Palpitations, syncope	Arrhythmia of almost any kind
Dullness to percussion at bases	Pleural effusion
Long smoking history, barrel chest	COPD
Recent anesthetic use, brown blood not improved with oxygen, clear lungs on auscultation, cyanosis	Methemoglobinemia
Burning building or car, wood-burning stove in winter, suicide attempt	Carbon monoxide poisoning

All of these will lack:

- Orthopnea/PND
- S_3 gallop

Diagnostic Tests

There is an enormous difference in the management of chronic CHF and pulmonary edema in office and ambulatory-based settings. The key is to identify the setting (ED versus office or clinic) and whether acute symptoms of dyspnea are seen at the time of presentation.

- Echocardiogram (**most important of all the CHF tests**)
  - All patients with CHF must undergo echocardiography to evaluate ejection fraction.
  - There is no way to distinguish systolic from diastolic dysfunction by history, physical examination, or other tests such as EKG, chest x-ray, BNP
- Transthoracic echocardiogram (TTE) (**best initial test**) to evaluate ejection fraction
- Multiple-gated acquisition scan (MUGA)
- Nuclear ventriculogram (**most accurate test/most precise for wall motion abnormalities**): used in rare cases, i.e., if you need to administer maximum amount of doxorubicin chemotherapy to a patient to cure his lymphoma but not so much as to cause cardiomyopathy
- Transesophageal echocardiogram (TEE) to evaluate heart valve function and diameter; TEE is not necessary for evaluating CHF
- Brain natriuretic peptide (BNP) level to evaluate acute shortness of breath when etiology is unclear and you cannot wait for an echo to be done; a normal BNP excludes CHF as a cause of the shortness of breath

Other tests that are used are *not to diagnose* CHF but rather to identify the **cause of CHF**. A diagnosis of CHF is a clinical diagnosis (based on history and physical) with the type of CHF determined by TTE.

> Chest x-ray misses nearly half of cardiomegaly.

Tests Used to Determine Etiology of CHF	
Test	**Etiology of CHF**
EKG	MI, heart block
Chest x-ray	Dilated cardiomyopathy
Holter monitor	Paroxysmal arrhythmias
Cardiac catheterization	Precise valve diameters, septal defects
CBC	Anemia
Thyroid function (T4/TSH)	Both high and low thyroid levels cause CHF
Endomyocardial biopsy	Rarely done; excludes infiltrative disease such as sarcoid or amyloid when other sites for biopsy inconclusive; biopsy is "most accurate test" for some infections
Swan-Ganz right heart catheterization	Distinguishes CHF from ARDS; rare, not routine

Treatment of Systolic Dysfunction

Systolic dysfunction (low ejection fraction) is managed as follows:

- ACEI or ARB for all patients at any stage of disease; any drug in the class has beneficial effects
  - Those with a cough from ACEI should be switched to an ARB or sacubitril + valsartan (sacubitril lowers mortality).
  - Patiromer or zirconium (for hyperkalemia) if an ACEI or ARB is needed to delay progression of renal failure or decrease mortality in CHF.
- Sacubitril/valsartan; the combination of an angiotensin receptor blocker neprilysin inhibitor (ARNI) is an alternative to ACEI or ARB
- Beta blockers; not proven that any drug in the class has beneficial effects
  - Only metoprolol, bisoprolol, and carvedilol have been proven to be effective.
  - Metoprolol and bisoprolol are beta-1 specific antagonists; carvedilol is a nonspecific beta blocker that also has alpha-1 receptor blocking activity.
  - Benefits of beta blockers likely stem from anti-ischemic effect, reduced heart rate leading to decreased oxygen consumption, and antiarrhythmic effect.
- Mineralocorticoid receptor antagonists (MRAs) (**first-line agents in CHF**): inhibit the effects of aldosterone.
  - Spironolactone
  - Eplerenone, an alternative to spironolactone, has no antiandrogenic side effects; also lowers mortality
- Digoxin (controls dyspnea but does not lower mortality)
  - No positive inotropic agent (digoxin, milrinone, amrinone, dobutamine) has been proven to lower mortality of CHF.
- Diuretics (control symptoms of CHF but do not lower mortality)
  - Initial therapy of CHF with low ejection fraction often includes a loop diuretic + an ACEI or ARB.
  - It does not matter whether the diuretic is furosemide, torsemide, or bumetanide.
  - Spironolactone, although a diuretic, is not used at the doses where it has a diuretic effect.

> Beta blockers used to treat systolic dysfunction are metoprolol, carvedilol, bisoprolol.

Which of the following is the most common cause of death from CHF?

a. Pulmonary edema
b. Myocardial infarction
c. Arrhythmia/sudden death
d. Emboli
e. Myocardial rupture

Answer: C. Ischemia provokes ventricular arrhythmia, leading to sudden death. Over 99.9% of patients with CHF are at home, not acutely short of breath. If they undergo sudden death, the physician never sees them. Beta blockers are antiarrhythmic and antiischemic, so they prevent sudden death. Do not give beta blockers in the acute treatment of CHF.

> What is the management of a patient with severe CHF who develops gynecomastia? Switch spironolactone to eplerenone.

What is the answer if the patient is still dyspneic after using ACE inhibitors, beta blockers, diuretics, digoxin, and mineralocorticoid inhibitors?

- **Hydralazine/nitrates**: Used when neither an ACE inhibitor nor an ARB can be used as vasodilator therapy. May add efficacy to ACE inhibitor or ARB in some patients.
- **Ivabradine**: SA nodal inhibitor of "funny channels" that slows the heart rate. Add it to systolic dysfunction if the pulse is >70 bpm or beta blockers can't be used. Ivabradine decreases symptoms. Side effects include transient visual disturbance.

▶ **TIP**

Don't walk into the USMLE Step 2 CK exam without being 100% clear on which drugs lower mortality in CHF.

Poor Prognostic Factors in Heart Failure	
Clinical	High NYHA class, hypotension, tachycardia at rest, JVD, S3
Labs	Hyponatremia, elevated BNP, renal insufficiency
EKG	QRS >120 milliseconds, LBBB
Echocardiogram	Severe reduction in EF, pulmonary hypertension, diastolic dysfunction, RV function impairment
Associated conditions	Anemia, atrial fibrillation, DM

Devices for CHF Treatment

Two other treatments are associated with a mortality benefit in CHF.

1. Implantable defibrillator: For those with ischemic cardiomyopathy and ejection fraction <35%, these devices have as much as a 25% relative reduction in the risk of death. Remember that arrhythmia leading to sudden death is the most common cause of death in CHF. A "life vest" is a temporary, externally wearable defibrillator.

2. Biventricular pacemaker: The biventricular pacemaker is indicated in those with dilated cardiomyopathy and ejection fraction <35% and wide QRS >120 milliseconds who have persistent symptoms. The wider the QRS, the greater the benefit.

The wider the QRS, the greater the benefit of a biventricular pacer.

Do not confuse the biventricular pacemaker with a dual-chamber pacemaker with a wire in both an atrium and a ventricle.

The biventricular pacemaker resynchronizes the heart when there is a conduction defect. Many patients who would otherwise be heading to a cardiac transplantation have had their symptoms markedly improved with the biventricular pacemaker.

> A 74-year-old African American man with a history of dilated cardiomyopathy secondary to MI is seen for routine evaluation. He is asymptomatic and is maintained on lisinopril, furosemide, metoprolol, aspirin, and digoxin. Lab tests reveal a persistently elevated level of potassium. EKG is unchanged. Patiromer and zirconium do not control the potassium. What is the best management?
>
> a. Switch lisinopril to candesartan
> b. Stop lisinopril
> c. Start polystyrene sulfonate
> d. Refer for dialysis
> e. Switch lisinopril to hydralazine and nitroglycerin
>
> Answer: **E.** Hydralazine is a direct-acting arteriolar vasodilator. There is a definite survival advantage with the use of hydralazine in combination with nitrates in systolic dysfunction. Hydralazine does not raise potassium. Candesartan is associated with hyperkalemia as well. Dialysis is used in hyperkalemia only if associated with renal failure as the cause.

Transplantation

When maximal medical therapy (ACEI, BB, spironolactone, diuretics, digoxin) and possibly the biventricular pacemaker fail to control symptoms of CHF, then the only alternative is to seek cardiac transplantation.

Routine anticoagulation with warfarin is always wrong in the absence of a clot in the heart.

> Do not confuse **diastolic dysfunction** due to hypertrophic cardiomyopathy with **HOCM,** a congenital condition where an asymmetrically enlarged (hypertrophic) septum leads to an obstruction of the left ventricular outflow tract. Diuretics are contraindicated in HOCM because they will increase the obstruction.

> Patiromer or zirconium keeps potassium levels low to allow more use of ACEIs/ARBs and spironolactone.

Systolic versus Diastolic Treatments		
	Systolic Dysfunction	**Diastolic Dysfunction**
Clearly beneficial	• ACEIs/ARBs • Sacubitril/valsartan • Beta blockers • Spironolactone/eplerenone • Hydralazine/nitrates • Implantable defibrillator	• Spironolactone • Diuretics
Clearly not beneficial	CCBs (some even raise mortality)	Digoxin
Benefit uncertain		• ACEIs • ARBs • Beta blockers

Diastolic Dysfunction

Diastolic dysfunction is CHF with preserved ejection fraction. Management is less clear.

- Spironolactone is useful in diastolic dysfunction.
- Beta blockers have no clear benefit and indicated only for another condition, i.e., CAD.
- Digoxin has no benefit and should not be used in diastolic dysfunction.
- Diuretics are used to control symptoms of fluid overload, as they are in any CHF patient.
- ACE inhibitors and ARBs have no clear benefit.

Pulmonary Edema

Pulmonary edema is the rapid onset of fluid accumulating in the lungs. It is the worst (i.e., most severe) form of CHF. Symptoms include an acute onset of shortness of breath associated with:

- Rales
- JVD
- S_3 gallop (**most specific**)
- Edema
- Orthopnea

There may also be ascites and enlargement of the liver and spleen if there has been sufficient time for the chronic passive congestion of the right side of the heart to prevent filling of the heart.

Diagnostic Tests

- Brain natriuretic peptide (BNP) if the etiology of the shortness of breath is not clear. A normal BNP level excludes pulmonary edema.
- Chest x-ray will show vascular congestion with filling of the blood vessels toward the head (cephalization of flow).
  - Ordinarily, most flow in the lungs is at the bases because of simple gravity.
  - In more chronic cases, there will be enlargement of the heart and pleural effusions.
- Oximetry/arterial blood gases
  - Hypoxia is expected.
  - There is usually respiratory alkalosis because of hyperventilation.
  - Because of the increased respiratory rate, carbon dioxide leaves more easily than oxygen enters the bloodstream.

- EKG (**most important test to do acutely** because it can effect immediate change in treatment)
  - If atrial fibrillation, atrial flutter, or ventricular tachycardia is the cause of pulmonary edema, the first thing to do is to perform rapid, synchronized cardioversion in order to restore atrial or ventricular systole and to return the atrial contribution to cardiac output. Normally, atrial systole contributes only 10–20% of cardiac output.
  - If the heart is diseased from dilated cardiomyopathy, decreased ejection fraction, or valvular heart disease, then the atrial contribution to cardiac output can be as much as 40–50% of cardiac output. If acute pulmonary edema is from an arrhythmia, the fastest way to fix it is with cardioversion.
- Echocardiogram in all patients to determine if there is systolic or diastolic dysfunction. (This makes no difference acutely if there is pulmonary edema because the initial treatment does not differ.)

> Echo is not needed to manage acute pulmonary edema.

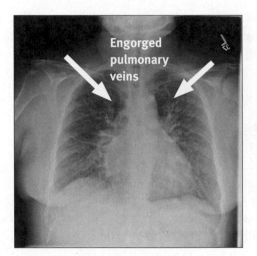

Figure 3.6 Pulmonary Edema with Cephalization of Flow and Engorged Pulmonary Veins. *Source: Saba Ansari, MD*

A 74-year-old woman comes to the ED with an acute onset of shortness of breath, respiratory rate of 38/min, rales to her apices, S_3 gallop, and jugulovenous distension. What is the best initial step in management?

a. Oximeter
b. Echocardiogram
c. IV furosemide
d. Ramipril
e. Metoprolol
f. Nesiritide

Answer: **C.** All of the answer choices can be used in the management of CHF, but the best initial step for acute pulmonary edema is removal of a large volume of fluid from the vascular space with a loop diuretic. Oximetry should be done, but oxygen is required first due to the patient's shortness of breath and hyperventilation. Echocardiogram should be done, but later. Ramipril, or any other form of ACEI or ARB, should be used if there is systolic dysfunction with low ejection fraction, but it makes no difference in an acutely unstable patient. The same is true of metoprolol. Nesiritide is an IV form of atrial natriuretic peptide which functions similarly to nitrates. There is no mortality benefit.

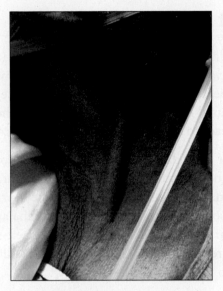

Figure 3.7 Jugulovenous Distention.
Source: Naveen Paddu, MD

Treatment

- **Preload reduction**
  - Oxygen
  - Loop diuretic such as furosemide or bumetanide
  - Nitrates (dangerous in reinfarction and AS)
  - Morphine
  - Loop diuretic such as furosemide or bumetanide (nesiritide is not more effective than diuretics and nitrates)
  - Remove 1–2 liters of fluid from the vascular space and the lungs to decrease symptoms

- **Positive inotropic agents**
  - When there is no response to preload reduction, use dobutamine (acute setting only)
  - Amrinone and milrinone are phosphodiesterase inhibitors that perform the same role; they increase contractility and decrease afterload
  - Digoxin (chronic setting only) increases contractility, but only after several weeks of use

- **Afterload reduction**
  - ACEIs and ARBs are used on discharge for long-term use in all patients with systolic dysfunction and low ejection fraction
  - Nitroprusside and IV hydralazine (acute setting only)

Heparin is always wrong for acute pulmonary edema management, in the absence of a clot.

> Furosemide is a pulmonary venodilator too!

Valvular Heart Disease

All valvular heart disease can be congenital in nature. Rheumatic fever can lead to any form of valve disease, but mitral stenosis is most common. Aging can automatically be associated with aortic stenosis. Regurgitant disease is most commonly caused by hypertension and ischemic heart disease. Infarction automatically leads to regurgitation, which automatically leads to dilation.

All forms of valvular heart disease are associated with shortness of breath and many of the signs and symptoms of CHF. Only the murmurs are specific in terms of presentation. Lesions on the right side of the heart (tricuspid and pulmonic valve) increase in intensity or loudness with inhalation. Inhalation will increase venous return to the right side of the heart. Left-sided lesions (mitral and aortic valve) increase with exhalation. Exhalation will "squeeze" blood out of the lungs and into the left side of the heart.

Diagnostic Tests

- For all valvular heart disease, echocardiogram is the **best initial test**. Transesophageal echo is more sensitive and more specific than transthoracic echo.
- Catheterization (**most accurate test**) allows the most precise measurement of valvular diameter, as well as the exact pressure gradient across the valve.

Even though EKG will show hypertrophy of chambers, it is not specific enough for valvular heart disease.

Similarly, even though chest x-ray will show hypertrophy and enlargement of various cardiac chambers, it will not provide a precise anatomic correlation. X-ray is neither the most accurate test nor the best initial test.

Treatment

All forms of valvular heart disease are associated with fluid overload in the lungs, so diuretics are always helpful.

- For **stenotic lesions** of the mitral and aortic valves: correction of the anatomy of the heart
  - Mitral stenosis needs dilation with a balloon.
  - Aortic stenosis needs surgical removal or replacement by catheter.
- For **regurgitant lesions**: vasodilator therapy with ACEIs/ARBs, nifedipine, or hydralazine
  - Surgical replacement must be done before the heart dilates too much; in other words, if the heart dilates excessively, valve replacement will not be able to correct the decrease in systolic function. If the myocardium "stretches" too much, it will not return to normal size and shape.
  - Ventricular size is based on the end-systolic diameter and the ejection fraction. When the end-systolic diameter expands, the valve must be replaced.

> Endocarditis prophylaxis is **not** indicated for any of these valve disorders unless the valve has actually been replaced or there has been previous endocarditis.

Mitral Stenosis

Mitral stenosis (MS) is most often caused by rheumatic fever. MS is extremely rare in the United States because of the very low incidence of acute rheumatic fever. Critical narrowing is defined as a valve surface area <1 cm², however, the main indication for treatment is the presence of symptoms. There is not much point in treating MS that is asymptomatic.

Most patients with mitral stenosis are immigrants to the United States coming from geographic regions in which acute rheumatic fever is still common.

Pregnancy is associated with a 50% increase in plasma volume which must traverse a narrow valve. In addition, during delivery, contraction of the uterus can "squeeze" as much as 500 mL of extra blood into the central circulation, thereby inducing pregnancy-related cardiomyopathy.

> Mitral stenosis often presents in **young adult** patients.

▶ **TIP**

Look for pregnancy and immigrant status in the history as a clue to answering "What is the most likely diagnosis?"

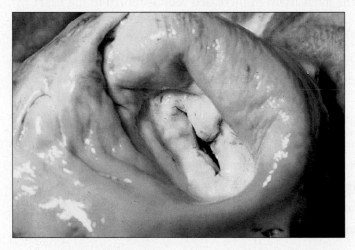

Figure 3.8 Mitral Stenosis. *Source: Wikicommons*

Besides the usual shortness of breath and CHF associated with all forms of valvular heart disease, MS has some unique symptoms:

- Dysphagia from left atrium (LA) pressing on the esophagus
- Hoarseness (LA pressing on laryngeal nerve)
- A-fib and stroke from enormous LA
- Hemoptysis

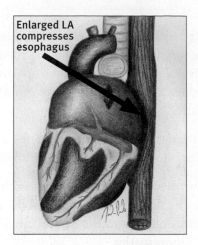 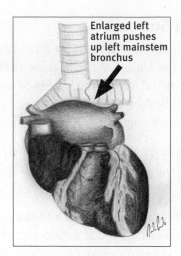

Figures 3.9, 3.10 Enlarged left atrium in mitral stenosis compresses the esophagus, causing dysphagia (left) as well as compression and displacement of the left mainstem bronchus.
Source: Andrew Peredo, MD

Murmur is in diastole, just after an opening snap. Squatting and leg raising increase the intensity from increased venous return to the heart.

Diagnostic Tests

- TTE (**best initial test**), with TEE more accurate than TTE.
- Catheterization (**most accurate test** for all valve diseases)
- EKG
  - Atrial rhythm disturbance, particularly A-fib (very common)
  - Left atrial hypertrophy, showing up as biphasic P wave in leads V1 and V2
- Chest x-ray: left atrial hypertrophy
  - Straightening of the left heart border
  - Elevation of the left mainstem bronchus
  - Second "bubble" behind the heart

Treatment

- Diuretics and sodium restriction when fluid overload is present in the lungs
- Balloon valvuloplasty done with a catheter
- Valve replacement if catheter procedure cannot be done or fails
- Warfarin for A-fib to an INR 2–3
- Rate control of A-fib with digoxin, beta blockers, or diltiazem/verapamil

> Mitral stenosis and metal heart valves are the two remaining indications for the use of **warfarin**. All others with A-fib and CHADS-VASc >2 use a NOAC.

Aortic Stenosis

Aortic stenosis (AS) can be caused by a congenital bicuspid valve or with increasing calcification as people age. Symptoms include:

- **Angina** (most common)
- **Syncope**

- **CHF** (poorest prognosis, with 2-year average survival)
- **Systolic, crescendo-decrescendo murmur** peaking in a diamond shape in mid-systole.
  - Murmur best heard at second right intercostal space, and radiates to the carotid artery
  - Valsalva and standing improve or decrease the intensity of the murmur from decreased venous return to the heart
  - Handgrip softens the murmur because of decreased ejection of blood

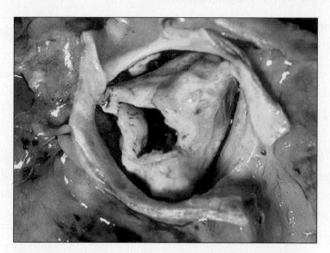

Figure 3.11 Aortic Stenosis. *Source: Wikicommons*

Diagnostic Tests

- TTE, then TEE, then catheterization
- EKG: left ventricular hypertrophy; S wave in V1 plus an R wave in V5 >35 mm
- Chest x-ray: left ventricular hypertrophy

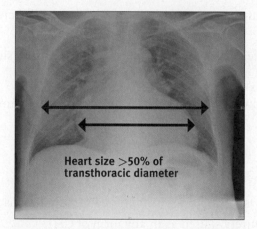

Heart size >50% of transthoracic diameter

Figure 3.12 Cardiac Enlargement (defined as heart diameter >50% than total transthoracic diameter). *Source: Nihar Shah, MD*

> Metal valves need warfarin:
> - Aortic INR 2–3
> - Mitral INR 2.5–3.5

> Transcatheter replacement is very effective for AS.

Treatment

Valve replacement is the only truly effective therapy for AS. Diuretics can be used to decrease CHF, but patients do not tolerate volume depletion very well.

- Surgical valve replacement
  - Has high risk of acute kidney injury and A-fib
- Transcatheter aortic valve replacement (TAVR) (valve replacement deployed through a catheter) is superior.
  - Not for use with regurgitant lesions

TAVR is not the same as balloon valvuloplasty.

- Balloon valvuloplasty is not routinely done for AS because the main mechanism for developing AS is calcification, which is not improved with balloon valvuloplasty.
- Balloon dilation is not replacement.

Mitral Regurgitation

Mitral regurgitation (MR) is an abnormal backward flow of blood through a mitral valve that does not fit together. Causes include hypertension, endocarditis, myocardial infarction with papillary muscle rupture, or any other reason that the heart dilates.

Symptoms include:

- Same signs and symptoms as CHF
- Murmur is the only unique finding
  - Pansystolic (holosystolic), obscuring both S1 and S2
  - Radiates to the axilla
  - Worsened by handgrip that pushes more blood backward through valve
  - Left-sided murmur (except MVP and HOCM) will increase with expiration
- Squatting and leg raising will also worsen MR by increasing venous return to the heart.

> Handgrip increases afterload and will worsen the murmurs of both AR and MR.

As with all murmurs, MR is diagnosed with echocardiogram.

Treatment
- Vasodilators
  - ACEIs or ARBs are best
  - No drug slows rate of progression of regurgitant lesions
- Digoxin and diuretics, used as in any form of CHF

- Valve replacement when heart starts to dilate
  - Do not wait for left ventricular end systolic diameter (LVESD) to become too large, because the damage will be irreversible. Do repair or replacement when LVESD >40 mm or ejection fraction drops <60%.
  - Valve repair means operative repair or with a catheter placing a clip or sutures across the valve to tighten it.

> Clipping the mitral valve by catheter is preferred to replacement.

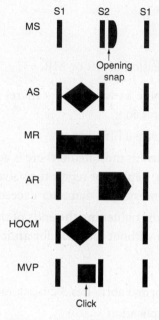

Figure 3.13 Timing of Each Murmur in Cardiac Cycle.
Source: Shawn Christian, MD

Aortic Regurgitation

Aortic regurgitation (AR) is caused by anything that makes the heart or aorta dilate in size:

- Myocardial infarction
- Hypertension
- Endocarditis
- Marfan syndrome or cystic medial necrosis
- Inflammatory disorder such as ankylosing spondylitis or Reiter syndrome
- Syphilis

Besides CHF, AR has a large array of specific physical findings:

- Wide pulse pressure
- Water-hammer (wide, bounding) pulse
- Quincke pulse (pulsations in nail bed)
- Hill sign (BP in legs as much as 40 mm Hg above BP in arms)

- Head bobbing (de Musset sign)
- Diastolic decrescendo murmur heard best at the lower left sternal border. Valsalva and standing make it better. Handgrip, which increases afterload by compressing the arteries of the arms, makes it worse.

Diagnostic Tests

Same as previous diagnostic tests mentioned. EKG and chest x-ray may show left ventricular hypertrophy.

Treatment

No drug delays the progression of AR or MR.

- ACEIs/ARBs or nifedipine as vasodilators increase forward flow of blood. They do not delay progression.
- Digoxin and diuretics have a little benefit.
- Surgical valve replacement is indicated if there is acute valve rupture, as with a myocardial infarction. Replace or repair the valve when EF falls below 55% or the left ventricular end systolic diameter exceeds 55 mm.
- Repair of the valve means tightening the ends of the valve with sutures. This decreases regurgitation without the need for anticoagulation.

Bicuspid Aortic Valve

- 1–2% of population (normal aorta has 3 cusps); most are asymptomatic
- AS most common complication
- Leads to aortic regurgitation with dilation of aortic root/ascending aorta
- Does not need endocarditis prophylaxis
- If asymptomatic age <30, monitor with echo every 1–2 years
- No treatment proven to delay progression; do **treat hypertension**
- If LV dysfunction and symptoms: surgical replacement

Mitral Valve Prolapse

Mitral valve prolapse (MVP) is so common (up to 5% of the population, mostly women) that it is considered a normal anatomic variant. Other causes are Marfan and Ehlers-Danlos syndrome.

MVP is most often asymptomatic. When symptoms do occur, it is **different from other forms of valvular heart disease**.

- Symptoms of CHF are usually absent
- Atypical chest pain
- Palpitations
- Panic attack

- Midsystolic click that, when severe, is associated with a murmur just after the click from mitral regurgitation
  - Auscultatory maneuvers have the opposite effect from the murmurs of the valvular disease described so far. Valsalva and standing, which decrease venous return to the heart, will worsen MVP.
  - Anything that increases left ventricular chamber size, such as squatting or handgrip, will improve or diminish the murmur of MVP.

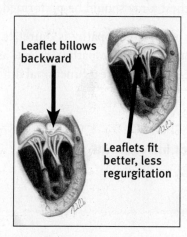

Leaflet billows backward

Leaflets fit better, less regurgitation

Figure 3.14 Redundant mitral valve leaflet does not seal, allowing regurgitation. *Source: Andrew Peredo, MD*

Diagnostic Tests

Echocardiogram is the best choice. Catheterization should rarely, if ever, be done. This is largely because an exact pressure gradient does *not* need to be determined, since valve replacement is rarely needed.

Treatment

- Beta blockers when patient is symptomatic
- Valve repair with a catheter (rarely needed) to place a clip to tighten the valve; a few stitches into the valve can markedly tighten up the leaflets
- Endocarditis prophylaxis is not recommended even in the presence of a murmur of mitral regurgitation.

Cardiomyopathy

Cardiomyopathy is an abnormal function of the heart muscle. Although valvular or auscultatory abnormalities are common, the origins of all the defects are an abnormally contracting or relaxing myocardium.

Cardiomyopathy can be dilated, hypertrophic, or restrictive.

- **Hypertrophic cardiomyopathy** is often called *diastolic dysfunction*, but the more accurate phrase is "cardiac failure with preserved ejection fraction."
- **Dilated cardiomyopathy, systolic dysfunction,** and **low ejection fraction** are often used interchangeably.

All forms of cardiomyopathy present with the following:

- Shortness of breath, particularly worsened by exertion
- Edema
- Rales
- JVD

Echocardiogram is the **best initial test** and also the **most accurate test**. Although an EKG and chest x-ray should be performed, they are nonspecific.

Treatment for all forms of cardiomyopathy is diuretics, plus additional treatment specific to the type of cardiomyopathy. In fact, aside from the etiology and physiology of the heart, the only real functional difference in management is the treatment.

Murmurs that do not increase with expiration:
- HOCM
- MVP

Dilated Cardiomyopathy

In addition to previous MI and ischemia, dilated cardiomyopathy can be caused by:

- Alcohol
- Postviral myocarditis
- Radiation
- Toxins such as doxorubicin
- Chagas disease

All the other aspects of the dyspnea, gallop, edema, and other symptoms are described in the section on CHF. The same is true for the evaluation of EF, first with echocardiography and the nonspecificity of the EKG and chest x-ray.

Many medications are available for the treatment of dilated cardiomyopathy.

- ACEIs, ARBs, and beta blockers (e.g., metoprolol, spironolactone) to lower mortality; if those cannot be used, give hydralazine + nitrates
- Diuretics and digoxin to control symptoms
- Biventricular pacemaker if QRS is wide (>120 milliseconds) to improve symptoms and survival. The wider the QRS, the greater the benefit of the biventricular pacemaker.
- Automated implantable cardioverter/defibrillator to improve mortality if there is low ejection fraction (success in <30% of cases)

Biventricular pacer
EF <35%
and
QRS >140: very strong
QRS >120: moderate

Hypertrophic Cardiomyopathy

Hypertrophic cardiomyopathy (HCM) is heart failure with preserved ejection fraction [HFpEF]). Hypertension is, by far, the most common cause.

- Reaction to stressors on the heart such as increased BP
- Heart hypertrophies to carry the load, but then develops difficulty "relaxing" in diastole
- If heart can't relax to receive blood, patient becomes short of breath
- Symptoms include S_4 gallop and fewer signs of right heart failure (e.g., ascites; enlargement of liver/spleen), unlike other forms of cardiomyopathy

Treatment of HFpEF is aimed at controlling hypertension.

- Spironolactone to decrease the rate of hospitalizations in diastolic dysfunction
- Use ACEIs and ARBs to manage hypertension (but they do not lower mortality as they do in dilated cardiomyopathy)
- Beta blockers only if there is an accompanying condition

Hypertrophic Obstructive Cardiomyopathy

It is important to distinguish between HCM and hypertrophic obstructive cardiomyopathy (HOCM). HOCM is a genetic disorder in which the septum of the heart is abnormally shaped. The asymmetrically hypertrophied septum literally forms an anatomic obstruction between the septum and valve leaflet, which blocks blood leaving the heart.

HCM is very distinct from HOCM.

- **HCM** is heart hypertrophy in response to stress: Inelastic muscle lets in less blood.
- **HOCM** arises from a genetic disorder: Abnormally shaped septum blocks outflow of blood.

Symptoms include:

- Systolic anterior motion (SAM) of the mitral valve (classic for HOCM); contributes to obstruction
- Dyspnea, as in any other form of cardiomyopathy
- Chest pain
- Syncope and lightheadedness
- Sudden death, particularly in healthy athletes

Symptoms are worsened by anything that increases heart rate (exercise, dehydration, diuretics) and anything that decreases left ventricular chamber size (ACEIs, ARBs, digoxin, hydralazine, Valsalva, sudden standing).

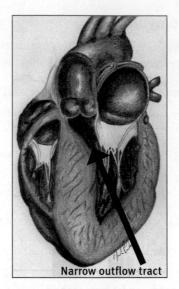

Narrow outflow tract

Figure 3.15 Thickened asymmetric septum obstructs the left ventricular outflow tract as the chamber becomes smaller. *Source: Andrew Peredo, MD*

Diagnostic testing for HOCM includes:

- Echocardiogram (**best initial test**): septum is 1.5 × the thickness of posterior wall
- EKG
  - May be normal in 25% of cases
  - Nonspecific ST and T wave changes (common)
  - LVH (common)
- Catheterization (**most accurate test** to determine precise gradients of pressure across chamber)

> Septal Q waves in the inferior and lateral leads are common in HOCM. They are **not** in MI.

Treatment is beta blockers (**best initial treatment**). Additionally:

- Agents with strong negative inotropic qualities (verapamil, disopyramide)
- Ablation of the septum, with a catheter placing absolute alcohol in the muscle causing small infarctions
- If all medical and catheter procedures fail, surgical myomectomy to remove part of the septum

Treatment of HCM versus HOCM

- For **both**, digoxin is always wrong.
- For **neither** do diuretics help.
- For **HOCM**, ACEIs and diuretics do not help and are contraindicated.
- For **HOCM with syncope**, use an implantable defibrillator.

Treatment for Hypertrophic versus Dilated Cardiomyopathy		
	Hypertrophic	**Dilated**
Beta Blockers	No	Yes
Diuretics	Yes	Yes
ACEI/ARB	Unclear benefit	Yes
Spironolactone	Yes	Yes
Digoxin	No	Yes

Restrictive Cardiomyopathy

Restrictive cardiomyopathy combines the worst aspects of both dilated and hypertrophic cardiomyopathy. The heart neither contracts nor relaxes normally because it is infiltrated with substances creating immobility. Causes are:

- Sarcoidosis
- Amyloid
- Hemochromatosis
- Endomyocardial fibrosis
- Scleroderma

Dyspnea is the most common complaint with signs of right heart failure such as ascites, edema, JVD, and enlargement of the liver and spleen.

Pulmonary hypertension is common because of an increase in wedge pressure.

▶ TIP

Kussmaul sign: An increase in jugulovenous pressure on inhalation is common.

Diagnostic testing includes:

- Echocardiogram (or cardiac MRI) (**best initial test**) shows amyloid with speckling of the septum
- Ejection fraction may be normal or elevated
- EKG shows low voltage
- Endomyocardial biopsy (**most accurate test**) is rarely done because the diagnosis is made from biopsy elsewhere in the body

Treat the underlying cause. Diuretics may relieve some of the pulmonary hypertension and signs of right heart failure. Cardiac maneuvers can simulate medical treatment, with the same effect: decrease venous return to the heart.

- **Standing** suddenly from a squatting position opens venous capacitance vessels of the legs
- **Valsalva** (exhalation against a closed glottis) increases intrathoracic pressure, making it harder for blood to return to right side of the heart

- **Stenotic and regurgitant murmurs will improve with diuretics** and/or salt restriction, and so are administered for all cases.
- **HOCM murmurs will improve with handgrip maneuver** because the heart is larger (more full), which decreases the obstruction.
- **MVP and HOCM murmurs will worsen with diuretics** because they decrease left ventricular chamber size.
- **MVP and HOCM will worsen with amyl nitrate** because the emptier heart is smaller, as it would be with diuretics, dehydration, or tachycardia.

More blood increases all murmurs except MVP and HOCM. Similarly, less blood decreases all murmurs except MVP and HOCM.

- **Handgrip** decreases left ventricular emptying
  - Ask patient to squeeze your hand; contraction of the arm muscles will compress arteries of the upper extremity (brachial, radial, ulnar arteries)
  - This will increase afterload by obstructing the ability of blood to empty the heart, leading to decreased ventricular emptying which will improve the lesions of MVP and HOCM (a bigger, fuller heart improves the obstruction of HOCM)

Additionally, inhalation of amyl nitrate, a direct arteriolar vasodilator, will increase emptying.

- Simulates the effect of ACEIs/ARBs on the heart
- Will improve any valvular disease that is treated with an ACEI/ARB ("improve" means a softer murmur)
- Will reduce the intensity of regurgitant lesions by increasing the forward flow of blood and decreasing the regurgitant, backward flow of blood (regurgitant lesions are treated with ACEIs, ARBs, and nifedipine as vasodilators).

Murmurs and the Effects of Maneuvers		
Lesion	Squatting/leg raising	Standing/Valsalva
Mitral and aortic stenosis	Increases both	Decreases both
Mitral and aortic regurgitation	Increases both	Decreases both
MVP	Decrease	Increase
HOCM	Decrease	Increase

▶ **TIP**

Handgrip = Fuller left ventricle

Amyl nitrate = ACEI = Emptier left ventricle

Myocarditis

Myocarditis is a global injury to the entire muscle of the heart. The cause can be an infection such as a virus, a toxin such as doxorubicin, or an autoimmune disorder.

There is no single symptom or physical finding that can diagnose myocarditis. Some patients are asymptomatic, some are dyspneic, and some present like MI, with chest pain and ST elevation.

Diagnostic testing includes:

- EKG can show any abnormality
- ESR and CRP may be elevated but those are nonspecific
- Echocardiogram will show decreased ejection fraction
- Biopsy of the heart (**most accurate test**) (rarely done)

Treatment is ACE inhibitors and beta blockers for those with low ejection fraction. Statins and antiplatelet medications are not indicated because the coronary arteries are normal. Steroids and IVIG do not help.

> Steroids worsen viral myocarditis.

Pericardial Disease

There is considerable overlap in the causes of all types of pericardial disease—pericarditis, pericardial tamponade, and constrictive pericarditis. For instance:

- If the etiology of pericarditis is associated with the extravasation of a great deal of fluid, then tamponade can occur.
- If the cause of pericarditis is chronic, then patients can develop the fibrosis and calcification of the pericardium that leads to constrictive pericarditis.

Pericarditis

Pericarditis can be caused by any infection, inflammatory disorder, connective tissue disorder, trauma to the chest, or cancer of an organ anatomically near the heart.

- Most common infection is viral, but *Staphylococcus*, *Streptococcus*, fungi, and other agents can cause pericarditis in same way that any infection can cause pneumonia
- Most common connective tissue disorder is SLE, but Wegener granulomatosis, Goodpasture, RA, polyarteritis nodosa, etc., can cause pericarditis

"What Is the Most Likely Diagnosis?"

Pericarditis is associated with sharp chest pain that changes in intensity with respiration as well as the position of the body. The pain is worsened by lying flat and improved by sitting up (probably from a change in the level of tension or "stretch" of the pericardium).

EKG shows ST segment elevation in all leads, but the most specific finding is PR segment depression.

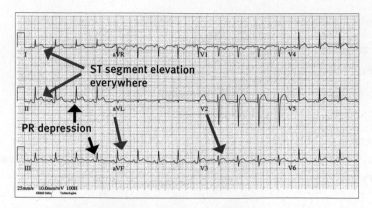

Figure 3.16 Pericarditis with ST Segment Elevation and PR Segment Depression Everywhere. *Source: Alejandro E. de la Cruz, MD*

Treat the underlying cause. For most cases, no clear cause is identified, and these "idiopathic" cases are presumed to be viral in etiology with Coxsackie B virus.

- NSAIDs
- Colchicine to decrease recurrences
- On the exam, if an answer choice includes an NSAID + colchicine, it is the correct answer.

Pericardial Tamponade

Any of the causes of pericarditis can extravasate enough fluid to cause tamponade. Compression of the chambers of the heart starts on the right side because the walls are thinner. As little as 50 mL of fluid accumulating acutely can cause tamponade. If accumulating over weeks to months, the pericardium will stretch to accommodate as much as 2 liters of fluid.

Tamponade can also result from trauma with a bleed into the pericardium; it requires emergent thoracotomy.

"What Is the Most Likely Diagnosis?"

- Hypotension
- Tachycardia
- Distended neck veins
- Clear lungs

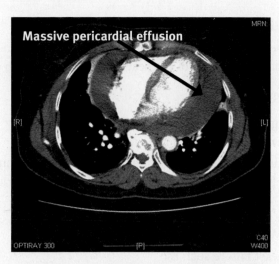

Figure 3.17 Pericardial Effusion. *Source: Birju Shah, MD*

A 78-year-old man with a history of lung cancer comes to the ED with several days of increasing shortness of breath. He also became lightheaded today. On physical examination, he has blood pressure is 106/70 mm Hg, pulse 112 bpm, and jugulovenous distention. The lungs are clear to auscultation. On inhalation, blood pressure drops to 92/58 mm Hg. Which of the following is the most appropriate to confirm the diagnosis?

a. EKG
b. Chest x-ray
c. Echocardiogram
d. Right heart catheterization
e. Cardiac MRI

Answer: **C.** The echocardiogram is most appropriate because the EKG often shows nothing except sinus tachycardia. Chest x-ray is normal in an acute tamponade (can show a "globular heart"). Although right heart catheterization is the most accurate to determine precise pressures, it would never be appropriate to do a catheterization to evaluate for tamponade without having done an echocardiogram first.

Diagnostic Tests

- EKG show electrical alternans (different heights of QRS complexes between beats)
- Chest x-ray shows enlarged cardiac shadow expanding in both directions ("globular heart")
- Echocardiogram shows right atrial and ventricular diastolic collapse
- Right heart catheterization shows equalization of pressures in diastole

Treatment

- Pericardiocentesis: needle drainage to rapidly re-expand the heart
- IV fluids
- A hole or "window" placed into the pericardium for recurrent cases

Diuretics will decrease intracardiac filling pressure and may markedly worsen the collapse of the right side of the heart.

Constrictive Pericarditis

Any cause of pericarditis can result in sufficient calcification and fibrosis to prevent filling of the right side of the heart if it is chronic, such as tuberculosis.

Physical findings may include:

- **Kussmaul sign**: increase in JVD on inhalation (normally the neck veins should go down on inhalation)
- **"Knock"**: This is an extra heart sound in diastole from ventricular filling. As the heart fills to its maximum, it hits the stiff, rigid pericardium with a "knock."

"What Is the Most Likely Diagnosis?"

Signs of right heart failure such as:

- Edema
- Ascites
- Enlargement of the liver and spleen
- JVD

Constrictive pericarditis is a combination of the physical findings described with calcification on chest x-ray.

Diagnostic testing includes:

- Chest x-ray (**best initial test**) will show calcification and fibrosis
- CT scan and MRI (**more accurate tests**) done only after chest x-ray
- Echocardiogram: indispensable for excluding right ventricular hypertrophy or cardiomyopathy as a cause; the myocardium moves normally in constrictive pericarditis

Treatment

- **Diuretics**: used first to decompress the filling of the heart and relieve edema and organomegaly
- **Surgical removal** of the pericardium

Peripheral Artery Disease

Peripheral artery disease (PAD) is the stenosis of peripheral arteries with the same causative factors as coronary and carotid disease such as:

- Tobacco smoking
- Diabetes mellitus
- Hyperlipidemia
- Hypertension

There is no routine screening for PAD since there is no mortality benefit to be obtained.

"What Is the Most Likely Diagnosis?"

The key to this question is leg pain in the calves on exertion, relieved by rest. PAD pain occurs when walking up or down hills. Severe disease is associated with loss of:

- Hair follicles
- Sweat glands
- Sebaceous glands

The skin becomes smooth and shiny.

Diagnostic testing includes:

- Ankle-brachial index (ABI) (**best initial test**); this is the ratio of BP in ankles to BP in brachial arteries
  - BP is normally equal, or slightly greater in ankles due to gravity
  - If difference between them >10% (ABI <0.9), then disease is present
- Angiogram (**most accurate test**) is not necessary unless specific revascularization will be done.

Treatment is as follows:

- Aspirin or vorapaxar
  - Vorapaxar: antiplatelet medication that is an alternative to aspirin and clopidogrel
  - Do not use when there is a history of stroke or TIA because it can cause bleeding
- Stopping smoking
- Cilostazol (**most effective medication**)
- Surgery to bypass stenosis if medical therapies are ineffective

Calcium blockers do not help PAD.

> **In all major vascular disease, control each of the following:**
> - BP (ACE inhibitor)
> - LDL goal 70 mg/dL, everyone on statins
> - Diabetes

> Spinal stenosis pain is worse when walking **down** hills, because of leaning back.

> - Beta blockers are not contraindicated in PAD.
> - Everyone with PAD should be on a statin.

Heart Disease in Pregnancy

Which of the following is the most dangerous condition in pregnancy?

a. Mitral stenosis
b. Peripartum cardiomyopathy
c. Eisenmenger phenomenon
d. Mitral valve prolapse
e. Atrial septal defect

Answer: **B.** The worst form of heart disease in pregnancy is peripartum cardiomyopathy with persistent ventricular dysfunction. If a woman with peripartum cardiomyopathy and persistent LV dysfunction becomes pregnant again, she has a very high chance of markedly worsening her cardiac function.

Peripartum Cardiomyopathy

It is unknown why antibodies against the myocardium arise in some pregnant women. The LV dysfunction is often reversible and short term. If the LV dysfunction does not improve, then the person must undergo cardiac transplantation.

The medical therapy consists of the same drugs as used for dilated cardiomyopathy of any cause, namely:

- ACEIs/ARBs
- Beta blockers
- Spironolactone
- Diuretics
- Digoxin

> Peripartum cardiomyopathy develops **after** delivery in most cases; that is why ACEIs/ARBs are acceptable to use.

Repeat pregnancy in a woman with peripartum cardiomyopathy will provoke enormous antibody production against the myocardium.

Eisenmenger Syndrome

Eisenmenger syndrome is the development of a right-to-left shunt from pulmonary hypertension. It is seen in those with a ventricular septal defect who have significant left-to-right shunting and then eventual development of pulmonary hypertension. When the pulmonary hypertension becomes very severe, then the shunt reverses and right-to-left shunting develops.

> Pregnancy increases plasma volume by 50%. Mitral stenosis will worsen in pregnancy, but **not** as much as peripartum cardiomyopathy or Eisenmenger syndrome.

▶TIP

If peripartum cardiomyopathy is not one of the choices for the question "What is the worst cardiac disease in pregnant women?", then look for Eisenmenger as one of the choices.

Pulmonology $\quad$ 4

Obstructive Lung Disease

Asthma

Asthma (or reactive airway disease) is an abnormal bronchoconstriction of the airways. Although asthma is very common, its etiology is unknown.

- It is reversible.
- Prevalence, incidence, and hospitalization rates are all increasing.
- It has an association with atopic disorders and obesity.

The main difference between asthma and COPD is that **asthma is reversible**, while **COPD is not**.

Acute exacerbation of asthma has many causes:

- Allergens (e.g., pollen, dust mites, cockroaches, cat dander)
- Infection and cold air
- Emotional stress or exercise
- Catamenial (related to menstrual cycle)
- Aspirin, NSAIDs, beta blockers, histamine, any nebulized medication, tobacco smoke
- GERD

> An oral temperature may not be accurately measured in patients breathing fast. Mouth breathing cools the thermometer.

Wheezing with the acute onset of shortness of breath, cough, and chest tightness make a "What is the most likely diagnosis?" question unlikely. Increased sputum production is common, although fever is not always present.

> Asthma can present exclusively as a cough.

"Which of the Following Is Most Likely to Be Seen in This Patient?"

- Symptoms worse at night
- Nasal polyps and sensitivity to aspirin
- Eczema or atopic dermatitis on physical examination
- Increased length of expiratory phase of respiration
- Increased use of accessory respiratory muscles (e.g., intercostals)

▶TIP

Make sure you can identify the sound of wheezing. This is a good multimedia question.

Diagnostic testing in asthma—especially the "best initial test"—is based on the severity of presentation.

<table><tr><td>

Peak flow is extremely dependent on height.

</td></tr></table>

- Peak expiratory flow (PEF) or arterial blood gas (ABG) (**best initial test in acute exacerbations**) to determine function
- Chest x-ray to exclude pneumonia as a cause of exacerbation (and in cases that aren't clear, to exclude other diseases such as pneumothorax and CHF)
- Chest x-ray is typically normal in asthma, but it may show hyperinflation

<table><tr><td>

In between exacerbations of acute asthma, PFTs will be normal.

</td></tr></table>

- PFTs (**most accurate test**): spirometry will show a decrease in ratio of FEV1 to FVC; FEV1 decreases more than FVC
  - Decreased FEV1 and decreased FVC
  - Increased FEV1 >12% and 200 mL with use of albuterol
  - Decreased FEV1 >20% with use of methacholine or histamine (methacholine is an artificial form of acetylcholine used in diagnostic testing; acetylcholine and histamine provoke bronchoconstriction and increased bronchial secretions)
  - Increased DLCO

<table><tr><td>

Asthma Diagnosis
- FEV1 ↑12%: albuterol
- FEV1 ↓20%: methacholine

</td></tr></table>

- CBC may show increased eosinophil count
- Skin testing to identify specific allergens that provoke bronchoconstriction
- Increased IgE level to suggest an allergic etiology (associated with allergic bronchopulmonary aspergillosis). IgE level may also help guide treatment, e.g., the use of the anti-IgE medication omalizumab.

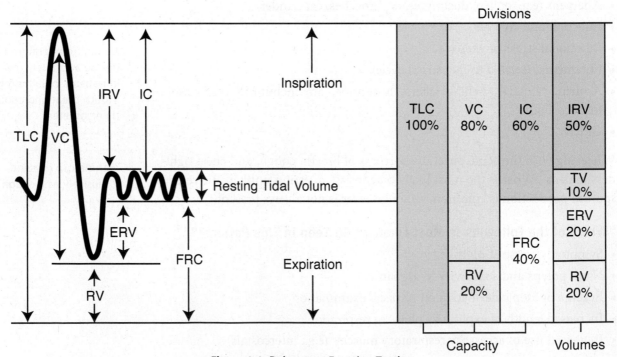

Figure 4.1 Pulmonary Function Testing

A 15-year-old boy presents with occasional shortness of breath every few weeks. Currently he feels well. He uses no medications and denies any other medical problems. Physical examination reveals pulse of 70 bpm and respiratory rate 12/min. Chest examination is normal. Which of the following is the most accurate diagnostic test?

a. Peak expiratory flow
b. Increased FEV1 with albuterol
c. Diffusion capacity of carbon monoxide
d. >20% decreased FEV1 with use of methacholine
e. Increased alveolar-arterial oxygen difference (A-a gradient)
f. Increased FVC with albuterol
g. Flow-volume loop on spirometry
h. Chest CT scan
i. Increased pCO_2 on ABG

Answer: **D.** When a patient is asymptomatic, it is unlikely to find increased FEV1 with the use of short-acting bronchodilators such as albuterol; when there are no symptoms, the test may be falsely negative. When a patient is asymptomatic, the most accurate test of reactive airway disease is a 20% decrease in FEV1 with the use of methacholine or histamine. Chest CT, like x-ray, shows nothing or hyperinflation. ABG and PEF are useful during an acute exacerbation. Flow-volume loop is best for fixed obstructions such as tracheal lesions or COPD.

> Methacholine challenge testing has 1–2% risk of inducing status asthmaticus.

Treatment of asthma is done in steps, i.e., treatment should be added progressively if there is no response.

- **Step 1**: Start with either:
  - An inhaled short-acting beta agonist (SABA), e.g., albuterol, pirbuterol, levalbuterol; or
  - Formoterol combined with a low-dose inhaled corticosteroid (ICS), used as needed (per 2021 recommendations)
- **Step 2**: Add a long-term control agent, e.g., a low-dose ICS.
  - Beclomethasone, budesonide, flunisolide, fluticasone, mometasone, triamcinolone
  - Leukotriene modifiers: montelukast, zafirlukast (hepatotoxic; associated with Churg-Strauss), zileuton (best for atopic patients)
- **Step 3**: Add a long-acting beta agonist (LABA), e.g., salmeterol or formoterol, or increase the dose of the ICS.
- **Step 4**: Increase the dose of the ICS to maximum in addition to the LABA and SABA. Add a long-acting anti-muscarinic receptor antagonist (LAMA).
- **Step 5**: If patient has elevated IgE or eosinophil count, add a monoclonal antibody against interleukin or IgE to the SABA, LABA, and ICS.
- **Step 6**: If symptoms are still not controlled, add an oral corticosteroid, e.g., prednisone.
  - Use steroids as a last resort because of harsh side effects, e.g., osteoporosis, cataracts, adrenal suppression/fat redistribution; hyperlipidemia, hyperglycemia, acne, hirsutism (particularly in women); thinning of skin, striae, and easy bruising).

> Never use LABAs first or alone!

> Side effects of inhaled steroids are dysphonia and oral candidiasis. However, high-dose inhaled steroids rarely lead to the side effects seen with prednisone.

> Influenza and pneumococcal vaccine are given to all asthma patients.

- To avoid steroid therapy in patients on SABAs, LABAs, inhaled steroids, leukotriene modifiers, or theophylline, try **monoclonal antibodies** (reslizumab/mepolizumab, benralizumab, or dupilumab) for anti-interleukin effect if eosinophil levels are elevated and omalizumab for anti-IgE. **Bronchial thermoplasty** (a heater probe removes constrictor muscles from around bronchi) is a last resort.

If SABAs, LABAs, and inhaled steroids are not sufficient, use an anticholinergic, which will dilate bronchi and decrease secretions. Anticholinergic inhalers have an effect in both COPD and asthma. They are used as a later choice in asthma.

Acute Asthma Exacerbation

Severity of an acute asthma exacerbation is quantified as follows:

- Decreased peak expiratory flow (PEF)
  - Approximation of the FVC, with no precise "normal" value; based mostly on height and age, not on weight
  - Used in acute assessment to compare PEF with usual PEF when patient is stable
- ABG with increased A-a gradient

> In extremely severe asthma, wheezing stops when there is loss of air movement.

Chest x-ray may be done to see if there is an infection leading to the exacerbation; asthma likewise predisposes patients to pneumothorax.

Treatment of acute exacerbation is as follows:

- Oxygen + inhaled short-acting beta agonist + bolus of steroids (**best initial treatment**)
  - Corticosteroids need 4–6 hours to become effective, so administer right away.
  - Albuterol
    ○ Ipratropium is used but works more slowly than albuterol.
    ○ Epinephrine injection (rarely used) is no more effective than albuterol but has more severe side effects
- Magnesium has some modest effect on bronchodilation.
- Endotracheal intubation for mechanical ventilation if there is no response to oxygen/albuterol/steroids or if respiratory acidosis (increased pCO_2) develops
- The following are **not effective in acute exacerbation**:
  - Theophylline
  - Cromolyn and nedocromil (best with extrinsic allergies, e.g., hay fever)
  - Leukotriene modifiers
  - Omalizumab or any of the interleukin inhibitors
  - LABAs (salmeterol, formoterol, olodaterol, vilanterol)

A 47-year-old man with a history of asthma comes to the ED with several days of increasing shortness of breath, cough, and sputum production. On physical examination his respiratory rate is 34/min. He has diffuse expiratory wheezing and a prolonged expiratory phase. Which of the following will best indicate the severity of his asthma?

a. Respiratory rate
b. Use of accessory muscles
c. Pulse oximetry
d. Pulmonary function testing
e. Pulse rate

Answer: **A.** Normal respiratory rate is 10–16/min. A respiratory rate of 34/min indicates severe shortness of breath. Accessory muscle use is hard to assess and is subjective. Pulse oximetry will not show hypoxia until the patient is nearly at the point of imminent respiratory failure. Oxygen saturation can be maintained above 90% by hyperventilating. PFTs cannot be done when a patient is acutely short of breath.

Chronic Obstructive Pulmonary Disease

Chronic obstructive pulmonary disease (COPD) is shortness of breath due to lung destruction, leading to decreased elastic recoil of the lungs.

- The ability to exhale primarily comes from elastin fibers in the lungs, passively allowing exhalation.
- In COPD this is lost; the result is a decrease in FEV1 and FVC and an increase in total lung capacity (TLC).
- COPD is not always associated with reactive airway disease such as asthma, although both are obstructive diseases.

Tobacco smoking leads to almost all COPD. Tobacco destroys elastin fibers. However, if the patient is young and a nonsmoker, the most likely cause is alpha-1 antitrypsin deficiency.

Symptoms of COPD include:

- Shortness of breath worsened by exertion
- Intermittent exacerbations with increased cough, sputum, and shortness of breath, often brought on by infection
- "Barrel chest" from increased air trapping
- Muscle wasting and cachexia

Diagnostic testing includes:

- Chest x-ray (**best initial test**)
  - Increased anterior-posterior (AP) diameter
  - Air trapping
  - Flattened diaphragms

- PFTs (**most accurate test**)
  - Decreased FEV1 (<80% predicted), decreased FVC, decreased FEV1/FVC ratio (<70%)
  - Increased TLC due to increased residual volume
  - Decreased DLCO (emphysema, not chronic bronchitis)
  - Incomplete improvement with albuterol
  - Little or no worsening with methacholine
- Plethysmography: increased residual volume
- CBCs: elevated hematocrit due to chronic hypoxia
- EKG
  - Right atrial and right ventricular hypertrophy
  - A-fib
  - Multifocal atrial tachycardia
- Echocardiogram
  - Right atrial and right ventricular hypertrophy
  - Pulmonary hypertension
- ABGs
  - Increased pCO_2 and hypoxia during acute exacerbations
  - Possible respiratory acidosis if there is insufficient metabolic compensation and bicarbonate level rises to compensate
  - In between exacerbations, not all those with COPD will retain CO_2

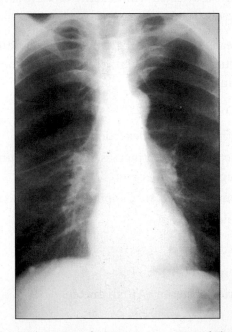

Figure 4.2 Chest X-ray of COPD. *Source: Conrad Fischer, MD*

Treatment is as follows:

- **Treatment that improves mortality and delays progression of disease**
  - Smoking cessation
  - Influenza and pneumococcal vaccinations
  - Oxygen if pO_2 ≤55 or saturation ≤88%; **mortality benefit is directly proportional to number of hours the oxygen is used**
    ○ Indicated if there are signs of right-sided heart disease/failure or elevated hematocrit, pO_2 <60 mm Hg, or oxygen saturation <90%.
    ○ Use only as much oxygen as is necessary to raise the pO_2 above 90% saturation.

- **Treatment that improves symptoms but does not improve mortality or delay progression of disease**
  - SABAs, e.g., albuterol
  - LABAs, e.g., salmeterol, formoterol, olodaterol
    ○ Never use LABAs alone
    ○ Always combine with inhaled steroids
  - Anticholinergic agents, e.g., tiotropium, ipratropium, aclidinium, umeclidinium, glycopyrrolate
  - Steroids
  - Pulmonary rehabilitation
  - Roflumilast (may decrease frequency of exacerbations)
  - Theophylline
  - Lung volume reduction surgery

- **Treatment of acute exacerbation of chronic bronchitis (AECB)**
  - Treatment is similar to the acute exacerbation of asthma
  - Bronchodilators and corticosteroids are combined with antibiotics (antibiotics are used because infection is by far the most commonly identified cause)
    ○ Patients have a broad range of response to inhaled bronchodilators, from no reversibility to full reversibility (defined as >12% and 200 mL increase in FEV1).
    ○ About 50% have some response.
  - Anticholinergic agents: only ipratropium for acute exacerbation
  - Although viruses cause 20–50% of episodes, coverage should be provided against *S. pneumoniae*, *H. influenzae*, and *Moraxella catarrhalis*.
    ○ Macrolides: azithromycin, clarithromycin
    ○ Cephalosporins: cefuroxime, cefixime, cefaclor, ceftibuten
    ○ Amoxicillin/clavulanic acid
    ○ Quinolones: levofloxacin, moxifloxacin, gemifloxacin
  - Second line agents: doxycycline, TMP/SMX

O₂ Use
pO_2 <55/sat ≤88% → **with pulmonary HTN, high HCT, or cardiomyopathy:** pO_2 <60/sat ≤90%

Use roflumilast or theophylline when patient has not responded to SABAs, LABAs, LAMAs, and inhaled steroids, and you would like to try something other than a long-term oral steroid.

- Inhaled anticholinergic agents such as ipratropium and tiotropium are helpful in both asthma and COPD. However, they are **most effective in COPD.**
- For **acute exacerbation of COPD,** only ipratropium is used.

> If you are asked, "What medication delays progression of COPD?", the answer is "Nothing."

> AECB treatment is identical to asthma treatment, just with less proven benefit.

> The idea of "eliminating hypoxic drive" is not accurate. Dyspneic, hypoxic patients with COPD must get oxygen.

- **Treatment that has no benefit in COPD**
  - Cromolyn
  - Leukotriene modifiers (e.g., montelukast)
  - Inhaled steroid monotherapy
  - IV aminophylline
  - Spirometry for an asymptomatic patient as a "screening method," even if there is a significant smoking history
  - Terbutaline, a beta-2 agonist (not better than albuterol)

When all medical therapy is insufficient, refer the patient for transplantation.

▶ **TIP**

- Asthma not controlled with albuterol → inhaled steroid
- COPD not controlled with albuterol → anticholinergic (e.g., tiotropium) → inhaled steroid

Lung volume reduction surgery helps some patients with severe disease and large bullae.

LABAs		LAMAs	
• Salmeterol	• Indacaterol	• Tiotropium	• Aclidinium
• Formoterol	• Vilanterol	• Ipratropium	• Glycopyrrolate
• Arformoterol	• Olodaterol	• Umeclidinium	

Sleep Apnea

Mild sleep apnea is 5–15 episodes/hr, while moderate sleep apnea is 15–30 episodes/hr. Severe is >30 episodes/hr.

- **Obstructive sleep apnea** (OSA) (far more common): caused by a narrowing or closure of the throat
- **Central sleep apnea** (CSA): caused by a change in breathing control and rhythm

Obstructive Sleep Apnea

Obesity is the most commonly identified cause of OSA. Patients present with daytime somnolence and a history of loud snoring. Other symptoms include:

- Headache, daytime sleepiness
- Impaired memory and judgment
- Depression
- Hypertension
- Erectile dysfunction
- "Bull neck"

Treatment is as follows:

- Weight loss
- Avoidance of alcohol and sedatives
- Oral appliances to keep the tongue out of the way
- Continuous positive airway pressure (CPAP)
- Surgical widening of the airway (uvulopalatopharyngoplasty) if that fails

Central Sleep Apnea

CSA symptoms are the same as those of OSA: daytime sleepiness, insomnia, inattention, erectile dysfunction, and snoring. In CSA, the respiratory drive is repetitively diminished from stroke, heart failure, or opiates. A unique feature of CSA is a lack of abdominal or thoracic movement during pauses in breathing.

Treatment is CPAP.

Polysomnography (sleep study) (**most accurate test**) will show >5 apnea/hypopnea episodes/hr. There is no daytime hypoventilation.

> With increased bicarbonate, sleep apnea is obesity/hypoventilation syndrome.

Bronchiectasis

Bronchiectasis is chronic dilation of the large bronchi—a permanent anatomic abnormality that cannot be reversed or cured. It is less common than it used to be, because of improved treatments for lung infections that cause weakening of the bronchial walls.

The single most common cause of bronchiectasis is cystic fibrosis (50% of cases). Other causes are:

- Infections: tuberculosis, pneumonia, abscess
- Panhypogammaglobulinemia and immune deficiency
- Foreign body or tumors
- Allergic bronchopulmonary aspergillosis
- Collagen-vascular disease such as rheumatoid arthritis

"What Is the Most Likely Diagnosis?"

- Recurrent episodes of very high-volume purulent sputum production (**key to diagnosis**)
- Possible hemoptysis
- Dyspnea and wheezing (most cases)
- Weight loss
- Anemia of chronic disease
- Crackles on lung exam
- Clubbing (uncommon)
- Dyskinetic cilia syndrome

Diagnosis of bronchiectasis requires an imaging study of the lungs, such as CT scan.

Diagnostic testing is as follows:

- Chest x-ray (**best initial test**) will show dilated, thickened bronchi, sometimes with "tram-tracks," (thickening of the bronchi)
- High-resolution CT scan (**most accurate test**)
- Sputum culture to determine the bacterial etiology of recurrent infections

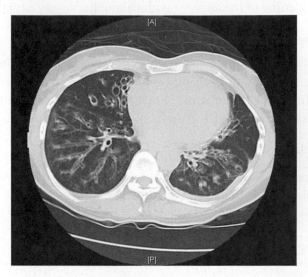

Figure 4.3 Bronchiectasis with Widening of the Bronchi in Multiple Areas
Source: Leyla Medinasab, MD

Treatment is as follows:

- Chest physiotherapy ("cupping and clapping") and postural drainage to dislodge plugged-up bronchi (**essential**)
- Antibiotics, rotated 1 weekly each month
- Possible surgical resection of focal lesions
- Dornase alfa, an enzyme which cleaves DNA in sputum, to reduce viscosity (for bronchiectasis arising from cystic fibrosis)
- Beta agonists and pulmonary rehabilitation are not clearly effective.

Treat each episode of bronchiectasis infection as it arises. Use the same antibiotics as for exacerbation of COPD. The only difference is that with bronchiectasis, inhaled antibiotics have some efficacy, and a specific microbiologic diagnosis is preferred since *Mycobacterium avium intracellulare* (MAI) can be found.

Cystic Fibrosis

Cystic fibrosis (CF) is an autosomal recessive disorder caused by a mutation in the genes that code for chloride transport (called the cystic fibrosis transmembrane conductance regulator [CFTR]).

- Mutations in the CFTR gene damage chloride and water transport across the apical surface of epithelial cells in exocrine glands throughout the body.
- This leads to abnormally thick mucus in the lungs, as well as damage to the pancreas, liver, sinuses, intestines, and genitourinary tract.
- Neutrophils in CF dump tons of DNA into airway secretions, clogging them up.
- Damaged mucus clearance decreases the ability to get rid of inhaled bacteria.

Presentation includes a young adult with chronic lung disease (cough, sputum, hemoptysis, bronchiectasis, wheezing, and dyspnea) and recurrent episodes of infection.

Other symptoms include:

- Sinus pain and polyps (common)
- GI involvement
  - Meconium ileus in infants with abdominal distention
  - Pancreatic insufficiency (90% of cases) with steatorrhea and vitamin A, D, E, and K malabsorption
  - Recurrent pancreatitis
  - Distal intestinal obstruction
  - Biliary cirrhosis
- GU involvement
  - Men: infertility; azoospermia (very common), vas deferens missing (20% of cases)
  - Women: infertility because chronic lung disease alters the menstrual cycle and thick cervical mucus blocks sperm entry

> In CF, lung disease accounts for 95% of deaths.

Diagnostic tests include:

- Increased sweat chloride test (**most accurate test**): pilocarpine increases acetylcholine, which increases sweat production
- Genotyping with CFTR (less accurate than sweat chloride level because there are so many types of mutation leading to CF)
- Chest x-ray and CT: no single abnormality on imaging of the chest will confirm diagnosis
  - Bronchiectasis
  - Pneumothorax
  - Scarring
  - Atelectasis
  - Hyperinflation
- ABGs may show hypoxemia and, in advanced disease, respiratory acidosis
- PFTs show mixed obstructive and restrictive patterns; decreased FVC and total lung capacity; and decreased DLCO
- Sputum culture
  - Nontypeable *Haemophilus influenzae*
  - *Pseudomonas aeruginosa*
  - *Staphylococcus aureus*
  - *Burkholderia cepacia*

> **Islets are spared. Beta cell** function is **normal** until much later in life.

Chloride levels in sweat >60 mEq/L on repeat testing establishes the diagnosis.

Treatment

- Antibiotics
  - Eliminating colonization is difficult, and sputum culture is essential to guide treatment.
  - Inhaled aminoglycosides as a treatment method are almost exclusively limited to CF.
- Inhaled recombinant human deoxyribonuclease (rhDNase) to break down the massive amounts of DNA in respiratory mucus that clogs up the airways
- Inhaled bronchodilators such as albuterol
- Pneumococcal and influenza vaccinations
- Pancreatic enzyme replacement
- Elexacaftor, tezacaftor and ivacaftor in combination will help the 90% of patients who have some type of mutation.
- Lung transplantation (only if no response to medical therapy)

Lung Infection

Pneumonia

Community-Acquired Pneumonia

Community-acquired pneumonia (CAP) is pneumonia occurring prior to hospitalization or within 48 hours of admission. It is among the top 10 causes of death in the United States.

The most common cause of CAP is *Streptococcus pneumoniae*. However, the environmental reservoir of *S. pneumoniae* and the method of acquisition are not known.

Other pathogens related to CAP are as follows:

Common Pathogens in CAP and Their Associations	
Pathogen	**Association**
Haemophilus influenzae	COPD
Staphylococcus aureus	Recent viral infection (influenza)
Klebsiella pneumoniae	Alcoholism, diabetes
Anaerobes	Poor dentition, aspiration
Mycoplasma pneumoniae	Young, healthy patients
Chlamydophila pneumoniae	Hoarseness
Legionella	Contaminated water sources, air conditioning, ventilation systems
Chlamydia psittaci	Birds
Coxiella burnetii	Animals at the time of giving birth, veterinarians, farmers

Presentation with all forms of pneumonia includes fever and cough. Rales, rhonchi, and crepitations are common auscultatory findings.

- Dyspnea (seen with severe infection)
- Chills or "rigors": a sign of bacteremia, often with bacterial pathogens
- Hypothermia: just as bad as fever, in terms of pathologic significance
- Abnormal vital signs (tachycardia, hypotension, tachypnea) or mental status (seen with severe infection)
- Cough from any etiology may be associated with hemoptysis
- Dullness to percussion if there is an effusion
- "Bronchial" breath sounds and egophony due to consolidation of air spaces
- Abdominal pain or diarrhea from infection in the lower lobes irritating the intestines through the diaphragm
- Chest pain from inflammation of the pleura
- Dry, nonproductive cough (seen with infection that preferentially involves the interstitial space and leaves the air spaces of the alveoli empty—explaining why there is less sputum production), e.g., *Mycoplasma*, viruses, *Coxiella*, *Pneumocystis*, *Chlamydia*

> Dyspnea, high fever, and abnormal chest x-ray are the main ways to distinguish pneumonia from bronchitis.

> Chest pain from pneumonia is often pleuritic, changing with respiration.

▶ **TIP**

USMLE Step 2 CK may play abnormal breath sounds as part of multimedia and ask you to recognize them.

Organism-Specific Associations on Presentation	
Pathogen	**Association**
Klebsiella pneumoniae	Hemoptysis from necrotizing disease, "currant jelly" sputum
Anaerobes	Foul-smelling sputum, "rotten eggs"
Mycoplasma pneumoniae	Dry cough, rarely severe, bullous myringitis
Legionella	GI symptoms (abdominal pain, diarrhea) or CNS symptoms such as headache and confusion
Pneumocystis	AIDS with <200 CD4 cells

Diagnostic testing is as follows:

- Chest x-ray (**best initial test**) (can be falsely negative in 10–20% of cases)

> It is impossible to identify the cause of pneumonia from the history and physical alone.

> The first chest x-ray can be falsely negative in 10–20% of cases.

- Leukocytosis (elevated WBCs) is often present but is nonspecific.
- Chest x-ray: bilateral interstitial infiltrates are seen with *Mycoplasma*, viruses, *Coxiella*, *Pneumocystis*, and *Chlamydia*
  - Same organisms that typically present with a nonproductive cough
  - X-ray lags behind clinical findings (in some cases, the first chest x-ray can be falsely negative)
- Chest CT and MRI show greater definition of abnormalities found on chest x-ray but will still not be able to identify microbiologic etiology
- Blood culture is positive in 5–15% of cases of CAP, particularly those with *S. pneumoniae*

Specific Diagnostic Tests by Organism	
Organism	**Diagnostic test**
Mycoplasma pneumoniae	PCR, cold agglutinins, serology, special culture media
Chlamydophila pneumoniae	Rising serologic titers
Legionella	Urine antigen, culture on charcoal-yeast extract
Chlamydia psittaci	Rising serologic titers
Coxiella burnetii	Rising serologic titers
Pneumocystis jiroveci (PCP)	Bronchoalveolar lavage (BAL)

> Severity of pneumonia, not etiology, drives initial treatment.

Treatment is often initiated without having a specific organism identified. It is the severity of disease, not the etiology, that drives initial treatment.

- If an exam question describes an organism on Gram stain, then direct treatment toward that organism.
- In the initial management of pneumonia, the most important step is usually determining the severity of disease so that it can be decided where to place the patient, i.e., inpatient or outpatient.

> New, large effusions secondary to pneumonia should be tapped.

- Bronchoscopy (rarely needed in CAP) if there is severe disease unresponsive to empiric treatment and requiring intensive care; an exception is pneumocystis pneumonia, where noninvasive testing rarely reveals a diagnosis, and precise confirmation of the etiology is critical to guide treatment.

The far majority of pneumonia cases can be treated outpatient with oral antibiotics. **Severe cases requiring hospitalization must have all of the following conditions**:

- Hypotension (systolic <90 mm Hg)
- Respiratory rate >30/min or pO_2 <60 mm Hg, pH <7.35
- BUN >30 mg/dL, sodium <130 mmol/L, glucose >250 mg/dL
- Pulse >125/min
- Confusion
- Temperature is >40 C (104 F)
- Age ≥65 with comorbidity such as cancer, COPD, CHF, renal failure, liver disease

Either hypoxia or hypotension alone is sufficient reason to hospitalize a patient.

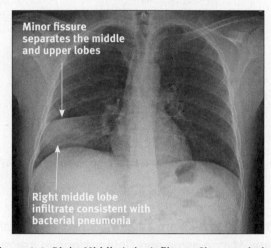

Figure 4.4 Right Middle Lobe Infiltrate Characteristic of Bacterial Pneumonia. *Source: Nirav Thakar, MD*

Lefamulin:

- Pleuromutilin antibiotic
- Inhibits ribosomes
- Use in community-acquired bacterial pneumonia = use of moxifloxacin in CAP

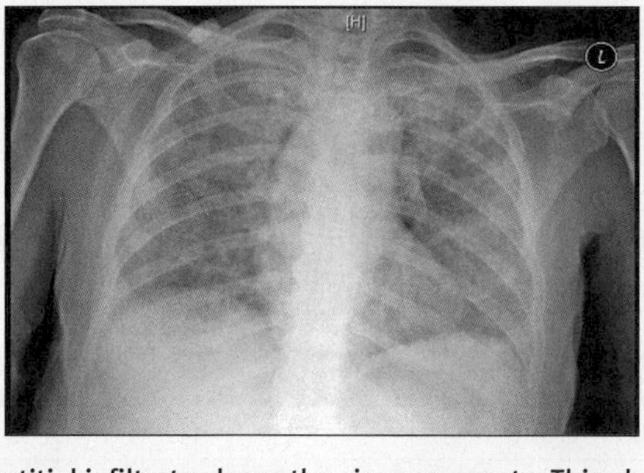

Figure 4.5 Interstitial infiltrates leave the air space empty. This chest x-ray can be consistent with PCP, mycoplasma, viruses, and chlamydia. *Source: Craig Thurm, MD*

Omadacycline

- Tetracycline derivative
- CAP and MRSA

▶ **TIP**

In infectious disease, the radiologic test is never the most accurate test.

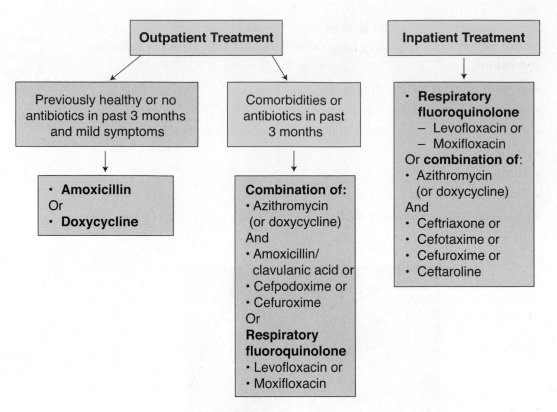

Figure 4.6 Outpatient and Inpatient Treatment of CAP

Chest x-ray **does not guide admission**. X-ray cannot reveal the severity of hypoxia.

▶**TIP**

Almost all infectious diseases are initially treated empirically, i.e., without a specific etiology. *Mycoplasma* and *Chlamydophila* are rarely confirmed because they are simply treated empirically.

Pleural Effusion

Exudate versus Transudate

- Pleural effusion with pH <7.2 or PMNs >1,000 suggests empyema and needs chest tube drainage.
- LDH >60% of serum (0.6) or protein >50% of serum (0.5) suggests an exudate; exudates are caused by infection and cancer

	Exudate	Transudate
Protein	>50% serum	<50% serum
LDH	>60% serum	<60% serum
Etiology	• Cancer • Infection • Connective tissue disease, e.g., SLE, RA, granulomatosis with polyangiitis (GPA), eosinophilic GPA, pancreatitis, PE, sarcoidosis	• CHF • Nephrotic syndrome • Atelectasis • Hypoalbuminemia

A 65-year-old woman is admitted to the hospital with CAP. Chest x-ray shows a lobar infiltrate and large effusion. She is placed on ceftriaxone and azithromycin. Thoracentesis reveals an elevated LDH and protein with 17,000 white blood cells per μL and pH 7.1. Blood cultures grow *Streptococcus pneumoniae* with a minimal inhibitory concentration (MIC) to penicillin <0.1 μg/mL. Oxygen saturation is 96% on room air. Blood pressure is 110/70 mm Hg, temperature is 38.8 C (102 F), and pulse 112 per minute. What is the most appropriate next step in management?

a. Repeat thoracentesis
b. Placement of chest tube for suction
c. Addition of ampicillin
d. Move patient to ICU
e. Pulmonary consultation

Answer: **B**. Infected pleural effusion or empyema will respond most rapidly to drainage by chest tube or thoracostomy. A large effusion acts like an abscess and is hard to sterilize. Each side of the chest can accommodate 2–3 liters of fluid. Adding ampicillin to ceftriaxone will have no benefit. A low MIC to penicillin automatically means that the organism is sensitive to ceftriaxone and, in fact, all cephalosporins. The ICU is not required for an effusion or chest tube drainage, unless the patient is unstable. Pulmonary consult will not add anything, although it may be commonly done in practice.

> **CURB65 = admission**
> - Confusion
> - Uremia
> - Respiratory distress
> - BP low
> - Age >65
>
> **CURB65 scoring**
> - 0–1 point: home
> - ≥2 points: admission

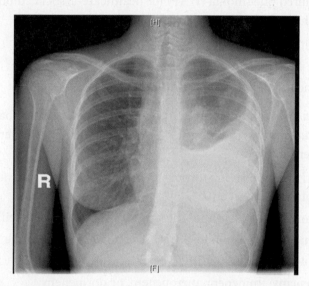

Figure 4.7 Pleural effusion with a large meniscus sign.
Only a fluid sample from thoracentesis can determine the specific cause.
Source: Craig Thurm, MD

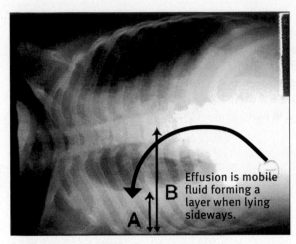

Figure 4.8 Effusion should be freely mobile and form a layer when the patient lies on her side.
Source: Nishith Patel, MD

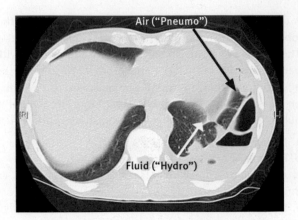

Figure 4.9 Hydropneumothorax is both abnormal air and fluid (effusion) in the pleural space. Chest tube drainage is the most effective way to remove this condition.
Source: Albert Takem, MD

Hospital-Acquired Pneumonia

Hospital-acquired pneumonia (HAP) (or healthcare-associated pneumonia) is pneumonia that occurs:

- After hospitalization in the last 90 days
- More than 48 hours after admission
- In association with a dialysis or infusion center

HAP patients have a much higher incidence of gram-negative bacilli such as *E. coli* or *Pseudomonas* as the cause of their infection. HAP differs from CAP in management approach:

- Unlike CAP, macrolides (azithromycin or clarithromycin) are not acceptable as empiric treatment.
- HAP treatment centers around therapy for gram-negative bacilli
  - **Antipseudomonal cephalosporins**: cefepime or ceftazidime
  - **Antipseudomonal penicillin**: piperacillin/tazobactam
  - **Carbapenems**: imipenem, meropenem, or doripenem

> Piperacillin and ticarcillin are always used in combination with a beta-lactamase inhibitor such as tazobactam or clavulanic acid.

Ventilator-Associated Pneumonia

Mechanical ventilation interferes with normal mucociliary clearance of the respiratory tract such as the ability to cough. Positive pressure is tremendously damaging to the normal ability to clear colonization. Ventilator-associated pneumonia (VAP) has an incidence as high as 5% per day in the first few days on a ventilator.

"What Is the Most Likely Diagnosis?"

Because of multiple concurrent illnesses such as CHF, even a diagnosis of VAP can be hard to establish. Look for:

- Fever and/or rising WBCs
- New infiltrate on chest x-ray
- Purulent secretions coming from the endotracheal tube

Diagnosis of a specific etiology is extremely difficult on a ventilator. Because of colonization of the endotracheal tube (ET), sputum culture is nearly worthless.

The following diagnostic tests are given in order from the **least accurate but easiest** to the **most accurate but most dangerous**:

- Tracheal aspirate: suction catheter is placed into the ET and aspirates the contents below the trachea when the catheter is past the end of the ET tube
- BAL: bronchoscope is placed deep into the lungs where there are not supposed to be any organisms; can be contaminated when passed through the nasopharynx
- Protected brush specimen: tip of the bronchoscope is covered when passed through the nasopharynx, then uncovered only inside the lungs; very specific because of decreased contamination
- Video-assisted thoracoscopy (VAT): scope is placed through the chest wall, and a sample of the lung is biopsied; allows a large piece of lung to be taken without needing to cut the chest open (thoracotomy); it is like sigmoidoscopy of the chest
- Open lung biopsy (**most accurate test**) has much greater morbidity and potential complications due to need for thoracotomy

> Culturing an endotracheal tube is like culturing urine with a Foley catheter in place: It will always grow something because of colonization.

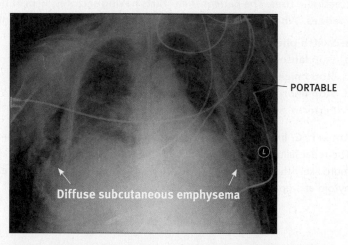

Figure 4.10 Subcutaneous emphysema is air abnormally leaking into the soft tissue of the chest wall. Chest tube placement may cause air to leak into soft tissues of the chest wall. *Source: Birju Shah, MD*

Treatment is a combination of 3 drug categories, i.e., use one from each category:

- Antipseudomonal beta-lactam (**choose one**)
  - Cephalosporin (ceftazidime or cefepime)
  - Penicillin (piperacillin/tazobactam)
  - Carbapenem (imipenem, meropenem, doripenem)
- Second antipseudomonal agent (**choose one**)
  - Aminoglycoside (gentamicin, tobramycin, amikacin)
  - Fluoroquinolone (ciprofloxacin, levofloxacin)
- Methicillin-resistant antistaphylococcal agent (**choose one**)
  - Vancomycin
  - Linezolid

For extended-spectrum beta lactamase (ESBL) producers (resistant to at least 3 classes of antipseudomonal drugs), use carbapenem.

What if the organism is carbapenem-resistant? Use one of these combinations:

- Meropenem/vaborbactam
- Imipenem/relebactam
- Ceftazidime/avibactam or ceftolozane/tazobactam

> No daptomycin for lungs! Daptomycin is inactivated by surfactant.

> If a specific etiology is identified, change the initial treatment.

A man who was admitted for head trauma and subdural hematoma is intubated for hyperventilation and a subsequent craniotomy. Several days after admission, he begins to vomit blood and is found to have stress ulcers of the stomach. Lansoprazole is started. VAP develops and the patient is placed on imipenem, linezolid, and gentamicin. Phenytoin is started prophylactically. Three days later, the creatinine rises. The patient then starts having seizures. Repeat head CT shows no changes. What is the most appropriate next step in management?

a. Switch phenytoin to carbamazepine
b. Stop lansoprazole
c. Stop imipenem
d. Stop linezolid
e. Perform an electroencephalogram

Answer: **C.** Imipenem can cause seizures. Imipenem is excreted through the kidneys. The renal failure has caused a rise in imipenem levels leading to toxicity. This is much more likely than a failure of phenytoin. Carbamazepine is no more effective than phenytoin at stopping seizures.

Pneumococcal vaccination recommendations are as follows:

- Everyone age >65 should receive vaccination with the 23 polyvalent vaccine.
- Regardless of age, everyone with chronic heart, liver, kidney, or lung disease (including asthma) should be vaccinated as soon as their underlying disease is apparent.
- Immunocompromised people should receive both the 13 and 23 polyvalent vaccines.
- If the first vaccination was given age <65 or with a condition previously described, give a second dose 5 years after the initial dose.
- Other reasons to vaccinate are:
  - Functional or anatomic asplenia (e.g., sickle cell disease)
  - Hematologic malignancy (leukemia, lymphoma)
  - Immunosuppression: DM, alcoholism, corticosteroid use, AIDS or HIV-positive
  - CSF leak and cochlear implantation

Healthcare workers do not need the pneumococcal vaccine.

Lung Abscess

Lung abscess is rare because aspiration pneumonia is now treated so promptly. It is seen in patients with large-volume aspiration of oral/pharyngeal contents, usually with poor dentition, who are not adequately treated.

Large-volume aspiration occurs from:

- Stroke with loss of gag reflex
- Seizures
- Intoxication
- Endotracheal intubation

> Aspiration pneumonia happens in the **upper** lobe **when lying flat.**

"What Is the Most Likely Diagnosis?"

Look for a person with a risk factor presenting with chronic infection over several weeks with large-volume sputum that smells foul because of anaerobes. Weight loss is common.

Diagnostic testing is as follows:

- Chest x-ray (**best initial test**) will show a cavity, possibly with an air-fluid level.
- Chest CT is more accurate than chest x-ray, but only lung biopsy (**most accurate test**) can establish the specific microbiologic etiology.

Treatment is clindamycin or penicillin.

> **Sputum culture** is the **wrong answer** for diagnosing a lung abscess. Everyone's sputum has anaerobes from mouth flora.

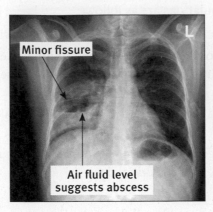 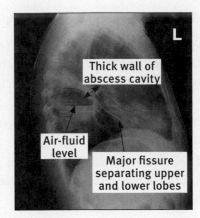

Figures 4.11, 4.12 Cavity Consistent with an Abscess with a Thick Wall and Air-Fluid Level. *Source: Alejandro de la Cruz, MD*

Pneumocystis Pneumonia

The agent causing pneumocystis pneumonia (PCP) is *P. jiroveci*. PCP occurs almost exclusively in patients with AIDS whose CD4 cell count has dropped below 200/µL and who are not on prophylactic therapy.

"What Is the Most Likely Diagnosis?"

Look for a patient with AIDS presenting with dyspnea on exertion, dry cough, and fever. The question will often suggest or directly state that the CD4 count is low (<200/µL) and that the patient is not on prophylaxis.

Diagnostic testing includes:

- Chest x-ray showing bilateral interstitial infiltrates or ABGs to look for hypoxia or increased A-a gradient (**best initial tests**)
- Elevated LDH (all cases)
- Bronchoalveolar lavage (**most accurate test**)
- Sputum stain for pneumocystis is quite specific if it is positive
  - If stain is positive, no further testing needed.
  - If stain is negative, do a bronchoscopy as the "**best diagnostic test**."

> You cannot distinguish PCP from *Mycoplasma*, *Chlamydophila*, or viruses by x-ray alone. However, in HIV, PCP is "most likely" with interstitial infiltrates.

▶ TIP

Normal LDH means you should not answer PCP as "the most likely diagnosis."

▶ TIP

Exam questions ask for the "most likely diagnosis," not the "for sure diagnosis."

Treatment is as follows:

- TMP/SMX (unquestionably the **best initial therapy both for treatment and prophylaxis**)
    - Atovaquone is an alternative if PCP is mild, i.e., mild hypoxia only.
    - If there is toxicity from TMP/SMX, switch to clindamycin + primaquine or pentamidine.
- Steroids to decrease mortality if PCP is severe (severe PCP is pO2 <70 or A-a gradient >35)

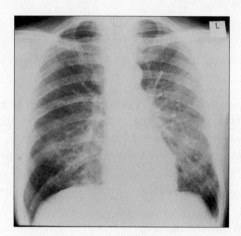

Figure 4.13 Another Example of Bilateral Interstitial Infiltrates.
Source: Conrad Fischer, MD

An HIV-positive African American man is admitted with dyspnea, dry cough, high LDH, and pO_2 63 mm Hg. He is started on TMP/SMX and prednisone. On hospital day 3 he develops severe neutropenia and a rash. He has anemia and there are bite cells visible on his smear. What is the most appropriate next step in management?

a. Stop TMP/SMX
b. Delay antiretroviral medications
c. Switch TMP/SMX to IV pentamidine
d. Switch TMP/SMX to aerosol pentamidine
e. Switch TMP/SMX to clindamycin and primaquine

Answer: **C.** Rash is the most common side effect of TMP/SMX, and bone marrow suppression the second most common. Although clindamycin and primaquine may have more efficacy than pentamidine, the patient seems to have G6PD deficiency, and primaquine is contraindicated in G6PD deficiency. He is an African American man, and there are bite cells suggestive of G6PD deficiency on his smear. For active disease, IV pentamidine is used, not aerosol. Antiretrovirals should be started immediately; they will help an acute opportunistic infection.

► **TIP**

On the exam, students often will see 2 correct treatments and think there is a mistake in the question. If you see 2 correct treatments, look for a contraindication to one of them.

PCP Prophylaxis

Start treatment to prevent PCP in those with AIDS whose CD4 count <200/µL.

1. TMP/SMX

If there is a rash or neutropenia from TMP/SMX, use:

2. Atovaquone or dapsone

Aerosol pentamidine is always the wrong answer. Aerosol pentamidine is not used as second-line therapy for prophylaxis because it has less efficacy than atovaquone or dapsone.

> Dapsone is contraindicated in those with glucose 6 phosphate dehydrogenase deficiency.

▶ TIP
Always choose therapy based first on efficacy, not adverse effects.

An HIV-positive woman with 22 CD4 cells/µL is admitted with PCP and is treated successfully with TMP/SMX. Prophylactic TMP/SMX is started. She is then started on antiretroviral medication and her CD4 rises to 420 cells; this CD4 count has remained steady for the last 6 months. What is the most appropriate next step in management?

a. Continue all medications
b. Stop TMP/SMX
c. Stop all medications and observe
d. Stop all medications if PCR-RNA viral load is undetectable

Answer: **B.** If the CD4 count is maintained >200/µL for several months, prophylactic TMP/SMX can be stopped. You cannot stop the antiretroviral medications because her CD4 count will drop. It is the antiretroviral medications that are maintaining her CD4 count. If the CD4 rises and is maintained high, there is no need for prophylactic medications. These cells are fully functional, and they will prevent opportunistic infections. The use of prophylactic medications is based on CD4 count, not viral load.

Tuberculosis

Tuberculosis (TB) is a bacterial infection caused by *Mycobacterium tuberculosis*. Almost all patients with TB have ≥1 established risk factor:

- Recent immigrant (in past 5 years)
- Prisoner
- HIV-positive
- Healthcare worker
- Close contact of someone with TB

- Steroid user
- Hematologic malignancy
- Alcoholic
- Diabetes mellitus

"What Is the Most Likely Diagnosis?"

Look for a person with a risk factor, presenting with fever, cough, sputum, weight loss, hemoptysis, and night sweats.

Diagnostic testing includes:

- Chest x-ray (**best initial test**)
- Sputum stain and culture specifically for acid-fast bacilli (mycobacteria) must be done 3 times to fully exclude TB
- Pleural biopsy (**most accurate test**)

For TB to be diagnosed, there must be a clear risk factor, cavity on chest x-ray, or positive smear.

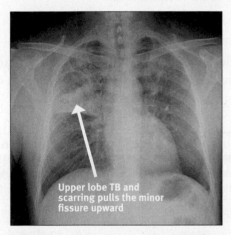

Upper lobe TB and scarring pulls the minor fissure upward

Figure 4.14 Chest X-ray Showing Upper Lobe Disease Consistent with Tuberculosis. *Source: Craig Thurm, MD*

▶**TIP**

In a symptomatic patient, PPD skin testing is never the best test for TB.

Treatment

When the smear is positive, begin with 4-drug therapy (**RIPE**). The standard of care is 6 months total.

- **R**ifampin
- **I**soniazid
- **P**yrazinamide (not for use in pregnancy)
- **E**thambutol (not needed only if it is known prior to treatment that the organism is sensitive to all TB medications)

After using RIPE for 2 months, stop pyrazinamide and ethambutol but continue rifampin and isoniazid for another 4 months.

Treatment is extended to >6 months for certain conditions:

- Osteomyelitis
- Miliary TB
- Meningitis
- Pregnancy or any other time pyrazinamide is not used
- Cavitary lesions

Failure to complete a full course of therapy is the most common cause of drug-resistance with TB. Therefore, **directly observed therapy** (DOT) is essential for ensuring compliance.

- Healthcare workers go to the patient's residence to ensure the medications are taken.
- For patients with mental health issues, DOT is especially critical.

Note the side effects of TB medications:

- All TB medications cause hepatoxicity, but should not be stopped unless transaminases rise to 3–5 × the upper limit of normal.
- Glucocorticoids decrease the risk of constrictive pericarditis in those with pericardial involvement. They also decrease neurologic complication in TB meningitis.

Side Effects of Antituberculosis Treatment		
Drug	**Toxicity**	**Management**
Rifampin	Red color to body secretions	None, benign finding
Isoniazid	Peripheral neuropathy	Use pyridoxine to prevent
Pyrazinamide	Hyperuricemia	No treatment unless symptomatic
Ethambutol	Optic neuritis/color vision	Decrease dose in renal failure

Latent TB testing is done with interferon gamma-release assay (IGRA) or PPD. These are not general screening tests for the population at large.

- Neither IGRA nor PPD is useful if patients have symptoms or abnormal chest x-ray (in those cases, use sputum acid-fast testing).
- **IGRA** is a blood test needing only a single visit.
  - Does not cross-react with BCG
  - Indications, risk of TB with a positive test, and treatment are identical to those for PPD

In the United States, TB continues to decline, but 70% of cases are recent immigrants from countries with poor control (including those patients who have previously received the bacillus Calmette-Guérin [BCG] vaccine). That is why previous BCG vaccination has no impact on latent TB infection (positive test for purified protein derivative of tuberculin, or PPD).

In other words, even if an immigrant who previously received the BCG vaccine has a positive PPD, you cannot assume that the TB has not reactivated. Basically, treat as if the patient never had a TB vaccination.

- **Positive PPD**: only induration is counted; erythema is irrelevant
  - **Induration >5 millimeters**: HIV-positive patients, glucocorticoid or anti-TNF users, close contacts of those with active TB, those with abnormal calcifications on chest x-ray, organ transplant recipients
  - **Induration >10 millimeters**: recent immigrants (past 5 years), prisoners, healthcare workers, close contacts of someone with TB, those with hematologic malignancy, alcoholics, those with diabetes mellitus
  - **Induration >15 millimeters**: those with no risk factors

Everyone with a reactive IGRA or PPD should have a chest x-ray to exclude active disease.

Treatment of positive IGRA or PPD is as follows:

- Isoniazid + rifapentine for 12 weeks (shortest possible treatment)
  - Both medications need only be given once a week, so it is only 12 total doses.
  - Use pyridoxine (B6) with isoniazid.

OR

- Rifampin for 4 months

OR

- Isoniazid for 9 months

A positive IGRA or PPD confers a 10% lifetime risk of TB; treatment will reduce this risk by 90%.

Neither the IGRA nor the PPD should be repeated once it is positive.

> ▶ **TIP**
> IGRA and PPD are among the hardest and most misunderstood tests on USMLE Step 2 CK. Reread the preceding section and forget what you have learned in the past.

Nontuberculous Mycobacteria (NTM) Infection

M. avium-intracellulare (MAI) Complex

In the absence of HIV, MAI presents as cough/sputum in an older person with COPD. A single positive sputum culture is considered colonization. Treat only if the colony grows repeatedly *and* respiratory symptoms are present *and* x-ray is abnormal. Use azithromycin (or clarithromycin) and rifampin (or rifabutin) and ethambutol.

Sidebar notes:

- IGRA and PPD are equal in sensitivity.
- **IGRA is preferred** because it requires only one visit.
- You are still required to understand PPD screening.

If the PPD is positive, the patient must be treated, regardless of past BCG immunization.

Only 1 month of treatment is needed before starting a TNF inhibitor.

12 doses (1 per week) of INH and rifapentine treats positive IGRA or PPD!

Rapidly Growing Mycobacteria

M. abscessus (*chelonae*) and *M. fortuitum*

- Infects skin and soft tissue, especially following surgery or trauma
- Grows in 5–10 days
- Lives in water and soil
- Look for a question describing a colonized water line in a dental unit.

M. kansasii

- Lung disease similar to TB
- 90% with cavitary lung disease
- Same medications as for MAI

ABPA

Allergic bronchopulmonary aspergillosis (ABPA) is hypersensitivity of the lungs to fungal antigens that colonize the bronchial tree. ABPA occurs almost exclusively in patients with asthma and a history of atopic disorders.

"What Is the Most Likely Diagnosis?"

Look for an asthmatic patient with recurrent episodes of brown-flecked sputum and transient infiltrates on chest x-ray. Cough, wheezing, hemoptysis, and sometimes bronchiectasis occur.

Diagnostic testing is as follows:

- Peripheral eosinophilia
- Skin test reactivity to *Aspergillus* antigens
- Precipitating antibodies to *Aspergillus* on blood test
- Elevated serum IgE
- Pulmonary infiltrates on chest x-ray or CT

Treatment is as follows:

- Oral steroids (prednisone) for severe cases
- Oral itraconazole for recurrent episodes
- Omalizumab to prevents exacerbations, particularly in those with asthma

Untreated ABPA causes progressive lung fibrosis or bronchiectasis.

An inhaler cannot deliver a high enough dose of steroids to be effective in ABPA. **Use oral steroids.**

COVID-19

In 2020, COVID-19 emerged and quickly escalated into a global pandemic. At the time of printing, management is not clear. Here's what is known:

- COVID-19 is an infectious disease caused by a coronavirus, SARS-CoV-2.
- While most coronaviruses cause minor respiratory illnesses (e.g., the common cold), SARS-CoV-2 is one of a few that can cause serious disease and death (the others are Middle East respiratory syndrome [MERS] and severe acute respiratory syndrome [SARS]).
- If the Step 2 CK exam addresses COVID-19 in the next year or two, the most likely question will be about diagnosis:
  - Fever, dry cough, and dyspnea *without* sneezing, runny nose, and sputum
  - Loss of smell and taste (central to answering the question)
- Testing
  - PCR (**most accurate test**)
  - Chest x-ray: will show abnormalities but is non-specific
  - Antibody testing: does not diagnose acute disease
  - Inflammatory markers, e.g., ferritin, D-dimer, LDH, and CRP
- Management
  - Respiratory isolation
  - Steroids such as dexamethasone for severely ill patients with hypoxia
  - No proven antiviral therapy at this time
  - Remdesivir, a broad-spectrum antiviral, has been approved for the treatment of hospitalized COVID-19 patients (age 12 or older) who require oxygen therapy or mechanical ventilation.

Solitary Pulmonary Nodule

When a patient has a solitary pulmonary nodule, the key issue for Step 2 CK regards biopsy.

When do you answer, "Biopsy the lung lesion"?

- Biopsy enlarging lung lesions, especially enlarging rapidly lung lesions.

For all lung lesions, the **best initial step** is to compare the size with old x-rays.

| Benign versus Malignant Pulmonary Nodule ||
Benign	**Malignant**
Age <30	Age >40
No change in size	Enlarging
Nonsmoker	Smoker
Smooth border	Spiculated (spikes)
Small, <1 cm	Large, >2 cm
Normal lung	Atelectasis
No adenopathy	Yes adenopathy
Dense, central calcification	Sparse, eccentric calcification
Normal PET scan	Abnormal PET scan

Biopsy all enlarging lung lesions, particularly if they are rapidly enlarging.

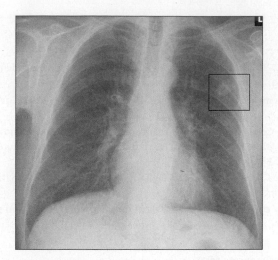

Figure 4.15 Chest X-ray Showing Solitary Lung Nodule.
Source: Conrad Fischer, MD

Diagnostic testing and treatment are as follows:

- **High-probability lesions**
  - **Resection of the lesion** when many of the "malignant" features described are present
  - Sputum cytology, needle biopsy, and PET scan are *not* used (negative tests are likely false negatives)
- **Intermediate-probability lesions** (the "gray" areas or inconclusive features of the solitary pulmonary nodule, e.g., age 30–40)
  - **Sputum cytology**; however, negative cytology does not exclude malignancy.
  - **Bronchoscopy or transthoracic needle biopsy** is the "**most appropriate next step**" in most patients with intermediate probability of malignancy.
    - Central lesions: use bronchoscopy
    - Peripheral lesions: use transthoracic biopsy
  - **PET scan** (sensitivity 85–95%) can identify without a biopsy whether the contents of the intermediate-risk lesion are malignant. Malignancy has increased uptake of tagged glucose. Negative PET scan points away from malignancy. It is most accurate with larger lesions.
  - **VATS** is more sensitive and more specific than all the other forms of testing. Frozen section in the operating room allows for immediate conversion to an open thoracotomy and lobectomy if malignancy is found.

▶ **TIP**
- On exam questions, remember that a clear answer must be present. So, if a question about the "best diagnostic test" for an intermediate lesion provides testing options that are not clear, the adverse effects will be clear.
- The most common side effect of a transthoracic biopsy is pneumothorax.

Lung cancer screening indications by chest CT:
- 20 pack-year tobacco history
- Age 50–80
- Not quit in the last 15 years

PET scan is most accurate with larger lesions (>1 cm).

Interstitial Lung Disease

Pulmonary Fibrosis

Pulmonary fibrosis (or idiopathic fibrosing interstitial pneumonia) is thickening of the interstitial septum of the lung between the arteriolar space and the alveolus. Fibrosis interferes with gas exchange in both directions.

Fibrosis can be idiopathic or secondary to a large number of inflammatory conditions, radiation, drugs, or from inhalation of toxins. All of them thicken the septum. Only some have white blood cell infiltrates with lymphocytes or neutrophils. Chronic conditions lead to fibrosis and thickening.

Causes of pulmonary fibrosis are as follows:

- Idiopathic; interstitial pulmonary fibrosis
- Radiation
- Drugs: bleomycin, busulfan, amiodarone, methysergide, nitrofurantoin, methotrexate

Types of Pneumoconioses	
Exposure	**Disease**
Coal	Coal worker's pneumoconiosis
Sandblasting, rock mining, tunneling	Silicosis
Shipyard workers, pipe fitting, insulators	Asbestosis
Cotton	Byssinosis
Electronic manufacture	Berylliosis
Moldy sugar cane	Bagassosis

All forms of pulmonary fibrosis, regardless of etiology, present with:

- Dyspnea, worsening on exertion
- Fine rales or "crackles" on examination
- Loud P_2 heart sound
- Clubbing of the fingers

Diagnostic testing includes:

- PFTs: restrictive lung disease with decrease of everything proportionately
  - FEV_1, FVC, TLC, and residual volume will all decrease, but since everything decreased, FEV_1/FVC ratio will be normal.
  - DLCO decreases in proportion to the severity of the thickening of the alveolar septum.
- Chest x-ray (**best initial test**)
- High resolution CT scan (**more accurate than chest x-ray**)
- Lung biopsy (**most accurate test**) shows granulomas in berylliosis
- Echocardiography often shows pulmonary hypertension and possibly right ventricular hypertrophy

> Inflammatory infiltration with white blood cells is reversible (treatable), whereas fibrosis is irreversible.

> Methotrexate causes fibrosis of both liver and lung.

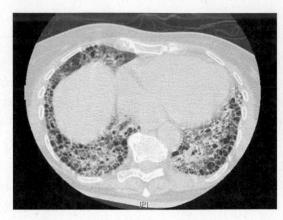

Figure 4.16 Severe, longstanding interstitial fibrosis produces thick walls between alveoli that give the appearance of "honeycombing."
Source: Craig Thurm, MD

Treatment

Most types of interstitial lung disease are untreatable. Treatment includes:

- Prednisone, if biopsy shows WBC or inflammatory infiltrate
- Steroids (of all the causes of pneumoconioses, berylliosis is the most likely to respond to steroids due to the presence of granulomas, a sign of inflammation)
  - If patients respond to steroids, switch to azathioprine for long-term treatment to get them off steroids.
  - If no response to steroids or azathioprine, try cyclophosphamide.
- Pirfenidone and nintedanib to slow the rate of fibrosis
  - Pirfenidone, an antifibrotic agent, inhibits collagen synthesis.
  - Nintedanib, a tyrosine kinase inhibitor, blocks fibrogenic growth factors and inhibits fibroblasts.

> N-acetylcysteine does not help lung disease.

Sarcoidosis

Sarcoidosis is an idiopathic inflammatory disorder predominantly of the lungs but can affect most of the body. It is common in African American women.

"What Is the Most Likely Diagnosis?"

Look for a young African American woman with shortness of breath on exertion and occasional fine rales on lung exam, but without the wheezing of asthma. Erythema nodosum and lymphadenopathy, either on examination or especially on chest x-ray, will hand you the diagnosis question.

Sarcoidosis also presents with:

- Parotid gland enlargement
- Facial palsy
- Heart block and restrictive cardiomyopathy
- CNS involvement
- Iritis and uveitis

> Although liver and kidney granulomas are very common on autopsy, they are rarely symptomatic.

▶ **TIP**

Answer sarcoidosis when a chest x-ray or CT shows hilar adenopathy in a generally healthy African American woman.

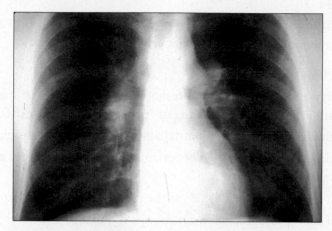

Figure 4.17 Sarcoidosis with Bilateral Hilar Adenopathy.
Source: Conrad Fischer, MD.

Diagnostic testing is as follows:

- Chest x-ray (**best initial test**) shows hilar adenopathy (almost all cases), parenchymal involvement, and lymphadenopathy.
- Lymph node biopsy (**most accurate test**): The granulomas are noncaseating.
- Hypercalcemia (5%): Granulomas in sarcoidosis make vitamin D.
- Elevated ACE level (60%)
- Hypercalciuria (20%)
- PFTs: restrictive lung disease (decreased FEV1, FVC, and TLC with normal FEV1/FVC ratio)

Treatment is prednisone (**drug of choice**). Few patients fail to respond.

Asymptomatic hilar adenopathy does not need to be treated.

> Bronchoalveolar lavage shows an elevated level of helper cells.

Pulmonary Hypertension

Pulmonary hypertension is a pulmonary systolic BP >20 mm Hg. Any chronic lung disease leads to back pressure into the pulmonary artery, obstructing flow out of the right side of the heart.

Pulmonary arterial hypertension is, by definition, idiopathic. Any form of chronic lung disease such as COPD or fibrosis elevates the pulmonary artery pressure. Hypoxemia causes vasoconstriction of the pulmonary circulation as a normal reflex in the lungs to shunt blood away from areas of the lung it considers to have poor oxygenation. This is why hypoxia leads to pulmonary hypertension, and pulmonary hypertension results in more hypoxemia.

> It is impossible to know that pulmonary hypertension is causing the dyspnea without testing.

Symptoms include:

- Dyspnea and fatigue
- Syncope
- Chest pain
- Wide splitting of S2 from pulmonary hypertension with a loud P2 or tricuspid and pulmonary valve insufficiency

Diagnostic testing includes:

- Chest x-ray and CT (**best initial tests**) will show dilation of the proximal pulmonary arteries with narrowing or "pruning" of distal vessels
- EKG: right axis deviation, right atrial and ventricular hypertrophy
- Echocardiography: RA and RV hypertrophy; Doppler estimates pulmonary artery pressure
- V/Q scan will identify chronic PE as the cause of pulmonary hypertension
- CBC will show polycythemia from chronic hypoxia
- Right heart or Swan-Ganz catheter (**most accurate test** and **most precise way to measure pressures by vascular reactivity**)

Treatment begins with correction of the underlying cause.

- Idiopathic disease is treated if there is vascular reactivity.
  - Prostacyclin analogues (PA vasodilators): epoprostenol, treprostinil, iloprost, beraprost, selexipag
  - Endothelin antagonists: bosentan, ambrisentan, macitentan
  - Phosphodiesterase inhibitors: sildenafil, tadalafil
  - cGMP stimulators: riociguat
  - CCBs
- Primary pulmonary hypertension has no clear treatment, i.e., it is uncertain which drug will open up or slow the closing of the pulmonary artery without right heart catheterization. When the catheter is in the pulmonary artery, you give each drug and see which one the patient's artery responds to.
- Oxygen to slow progression, particularly with COPD (most effective when etiology of pulmonary hypertension is lung disease that causes hypoxia)
- Lung transplant (curative only for idiopathic pulmonary hypertension)

BOOP/COP

Previously called *bronchiolitis obliterans organizing pneumonia* (BOOP), cryptogenic organizing pneumonia (COP) is caused by infections and autoimmune disorders. It presents as a patchy process with proliferation of granulation tissue in small airways and ducts. Symptoms are similar to those of CAP, with cough, dyspnea, fever, malaise, and weight loss.

There is no specific finding on x-ray or CT.

The **most accurate test** is lung biopsy.

Treatment is glucocorticoids. It does not respond to antibiotics.

Hypersensitivity Pneumonitis

Hypersensitivity pneumonitis is an exaggerated immunological response to repeated administration of antigens such as *Actinomyces*, fungi, molds, and bird droppings. In addition to cough and dyspnea, there are symptoms of acute inflammatory response such as chills, malaise, myalgia, and rash.

Symptoms markedly decrease a few days after the end of the exposure (unlike interstitial fibrosis). Chest x-ray and CT show bilateral hazy opacities. Patients with persistent, severe post-exposure symptoms are given glucocorticoids.

	Interstitial lung disease	**Hypersensitivity pneumonitis**
Symptoms	• Lung only (no fever) • No fever • Chronic/progressive	• Fever, chills, myalgia • Symptoms arise 1–2 days after exposure begins
Treatment	If idiopathic, pirfenidone or nintedanib	• Glucocorticoids • Azathioprine or mycophenolate if chronic steroids needed

Eosinophilic Pneumonia

This form of pneumonia presents as 1–2 weeks of fever, cough, and shortness of breath that progresses to respiratory failure. Look for these in the patient history:

- Cancer
- Medications: amiodarone, NSAIDs, nitrofurantoin, phenytoin, daptomycin
- Parasitic infections: strongyloidiasis, ascariasis, trichinellosis, schistosomiasis

The **most accurate test** is presence of eosinophils on bronchoalveolar lavage (BAL) or lung biopsy. Treat with steroids.

Thromboembolic Disease

Pulmonary embolism (PE) and **deep vein thrombosis (DVT)** are addressed as a spectrum of the same disease. The risks and treatment are the same for both conditions.

- PE derives from DVT of the large vessels of the legs (70%) and pelvic veins (30%)
- DVT is caused by stasis from immobility, surgery, trauma, joint replacement, or thrombophilia such as factor V Leiden mutation and antiphospholipid syndrome. Additionally, malignancy of any kind can lead to DVT.

> The highest risk of clot is with ankle replacement.

"What Is the Most Likely Diagnosis?"

Look for the sudden onset of shortness of breath with clear lungs on examination and a normal chest x-ray.

Other findings are:

- Tachypnea, tachycardia, cough, and hemoptysis
- Unilateral leg pain from DVT
- Pleuritic chest pain from lung infarction
- Fever (can arise from any cause of clot or hematoma)
- Hypotension (produced by extremely severe emboli)

► **TIP**

The main issue is to know "What is the most common finding?" and "What is the most common abnormality?"

Diagnostic testing includes:

- PE: no single, uncomplicated diagnostic test
  - Chest x-ray, EKG, and ABG (**best initial tests**); after these have been done, the "**best next step**" is usually CT angiogram
    - Chest x-ray is usually normal; **most common abnormality is atelectasis**; much less common are wedge-shaped infarction, pleural-based lesion (Hampton hump), and oligemia of one lobe (Westermark sign)
    - EKG usually shows sinus tachycardia; **most common abnormality is nonspecific ST-T wave changes**; much less common are right axis deviation, RV hypertrophy, and right bundle branch block
    - ABG shows hypoxia and respiratory alkalosis (high pH and low p CO_2) (**with normal chest x-ray, extremely suggestive of PE**)
  - **CT angiogram** (**standard of care to confirm a PE after x-ray, EKG, and ABG**) has excellent specificity (>95%) and sensitivity for clinically significant clots.
  - **Ventilation/perfusion (V/Q) scan** for patients with borderline renal function, in whom the contrast for the CT angiogram should be avoided, i.e., in pregnancy. V/Q is most accurate only in chronic thromboembolic disease.
    - High-probability scan has no clot (false positive) in 15%.
    - Low-probability scan has a clot (false negative) in 15%.
    - Completely normal scan essentially excludes a clot.
  - D-dimer has very high sensitivity (>97% negative predictive value) but very poor specificity since any cause of clot or increased bleeding can elevate the d-dimer; a negative test excludes a clot, but a positive test means little.

> The most common **wrong** answer is to choose S1, Q3, T3 as the most common abnormality that will be found on EKG.

– Lower extremity (LE) Doppler study: If LE Doppler is positive, no further testing is needed.

○ CT or V/Q scan is not needed to confirm a PE if there is a clot in the legs because they would not change treatment; patient will still need anticoagulation for 6 months.

> What to do is not always clear. However, the **side effects of angiogram** (allergy, renal toxicity) are very clear.

A 65-year-old woman who recently underwent hip replacement comes to the ED with an acute onset of shortness of breath and tachycardia. Chest x-ray is normal, with hypoxia on ABG, an increased A-a gradient, and EKG with sinus tachycardia. What is the most appropriate next step in management?

a. Enoxaparin
b. Thrombolytics
c. Inferior vena cava filter
d. Embolectomy
e. Spiral CT scan
f. Ventilation/perfusion (V/Q) scan
g. Lower-extremity Doppler studies
h. D-dimer

Answer: **A.** When the history and initial labs are suggestive of PE, it is far more important to start therapy (with LMW heparin or enoxaparin or with a NOAC) than to wait for the results of confirmatory testing such as the spiral CT or V/Q scan. Embolectomy with a catheter is done only if there is persistent hypotension, hypoxia, and tachycardia and thrombolytics are contraindicated or ineffective. There is no benefit of IV unfractionated heparin except a short half-life. D-dimer is a poor choice when the presentation is clear because it has poor specificity.

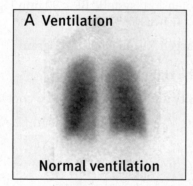 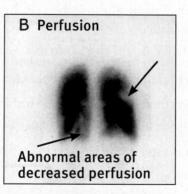

Figure 4.18 Ventilation/perfusion scanning (V/Q scanning) is still very useful in evaluating pulmonary emboli. A positive test is an area that is ventilated with decreased perfusion. *Source: Nishith Patel, MD*

> Chest x-ray must be normal for the V/Q scan to have any degree of accuracy.

▶**TIP**

D-dimer is the answer when the pretest probability of PE is low and you need a simple, noninvasive test to exclude thromboembolic disease.

> The USMLE Step 2 CK exam will not ask you to choose between two acceptable forms of treatment.

> Andexanet alfa reverses NOACs.

Treatment is as follows:

- NOAC or low-molecular-weight (LMW) heparin (enoxaparin) followed by warfarin
  - NOACS (oral agents) include rivaroxaban, apixaban, edoxaban, and dabigatran
  - **NOACs are as effective as enoxaparin and warfarin for PE and DVT** and have fewer complications: less intracranial bleeding than warfarin; require no INR monitoring; need no enoxaparin beforehand; reach a therapeutic effect in several hours instead of days like warfarin
  - Hemodynamically stable patients can be treated with a NOAC
- Fondaparinux, an alternative to heparin, is safe to use with heparin-induced thrombocytopenia (HIT). It is easier to monitor than argatroban.

What agents reverse anticoagulation?

- Andexanet alfa reverses rivaroxaban, apixaban, and edoxaban.
- Idarucizumab reverses dabigatran.
- Prothrombin complex concentrate (PCC) reverses warfarin.

When is an inferior vena cava (IVC) filter the right answer?

- When there is a DVT and a contraindication to the use of anticoagulants (e.g., melena, CNS bleeding)
- Recurrent emboli while on a NOAC or fully therapeutic warfarin (INR 2–3)

When are thrombolytics the right answer?

- Hemodynamically unstable (e.g., hypotension [systolic BP <90 mm Hg] and tachycardia)
- Acute RV dysfunction such as an enlarged RV on echocardiogram

> There is no specific time limit in which to use thrombolytics as there is in stroke or MI.

When is catheter removal of the clot the right answer?

- When there is hemodynamic instability and thrombolytics are contraindicated or ineffective

> Thrombolytics in PE:
> - Hypotensive
> - Acute right heart strain

When is aspirin the answer?

- Never

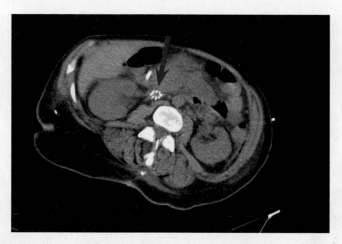

Figure 4.19 Chest CT of IVC Filter.
Source: Pramod Theetha Kariyanna, MD.

Acute Respiratory Distress Syndrome

Acute respiratory distress syndrome (ARDS) is respiratory failure from overwhelming lung injury or systemic disease leading to severe hypoxia. Chest x-ray is suggestive of congestive failure but has normal cardiac hemodynamic measurements.

- ARDS decreases surfactant and makes the lung cells "leaky" so that the alveoli fill up with fluid.
- ARDS is idiopathic. A large number of illnesses and injuries are associated with alveolar epithelial cell and capillary endothelial cell damage.

Illnesses associated with developing ARDS include sepsis/aspiration, lung contusion/trauma, near-drowning, and burns/pancreatitis.

ARDS is defined as **pO_2/FIO_2 ratio <300** (i.e., ratio of arterial oxygen partial pressure to fractional inspired oxygen).

- FIO_2 is expressed as a decimal, so room air with 21% oxygen is 0.21.
- If pO_2 is 105 on room air (21% oxygen or 0.21), the ratio of pO_2/FIO_2 is 500 (105/0.21).
- If pO_2 (as measured on ABG) is 70 while breathing 50% oxygen, the ratio is 70/0.5 or 140.

Testing includes:

- Chest x-ray shows bilateral infiltrates that quickly become confluent ("white out")
- Air bronchograms (common)
- Right heart catheterization will have normal findings
- Wedge pressure is normal, but not necessary to measure

> If **pO_2/FIO_2 <300**, the diagnosis is ARDS.
> - If <200, it is **moderately severe**.
> - If <100, it is **severe**.

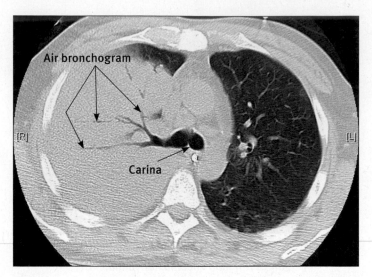

Figure 4.20 Air bronchograms are a sign of dense consolidation of the lung air space. This is a case of pneumococcal pneumonia that left only the air space in the larger bronchi open or air bronchograms. *Source: Omid Edrissian, MD*

There is no treatment to reverse ARDS. Treat the underlying cause.

- Low tidal-volume mechanical ventilation (best support while waiting to see if lungs will recover), i.e., tidal volume at 6 mL/kg of ideal body weight
- PEEP to decrease FIO_2 when patient is on mechanical ventilation (FIO_2 >50% is toxic to lungs); maintain plateau pressure is <30 cm of water (measured on ventilator)
- Prone positioning

Steroids are not clearly beneficial in most cases. They may help in late-stage disease if pulmonary fibrosis develops.

- Steroids are not clearly helpful in ARDS.
- N-acetylcysteine (NAC) is never helpful in pulmonary disease. When NAC is an answer choice on the exam, it is always wrong.

Infectious Diseases 5

Management of Infectious Disease

When answering questions about infectious disease, note the following principles:

- The radiologic test is never "the most accurate test."
- Risk factors for an infection are not as important as the individual presentation.
- Beta-lactam antibiotics have greater efficacy than other classes.

Regarding antibiotics, while the organisms associated with particular infections do not change over time, the antibiotics that treat the infections do change.

The most important thing to learn is the antibiotics associated with each group of organisms.

Treatment of *Staphylococcus*

The first step is to figure out whether the question is describing a sensitive organism or a resistant organism. Although methicillin is never used clinically, the terms "methicillin-sensitive *Staphylococcus aureus*" (MSSA) and "methicillin-resistant *Staphylococcus aureus*" (MRSA) are standard. If you use medications for a resistant organism when the organism is really sensitive, there is a higher treatment failure rate, particularly with the use of vancomycin for sensitive staphylococci in the blood.

Sensitive Staphylococcal Isolates

First agents:

- Intravenous: oxacillin, nafcillin, cefazolin
- Oral: dicloxacillin, cephalexin, cefadroxil

Additional agents:

- Intravenous: any cephalosporin, any carbapenem, beta-lactam/beta lactamase combinations
- Oral: amoxicillin/clavulanate, any oral cephalosporin

> **MRSA drugs:**
> - Ceftaroline
> - Dalbavancin
> - Daptomycin
> - Linezolid
> - Oritavancin
> - Tedizolid
> - Telavancin
> - Vancomycin

Resistant Staphylococcal Isolates

First agents:

- Intravenous: vancomycin, linezolid, daptomycin, ceftaroline, oritavancin, telavancin, dalbavancin
- Oral: linezolid, TMP/SMX, doxycycline

Additional agents:

- Oral: tedizolid, delafloxacin

> Delafloxacin is the only quinolone to cover MRSA.

You are called by the laboratory, which reports gram-positive cocci in clusters growing from the blood culture bottles. What is the best next step in management?

a. Start oxacillin
b. Start erythromycin
c. Start vancomycin
d. Start doxycycline
e. Consult infectious diseases
f. Wait for speciation and sensitivity of the organism
g. It is contamination; no treatment is needed

Answer: **C.** The **best empiric therapy** for gram-positive cocci growing from blood cultures is vancomycin. If there is intolerance or allergy to vancomycin, the correct answer is linezolid, daptomycin, or ceftaroline. Oxacillin is not first because it *will not cover MRSA*, and you must cover for resistance until you have the results of sensitivity testing. Erythromycin and macrolides are not adequate to cover any form of staphylococcal bacteremia. Doxycycline could be used for minor infections of the skin. Do not wait for speciation or to consult anyone; you should know how to initiate treatment for *Staphylococcus*.

Adverse effects of MRSA drugs:

- Linezolid: thrombocytopenia, interaction with MAO inhibitors
- Daptomycin: causes CPK elevation, not effective in the lung
- Tigecycline: should not be used for MRSA in blood
- Quinupristin/dalfopristin: *no longer correct* for anything

---

Minor MRSA infections of the skin are treated with:

- TMP/SMX
- Clindamycin
- Doxycycline
- Linezolid
- Delafloxacin

Beta-Lactam Antibiotics

Penicillins

Penicillin (G, VK, benzathine): viridans group streptococci, *Streptococcus pyogenes*, oral anaerobes, syphilis, *Leptospira*

Ampicillin and amoxicillin: cover the same organisms as penicillin, as well as *E. coli*, Lyme disease, and a few other gram-negative bacilli.

> There is no cross-reaction in allergies to aztreonam and penicillin.

Which of the following is the most accurate test for an infectious disease?

a. Protein level of fluid
b. Culture
c. IgM levels
d. IgG levels
e. Gram stain
f. Response to specific therapy

Answer: **B.** When an organism can be grown in culture, culture is definitely the **most accurate diagnostic test** for infectious diseases. This is true of almost all bacteria and certainly for *Staphylococcus*, *Streptococcus*, and gram-negative bacilli. A few infectious disease agents do not grow in culture, such as those that cause pneumocystis and syphilis. But for everything else, the accuracy of the test is compared with the accuracy of culture.

Amoxicillin is the "**best initial therapy**" for:

- Otitis media
- Dental infection and endocarditis prophylaxis
- Lyme disease limited to rash, joint, or seventh cranial nerve involvement
- Urinary tract infection (UTI) in pregnant women (or nitrofurantoin)
- *Listeria monocytogenes*
- Enterococcal infections

Penicillinase-resistant penicillins (PRPs): oxacillin, cloxacillin, dicloxacillin, and nafcillin.

These drugs are used to treat:

- Skin infections: cellulitis, impetigo, erysipelas
- Endocarditis, meningitis, and bacteremia from staphylococci
- Osteomyelitis and septic arthritis only when the organism is proven sensitive

They are not active against methicillin-resistant *Staphylococcus aureus* (MRSA) or *Enterococcus*.

"Methicillin sensitive or resistant" really means "oxacillin sensitive or resistant."

▶ **TIP**

Methicillin is never the right answer. It causes renal failure from allergic interstitial nephritis.

Piperacillin, ticarcillin, azlocillin, mezlocillin: These agents cover gram-negative bacilli (e.g., *E. coli, Proteus*) from the large Enterobacteriaccac group as well as pseudomonads. They and cephalosporins are the "best initial therapy" for:

- Cholecystitis and ascending cholangitis
- Pyelonephritis
- Bacteremia
- Hospital-acquired and ventilator-associated pneumonia
- Neutropenia and fever

Although these agents cover streptococci and anaerobes, they are not the answer when the infection is exclusively from these single organisms; you would use a narrower agent. They are nearly always used in combination with a beta-lactamase inhibitor such as tazobactam or clavulanic acid.

> Which of the following antibiotics covers methicillin-resistant *Staphylococcus aureus* (MRSA)?
>
> a. Nafcillin
> b. Cefazolin
> c. Piperacillin-tazobactam
> d. Ceftaroline
> e. Azithromycin
>
> Answer: **D.** The only cephalosporin that will cover MRSA is ceftaroline. None of the others covers MRSA. No macrolide (azithromycin, clarithromycin, erythromycin) will cover MRSA. The medications that do cover MRSA are vancomycin, daptomycin, ceftaroline, linezolid, tedizolid, dalbavancin, telavancin, and tigecycline.

Cephalosporins

Listeria, MRSA, and *Enterococcus* are resistant to all forms of cephalosporins. Ceftaroline is the only cephalosporin to cover MRSA.

The amount of cross-reaction between penicillin and cephalosporins is very small (<3%). All cephalosporins, in every class, will cover group A, B, and C streptococci, viridans group streptococci, *E. coli*, *Klebsiella*, and *Proteus mirabilis*. No cephalosporin covers the multidrug-resistant (MDR) gram-negative rods that are known as extended-spectrum beta lactamase–producing (ESBL-producing) bacteria. ESBL-producing MDROs are treated with carbapenems.

▶ **TIP**

If the case describes a rash to penicillin: Answer cephalosporins.

If the case describes anaphylaxis, you must use a non-beta-lactam antibiotic.

Answer **delafloxacin** for:
- MRSA of skin/soft tissue
- Gram-negative rods

First Generation: Cefazolin, Cephalexin, Cephradine, Cefadroxil

First-generation cephalosporins are used to treat:

- Staphylococci: methicillin sensitive = oxacillin sensitive = cephalosporin sensitive
- Streptococci (except *Enterococcus*)
- Some gram-negative bacilli such as *E. coli*, but not *Pseudomonas*
- Osteomyelitis, septic arthritis, endocarditis, cellulitis

Second Generation: Cefotetan, Cefoxitin, Cefaclor, Cefprozil, Cefuroxime

These agents cover all the same organisms as first-generation cephalosporins and add coverage for anaerobes and more gram-negative bacilli.

- Cefotetan or cefoxitin: **best initial therapy** for pelvic inflammatory disease (PID) combined with doxycycline. Warning: Cefotetan and cefoxitin increase the risk of bleeding and give a disulfiramlike reaction with alcohol.
- Cefuroxime, cefprozil, cefaclor: respiratory infections such as bronchitis, otitis media, and sinusitis

> Of the cephalosporins, only cefotetan and cefoxitin cover anaerobes.

Third Generation: Ceftriaxone, Cefotaxime, Ceftazidime

- Ceftriaxone: first-line for pneumococcus, including partially insensitive organisms
  - Meningitis
  - Community-acquired pneumonia (in combination with macrolides)
  - Gonorrhea
  - Lyme involving the heart or brain
  - Avoid in neonates because of impaired biliary metabolism.
- Cefotaxime
  - Superior to ceftriaxone in neonates
  - Spontaneous bacterial peritonitis
- Ceftazidime has pseudomonal coverage.

> Ceftaroline is the only cephalosporin to cover MRSA!

Fourth Generation: Cefepime

Cefepime has better staphylococcal coverage compared with the third-generation cephalosporins. It is used to treat:

- Neutropenia and fever
- Ventilator-associated pneumonia

Fifth Generation: Ceftaroline

- Gram-negative bacilli and MRSA, not *Pseudomonas*.

> Cefiderocol is a "siderophore" (iron-binding) cephalosporin for multi-resistant gram-negative rods causing urinary infections.

> **Adverse Effects of Cephalosporins**
>
> Cefoxitin and cefotetan deplete prothrombin and increase risk of bleeding. With ceftriaxone, there is inadequate biliary metabolism.

Carbapenems

> Ertapenem differs from the other carbapenems. It does not cover *Pseudomonas*.

Carbapenems cover gram-negative bacilli, including many that are resistant, anaerobes, streptococci, and staphylococci. They are used to treat neutropenia and fever. Carbapenems are the **"best therapy"** for ESBL-producing gram-negative bacteria.

Aztreonam

This is the only drug in the class of monobactams.

- Exclusively for gram-negative bacilli including *Pseudomonas*
- No cross-reaction with penicillin

Which of the following is most likely to be effective for *Morganella* or *Citrobacter*?

a. Tedizolid

b. Dalbavancin

c. Ertapenem

d. Oritavancin

e. Erythromycin

Answer: **C.** Ertapenem is a carbapenem antibiotic. All carbapenems are highly active against gram-negative bacilli. *Morganella* and *Citrobacter* are gram-negative bacilli in the same family as *E. coli*. Ertapenem covers most gram-negative rods and bacilli except *Pseudomonas*. Tedizolid, dalbavancin, and oritavancin are exclusively for gram-positive cocci and MRSA, such as would be found in skin and soft tissue infections. Erythromycin has no meaningful gram-negative coverage.

Fluoroquinolones

The fluoroquinolones include ciprofloxacin, gemifloxacin, levofloxacin, and moxifloxacin. Fluoroquinolones are used for:

- Community-acquired pneumonia, including penicillin-resistant pneumococcus (except ciprofloxacin)
- Gram-negative bacilli including most pseudomonads
- Diverticulitis and GI infections, but ciprofloxacin, gemifloxacin, and levofloxacin must be combined with metronidazole because they don't cover anaerobes; the exception is moxifloxacin. Moxifloxacin can be used as a single agent for diverticulitis and does not need metronidazole.

Other specific applications and exceptions:

- Ciprofloxacin is used for cystitis, pyelonephritis, and ventilator-associated pneumonia.
- Delafloxacin is the only quinolone to cover MRSA and the only quinolone that does not prolong QT. It equals ceftriaxone and vancomycin.

> Quinolones cause:
> - Bone growth abnormalities in children and pregnant women
> - Tendonitis and Achilles tendon rupture
>
> Gatifloxacin has been removed from use because of glucose abnormalities.

Aminoglycosides

The aminoglycosides include gentamicin, tobramycin, and amikacin.

- Gram-negative bacilli (bowel, urine, bacteremia)
- Synergistic with beta-lactam antibiotics for enterococci and staphylococci
- No effect against anaerobes, since they need oxygen to work
- Adverse effects: nephrotoxic and ototoxic

> Plazomicin is an aminoglycoside used for complicated UTI.

Doxycycline

- Bronchitis
- Lyme disease limited to rash, joint, or seventh cranial nerve palsy
- *Rickettsia*
- MRSA of skin and soft tissue (cellulitis)
- Primary and secondary syphilis in those allergic to penicillin
- *Borrelia, Ehrlichia, Anaplasma,* and *Mycoplasma*
- *Chlamydia*
- Adverse effects: Fanconi syndrome (type II RTA proximal), photosensitivity, esophagitis/ulcer

> Nitrofurantoin has one indication: cystitis, especially in pregnant women.

New Tetracyclines

- Omadacycline: pneumonia and MRSA
- Eravacycline: intra-abdominal infections

Trimethoprim/Sulfamethoxazole

- Cystitis
- Pneumocystis pneumonia treatment and prophylaxis
- MRSA of skin and soft tissue (cellulitis)
- Adverse effects: rash, hemolysis with G6PD deficiency, bone marrow suppression (folate antagonist)

Beta-Lactam/Beta-Lactamase Combinations

- Amoxicillin/clavulanate
- Ampicillin/sulbactam
- Ticarcillin/clavulanate
- Piperacillin/tazobactam
- Ceftazidime/avibactam (treats ESBL producers that carbapenems fail to clear)
- Ceftolozane/tazobactam
- Meropenem/vaborbactam and imipenem/relebactam (treats carbapenemase-producing gram-negative rods)

Beta-lactamase adds coverage against sensitive staphylococci to these agents. They cover anaerobes and are a first choice for mouth and GI abscess.

A patient has a perforation of an abdominal portion of the bowel and leakage into the peritoneum. There is fever and hypotension. The report on the anaerobic bottle of blood cultures states that it is growing an organism. Which of the following is most appropriate to start while waiting for the speciation and sensitivity testing?

a. Aztreonam
b. Piperacillin/tazobactam
c. Oxacillin
d. Cefepime
e. Doxycycline
f. Vancomycin

Answer: **B.** Piperacillin/tazobactam is the only medication of those listed that covers anaerobes. All the beta-lactam/beta-lactamase inhibitors cover anaerobes with equal efficacy to metronidazole. Carbapenems (such as ertapenem, doripenem, meropenem, and imipenem) cover the GI tract quite well because they cover the anaerobes as well as gram-negative bacilli.

Anaerobes

Oral (above the diaphragm)

- Penicillin (G, VK, ampicillin, amoxicillin)
- Clindamycin

Abdominal/gastrointestinal

- Metronidazole, beta-lactam/lactamase combinations, carbapenems

> Piperacillin, carbapenems, and second-generation cephalosporins also cover anaerobes.

Gram-Negative Bacilli *(E. coli, Klebsiella, Proteus, Pseudomonas, Enterobacter, Citrobacter)*

These organisms cause infections of the bowel (peritonitis, diverticulitis); urinary tract (pyelonephritis); and liver (cholecystitis, cholangitis).

All of these agents cover gram-negative bacilli:

- Quinolones
- Aminoglycosides
- Carbapenems
- Piperacillin, ticarcillin
- Aztreonam
- Cephalosporins
- Polymyxin (used last because of renal toxicity)

> Use polymyxin when an ESBL is resistant to carbapenem.

> Vancomycin in combination with piperacillin increases risk of AKI.

A man is admitted with *E. coli* bacteremia. Which of the following is the most appropriate treatment?

a. Vancomycin
b. Linezolid
c. Quinolones, aminoglycosides, carbapenems, piperacillin, ticarcillin, or aztreonam
d. Doxycycline
e. Clindamycin
f. Oxacillin

Answer: **C.** All of the agents listed under "gram-negative bacilli" could be the right answer. This question is like an IQ test: "Which of these is different from the other choices?" Choice (C) is the only one covering gram-negative bacilli.

ESBL-Producing Organisms

Extended-spectrum beta-lactamase–producing organisms (ESBL-producing organisms) are resistant to multiple classes of medications, such as quinolones, cephalosporins, monobactams (aztreonam), and penicillins. Treat with carbapenems. If the organism is resistant to carbapenems, the answer is:

- Ceftolozane/tazobactam
- Ceftazidime/avibactam
- Meropenem/vaborbactam and imipenem/relebactam (treats carbapenemase-producing gram-negative rods)
- Polymyxin (causes more renal injury)

Central Nervous System Infections

All central nervous system (CNS) infections may present with fever, headache, nausea, and vomiting. All of them can lead to seizures.

Clues to Answering the "Most Likely Diagnosis" Question	
Symptom	**Diagnosis**
Stiff neck, photophobia, meningismus	Meningitis
Confusion	Encephalitis
Focal neurological findings	Abscess

Meningitis

Meningitis is an infection or inflammation of the covering, or meninges, of the CNS. While virtually any infection can cause this, the great majority of cases have the following etiology:

- *Streptococcus pneumoniae* (60% of cases)
- Group B streptococci (14%)
- *Haemophilus influenzae* (7%)
- *Neisseria meningitidis* (15%)
- *Listeria* (2%)
- *Staphylococcus* is seen in those with recent neurosurgery.

Look for a fever, headache, neck stiffness (nuchal rigidity), and photophobia. Acute bacterial meningitis develops over several hours. Focal neurological abnormalities occur in up to 30% of patients.

If confusion occurs, you will not be able to answer "What is the most likely diagnosis?" without a CT and lumbar puncture (LP). Cryptococcal meningitis may be present for several weeks.

Organism Specific Presentations/"What Is the Most Likely Diagnosis?"	
Presentation	**The most likely diagnosis is...**
AIDS with <100 CD4 cells/µL	*Cryptococcus*
Camper/hiker, **rash shaped like a target**, joint pain, facial palsy, tick remembered in **20%**	Lyme disease
Camper/hiker, **rash moves from arms/legs to trunk**, tick remembered in **60%**	Rocky Mountain spotted fever (*Rickettsia*)
Pulmonary TB in **85%**	Tuberculosis
None	Viral
Adolescent, petechial rash	*Neisseria*

Diagnostic Tests

- LP (**best initial and most accurate test**)
- If immediate LP is contraindicated, give antibiotics (**best initial step in management**)
- Head CT is needed before an LP only if there is a chance that a space-occupying lesion may cause herniation, i.e., with papilledema, seizures, focal neurological abnormalities, or confusion interfering with the neurological exam.
  - An accurate neurological exam requires a cooperative patient who can understand, follow instructions, and answer questions.
  - If the patient is severely confused, you cannot do an accurate neurological exam.

Better to treat and decrease the accuracy of a test than to risk permanent brain damage.

- Bacterial antigen-detection (latex agglutination) tests (rarely indicated) are similar to a Gram stain. These tests by themselves are not sufficiently sensitive to exclude bacterial meningitis, i.e., if positive they are extremely specific, but if negative the patient could still have the infection. Sensitivity ranges from 50–90% depending on the organism.

CSF Evaluation				
	Bacterial meningitis	***Cryptococcus*, Lyme, *Rickettsia***	**Tuberculosis**	**Viral**
Cell count	1000s, neutrophils	10s–100s lymphocytes	10s–100s lymphocytes	10s–100s lymphocytes
Protein level	Elevated	Possibly elevated	Markedly elevated	Usually normal
Glucose level	Decreased	Possibly decreased	May be low	Usually normal
Stain and culture	Stain: 50–70%; culture: 90%	Negative	Negative	Negative

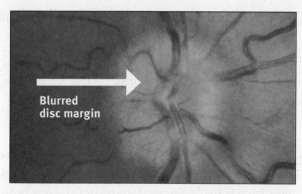

Figure 5.1 Papilledema is a blurred, fuzzy disc margin
from increased intracranial pressure. *Source: Conrad Fischer, MD*

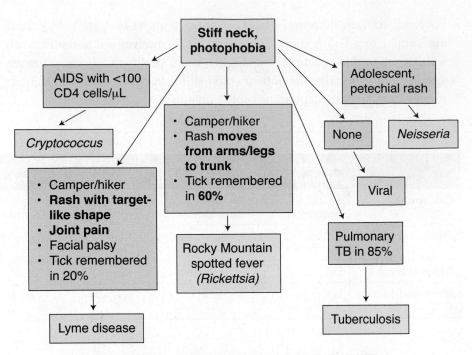

Figure 5.2 CNS Infections "Most Likely Diagnosis" Algorithm

When is a **bacterial antigen test** indicated?

- When patient has received antibiotics prior to the LP and the culture may be falsely negative

Treatment

Ceftriaxone, vancomycin, and steroids (**best initial treatment**) should be given based on cell count. Culture takes 2–3 days and is never available at the time that a treatment decision is made. Gram stain is useful if it is positive; however, the false-negative rate is 30–50%. Protein and glucose levels are too nonspecific to allow for a treatment decision.

Although steroids (dexamethasone) have been proven to lower mortality only in *S. pneumoniae* infection, you must give them when you see thousands of neutrophils because you will not know the culture results for several days. *Cryptococcus* is treated with amphotericin and 5FC.

Listeria monocytogenes

Listeria is resistant to all cephalosporins but sensitive to penicillins. You must add ampicillin to ceftriaxone and vancomycin if the case describes risk factors for *Listeria*:

- Elderly or neonate age
- Steroid use
- AIDS or HIV
- Immunocompromised, including alcoholism
- Pregnancy

> Thousands of neutrophils on CSF means treat with ceftriaxone, vancomycin, and steroids. Add ampicillin for *Listeria* if the patient is immunocompromised.

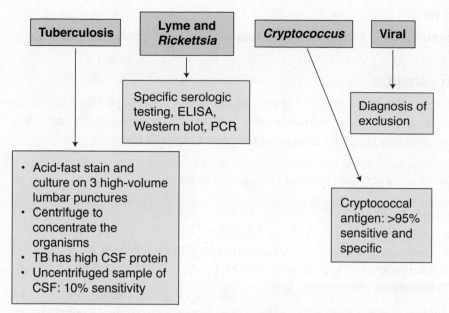

Cryptococcal Meningitis

Low CSF WBC count = High risk of death

Figure 5.3 CNS Infections "Most Accurate Diagnostic Test" Algorithm

Neisseria meningitidis: Additional Management

- Droplet isolation
- Rifampin, ciprofloxacin, or ceftriaxone to the close contacts to decrease nasopharyngeal carriage
    - "Close contacts" means those who have major respiratory fluid contact, such as household contacts, kissing, or sharing cigarettes or eating utensils.
    - Routine school and work contacts are not close contacts. Sitting in class with someone with *Neisseria* infection does not make them a close contact.
    - Healthcare workers qualify only if they have contact with respiratory secretions (e.g., intubation or suctioning).

What is the most common neurological deficit of untreated bacterial meningitis? Eighth cranial nerve deficit or deafness.

A man comes to the ED with fever, severe headache, neck stiffness, and photophobia. On physical examination he is found to have weakness of his left arm and leg. What is the most appropriate next step in management?

a. Ceftriaxone, vancomycin, and steroids
b. Head CT
c. Ceftriaxone
d. Neurology consultation
e. Steroids

Answer: **A.** When there is a contraindication to an immediate LP, the most important step is to initiate treatment. Ceftriaxone or steroids alone would not be sufficient. This patient's presentation is clear for meningitis. Although antibiotics may decrease the sensitivity of the CSF culture, it is more important to prevent neurological damage from untreated meningitis than it is to have a specific microbiological diagnosis. You can also still use the Gram stain and bacterial antigen detection methods to establish a diagnosis after the start of antibiotics, although they cannot tell sensitivity patterns. Head CT is important for this patient because of focal neurological deficits, but it is more important to initiate treatment. In addition, if the head CT shows a mass lesion, you may never be able to perform an LP.

▶ **TIP**

Consultation is almost always a wrong answer on USMLE Step 2 CK.

Encephalitis

Look for the acute onset of fever and confusion. Although there are many causes of encephalitis, herpes simplex is by far the most common cause. You must do a head CT first because of the presence of confusion.

What is the most accurate test of herpes encephalitis?

a. Brain biopsy
b. PCR of CSF
c. MRI
d. Viral culture of CSF
e. Tzanck prep
f. Serology for herpes (IgG, IgM)

Answer: **B.** PCR is more accurate than a brain biopsy. Viral culture is a test of skin and genital lesions, but it is not as accurate as PCR. Tzanck prep is not sensitive or specific for anything. Serology for herpes is useless; 95% of the population will be positive, since blood serology cannot distinguish oral herpes from a routine cold sore, genital herpes, or encephalitis.

> Herpes encephalitis gives red cells on CSF.

Treatment

Acyclovir is the best initial treatment for herpes encephalitis. Famciclovir and valacyclovir are not available as IV formulations. For acyclovir-resistant herpes, use foscarnet.

A woman is admitted for herpes encephalitis confirmed by PCR. After 4 days of acyclovir her creatinine level begins to rise. What is the most appropriate next step in management?

a. Stop acyclovir
b. Reduce the dose of acyclovir and hydrate
c. Switch to oral famciclovir or valacyclovir
d. Switch to foscarnet

Answer: **B.** Oral medications such as famciclovir and valacyclovir are insufficient for herpes encephalitis. While acyclovir is occasionally renally toxic because the medication precipitates in the renal tubules, foscarnet has far more renal toxicity.

Brain Abscess

A brain abscess is a collection of infected material within the parenchyma of the brain tissue, acting as a space-occupying lesion.

Anything that leads to bacteremia (e.g., pneumonia and endocarditis) can allow infected material to lodge in the brain. Brain abscess can spread from contiguous infection in the sinuses, mastoid air cells, or otitis media.

Presentation is nonspecific, and without a biopsy there is no way to distinguish a brain abscess from cancer. Look for the following:

- Headache
- Nausea/vomiting
- Fever (cancer can produce fever)
- Seizures
- Focal neurological findings

Diagnostic testing is as follows:

- Head CT or MRI (**best initial test**) will show a "ring" or contrast-enhancing lesion with surrounding edema and mass effect.
- Brain biopsy (**most accurate test**) is indicated because cancer and infection are indistinguishable based on imaging alone.
  - Determines the precise organism and its sensitivity pattern.
  - Abscess can result from staphylococci, streptococci, gram-negative bacilli, or anaerobes. Infections are also frequently mixed, so a precise microbiologic diagnosis is important given that the duration of treatment is very long (6–8 weeks intravenously, followed by 2–3 more months orally).
- CSF is not used to diagnose brain abscess (would have no added value).
- LP is contraindicated because of possible herniation.

Empiric treatment should be started while waiting for the results of the culture.

- Penicillin + metronidazole + ceftriaxone (or cefepime)
- If there has been recent neurosurgery and the risk of staphylococci (especially resistant staphylococci) is increased, use vancomycin instead of penicillin.

> Biopsy for culture is indispensable in precise treatment of brain abscess. Avoid prolonged empiric therapy.

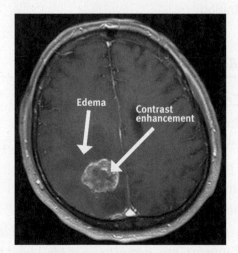

Figure 5.4 Both cancer and infection enhance with contrast.
You cannot distinguish them based on CT scan appearance alone.
Source: Nishith Patel, MD

Head and Neck Infections

Influenza (The "Flu")

Influenza presents with:

- Arthralgias/myalgias
- Cough
- Fever
- Headache and sore throat
- Nausea, vomiting, or diarrhea, especially in children

The "most appropriate next step in management" depends on the time course from presentation. If it is ≤48 hours since the onset of symptoms, perform a nasopharyngeal swab or wash in order to rapidly detect the antigen associated with influenza.

Treatment

Treatment is the same for both influenza A and B.

- **Symptoms <48 hours:**
  - Oseltamivir or zanamivir or baloxavir
    - Does not minimize complications of influenza, e.g., pneumonia
    - Peramivir is IV version of oseltamivir
  - Neuraminidase inhibitors or baloxavir to shorten duration of symptoms; if patient needs to be hospitalized, give one of these even if >48 hrs since onset of symptoms
- **Symptoms >48 hours:** symptomatic treatment only, i.e., analgesics, rest, antipyretics, hydration

> Baloxavir
> - Endonuclease cap inhibitor
> - Different mechanism from oseltamivir, same efficacy

Infectious Diarrhea

Blood and WBCs in Stool

- *Salmonella*: poultry
- *Campylobacter*: most common cause, associated with GBS
- *E. coli* 0157:H7—hemolytic uremic syndrome (HUS)
- *Shigella*: second most common association with HUS
- *Vibrio parahaemolyticus*: shellfish and cruise ships
- *Vibrio vulnificus*: shellfish, history of liver disease, skin lesions
- *Yersinia*: high affinity for iron, hemochromatosis, blood transfusions
- *Clostridiodes difficile*: white and red blood cells in stool

> Tests for CMV Colitis
> - Biopsy: yes
> - Stool PCR: no

The **best initial test** is for blood and/or fecal leukocytes, but this will not determine a specific organism. Stool lactoferrin has greater sensitivity and specificity compared with stool leukocytes. Lactoferrin is a better answer than fecal leukocytes if it is one of the choices. The most accurate test is stool culture.

No Blood or WBCs in Stool

- Viral
- *Giardia*: camping/hiking and unfiltered fresh water
- *Cryptosporidium*: AIDS with <100 CD4 cells; detect with modified acid-fast stain
- *Bacillus cereus*: vomiting
- *Staphylococcus*: vomiting

Scombroid

- Most rapid onset
- Wheezing, flushing, rash
- Found In fish
- Treat with antihistamines

Treatment

- Oral fluid replacement for mild disease
- Fluid replacement and oral antibiotics such as ciprofloxacin for severe disease

Which of the following is the most accurate in determining the etiology of infectious diarrhea?

a. Recent history of eating chicken
b. Frequency of bowel movements
c. Blood in stool
d. Odor of stool
e. Recent interstate travel

Answer: **C.** Blood in the stool means there has to be an invasive pathogen such as *Salmonella, Shigella, Yersinia,* or *E. coli.* The other choices—such as what food was eaten, bowel movement frequency, and smell—are useless. Stop smelling stool. It all smells bad!

"Severe" infectious diarrhea means:

- Hypotension
- Tachycardia
- Fever
- Abdominal pain
- Bloody diarrhea
- Metabolic acidosis

Disease-Specific Treatment	
Organism	**Treatment**
Giardia	Metronidazole, tinidazole
Cryptosporidium	Treat underlying AIDS, nitazoxanide
Viral	Fluid support as needed
B. cereus, Staphylococcus	Fluid support as needed
Strongyloides	Ivermectin

Sexually Transmitted Diseases

Urethritis

Urethritis (inflammation of the urethra) is often caused by *N. gonorrhoeae* and *Chlamydia*. Other causes include *Mycoplasma genitalium* and *Ureaplasma*.

Both urethritis and cystitis cause dysuria with urinary frequency and burning, but **with cystitis there is no urethral discharge**. Look for *urethral discharge* to answer, "What is the most likely diagnosis?"

Testing for urethritis is as follows:

- Urine testing for nucleic acid amplification (NAAT); can detect both gonorrhea and chlamydia
- WBCs, which will be elevated; if intracellular gram-negative diplococci are seen, that is sufficient evidence of *N. gonorrhoeae* to initiate treatment

NAAT can be accurately done on voided urine, so a urethral swab is not necessary.

> Oral cefixime is not used for gonorrhea.

Treatment is a combination of one drug for gonorrhea (IM ceftriaxone) and one for chlamydia (oral azithromycin). Quinolones are not the best initial treatment because of resistance.

Cervicitis

Cervicitis presents with cervical discharge and an inflamed "strawberry" cervix on physical examination. Diagnose with self-administered swab for NAAT. The **most accurate test** for *Trichomonas* is NAAT.

Treatment is ceftriaxone and azithromycin as a single dose. Doxycycline is equal in efficacy to azithromycin but harder to use. You should routinely test for cure of gonorrhea and chlamydia.

Epididymitis

Epididymitis presents with scrotal pain superior and lateral to the testicle. Look for pain developing "over a few days" and "very severe point tenderness" of the testicle. Younger men (<35) are generally treated for gonorrhea and chlamydia with ceftriaxone and doxycycline. Older men are treated for the gram-negative rods that would cause a urinary tract infection, such as *E.coli*, with TMP/SMX or a quinolone.

	Epididymitis	**Torsion**	**Varicocele**
Presentation	Point tenderness	Elevated testicle in transverse (horizontal) position	• "Bag of worms" feeling on palpation • Worse on standing
Diagnosis	Clinical	Doppler U/S	Abdominal CT
Treatment	Antibiotics	Emergency surgery	• None if few symptoms • Surgical ligation if bothersome or infertility develops

Pelvic Inflammatory Disease

Pelvic inflammatory disease (PID) presents with:

- Lower abdominal tenderness and pain
- Fever
- Cervical motion tenderness
- Leukocytosis

If all the symptoms are present, the most appropriate first step is to exclude pregnancy.

Diagnostic testing includes:

- Cervical swab (self-administered) for culture, DNA probe, or NAAT to confirm the etiology so that precise treatment decisions can be made (i.e., for partner if an STD or for precise treatment choice if organism is resistant)
- Laparoscopy (**most accurate test**) is needed only if the diagnosis is unclear, symptoms persist, or there is recurrence for unclear reasons.

Treatment is a combination of medications for gonorrhea and chlamydia.

- **Inpatient**: cefoxitin or cefotetan + doxycycline (if penicillin-allergic, use clindamycin, gentamicin, or doxycycline)
- **Outpatient**: ceftriaxone + doxycycline (possibly + metronidazole) (if penicillin-allergic, use levofloxacin or metronidazole)

> Cervical testing is not the "most accurate test" for PID.

Ulcerative Genital Disease

"What Is the Most Likely Diagnosis?"

▶ **TIP**

It is often impossible to determine the diagnosis of genital ulcers by physical examination characteristics alone, but if this topic appears on the USMLE exam, the question will provide sufficient clues.

All ulcerative genital disease can have inguinal adenopathy.

> If dark-field is positive for spirochetes, no further testing for syphilis is necessary.

Presentation of STDs	
History and physical findings	**Most likely diagnosis**
Painless ulcer, painless nodes	Syphilis
Painful ulcer	Chancroid (*Haemophilus ducreyi*)
Lymph nodes tender and suppurating	Lymphogranuloma venereum
Vesicles prior to ulcer and painful	*Herpes simplex*

Diagnostic Testing and Treatment of STDs		
Diagnosis	**Diagnostic Test**	**Treatment**
Syphilis	Dark-field microscopy VDRL or RPR (75% sensitive in primary syphilis) FTA or MHA-TP (confirmatory)	Single dose of intramuscular benzathine penicillin Doxycycline if penicillin allergic
Chancroid (*Haemophilus ducreyi*)	Stain and culture on specialized media	Azithromycin (single dose)
Lymphogranuloma venereum	Complement fixation titers in blood Nucleic acid amplification testing on swab	Doxycycline
Herpes simplex	PCR is the most accurate test; if PCR is not among the choices, answer viral culture	Acyclovir, valacyclovir, famciclovir Foscarnet for acyclovir-resistant herpes

A woman comes to clinic with multiple painful genital vesicles. What is the next step in management?

a. Valacyclovir orally
b. Acyclovir topically
c. Tzanck prep
d. Viral culture
e. Serology
f. PCR

> Tzanck prep is not sensitive or specific enough to help.

> Herpes
> - PCR most accurate
> - Viral culture allows sensitivity testing

Answer: **A.** If the presentation is clear for herpes with multiple vesicles of the mouth or genitals, diagnostic testing is not necessary. Acyclovir, famciclovir, and valacyclovir are all equal in efficacy, so any one of them could be correct. Topical acyclovir is worthless. PCR is the most accurate test, but not necessary if the vesicles are obvious. Serology is always worthless, since it cannot distinguish an acute genital infection from an oral herpes infection in the past.

Syphilis

Primary syphilis:

- Painless genital ulcer with heaped-up indurated edges (it becomes painful if it becomes secondarily infected with bacteria)
- Painless adenopathy

Secondary syphilis:

- Rash (palms and soles)
- Alopecia areata
- Mucous patches
- Condylomata lata

Tertiary syphilis:

- Neurosyphilis
    - **Meningovascular** (stroke from vasculitis)
    - **Tabes dorsalis** (loss of position and vibratory sense, incontinence, cranial nerve)
    - **General paresis** (memory and personality changes)
    - **Argyll Robertson pupil** (reacts to accommodation, but not light)
- Aortitis (aortic regurgitation, aortic aneurysm)
- Gummas (skin and bone lesions)

> **Chancres heal spontaneously** even without treatment. Penicillin prevents later stages.

Sensitivity of Diagnostic Tests by Stage			
Test	**Primary**	**Secondary**	**Tertiary**
VDRL or RPR	75%–85%	99%	95%
FTA-ABS	95%	100%	98%

Which of the following is the most sensitive test of CSF for neurosyphilis?

a. VDRL
b. RPR
c. FTA
d. Stain
e. Dark field
f. Culture

Answer: **C.** FTA is nearly 100% sensitive in CSF. A negative fluorescent treponemal antibody (FTA) test of the CSF effectively excludes neurosyphilis. VDRL and RPR are positive only in 50% of patients, and if they are negative, it means nothing because they do not rule out neurosyphilis. A negative FTA means "not neurosyphilis." Everyone NOT reading this book will be wrong on this question on USMLE. VDRL and PCR are specific tests of CSF. If these are positive, the patient is positive for neurosyphilis.

> MHA-TP = FTA for syphilis diagnostics

> **False positive VDRL/RPR in blood**
> - Infection, older age, injection drug use and AIDS, malaria, antiphospholipid syndrome, and endocarditis

Treatment is as follows:

- **Primary and secondary syphilis**: single intramuscular injection of penicillin; if penicillin-allergic, use oral doxycycline
  - Late secondary syphilis is most often asymptomatic, with just positive serology. It is the stage is after the chancre and rash of primary and secondary syphilis have resolved.
  - Treat with penicillin 1×/ week for 3 weeks
- **Tertiary syphilis**: IV penicillin; if penicillin-allergic, desensitize to penicillin

> Titers of VDRL or RPR are reliable at >1:8.
> - Lower titers are more often falsely positive.
> - High titers (>1:32) are rarely falsely positive.

> **Jarisch-Herxheimer reaction**
> - Fever and worse symptoms after treatment
> - Give aspirin and antipyretics; it will pass.

▶ **TIP**

Desensitization is the answer for neurosyphilis and pregnant women.

Genital Warts (Condylomata Acuminata)

Condylomata acuminata from papillomavirus is diagnosed simply based on the visual appearance. Wrong answers include biopsy, serology, stain, smear, and culture. Remove them by physical means such as cryotherapy with liquid nitrogen, surgery for large ones, laser, or "melting" them with podophyllin or trichloroacetic acid. Imiquimod is a locally applied immunostimulant that leads to the sloughing off of the lesion. Imiquimod also works for actinic keratosis and basal cell cancer. Imiquimod does not burn or damage the skin.

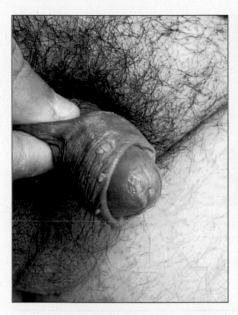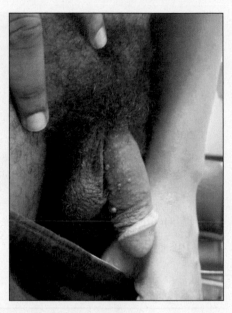

Figure 5.5 Condylomata Acuminata (Genital Warts).
Source, left: Farshad Bagheri, MD. Source, right: Pramod Theetha Kariyanna, MD

Pediculosis (Crabs)

- Found on hair-bearing areas (axilla, pubis)
- Causes itching
- Visible on the surface
- Treat with permethrin or malathion

Scabies

- Found in web spaces between fingers and toes or at elbows or genitalia
- Found around the nipples or near the genitals
- Burrows visible (they dig) but smaller than pediculosis
- Scrape and magnify
- Treat with permethrin or malathion
- Widespread disease is "crusted" or hyperkeratotic and responds to ivermectin; severe disease needs repeat dosing

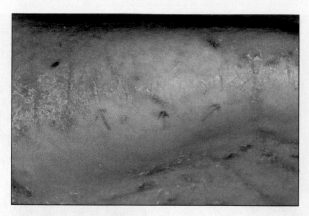

Figure 5.6 Scabies burrow under the skin and must be scraped out to establish a diagnosis. *Source: Conrad Fischer, MD*

Urinary Tract Infection

Urinary tract infection (UTI) refers to any bacterial infection of the urinary tract. The most common cause of UTI is *E. coli*, but other causes include:

- Anatomical defect: stones, strictures, tumor, or prostate hypertrophy (men who get frequent UTI are found to have many more anatomic defects than women)
- Obstruction in urinary system, e.g., neurogenic bladder
- Foreign body in urinary system, e.g. Foley catheter
- Diabetes

The most common symptom for all UTIs is dysuria (frequency, urgency, burning), but fever is possible.

> *Frequency* means multiple episodes of micturition. *Polyuria* is an increase in the volume of urine.

Testing is urinalysis with >10 WBCs (**best initial test**) and urine culture (**most accurate test**).

Cystitis

Cystitis (lower UTI, i.e., inflammation of the bladder) presents with:

- Dysuria
- Suprapubic pain/discomfort
- Mild or absent fever

Urine culture should be done only if there are WBCs.

> Pentosan relieves bladder pain.

Treat with:

- Nitrofurantoin or fosfomycin
- TMP/SMX if local resistance is low
- Ciprofloxacin (not used routinely to avoid resistance)
- Cefixime
- Pentosan to relieve bladder pain (also used for interstitial cystitis)

> All beta-lactam antibiotics are considered safe in pregnancy.

A 36-year-old generally healthy woman presents with urinary frequency and burning. Urinalysis shows >50 WBC per high-power field. What is the most appropriate next step in management?

a. Nitrofurantoin for 3 days
b. TMP/SMX for 7 days
c. Urine culture
d. U/S of urinary system
e. CT scan of urinary system

Answer: **A.** When symptoms of cystitis are clear and there are WBCs in the urine, there is no need for urine culture or imaging; those are done only when there is frequent cystitis or failure to respond to treatment. For uncomplicated cystitis, 3 days is sufficient. If there is an anatomic abnormality, 7 days is standard.

> Phenazopyridine is a urinary tract anesthetic taken orally. It brings instant pain relief from UTI.

Pyelonephritis

Pyelonephritis (upper UTI, i.e., inflammation of the kidney) presents with:

- Dysuria
- Flank or costovertebral angle tenderness
- High fever
- Occasional abdominal pain from inflamed kidney

> Ceftriaxone is first for pyelonephritis.

Urinalysis shows increased WBCs. Imaging studies (CT or sonogram) are done to determine if there is an anatomic abnormality causing the infection.

Quinolone antibiotics are the **best initial treatment**. Change antibiotics when culture results are known.

- Ceftriaxone (**first-line**) or ertapenem
- Ampicillin and gentamicin
- Ciprofloxacin (oral for outpatient)

Perinephric Abscess

One complication of UTI is perinephric abscess, an anatomic collection of infected material. When both the choice of drug and the dosage for UTI are correct, failure of an infection to resolve is often due to an anatomic problem.

> Any of the drugs for gram-negative bacilli would be effective for pyelonephritis.

Look for pyelonephritis associated with fever that does not resolve with 5–7 days of treatment. Perform an imaging study such as a sonogram or CT scan.

Drainage of the fluid collection is mandatory. Culture of the infected fluid is essential to guide treatment.

Acute Prostatitis

Acute prostatitis (i.e., inflammation of the prostate gland) presents with:

- Dysuria
- Perineal pain
- Tender prostate on examination

Testing is urine culture; prostate massage should be done to improve the diagnostic yield of the culture.

Treatment is as follows:

- **Acute prostatitis**: quinolone antibiotics (**best initial treatment**); change antibiotics when culture results are known
  - Ceftriaxone (first-line) or ertapenem
  - Ampicillin and gentamicin
  - Ciprofloxacin (oral for outpatient)
- **Chronic prostatitis**: ciprofloxacin or TMP/SMX for 6–8 weeks

In a 60-year-old man, what is the single biggest difference between the treatment of prostatitis and cystitis?

a. Causative organism
b. Duration of treatment
c. Use of urinalysis
d. Efficacy of TMP/SMX
e. Efficacy of IV medications

Answer: **B.** Duration of treatment is the key difference. Prostatitis (seen in elderly men) needs 2–6 weeks of treatment based on the chronicity of the infection in men, while cystitis in men is treated for 7 days. Both conditions will show WBCs in urinalysis. IV antibiotics are not needed in either condition.

Endocarditis

Endocarditis is an infection of the heart valve, leading to fever and a murmur. The risk of endocarditis is directly proportional to the degree of damage on the valves.

On normal heart valves it is very rare for endocarditis to develop; however, it is possible if there is bacteremia with highly pathogenic organisms. For instance:

- Prosthetic valves (**highest risk**)
- Injection drug use (users damage their valves by injecting impurities)
- *Staphylococcus aureus*
- Regurgitant and stenotic lesions

Dental procedures confer an increased (yet small) risk of endocarditis. Even surgery of the mouth or respiratory tract confers no risk unless there is a severe valvular disorder. Less invasive procedures such as endoscopy confer no increased risk, even with a biopsy.

Diagnosis of endocarditis is made with echocardiogram showing vegetations, plus positive blood cultures. Look for fever and a new murmur (or change in a murmur).

Diagnostic tests include:

- Blood culture (95–99% sensitive) (**best initial test**); if negative, establish diagnosis with the following:
  - Oscillating vegetation on echocardiogram
  - Three minor criteria: fever >38 C (>100.4 F) high risk, i.e., prosthetic valve; and signs of embolic phenomena
- Transthoracic echocardiogram (60% sensitive but 95–100% specific)
- Transesophageal echocardiogram (95% sensitive and specific)
- EKG may show AV block if there is dissection of the conduction system (<5–10% sensitive).

Complications of endocarditis include:

- Splinter hemorrhage
- Janeway lesions (flat and painless)
- Osler nodes (raised and painful)
- Roth spots in the eyes
- Brain (mycotic aneurysm)
- Kidney (hematuria, glomerulonephritis)
- Conjunctival petechiae
- Splenomegaly
- Septic emboli to the lungs

The **best initial empiric treatment** is vancomycin. When culture results are available, treat as indicated in the table. Right-sided endocarditis can be treated for only 2 weeks.

> Endocarditis = Fever + Murmur

Treatment of Culture-Positive Endocarditis	
Organism	**Treatment**
Viridans streptococci	Ceftriaxone for 4 weeks
Staphylococcus aureus (sensitive)	Oxacillin, nafcillin, or cefazolin for 6 weeks
Fungal	Amphotericin and valve replacement
Staphylococcus epidermidis or resistant *Staphylococcus*	Vancomycin or daptomycin for 6 weeks
Enterococci	Ampicillin and gentamicin
For resistant organisms	Add an aminoglycoside and extend duration of treatment

Two features are needed to establish the need for prophylaxis in endocarditis, i.e., both features are required.

- **Significant cardiac defect**
  - Prosthetic valve (add rifampin for prosthetic valve endocarditis with *Staph*)
  - Previous endocarditis
  - Cardiac transplant recipient with valvulopathy
  - Unrepaired cyanotic heart disease
- **Risk of bacteremia**
  - Dental work with blood
  - Respiratory tract surgery that produces bacteremia
  - Prior to bacteremia-causing procedures, give patients amoxicillin (if penicillin-allergic, use clindamycin, azithromycin, or clarithromycin)

Endoscopic and genitourinary procedures do not need prophylaxis.

Surgical treatment is required under certain circumstances:

- Acute valve rupture and CHF (**strongest indications for surgery**)
- Prosthetic valves
- Fungal endocarditis
- Abscess
- AV block
- Recurrent emboli while on antibiotics

> Colon pathology is associated with both *Streptococcus bovis* and *Clostridium septicum*.

> Use the acronym **HACEK** to remember organisms that are difficult to culture but that cause endocarditis.
> - *Haemophilus aphrophilus*
> - *Haemophilus parainfluenzae*
> - *Actinobacillus*
> - *Cardiobacterium*
> - *Eikenella*
> - *Kingella*
>
> Treatment for these is ceftriaxone.

A man comes to the ED with fever and a murmur. Blood cultures grow *Clostridium septicum*. Transthoracic echocardiography shows a vegetation. What is the most appropriate next step in management?

a. Colonoscopy
b. Transesophageal echocardiogram
c. CT of the abdomen
d. Repeat blood cultures
e. Surgical valve replacement

Answer: **A.** *Clostridium septicum* is associated with colonic pathology ranging from diverticula to polyps to colon cancer. If *Streptococcus bovis* grows, perform colonoscopy. CT scan will not show diverticula. There is no point in repeating the blood culture if it is already positive. Valve replacement is premature. *C. septicum* has an even greater association with colon pathology than *S. bovis*.

Lyme Disease

Lyme disease is an arthropod-borne disease from the spirochete *Borrelia burgdorferi*. It is transmitted by the deer tick (*Ixodes scapularis*).

Symptoms most often include a fever and rash. Untreated infection can recur as joint pain, cardiac disease, or neurological disease.

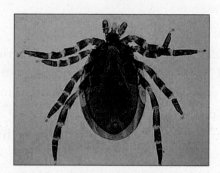

Figure 5.7 *Ixodes scapularis* Tick (Deer Tick).
Source: Wikicommons

Only 20% of patients recall the bite of the tick. Many cases will describe the patient as having recently been hiking or camping.

The tick must be attached for at least 24 hours in order to transmit the organism. The *Ixodes* tick is not present everywhere in the United States. Lyme typically occurs only in northeast states such as Connecticut (where the town of Lyme gave the disease its name), Massachusetts, New York, and New Jersey.

Symptoms include:

- Rash (or erythema migrans) (**most common manifestation**), which is a round red lesion with a pale area in the center (resembling a "target" or "bull's-eye")
- Fever (common)
- Joint pain (**most common long-term manifestation**) affects "a few joints" (oligoarthritis). Joint fluid will have ~25,000 WBCs/µL (although this does not distinguish it from other causes of joint inflammation or infection).
- Neurological manifestations (uncommon) include CNS or PNS symptoms, e.g., meningitis, encephalitis, or cranial nerve palsy.
- Cardiac manifestations (uncommon) may include damage to any part of the myocardium or pericardium, e.g., myocarditis or ventricular arrhythmia.

> The knee is the most commonly affected joint in Lyme disease.

> - **Most common cardiac manifestation** in Lyme: transient AV block
> - **Most common neurologic manifestation** of Lyme: seventh cranial nerve palsy (Bell palsy)

Diagnostic testing is with IgM, IgG, ELISA, Western blot, and PCR.

- If there is a **lesion typical of Lyme**: no confirmatory testing with serology is needed to start treatment

- If there are **other manifestations such as joint, neurologic, and cardiac**: testing with serology (Western blot) is required (since most cases of seventh cranial nerve palsy, arthralgia, and AV block are *not* caused by Lyme)

Treatment is as follows:

- Asymptomatic tick bite: no prophylactic treatment
  - However, if *Ixodes scapularis* **is identified as the tick causing the bite; tick is attached >24–48 hrs; tick is engorged, nymph-stage; or area is endemic**: doxycycline (single dose) is indicated within 72 hours of tick bite
- Rash: doxycycline or amoxicillin or cefuroxime
- Joint pain, seventh cranial nerve palsy: doxycycline or amoxicillin/cefuroxime
- Cardiac and neurologic manifestations other than seventh cranial nerve palsy: IV ceftriaxone

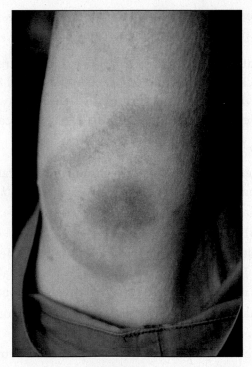

Figure 5.8 Target-Shaped Rash of Lyme Disease or Erythema Migrans.
Source: Nishith Patel, MD

HIV/AIDS

HIV is a retrovirus infecting the CD4 (T-helper) cell. If untreated, CD4 cells will drop from 600–1,000 per µL (normal level) at a rate of 50–100 per year.

Risk of Transmission of HIV Without Prophylactic Treatment	
Mode of transmission	**Percentage of risk with each event**
Vaginal transmission	1:3,000–1:10,000 for insertive intercourse 1:1,000 for receptive intercourse
Oral sex	1:1,000 for receptive fellatio with ejaculation Unclear for insertive fellatio or cunnilingus
Needle stick injury	1:300
Anal sex	1:100 for receptive anal intercourse
Mother to child	25%–30% perinatal transmission without medication

It takes 5–10 years of CD4 cell depletion before clinical manifestations occur; the depletion leads to opportunistic infections, which then lead to illness.

- When **CD4 count <50/µL**, infections occur with profound immunosuppression. PCP occurs when CD4 count <200/µL.
- When **CD4 count >200/µL**, few infections occur. However, the following infections are seen more frequently:
  - Varicella zoster (shingles)
  - Herpes simplex
  - Tuberculosis
  - Oral and vaginal candidiasis
  - Bacterial pneumonia

Conversely, HIV can cause a falsely negative hepatitis C test.

Diagnostic testing is as follows:

- HIV-1/2, p24 test (**best initial test**)
- Viral load testing (PCR-RNA level) to measure response to therapy (decreasing levels are good), detect treatment failure (rising levels are bad), and diagnose HIV in babies
- PCR for infected infants (ELISA testing is unreliable in infants because maternal HIV antibodies may be present for up to 6 months after delivery)
- Viral resistance testing (genotyping)
  - Reduces chance of resistance to ART (should be done before initiating ART)
  - Helps if there is evidence of treatment failure (treatment can then be tailored to select 3 drugs from different classes to which the patient's virus is susceptible)

The life expectancy for a person with HIV whose viral load is undetectable by PCR-RNA is equal to that of an HIV-negative person.

Bictegravir
- 99% go undetectable
- Use with 2 nucleosides

Kissing does not transmit HIV.

HIV testing combines HIV 1/2 with P24.

Treatment

The goal of treatment is to drive down the viral load. Undetectable levels (<20/ μL) indicate that the CD4 will rise. When viral load is undetectable and the CD4 rises, opportunistic infections don't occur.

Treating everyone, no matter how high the CD4 count, is encouraged.

First-Line Agents

- **Antiretroviral therapy (ART)** for all patients who are HIV-positive and have detectable levels of the virus of PCR-RNA viral load testing (even if CD4 is normal)
- Two nucleoside reverse-transcriptase inhibitors (NRTIs) and an integrase inhibitor
  - NRTIs: preferred combinations are tenofovir alafenamide + emtricitabine or abacavir + lamivudine
    ○ Tenofovir has 2 formulations: disoproxil version (associated with RTA and bone demineralization) and alafenamide version (absorbed into CD4 cell and has lower plasma level, thus fewer side effects)
    ○ Abacavir use requires prior testing for HLA B5701 mutation; those who have it are at risk for life-threatening skin reactions such as Stevens-Johnson
  - Integrase inhibitor: bictegravir, dolutegravir, raltegravir, or elvitegravir
    ○ Superior to protease inhibitors and the nonnucleoside efavirenz. Efavirenz does not interfere with TB medications; active TB is the only circumstance in which efavirenz is truly preferred.
    ○ Greater long-term viral suppression and fewer side effects
    ○ Use elvitegravir in combination with cobicistat, which increases its blood level (cobicistat inhibits metabolism of darunavir and elvitegravir, boosting levels). Cobicistat can increase the serum creatinine without damaging GFR.
- If treatment drives the HIV viral load to an undetectable level, it cannot be transmitted to others.

> Treat with ART as soon as possible after an HIV diagnosis. The only reason to delay is if there is Cryptococcus.

Postexposure Prophylaxis (PEP)

All significant needle-stick injuries and sexual exposures are given 4 weeks of combination therapy with an integrase inhibitor and 2 nucleosides.

- Exposure to urine or stool is not an indication for PEP unless it contains blood.
- Unknown HIV status in a needle-stick injury is not an indication for PEP.
- Bites from an HIV-positive person are an indication for PEP.

Prevention of Perinatal Transmission

- If HIV-positive patient is already on ART that is effective at the time of pregnancy, continue the same regimen to prevent perinatal transmission.

- With the pregnant patient who is HIV-positive, do not wait for the genotype; treat immediately.

- Protease inhibitors are safe during pregnancy. Even if the pregnant woman has a high CD4 ($\geq$500), treatment with combination ARTs should still be given to prevent perinatal transmission.

- Baby should be given zidovudine for 6 weeks afterward to help prevent transmission.

- Intrapartum IV with zidovudine is routinely administered in every pregnant HIV-positive patient if the viral load is detectable. HIV-positive women should be treated with ART during the entire pregnancy. Do not wait for the second trimester, and always use at least 3 drugs.

- Begin ART even in first trimester, no matter how low the viral load or how high the CD4 count. Viral load and CD4 cell count have no bearing on the use of ARTs for HIV in pregnancy.

- If viral load is high at time of delivery ($>$1,000/μL), do a cesarean delivery. Make sure viral load is controlled by the time of parturition.

> Intrapartum zidovudine is given only if the viral load is detectable at the time of delivery.

Pre-Exposure Prophylaxis (PrEP)

Pre-exposure prophylaxis (PrEP) is for people uninfected with HIV who want to protect themselves from high-risk practices with potentially HIV-infected contacts.

- Start emtricitabine-tenofovir before the exposure to HIV and continue for a month after the last exposure (continue long-term if the HIV-risk behavior is expected to continue).

- PrEP stops a significant amount of transmission.

- On the Step 2 exam, you might be asked about a person who is HIV negative but who engages in unprotected sex with someone who is potentially HIV-positive. Prescribe emtricitabine-tenofovir to prevent the HIV.

- If the PreP is stopped (or used intermittently) in those who are surface antigen-positive, that can lead to the reactivation of hepatitis B. Tenofovir treats and suppresses hepatitis B.

▶**TIP**

USMLE Step 2 CK does not test dosing.

Ritonavir in a small dose is used to "boost" darunavir or atazanavir levels.

Antiretroviral First-line Medications by Class			
Nucleoside reverse transcriptase inhibitors (NRTIs)	**Integrase inhibitors**	**Non-nucleoside RTIs**	**Protease inhibitors**
• Emtricitabine • Tenofovir • Zidovudine • Lamivudine • Abacavir	• Elvitegravir • Raltegravir • Dolutegravir • Bictegravir	• Efavirenz • Etravirine • Nevirapine • Rilpivirine	• Darunavir • Atazanavir • Ritonavir

Pregnant? Do not wait for genotype to start ART.

If the mother's viral load is undetectable at the time of delivery, intrapartum zidovudine is not needed. Fully controlled HIV (viral load undetectable) leads to <1% transmission.

Side Effects of HIV Medications	
Drug	**Adverse effect**
Zidovudine	Anemia
Stavudine and didanosine	Peripheral neuropathy and pancreatitis
Abacavir (HLA B5701)	Hypersensitivity, Stevens-Johnson reaction
Protease inhibitors	Hyperlipidemia, hyperglycemia
Indinavir	Nephrolithiasis
Tenofovir disoproxil	Renal insufficiency, bone demineralization

Fungal Diseases

Dimorphic fungi are those that exist as a spore at cold temperatures near 20 C (68 F) but transform into a yeast in the warm (37 C; 98.6 F) and moist environment of the body. Examples of diseases caused by dimorphic fungi are coccidioidomycosis, histoplasmosis, cryptococcosis, and blastomycosis. All of these enter the body primarily as inhaled spores.

Most infected patients are asymptomatic, but when they do occur, symptoms include cough, headache, fever, arthralgia, and myalgia, along with a self-limited pneumonia. In symptomatic patients, a chest x-ray is often abnormal. In a small number of cases (particularly immunocompromised or HIV-positive patients), there is dissemination of the infection to the brain, skin, and bones.

Culture on fungal media is very sensitive and specific, though for cryptococcosis and histoplasmosis, antigen detection methods can be faster. Most cases need no treatment and resolve spontaneously. Mild to moderate disease is treated with antifungal medication such as fluconazole. The most severe disease, such as meningitis, is treated with amphotericin.

Coccidioidomycosis

This spore is more common in hot, dry areas such as the desert; it is sometimes called "valley fever."

- Clues to diagnosis: joint pain ("desert rheumatism") is common; erythema nodosum
- **Most accurate test**: sputum culture, serology
- Treatment:
  - Moderate disease: fluconazole or itraconazole
  - Severe disease: amphotericin
  - Echinocandins such as caspofungin are not effective.

Histoplasmosis

- *Histoplasma* fungus found in moist soil containing bird and bat feces (e.g., caves, river valleys)
- Disease can resemble tuberculosis with lung cavities
- Involves bone marrow (pancytopenia) as well as the spleen and lymph nodes
- **Most accurate test**: culture of sputum, blood, or affected organs
- Urine and serum antigen highly specific
- Treatment: severe illness gets amphotericin followed by oral itraconazole (superior to fluconazole)

> Anything TB can do, histoplasmosis can do.

Blastomycosis

- *Blastomyces* fungus found in soil and rotten wood near water
- Besides the lung, can involve bone, skin, and prostate
- Culture is definitive; no serum or urine antigen testing
- Treatment: itraconazole; rarely, severe cases need amphotericin

▶ TIP

A blastomycosis question on Step 2 CK will describe a "broad, budding yeast" found on smear.

Mucormycosis (Zygomycosis)

This mold occurs exclusively in immunocompromised patients, especially diabetics in DKA. Deferoxamine increases the risk of mucormycosis by mobilizing iron. Mucormycosis is hard to grow in culture. It can be seen on biopsy.

The organism rapidly dissects the nasal canals and eyes on through to the brain. Mortality is very high. Mucormycosis is a **surgical emergency**: You must quickly resect necrotic areas. It is one of the few indications to **use amphotericin as the best initial therapy**. Should the patient survive, follow up therapy with posaconazole or isavuconazole.

Invasive Aspergillosis

Although allergic bronchopulmonary aspergillosis can occur in a relatively normal host, invasive disease occurs exclusively in severely immunocompromised patients, most frequently patients with neutropenia and leukemia. Invasive aspergillosis progresses rapidly, with lung infiltrates visible on x-ray and CT.

There are 3 noninvasive tests for invasive aspergillosis:

- Serum galactomannan assay
- β-D-glucan level
- PCR

If any 2 of these are positive, there is >95% specificity for the disease. Because sputum testing lacks sensitivity, however, diagnosis often needs a lung biopsy. The best initial treatment is voriconazole, isavuconazole, or caspofungin. Amphotericin is inferior to these medications and is the most common wrong answer.

Candida auris

- Bloodstream fungal infection
- Immunocompromised host
- Isolated from blood cultures
- Resistant to fluconazole and voriconazole
- Sensitive to echinocandins (e.g., caspofungin, micafungin)

> *Candida krusei* and *C. glabrata* are routinely resistant to fluconazole. Treat them with an echinocandin.

Tropical Diseases

Cholera

Patients with cholera present with massive watery, **nonbloody** diarrhea ("rice-water" diarrhea), along with vomiting, muscle cramps, sunken eyes, and loose skin.

Without treatment, hypokalemia and acidosis result in 50% mortality. Treatment is massive hydration, with the patient continuing to eat food. Although hydration solves most cases, doxycycline treats severe infection.

Vaccination is appropriate for travel to cholera-affected areas but not for most tourists.

Malaria

Malaria is a mosquito-borne disease presenting with fever, headache, fatigue, and hemolysis. Diagnose with a **thick** smear for detection, **thin** smear for speciation.

Treatment for mild to moderate malaria is as follows:

- Infection with *Plasmodium falciparum*: mefloquine or atovaquone/proguanil
- Non-*falciparum* infection: chloroquine or (*P. vivax* and *P. ovale* only) primaquine

Manifestations of severe malaria include:

- Parasitemia >5%
- CNS abnormalities (confusion, seizure, coma)
- Hypotension/shock or pulmonary edema
- Renal injury, acidosis, or hypoglycemia

Treatment for severe malaria is artemisinins (artemether, artesunate).

> Test for G6PD before using primaquine!

> Severe malaria gets an artemisinin.

Malaria prophylaxis:

- Mefloquine or atovaquone/proguanil
- Avoid mefloquine with history of neuropsychiatric illness.
- Tafenoquine is prophylaxis against multiresistant malaria.

Mosquito-Transmitted Viral Syndromes

While many mosquito-transmitted viral syndromes exist, only a few will be tested on the Step 2 CK exam. The likelihood of testing is based on the likelihood that the syndrome will be brought to the United States by travelers, tourists, or immigrants.

Zika, dengue, and chikungunya are all transmitted by *Aedes* mosquitoes. Ebola is not transmitted by a mosquito. All cause fever, headache, and malaise. All are diagnosed by serology such as ELISA or PCR. None has a specific antiviral therapy or an effective vaccine.

What are the differences between these viruses to answer the single question, "What is the most likely diagnosis?"

Zika

- Most dangerous viral syndrome in pregnancy because it causes microcephaly
- Associated with Guillain-Barré

Chikungunya

- Caused by a single-stranded RNA of African origin
- Symptoms include intense joint pain that may persist for months, periarticular edema, and rash (<50% of cases)

Dengue

- Symptoms include bone pain (*not* joint pain)—where the second episode is worse—plus severe thrombocytopenia that can lead to petechiae and GI bleeding (with possible fatal hemorrhage and shock)
- Look for low WBC count and high transaminases
- Fluids with blood and platelet transfusion may be needed

> There is a vaccine against dengue and Ebola.

Ebola

- Not airborne or transmitted by mosquito
- Transmissible only by direct contact with body fluids from a person in whom symptoms are present
- Symptoms include nonspecific viral symptoms followed by severe GI distress with high-volume diarrhea
- Look for low WBC count, high transaminases, and thrombocytopenia
- Encephalitis often develops before patients succumb to hypovolemic shock and death
- Even with rehydration, mortality is 70%

Familial Mediterranean Fever (FMF)

- Symptoms include recurrent episodes of abdominal pain, tenderness, and fever
- Look for elevated ESR, CRP, WBC, and fibrinogen
- Abdominal ultrasound, CT scan, stool studies, and colonoscopy are normal
- Treatment is colchicine
- Amyloidosis is a long-term complication

> The MEFV gene supports diagnosis of FMF.

Animal-Borne Diseases

Anthrax

Bacillus anthracis is a gram-positive, spore-forming bacterium that occurs in sheep, cattle, horses, and goats. The 3 forms known to occur in the United States are as follows:

- **Cutaneous anthrax** is characterized by a painless black eschar at site of contact. The disease is often self-limited.
- **Gastrointestinal anthrax** occurs as an ulcerative lesion that produces abdominal pain, vomiting, and diarrhea; the lesion may perforate.
- **Inhalation anthrax** can be rapidly fatal. Look for a widened mediastinum with hemorrhagic lymphadenitis and pleural effusion.

Diagnose with culture showing boxcar-shaped, encapsulated rods. Treat with quinolone or doxycycline.

Babesiosis

Babesia is a protozoan, originally from cattle and transmitted by ticks. It infects red blood cells, causing hemolysis. Babesiosis is life-threatening in asplenic patients.

Blood smear showing red blood cell inclusions is the **best initial test**. PCR is the **most accurate test**.

Treatment is azithromycin plus atovaquone.

Bartonellosis

Cat-scratch disease:

- Caused by *Bartonella henselae*, producing enlarged and tender regional lymph nodes.
- Diagnosis: clinical, supported by serology
- Treatment:
  - Usually none needed, but azithromycin speeds resolution
  - Doxycycline or azithromycin + rifampin for hepatosplenic involvement or neuroretinitis

Endocarditis:

- Caused by *B. quintana*
- Look for a patient who is homeless and/or has flea bites.
- Diagnosis: serology/PCR
- Treatment: ceftriaxone, doxycycline, gentamicin until *Bartonella* is confirmed; then doxycycline and gentamicin

Brucellosis

Infection with *Brucella* may present as fever for weeks/months, hepatosplenomegaly, endocarditis, osteomyelitis, meningitis, or chronic joint pain. Look for:

- Patient from outside the United States
- Exposure to unpasteurized milk or uninspected meat
- "Returning war veteran" in medical history

Diagnose with culture of blood, CSF, urine, marrow. Treatment is doxycycline and gentamicin. Add rifampin for bone and heart infection.

> *Brucella* needs long periods to grow—weeks to months.

Echinococcosis

- Animal source: dogs and sheep shedding *Echinococcus* eggs
- Eggs ingested by human
- Spreads to liver, lung, and brain, forming hydatid cysts
- Diagnosis: detect cysts with sonogram, CT, or MRI; confirm with ELISA
- Treatment:
  - Do not aspirate cysts—can spread the infection
  - Oral albendazole, injection of alcohol into the cysts

Ehrlichiosis (Monocytic) and Anaplasmosis (Granulocytic)

Ehrlichia and *Anaplasma* are obligate intracellular parasites similar to *Rickettsia*. *Anaplasma* is transmitted from the bite of the *Ixodes scapularis* tick, just like Lyme and Babesia. *Ehrlichia* is transmitted by the lone star tick, which also transmits *Rickettsia*.

Infection presents with fever, headache, malaise, and chills; rash is uncommon. Also look for a low WBC, low platelets, and high transaminases (AST, ALT). The **most accurate test** is serology. The blood smear will show morulae in WBCs. Treat both *Ehrlichia* and *Anaplasma* with doxycycline.

> *Ehrlichia* and *Anaplasma* are transmitted by different ticks in different parts of the country, but they are clinically indistinguishable and receive the same treatment.

Leptospirosis

Infection with *Leptospira* most often occurs by ingestion of food contaminated with the urine of an infected animal, usually a rodent. The kidneys (oliguria) and liver are affected, and possibly the CNS as well. Look for conjunctival suffusion, muscle pain, and CK elevation.

Diagnose with blood titers. Treat with amoxicillin or doxycycline.

> Leptospirosis is caused by a spirochete and gives the Jarisch-Herxheimer reaction.

Leishmaniasis

- Caused by *Leishmania* protozoan, spread by sandflies
- Two forms: skin/mucosal and visceral (liver and spleen involvement with fever)
- Diagnosis: direct visualization on aspirates of liver, spleen, or marrow or in white blood cells; confirm with PCR and culture
- Treatment:
  - Liposomal amphotericin, miltefosine, or antimonials (stibogluconate)
  - Miltefosine for cutaneous, mucosal, and visceral leishmaniasis

Plague

Infection with *Yersinia pestis* presents with sudden-onset high fever, intense headache, and severe myalgia. The bubonic form also has massively enlarged lymph nodes (buboes). The pneumonic (lung) form can be fatal in 24 hours. Look for rodent exposure and the American Southwest region in the patient history.

- **Best initial test**: smear of node aspirate showing gram-negative rods
- **Most accurate test**: culture
- Treatment: streptomycin, gentamicin, or doxycycline

Tularemia

- Routes of infection with *Francisella tularensis* include contact with infected rabbits/muskrats/prairie dogs and bites from ticks or flies.
- Symptoms include skin ulcers, glandular enlargement, and/or conjunctivitis from a tick bite.
- Inhalation of spores (bioterrorism) causes rapidly fatal pneumonia.
- Culture gives dangerous spores; diagnose with serology.
- Treatment is streptomycin, gentamicin, or doxycycline.

Allergy and Immunology 7

Anaphylaxis

Anaphylaxis is defined as the worst form of allergic condition or acute event. It is synonymous with the term *immediate hypersensitivity*.

Anaphylaxis is defined by the *severity*, not the cause, of the reaction.

- Patient must already have been sensitized to the antigen.
- IgE binds to mast cells, leading to the release of their granules (e.g., histamine, prostaglandins, and leukotrienes), which results in the abnormalities that essentially define anaphylaxis.
- Anaphylactoid reactions are non-IgE related, are clinically identical and treated the same way, and do not need preceding sensitization to the antigen.
  - Respiratory
  - Hemodynamic

The causes of anaphylaxis are the same as the causes of any allergic event, such as:

- Insect bites and stings
- Medications: penicillin, phenytoin, lamotrigine, quinidine, rifampin, sulfa
- Foods

> Latex is a very important cause of anaphylaxis in healthcare workers.

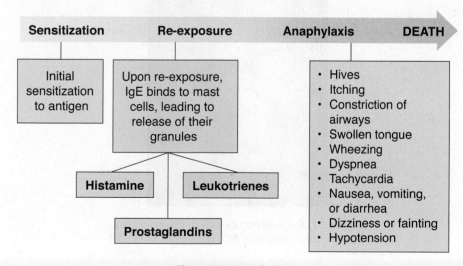

Figure 7.1 Anaphylaxis

> Urticaria is considered part of anaphylaxis, not just an allergy.

Symptoms include:

- Rash (present with any allergic reaction)
- Hypotension, tachycardia
- Respiratory distress: shortness of breath; wheezing; swelling of the lips, tongue, or face; stridor

There is no specific diagnostic test to define anaphylaxis.

Treatment is as follows:

- Epinephrine
- Antihistamines such as diphenhydramine (H1-blocker) and ranitidine (H2-blocker)
- Glucocorticoids such as methylprednisolone or hydrocortisone
- Emergent airway protection if needed: intubation or cricothyroidotomy

Angioedema

Angioedema is sudden swelling of the face, tongue, eyes, and airway, commonly due to a deficiency of C1 esterase inhibitor. There is a characteristic association with the onset with minor physical trauma or the recent start of ACE inhibitors.

- Angioedema often has an idiopathic origin.
- Hereditary angioedema is characterized by sudden facial swelling and stridor with the absence of pruritus and urticaria. Hereditary angioedema does not respond to glucocorticoids or epinephrine.

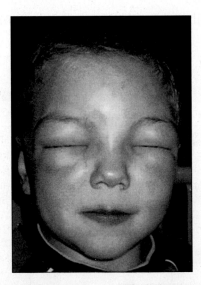

Figure 7.2 Angioedema can swell the eyes shut.
Source: James Heilman, MD, Wikipedia, CC-BY-SA

The **best initial tests** are decreased C2 and C4 in the complement pathway and deficiency of C1 esterase inhibitor.

Treatment is as follows:

- Ensure the airway first, as the process can evolve rapidly.
- Acute attack: fresh frozen plasma, ecallantide, or icatibant
- Urticaria and early respiratory compromise: epinephrine, antihistamine, steroids
- Hereditary angioedema with severe laryngeal involvement: C1 esterase inhibitor concentrate (or recombinant C1 inhibitor concentrate)
- Bradykinin B2 receptor antagonist: icatibant
- Kallikrein inhibitor: ecallantide
- Lanadelumab: antibody against kallikrein
- Prophylaxis for surgical and dental procedures, which can precipitate angioedema:
  - Antifibrinolytics (e.g., tranexamic acid): decrease C1 protein and therefore decrease the production of bradykinin
  - Androgens (danazol, stanozolol)
  - Infusions of C1 esterase inhibitor (recombinant or plasma-derived)

Antihistamines, glucocorticoids, and epinephrine are not effective for angioedema. They are helpful for anaphylaxis—not for C1 esterase inhibitor deficiency.

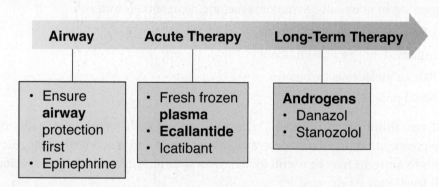

Figure 7.3 Angioedema Treatment

Urticaria

Urticaria is an allergic reaction that causes sudden swelling of the superficial layers of the skin. Causes include insects, medications, and physical agents such as pressure (dermatographism); cold; and vibration.

Treatment is as follows:

1. Antihistamines: hydroxyzine, diphenhydramine, fexofenadine, loratadine, or cetirizine plus ranitidine
2. Leukotriene receptor antagonists: montelukast or zafirlukast

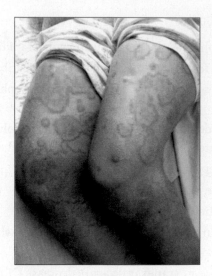

Figure 7.4 Urticaria, Localized Anaphylaxis with a "Wheal and Flare."
Source: Farshad Bagheri, MD

Allergic Rhinitis

Seasonal allergies such as "hay fever" are common. This is an IgE-dependent triggering of mast cells. Symptoms include recurrent episodes of:

- Watery eyes, sneezing, itchy nose, and itchy eyes
- Inflamed, boggy nasal mucosa
- Pale or violaceous turbinates
- Nasal polyps

Allergic rhinitis is most often a clinical diagnosis with recurrent episodes of the presentation previously described. Skin testing and blood testing for reactions to antigens may be useful to identify a specific etiology. Allergen-specific IgE levels may be elevated.

> Nasal smear may show large numbers of eosinophils.

Treatment

- Prevention, with avoidance of the precipitating allergen
    - Close windows and use air conditioning to avoid pollen
    - Get rid of animals to which the patient is allergic
    - Cover mattresses and pillows
    - Use air purifiers and dust filters
- Intranasal corticosteroid sprays
- Antihistamines: loratadine, clemastine, fexofenadine, brompheniramine
- Intranasal anticholinergic medications: ipratropium
- Desensitization to allergens that cannot be avoided

Primary Immunodeficiency Disorders

Common Variable Immunodeficiency (CVID)

In CVID, B cells are present in normal numbers, but they do not make sufficient amounts of immunoglobulins. There is a decrease in all the subtypes: IgG, IgM, and IgA. There is also a decreased response to antigen stimulation of B cells.

CVID presents with recurrent sinopulmonary infections in adults. Rates of incidence are equal in men and women. Bronchitis, pneumonia, sinusitis, and otitis media are common, as are:

- Giardiasis
- Spruelike intestinal malabsorption
- Increases in autoimmune diseases such as pernicious anemia and seronegative rheumatic diseases

▶ TIP

The clues to CVID are a reduced output of B lymphocytes, a normal number of B cells, and a normal amount of lymphoid tissue (e.g., nodes, adenoids, and tonsils).

Treat each infection as it arises with antibiotics. Chronic maintenance for CVID is with regular **infusions of IV immunoglobulins**.

X-Linked (Bruton) Agammaglobulinemia

X-linked agammaglobulinemia presents in male children with increased sinopulmonary infections. B cells and lymphoid tissues are diminished. There is a decrease or absence of the tonsils, adenoids, lymph nodes, and spleen. T cells are normal.

Treatment is management of the infections as they arise. Long-term, regular administration of IVIG keeps these children healthier.

Severe Combined Immunodeficiency

The word "combined" in severe combined immunodeficiency (SCID) means that there is deficiency in both B and T cells. This results in infections related to both deficiencies.

- **B cells**: decreased immunoglobulin production leads to recurrent sinopulmonary infection beginning as early as age 6 months
- **T cells**: markedly decreased numbers of T cells give many of the infections that you would see with AIDS patients, e.g., PCP, varicella, and *Candida*

Treat the infections as they arise; in addition, these patients should undergo a bone marrow transplant, which can be curative.

IgA Deficiency

These patients also present with recurrent sinopulmonary infections. The difference between this syndrome and the others is:

- Atopic diseases
- Anaphylaxis to blood transfusion when blood is given from a patient who has normal levels of IgA
- Spruelike condition with fat malabsorption
- Increase in the risk of vitiligo, thyroiditis, and rheumatoid arthritis

Treatment is management of the infections as they arise.

- Use only blood that is from IgA-deficient donors or has been washed.
- IVIG injection will not work because the amount of IgA is too low to be therapeutic.
- Trace amounts of IgA in IVIG may provoke anaphylaxis in the same way that a blood transfusion does.

Hyper IgE Syndrome

This presents with recurrent skin infections with *Staphylococcus*. Treat these infections as they arise and consider prophylactic antibiotics such as dicloxacillin or cephalexin.

Wiskott-Aldrich Syndrome

This is an immunodeficiency combined with thrombocytopenia and eczema. T lymphocytes are markedly deficient in the blood and the lymph nodes. Bone marrow transplantation is the only definitive treatment.

Chronic Granulomatous Disease

Test for dihydrorhodamine in chronic granulomatous disease.

Chronic granulomatous disease (CGD) is a genetic disease resulting in extensive inflammatory reactions. The result is lymph nodes with purulent material leaking out.

Aphthous ulcers and inflammation of the nares are common. Granulomas may become obstructive in the GI or urinary tract.

"What Is the Most Likely Diagnosis?"

Look for infections with the odd combination of:

- *Staphylococcus*
- *Burkholderia*
- *Nocardia*
- *Aspergillus*

Diagnostic testing:

- Abnormal results of nitroblue tetrazolium testing or dihydrorhodamine testing detect the decrease in the respiratory burst that produces hydrogen peroxide.
- This is a decrease in NADPH oxidase, which generates superoxide.

Primary Immunodeficiency Disorders	
Common variable immunodeficiency (CVID)	• Low B cell output • Normal T cells
X-linked (Bruton) agammaglobulinemia	Low B cells, normal T cells in young male children
Severe combined immunodeficiency (SCID)	• Low B cells and T cells • Analogous to HIV
IgA deficiency	• Atopic disorders • Anaphylaxis
Hyper IgE syndrome	Skin infections (e.g., *Staphylococcus*)
Wiskott-Aldrich syndrome	• Low T cells • Normal B cells • Low platelets • Eczema

Chronic granulomatous disease	• Lymph nodes with purulent material
	• Infections, combined with:
	  – *Staphylococcus*
	  – *Burkholderia*
	  – *Nocardia*
	  – *Aspergillus*

Joint Diseases

Osteoarthritis

Osteoarthritis (OA), or degenerative joint disease (DJD), is a chronic, slowly progressive, erosive damage to joint surfaces. The loss of articular cartilage causes increasing pain with minimal or no inflammation.

- Incidence of OA is directly proportional to increasing age and trauma to the joint.
- Risk factors include playing contact sports with trauma, obesity, and developmental deformities.
- Modest recreational running is not a risk factor. It does not cause OA.

> OA is, by far, the most common cause of joint disease.

Symptoms of OA most commonly affect the weight-bearing joints (knee, hip, ankle).

- The hand is affected but is not as great a cause of disability.
  - In the hand, distal interphalangeal (DIP) joints are more commonly affected than the proximal interphalangeal (PIP) and metacarpophalangeal joints (MCP).
  - DIP enlargement: Heberden nodes
  - PIP enlargement: Bouchard nodes
- Crepitations of the involved joints are common.
- Effusion is rare.
- Stiffness is brief (<15 minutes).

> OA falsely elevates the T-score on DEXA scan.

Diagnostic testing is as follows:

- Normal lab tests: CBC; ESR; antinuclear antibody (ANA); and rheumatoid factor
- X-ray of the affected joint (**most accurate test**) will show:
  - Joint space narrowing
  - Osteophytes
  - Dense subchondral bone
  - Bone cysts

> An absence of inflammation, normal lab tests, and short duration of stiffness distinguish OA from rheumatoid arthritis.

Glucosamine and chondroitin sulfate are no more effective than placebo.

Topical NSAIDs can avoid systemic toxicity.

The key to diagnosis of RA is **morning stiffness** of multiple small, inflamed joints.

- In RA, tarsal tunnel syndrome (at the ankle) is increased.
- In RA, the DIP joints are spared (unlike DJD, where there is DIP involvement).

Treatment is as follows:

- Weight loss and moderate exercise (swimming, tai chi, yoga)
- Acetaminophen (less toxic but less effective than NSAIDs)
- NSAIDs alone or with acetaminophen (**best initial therapy**)
- Capsaicin cream
- Intraarticular steroids if other medical therapy does not control pain
- Joint replacement if function is compromised
- Duloxetine for knee pain

Rheumatoid Arthritis

Rheumatoid arthritis (RA) is an autoimmune disorder mainly of the joints but with many systemic manifestations of chronic inflammation. There is an association with specific HLA types.

- Women > men (as with most autoimmune diseases)
- Chronic synovitis leads to overgrowth, or pannus formation, which damages all the structures surrounding the joint (bone, ligaments, tendons, and cartilage).

Symptoms include:

- Bilateral, symmetrical joint involvement: PIP joints of the fingers, MCP joints of the hands, and the wrists, knees, and ankles
- Morning stiffness lasting at least 30 minutes, but often much longer
- Rheumatoid nodules (20%), most often over bony prominences (**most common** extra-articular manifestation)
- Ocular symptoms: episcleritis
- Lung involvement: pleural effusion with low glucose and nodules of lung parenchyma
- Vasculitis: skin, bowel, and peripheral nerves
- Cervical joint involvement, particularly at C1 and C2, which can lead to subluxation
- Baker cyst may rupture and mimic a DVT
- Pericarditis and pleural disease
- Carpal tunnel syndrome
- Hoarseness from cricoarytenoid joint damage

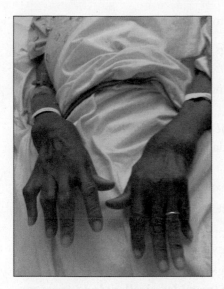 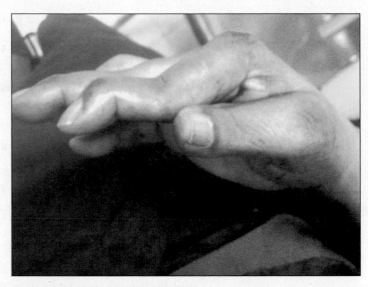

Figures 8.1, 8.2 Boutonnière (left) and swan neck (right), are classic deformities of the hands in RA. *Sources: left: Nirav Thakur, MD, right: Raphael Shaw*

Diagnostic testing includes:

- Rheumatoid factor (RF) (70–80% of cases) but is nonspecific
- Anti-cyclic citrullinated peptide (anti-CCP) is >80% sensitive and >95% specific
- X-rays show erosion of joints and osteopenia
- Elevated ESR or C-reactive protein
- Anemia: normocytic
- Arthrocentesis (if diagnosis not clear) to exclude crystal disease; infection will show modest elevation in lymphocytes

Diagnostic criteria are assessed with "points": ≥6 points diagnoses RA (abnormal x-ray is not needed)

- Joint involvement (up to 5 points)
- ESR or CRP (1 point)
- Duration for >6 weeks (1 point)
- RF or anti-CCP (1–3 points)

- **Sicca syndrome** affects dry eyes, mouth, and other mucous membranes
- **Felty syndrome** causes RA, splenomegaly, and neutropenia
- **Caplan syndrome** causes RA, pneumoconiosis, and lung nodules

The most common cause of death in RA is coronary artery disease.

Treatment is RA is as follows. The goal is to stop progression of the disease.

- Disease modifying antirheumatic drugs (DMARDs) for all patients with erosive RA
  - Start with methotrexate (side effects include liver and pulmonary toxicity plus bone marrow suppression)
  - If no response or intolerance to methotrexate, use a tumor necrosis factor (TNF) inhibitor (infliximab, adalimumab, etanercept, golimumab, certolizumab)
    - ° Consider combining with methotrexate to prevent disease progression
    - ° Side effects include infection and reactivation of TB, so screen with a PPD prior to use
    - ° TNF inhibitors are safe in pregnancy
  - Rituximab (developed for non-Hodgkin lymphoma) to remove CD20 positive lymphocytes from circulation (**provides excellent long-term control of RA**); consider combining with methotrexate if there is no response to anti-TNF medication
  - Hydroxychloroquine for mild disease that doesn't require the strength of methotrexate
    - ° Consider combining with methotrexate
    - ° Side effects include toxicity to the retina, so do a dilated eye exam prior to use
    - ° Hydroxychloroquine is safe in pregnancy
- Alternatives to DMARDs include sulfasalazine, abatacept, and anakinra. Consider adding to methotrexate if anti-TNF agents do not control disease.
  - Side effects of sulfasalazine include bone marrow toxicity, hemolysis with G6 PD deficiency, oligospermia, and rash.

> Methotrexate can give stomatitis or oral ulcers. If there is toxicity, leflunomide is the alternative.

> **"Erosive"** disease means:
> - Joint space narrowing
> - Physical deformity of joints
> - X-ray abnormalities

A patient with long-standing RA is to have coronary bypass surgery. Which of the following is most important prior to surgery?

a. Cervical spine x-ray
b. Rheumatoid factor
c. Extra dose of methotrexate
d. ESR
e. Pneumococcal vaccination

Answer: A. RA is associated with C1/C2 subluxation. Cervical spine imaging to detect possible instability of the vertebra is essential prior to the hyperextension of the neck that typically occurs with endotracheal intubation. Methotrexate does not work acutely, and additional doses are not useful. Although pneumococcal vaccination is useful in any immunocompromised person, there is no particular indication for vaccination surrounding surgical procedures.

Rheumatoid Arthritis Medications			
Biological agent	**Mechanism**	**Uses**	**Special notes**
Adalimumab	TNF-a antibody	• RA • Ankylosing spondylitis • IBD	• **Check TB status** • **Contraindicated in CHF**
Certolizumab			
Golimumab			
Infliximab			
Etanercept	**TNF-a decoy receptor**		**Not good for IBD arthritis**
Abatacept	T cell inhibitor	RA	
Rituximab	Anti-CD 20	• RA • Psoriatic arthritis • IBD	**Decreases response to vaccines**
Tocilizumab	Anti-IL 6	RA	
Belimumab	BAFF inhibitor	SLE	
Tofacitinib	JAK inhibitor	RA	
Ustekinumab	Anti-IL 12/23	Psoriatic arthritis	
Anakinra	Anti-IL 1	• RA • Psoriatic arthritis	
Rilonacept	Anti-IL 1b	RA	
Canakinumab			

Treatment for the symptoms of RA is as follows. Neither NSAIDs nor steroids prevent progression of disease.

- NSAIDs (**best initial treatment for pain**) work immediately to improve inflammation.
- When there is no response to NSAIDs, use steroids to control the pain of RA secondary to inflammation; additionally, use steroids as a bridge when waiting for DMARDs to take effect. (DMARDs have much slower onset of action than steroids.)

Adverse Effects of RA Medications	
Drug	**Adverse effect**
Anti-TNF	Reactivation of tuberculosis
Hydroxychloroquine	Ocular
Sulfasalazine	Rash, hemolysis
Rituximab	Infection
Methotrexate	Liver, lung, marrow

▶ **TIP**

The Step 2 CK exam is unlikely to ask which DMARD to use in combination with methotrexate or after methotrexate fails, because the answer is not clear. However, the side effects of drugs are mandatory to know.

Gout

Gouty arthritis (90% of cases in men) is caused by an overproduction or underexcretion of uric acid.

Overproduction causes:

- Idiopathic
- Increased turnover of cells (cancer, hemolysis, psoriasis, chemotherapy)
- Enzyme deficiency (Lesch-Nyhan syndrome, glycogen storage disease)
- Ethanol

Underexcretion causes:

- Renal insufficiency
- Ketoacidosis or lactic acidosis
- Thiazides and aspirin

"What Is the Most Likely Diagnosis?"

Look for a man who develops sudden, excruciating pain, redness, and tenderness of the big toe at night after binge drinking with beer. Fever is common, and it can be hard to distinguish the initial gouty attack from infection without the use of arthrocentesis.

Although the metatarsal phalangeal (MTP) joint of the great toe is the most frequently affected site, gout can also be symptomatic in the ankle, feet, and knees.

Chronic gout often has long asymptomatic periods. The following can result:

- **Tophi**: tissue deposits of urate crystals with foreign body reaction
  - Commonly occur in cartilage, subcutaneous tissue, bone, and kidney
  - Often take years to develop
- **Uric acid kidney stones** (5–10% of patients)

Diagnostic testing is as follows:

- Aspiration of the joint (**most accurate test**), showing needle-shaped crystals with negative birefringence on polarized light microscopy
- Elevated WBC count on joint fluid (2,000–50,000/μL), predominantly neutrophilic
- Tapping of the joint to exclude infection, because gout can look like an infected joint (red, warm, and tender)
- Elevated uric acid: a single level during an acute gouty attack is normal in 25%
- Elevated ESR and leukocytosis (in acute attacks)
- X-ray: normal in early disease; erosions of cortical bone in later disease

▶ **TIP**

Protein and glucose levels in synovial fluid don't help answer the "most likely diagnosis" question.

Treatment for **acute attack** is as follows:

- NSAIDs (**best initial treatment**); superior to colchicine
- Corticosteroids, e.g., triamcinolone, when no response or contraindications to NSAIDs; use injection in a single joint or orally for multiple joints
- Colchicine when NSAIDs and steroids cannot be used

Do not start uricosuric agents or allopurinol during an acute attack of gout. If the patient is already on allopurinol, it can safely be continued.

Treatment for **chronic disease** is as follows:

- Management between attacks prevents recurrences.
  - Reduce alcohol (especially beer), weight, and high-purine foods (meat, seafood)
  - Stop thiazides, aspirin, and niacin; use losartan first for hypertension
  - Medications:
    ◦ Colchicine (low dose): effective at preventing second attacks of gout and attacks brought on by sudden fluctuations in uric acid due to probenecid or allopurinol
    ◦ Allopurinol: decreases production of uric acid
    ◦ Febuxostat (xanthine-oxidase inhibitor): used if allopurinol is contra-indicated
    ◦ Pegloticase: dissolves uric acid (uric acid metabolism is accelerated by pegloticase); contraindicated in G6PD deficiency
    ◦ Probenecid and sulfinpyrazone (rarely used) increase uric acid excretion in the kidney (uricosuric)
    ◦ Anakinra (IL1 inhibitor): used when multiple agents fail to control gout

Losartan (ARB) lowers uric acid. It is the best drug for BP in gout.

Probenecid, NSAIDs, and sulfinpyrazone are contraindicated in renal insufficiency.

- Side effects of medications include:
  - Uricosuric agents and allopurinol: hypersensitivity (rash, hemolysis, allergic interstitial nephritis); TEN; SJS
  - Colchicine (high dose): diarrhea and bone marrow suppression (neutropenia)

Note that chronic treatment can have some side effects.

- Uricosuric agents and allopurinol: hypersensitivity (rash, hemolysis, allergic interstitial nephritis); TEN or Stevens-Johnson
- Colchicine (high dose): diarrhea and bone marrow suppression (neutropenia)

Pseudogout

Calcium pyrophosphate deposition disease (CPPD) (or "pseudogout") is caused by calcium-containing salts depositing in the articular cartilage.

- Hemochromatosis and hyperparathyroidism (most common risk factors)
- Associated with diabetes, hypothyroidism, and Wilson disease
- **Unlike gout**: large joints (e.g., the knee and wrist) are affected, but not particularly the first MCP of the foot
- **Unlike OA**: DIP and PIP are not affected

Testing includes:

- Uric acid: normal
- X-ray shows linear calcification or chondrocalcinosis of the cartilaginous structures of the joint and DJD
- Arthrocentesis (**most accurate test**) reveals positively birefringent rhomboid-shaped crystals
- Synovial fluid: elevated WBCs between 2,000 and 50,000/μL (but will not distinguish CPPD from gout or other inflammatory disorders of the joint such as RA)

Treatment is as follows:

- NSAIDs (**best initial treatment**)
- Intraarticular steroids such as triamcinolone for severe disease or if no response to NSAIDs
- Colchicine (low dose) as prophylaxis between attacks

> You cannot confirm a diagnosis of CPPD without aspiration of the joint.

Disease	DJD	Gout	CPPD	Rheumatoid arthritis	Septic arthritis
Characteristic history	Older, slow, worse with use	Men, acute, binge drinking	Hemochromatosis Hyperparathyroidism	Young, female, morning stiffness better with use	High fever, very acute
Physical findings	DIP, PIP, hip, and knees	1st big toe	Wrists and knees	Multiple joints of hands and feet	Single hot joint
Synovial fluid analysis	<200 WBCs, osteophytes and joint space narrowing	2,000–50,000 WBCs, negatively birefringent needles	2,000–50,000 WBCs, positively birefringent rhomboids	Anti-cyclic citrullinated peptide (anti-CCP) in blood, 10,000–20,000 WBC in fluid	>50,000 neutrophils, culture of fluid

Seronegative Spondyloarthropathies

The seronegative spondyloarthropathies are common in men age <40. Symptoms include joint pain, specifically:

- Involvement of the spine and large joints
- Negative rheumatoid factor (hence the name *seronegative*)
- Enthesopathy (inflammation where tendons and ligaments attach to bones)
- Uveitis
- HLA-B27

Corticosteroids are not helpful in the treatment of seronegative spondyloarthropathy.

▶ TIP

Despite the association with HLA-B27, this is never the "best initial" or "most accurate" test for seronegative spondyloarthropathies.

Ankylosing Spondylitis—"What Is the Most Likely Diagnosis?"

Look for a young man with low backache and stiffness of his back and pain that radiates to the buttocks, with flattening of the normal lumbar curvature and decreased chest expansion. Eventually the spine will not expand in any direction. Enthesopathy occurs at the Achilles tendon.

Other findings include:

- Transient peripheral arthritis of knees, hips, and shoulders (50%)
- Cardiac: atrioventricular block (3–5%; aortic insufficiency)
- Uveitis
- "Bamboo spine," fusion of vertebral joints (late finding)

Diagnostic testing includes:

- X-ray of the sacroiliac (SI) joint (**best initial test**)
- MRI (**most accurate test**) detects abnormalities years before the x-ray becomes abnormal

> Look for back pain **worsened by rest** and relieved by activity.

- ESR (elevated in 85%)
- HLA B27 (not a confirmatory test since 8% of general population is positive)

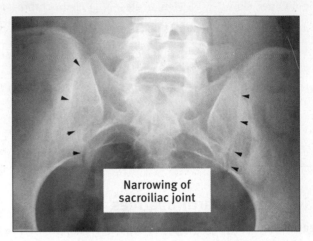

Figure 8.3 The best initial test for seronegative spondyloarthropathies is an x-ray of the sacroiliac joint. *Source: Conrad Fischer, MD*

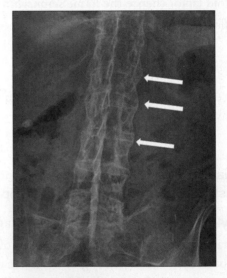

Figure 8.4 Bamboo spine is a late finding of ankylosing spondylitis. The vertebral bodies are fused by bridging syndesmophytes. *Source: Shreya Patel, MD, and Nishith Patel, MD*

Treatment is exercise and NSAIDs. If there is no response, use an anti-TNF drug such as etanercept, adalimumab, or infliximab.

Psoriatic Arthritis

In patients with psoriatic arthritis, 80% will have preceding psoriasis. It is more common with severe skin disease. Besides SI joint involvement, characteristic findings are:

- Sausage digits from enthesopathy
- Nail pitting

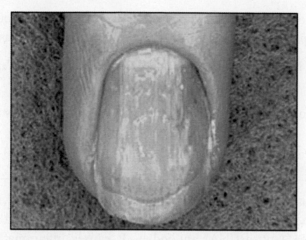

Figure 8.5 Arthritis with Nail Pitting (10% of psoriasis patients).
Source: Conrad Fischer, MD.

Testing includes:

- ESR is elevated in almost all patients but nonspecific
- X-ray of the joint (**best initial test**) shows a "pencil in a cup" deformity plus bony erosions and irregular bone destruction
- Uric acid level is elevated from increased skin turnover

Treatment starts with NSAIDS. If there is no response or if there is severe disease, use methotrexate.

- If methotrexate does not control disease, use anti-TNF agents.
- If anti-TNF agents cannot be used, use anti-IL17 medications (secukinumab or ixekizumab).
- Apremilast, an oral phosphodiesterase inhibitor, can be helpful.
- Steroids are a wrong choice.

> Ustekinumab is an anti-IL12/IL23 drug used if anti-TNF meds fail.

Reactive Arthritis (Reiter Syndrome)

Reactive arthritis occurs secondary to:

- Inflammatory bowel disease (equal sex incidence)
- Sexually transmitted infection (far greater in men)
- Gastrointestinal infection (*Yersinia, Salmonella, Campylobacter*)

"What Is the Most Likely Diagnosis?"

Look for the triad of:

- Joint pain
- Ocular findings (uveitis, conjunctivitis)
- Genital abnormalities (urethritis, balanitis)

> Keratoderma blennorhagicum is a skin lesion unique to reactive arthritis that looks like pustular psoriasis.

There is no specific test for reactive arthritis. Hot, swollen joints should be tapped to rule out septic joint. The diagnosis is based on the triad previously described.

Treatment is NSAIDs. When there is no response, use sulfasalazine. Steroid injections into the joints can help.

Antibiotics do not reverse reactive arthritis once joint pain has started.

Systemic Lupus Erythematosus

Systemic lupus erythematosus (SLE) is an autoimmune disorder with a number of autoantibodies, including antinuclear antibodies (ANA) and anti-double-stranded DNA (anti-dsDNA) antibodies. It causes inflammation diffusely through the body (skin, brain, kidneys, joints) and the blood.

SLE has numerous abnormal blood tests associated with it (anemia, anti-Sm, antiphospholipid antibodies), but this is not the same thing as knowing what causes SLE. Its cause is a mystery.

Diagnosis is based on the presence of ≥4 of 11 known manifestations of the disease.

1. Malar rash
2. Discoid rash
3. Photosensitivity
4. Oral ulcers
5. Arthritis (90% of patients)
   - Often the first symptom that brings patients to seek medical attention
   - Joint pain of SLE is without deformation or erosion, explaining why the x-ray is normal.
6. Serositis: inflammation of pleura and pericardium creates chest pain with possible pericardial and pleural effusion
7. Renal disorder (any degree, even mild proteinuria): membranous glomerulonephritis most common; RBC casts and hematuria occur
8. Neurologic disorder including psychosis, seizures, or stroke from vasculitis
9. Hemolytic anemia is part of the diagnostic criteria, but the anemia of chronic disease is more commonly found. Lymphopenia, leukopenia, and thrombocytopenia are also seen.
10. ANA abnormality (positive ANA)
11. Immunologic disorder (any of the following):
    - Anti-dsDNA
    - Anti-Sm
    - False positive test for syphilis
    - Positive LE cell preparation

Drug-induced lupus spares the kidney and brain. Antihistones are present, but anti-dsDNA antibodies are absent.

Additional findings include mesenteric vasculitis, Raynaud phenomenon, and antiphospholipid syndromes.

Diagnostic testing is as follows:

- ANA (95–99% of cases)
  - Negative ANA is extremely sensitive for lupus, but positive ANA has little specificity
  - Many rheumatologic diseases are associated with positive ANA
  - Do not treat asymptomatic ANA
- Anti-dsDNA (60%) and anti-Sm (30%)
  - Found only in SLE
  - Extremely specific for SLE
- Decreased complement levels: correlate with disease activity; drop even further with acute disease exacerbations
- Anti-SSA (anti-Ro) and anti-SSB (anti-La) (10–20% of cases)
  - Add little to the diagnosis if the DNA is positive
  - Most often found in Sjögren syndrome (65% of cases)
  - A finding of anti-SSA or anti-Ro in the mother's blood predicts who is at risk of passing on neonatal SLE. If the mother is anti-Ro positive, answer "check baby EKG" or "baby at risk of heart block" on the exam.
- Ribosomal P indicates risk or presence of cerebral lupus.

> These features may be seen in SLE but are not criteria for diagnosis:
> - **Alopecia** (common)
> - **Pulmonary findings:** pneumonia, alveolar hemorrhage, and restrictive lung disease
> - **Ocular findings:** photophobia, retinal lesions (cotton wool spots), and blindness

A 34-year-old woman with a history of SLE is admitted with pneumonia and confusion. You need to determine if this is a flare of lupus or simply an infection with sepsis causing confusion, and you must decide whether to give a bolus of high-dose steroids in someone with an infection. Which of the following will provide the most useful information?

a. Elevated anti-Sm
b. Elevated ANA
c. Decreased complement
d. Decreased complement and rise in anti-dsDNA
e. Brain MRI
f. Response to steroids

Answer: **D.** Although anti-Sm is specific for SLE, the level does not change in an acute flare. ANA level does not tell severity of disease. Brain MRI is most often normal in lupus cerebritis unless there has been a stroke. In an acute lupus flare, complement levels drop and anti-dsDNA levels rise. SSA, SSB, and anti-Sm tests are most useful when the ANA is positive and dsDNA test is negative.

Treatment is as follows:

- **Acute lupus flare**: high-dose boluses of steroids
- **Mildly chronic disease** limited to skin/joins: hydroxychloroquine

- **Lupus nephritis**: steroids +/− cyclophosphamide or mycophenolate
  - Kidney biopsy is the only way to determine severity of disease, i.e., is there simple glomerulosclerosis or scarring of the kidney (which will not respond to therapy)?
  - Urinalysis is insufficient to determine severity.
- Belimumab controls progression of the disease.

> Belimumab inhibits B cell action to control SLE.

In young patients, infection is the most common cause of death. In older patients, accelerated atherosclerosis makes myocardial infarction the most common cause of death.

Antiphospholipid Syndrome

Most cases of antiphospholipid syndrome (APS) are not associated with SLE. APS is an idiopathic disorder with IgG or IgM antibodies made against negatively charged phospholipids, commonly:

- Lupus anticoagulant
- Anticardiolipin antibodies
- Beta 2 glycoprotein

APS presents with thromboses of both arteries and veins as well as recurrent spontaneous abortion. Additionally:

- Elevated aPTT, normal PT, and normal INR (unlike other causes of thrombophilia)
- False-positive VDRL or RPR with normal FTA (because the antibody reacts with the reagent in the lab, which is a cardiolipin); anticardiolipin antibodies more often give spontaneous abortion, and the lupus anticoagulant is more often associated with elevated aPTT

> APS = clotting + **elevated aPTT** + normal PT

Diagnostic testing includes:

- Mixing study (**best initial test**) where patient's plasma is mixed with an equal amount of normal plasma
  - If elevated aPTT is due to a clotting factor deficiency, the aPTT will come down to normal
  - If antiphospholipid antibody is present in plasma, the aPTT will remain elevated.
  - Russell viper venom test (RVVT) (**most specific test for lupus anticoagulant**): RVVT is prolonged with antiphospholipid antibody and does not correct on mixing with normal plasma. The use of heparin interferes with the RVVT.

Treatment is as follows:

- Thromboses (DVT or PE) are treated with heparin, then warfarin.
- Thrombotic episodes are treated lifelong.
- No treatment is needed for asymptomatic antiphospholipid antibody.

Spontaneous Abortion

There is no treatment for a spontaneous abortion that is in the process of occurring. It is too late. The most commonly asked questions are:

- **What should be investigated for anticardiolipin antibody as a cause of spontaneous abortion?**
  - Answer: two or more first-trimester events or a single second-trimester event
- **What is the treatment to prevent a recurrence?**
  - Answer: heparin and aspirin

▶ **TIP**

Warfarin and steroids are wrong answers for preventing spontaneous abortion. Warfarin is contraindicated in the first trimester of pregnancy and steroids are not effective.

Sjögren Syndrome

Sjögren syndrome is an idiopathic autoimmune disorder secondary to antibodies predominantly against lacrimal and salivary glands; 90% of those affected are women.

Sjögren is associated with the following:

- Rheumatoid arthritis
- SLE
- Primary biliary cirrhosis
- Polymyositis
- Hashimoto thyroiditis

Symptoms include:

- Joint pain (90% of patients)
- Dryness of the mouth and eyes
  - Produces the need to constantly drink water
  - Causes difficulty swallowing, especially dry foods
  - Causes rampant dental caries +/− tooth loss as a result of reduced saliva (whose main function is to physically wash food off teeth and neutralize acid)
- Ocular abnormalities, giving a feeling of "sand in the eyes" plus burning and itching (called *keratoconjunctivitis sicca*)
- Loss of vaginal secretions, leading to dyspareunia

> The vast majority of Sjögren patients have joint pain.

Less common symptoms include:

- Vasculitis
- Lung disease
- Pancreatitis
- Renal tubular acidosis (20%)

▶ **TIP**

When asked what is the "most dangerous" complication of Sjögren, answer **lymphoma**.

Diagnostic testing is as follows:

- Schirmer test (**best initial test**) observing the amount of tears, i.e., wetness, a piece of filter paper gets when placed against the eye where a piece of filter paper is placed against the eye
- Lip or parotid gland biopsy (**most accurate test**) reveals lymphoid infiltration in the salivary glands
- SS-A and SS-B (also called "Ro" and "La") (**best initial test on blood**) (65% of cases); SLE is associated with SS-A and SS-B in 10–20% of cases
- Rose bengal stain shows abnormal corneal epithelium
- ANA, RF, anemia, leukopenia, and eosinophilia, but all are nonspecific

Treatment is as follows:

- Hydrate the mouth (**best initial therapy**) with frequent sips of water, sugar-free gum, and fluoride treatments
- Artificial tears to avoid corneal ulcers, topical lifitegrast or cyclosporine to reduce ocular inflammation
- Pilocarpine and cevimeline increase acetylcholine, the main stimulant to the production of saliva; cevimeline increases saliva production
- There is no cure, but lifespan is not shortened. Evaluate for lymphoma (seen in up to 10% of patients).

> Steroids are always a wrong answer for Sjögren syndrome.

Scleroderma (Systemic Sclerosis)/CREST

Scleroderma is diffuse in 20% of cases and limited in 80%. Limited scleroderma is also known as **CREST** syndrome (**C**alcinosis, **R**aynaud, **E**sophageal dysmotility, **S**clerodactyly, **T**elangiectasia).

"What Is the Most Likely Diagnosis?"

Look for a young (20s to 40s) woman (3 times more likely than men) with fibrosis of the skin and internal organs such as the lung, kidney, and GI tract.

Symptoms include:

- Raynaud syndrome: increased vascular reactivity of the fingers, beginning with pain and pallor (white) or cyanosis (blue) followed by reactive hyperemia (red)
  - Precipitated by cold and emotional stress
  - Some cases lead to ulceration and gangrene
- Skin manifestations: fibrosis of the hands, face, neck, and extremities; telangiectasia and abnormalities of pigmentation
- Gastrointestinal: esophageal dysmotility with GERD, large-mouthed diverticula of small and large bowel; diarrhea
- Renal: sudden hypertensive crisis
- Lung: fibrosis leading to restrictive lung disease and pulmonary hypertension
- Cardiac: myocardial fibrosis, pericarditis, and heart block; lung disease gives right ventricular hypertrophy

> Scleroderma causes diarrhea because of bacterial overgrowth in large diverticula.

> CREST gives primary pulmonary hypertension, but the lungs are normal.

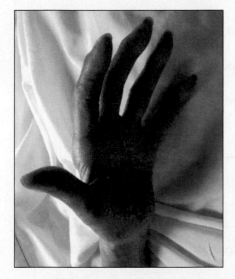

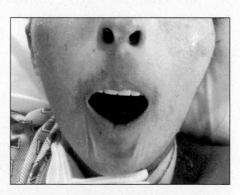

Figures 8.6, 8.7 Manifestations of Scleroderma. Left: Classic sclerodactyly.
Right: Note the tightening of the face, especially around the lips.
Source: Pramod Theetha Kariyanna, MD

Limited scleroderma	Diffuse scleroderma
• Distal to elbows and knees	• Proximal to elbows and knees
• Can involve face and neck	• Can involve face and neck
• Anti-centromere +	• Anti-SCL-70 +
• Pulmonary hypertension	• Pulmonary fibrosis

Diagnostic testing includes:

- ANA positive in 85–90%, but nonspecific
- ESR usually normal

> Anticentromere antibodies are extremely specific for CREST syndrome.

- SCL-70 (anti-topoisomerase) (**most accurate test**) but present in only 30% with diffuse disease (scleroderma) and 20% with limited disease
- Anticentromere present in 50% of those with CREST syndrome

Treatment is as follows:

- Methotrexate to slow the underlying disease (penicillamine is not effective)
- Renal crisis: ACE inhibitors (even if creatinine is elevated)
- Esophageal dysmotility: PPIs for GERD
- Raynaud: CCBs
- Pulmonary fibrosis: cyclophosphamide improves dyspnea and PFTs
- Pulmonary hypertension: bosentan ambrisentan (endothelin antagonist); sildenafil; prostacyclin analogs (iloprost, treprostinil, epoprostenol)
- Thromboembolic disease: riociguat (cGMP stimulator)

CREST versus Scleroderma

Scleroderma has the same presentation as CREST but adds more organ dysfunction.

- CREST syndrome is **C**alcinosis, **R**aynaud phenomenon, **E**sophageal dysmotility, **S**clerodactyly, and **T**elangiectasia.
- When the lungs, heart, and kidney are also involved, it is scleroderma.
- CREST can cause primary pulmonary hypertension, although the lungs themselves are normal.

Myositis

Myositis is inflammation of the body's connective tissues and muscles.

Polymyositis

Inflammatory myopathies present with proximal muscle weakness, which over time causes difficulty getting up from a seated position or walking up stairs.

- Facial or ocular muscles are not affected (as in myasthenia gravis).
- Proximal muscles are weak, but only 25% of cases have pain and tenderness.
- Dysphagia occurs from involvement of the striated muscles of the pharynx, making it difficult to initiate swallowing.
- Cardiac muscles are rarely affected
- CK-MB level may be elevated.
- Anti-Mi-2 antibodies are present.

Dermatomyositis

Dermatomyositis is characterized by inflammatory and degenerative changes in the muscles and skin. Symptoms include:

- Malar involvement
- Shawl sign: erythema of the face, neck, shoulders, upper chest, and back
- Heliotrope rash: edema and purplish discoloration of the eyelids
- Gottron papules: scaly patches over the back of the hands, particularly PIP and MCP joints

> Dermatomyositis is associated with cancer (25% of cases), often seen in the ovary, lung, GI, and lymphatic system.

Diagnostic testing is as follows:

- CPK and aldolase (**best initial test**)
- Muscle biopsy (**most accurate test**)
- ANA often positive but nonspecific
- Anti-Jo-1 antibodies associated with lung fibrosis
- MRI detects patchy muscle involvement
- Electromyography often abnormal
- ESR, C-reactive protein, and rheumatoid factor may be abnormal but are nonspecific.

> In dermatomyositis, anti-Jo-1 antibodies suggest lung involvement.

Treatment is steroids, which are usually sufficient. When there is no response or intolerance to steroids, use:

- Methotrexate
- Azathioprine
- IV immunoglobulin
- Mycophenolate

Hydroxychloroquine helps the skin lesions.

Inclusion Body Myositis

Inclusion body myositis is slowly progressive weakness of both distal and proximal muscles, which affects distal upper extremity flexors in particular.

On examination, both quadriceps *and* the ability to make a fist are weak at the same time.

- Muscle biopsy is the **most accurate test**.
- Creatinine kinase is elevated.
- There is no treatment.

Mixed Connective Tissue Disease

Mixed connective tissue disease (MCTD) is the overlap between SLE, scleroderma, and polymyositis. The condition is characterized by joint pain with:

- Hand edema and synovitis on presentation
- Myositis and pulmonary hypertension
- Sclerodactyly, calcinosis, malar rash
- Gottron rash
- Kidney involvement (25%)
- Serositis and sicca symptoms (50%)

Testing is anti-U1 ribonuclear protein (RNP) (**most specific test**). If positive for anti-Sm or anti-dsDNA, the more likely the diagnosis is SLE.

Treatment is steroids, azathioprine, or methotrexate. Cyclophosphamide is for interstitial lung disease.

Low Back Pain

Low back pain is extremely common over a lifetime (80% of population). The goal is to identify those few patients with serious pathology that requires radiologic testing and possible surgical treatment.

Degenerative joint disease (DJD) on an x-ray or MRI of the spine is nearly universal in those age >50 and has no meaning when it is found.

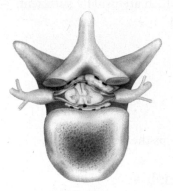

Figure 8.8 Vertebra. *Source: Oleg Reznik*

▶ **TIP**

On the exam, the most frequently tested question about low back pain is "Who should get an imaging study?"

"What Is the Most Likely Diagnosis?"

If all of the diseases described in the following sections are excluded, the patient has simple low back pain from "lumbosacral strain" or idiopathic cause. Imaging and treatment beyond NSAIDs are not needed.

Compression of the Spinal Cord

Malignancy or infection compressing the spinal cord is a **neurological emergency** that needs urgent identification and treatment. Look for a history of cancer combined with the sudden onset of focal neurological deficits such as a sensory level.

- Compression at the level of the 4th thoracic vertebra would lead to sensory loss below the nipples.
- Compression at the 10th thoracic vertebra would lead to sensory loss below the umbilicus.
- Point tenderness at the spine with percussion of the vertebra is highly suggestive of cord compression.
- Hyperreflexia is found below the level of compression.
- Epidural abscess (most often from *Staphylococcus aureus*) presents in the same way as cord compression from cancer, but there is a high fever and markedly elevated ESR.

Disk Herniation (Sciatica)

Herniation at the L4/5 and L5/S1 level accounts for 95% of all disk herniations.

- The straight leg raise (SLR) test is positive if the patient has pain going into the buttock and below the knee when the leg is raised above 60°.
- Although only 50% of those with a positive SLR actually have a herniated disk, the sensitivity is excellent. A negative SLR excludes herniation with 95% sensitivity.

Nerve Root Innervation			
Nerve root	Motor deficit	Reflex affected (lost)	Sensory area affected
L4	Dorsiflexion of foot	Knee jerk	Inner calf
L5	Dorsiflexion of toe	None	Inner forefoot
S1	Eversion of foot	Ankle jerk	Outer foot

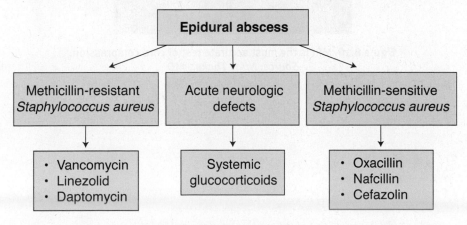

Figure 8.9 Low Back Pain Treatment

Diagnostic testing is as follows:

- Imaging (required) for cord compression, epidural abscess, ankylosing spondylitis, and cauda equina syndrome
- Plain x-ray (**best initial test** for cancer with compression, infection, and fracture)
- MRI (**most accurate test**)
- CT scan (**most accurate test if MRI is contraindicated**, i.e., pacemaker); intrathecal contrast must be given to increase accuracy (CT myelogram)

Imaging in disk herniation is controversial. It is not clear that it actually changes management. On the exam, we recommend that you answer as follows:

- "No MRI" for low back pain and a positive SLR alone
- "Yes MRI" for severe or progressive neurological deficits (paralysis, weakness)

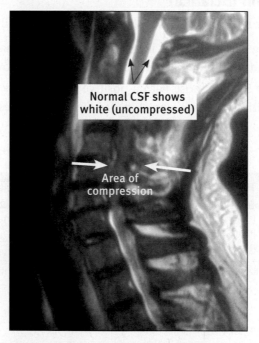

Normal CSF shows white (uncompressed)

Area of compression

Figure 8.10 MRI is the most accurate test of cord compression.
Source: Nirav Thakur, MD

Classification of Back Pain					
Diagnosis	**Cord compression**	**Epidural abscess**	**Cauda equina**	**Ankylosing spondylitis**	**Disk herniation**
History to answer "most likely diagnosis"	History of cancer	Fever, high ESR	Bowel and bladder incontinence, erectile dysfunction	Under age 40, pain worsens with rest and improves with activity	Pain/numbness of medial calf or foot
Physical findings	Vertebral tenderness, sensory level, hyperreflexia	Same as cord compression	Bilateral leg weakness, saddle area anesthesia	Decreased chest mobility	Loss of knee and ankle reflexes, positive straight leg raise

Treatment is as follows:

- Cord compression:
  - Systemic glucocorticoids, chemotherapy for lymphoma, radiation for many solid tumors
  - Surgical decompression if steroids and radiation are not effective
- Epidural abscess:
  - Steroids for acute neurological deficits
  - Antistaphylococcal antibiotics, e.g., vancomycin or linezolid, until sensitivity of the organism is known; if a sensitive *Staphylococcus* is found, switch to beta-lactam antibiotics, e.g., oxacillin, nafcillin, or cefazolin (have greater efficacy when organism is sensitive)
  - Gentamicin is added for synergy with *Staphylococcus* as is done for endocarditis
  - Surgical drainage for larger collections of infected material
- Cauda equina syndrome: surgical decompression
- Disk herniation (sciatica)
  - NSAIDs with continuation of ordinary activities (conservative management); superior to bed rest
  - Yoga (just as effective as a more regimented exercise program for the back)
  - Steroid injection into the epidural space (produces rapid/dramatic benefit for those who do not respond to conservative treatment)
  - Surgery (rarely needed) only if focal neurological deficits develop or progress

> Spine trauma: Steroids are not clearly effective.

> Using glucocorticoids to relieve compression is more important than waiting for test results.

> The most common **wrong answer** for sciatica is **bed rest**. Patients should take NSAIDs and continue their daily activities.

Approach epidural abscess like endocarditis:
- Use vancomycin as initial empiric therapy.
- Switch to oxacillin if it is sensitive.
- Drain it if the infection is large enough to produce neurological deficits or it does not respond to antibiotics alone.

A man with a history of prostate cancer comes to the ED with severe back pain and leg weakness. He has tenderness of the spine, hyperreflexia, and decreased sensation below his umbilicus. What is the most appropriate next step in management?

a. Dexamethasone

b. MRI

c. X-ray

d. Radiation

e. Flutamide

f. Ketoconazole

g. Finasteride

h. Leuprolide (GnRH agonist)

i. Biopsy

j. Orchiectomy

Answer: A. When there is obvious cord compression, the most important step is to begin steroids urgently in order to decrease the pressure on the cord. Radiation is necessary in those with metastatic cancer to the cord, but it does not work as fast as giving steroids. X-ray may show vertebral damage, and MRI is the most accurate imaging study, but preventing permanent paralysis with steroids is more important to do first. Leuprolide is actually dangerous without first blocking the peripheral receptors to testosterone with flutamide. GnRH agonists will give a transient burst up in testosterone levels. Finasteride is a 5-alpha reductase inhibitor that is not helpful for prostate cancer. Finasteride is used for benign prostatic hypertrophy and male pattern hair loss. Ketoconazole is no longer used to inhibit androgens. The fastest way to lower androgen levels is with orchiectomy, but this step is rarely necessary. Biopsy is done if the etiology is not clear. The key issue in this question is timing: What decompresses the spine fastest? The answer is glucocorticoids like dexamethasone.

▶ TIP

Most commonly tested point: In patients without focal neurological abnormalities and patients with simple lumbosacral strain, *do not do imaging studies*.

Lumbar Spinal Stenosis

Narrowing of the spinal canal leading to pressure on the cord is idiopathic. Pain occurs when the back is in extension and the cord presses backward against the ligamentum flavum.

Exertion with leaning back leads to worse pain because of pressure on the cord.

"What Is the Most Likely Diagnosis?"

Look for a person age >60 with back pain while walking, radiating into the buttocks and thighs bilaterally.

- Pain is worse when walking downhill and alleviated when sitting or leading forward (e.g., cycling).
- Pedal pulses and ankle/brachial index are normal.
- Unsteady gait and leg weakness occur when walking.
- Lower extremity reflexes are diminished (25% of cases).

Spinal stenosis can simulate peripheral arterial disease, but the vascular studies are normal.

Diagnostic testing and treatment are as follows:

- MRI is the **most accurate test**.
- Treatment is weight loss and pain meds (NSAIDs, opiates, aspirin) first.
- Steroid injection into the lumbar epidural space (25–50% success rate)
- Physical therapy and exercise such as bicycling or swimming (very effective)
- Surgical correction to dilate the spinal canal (needed in 75% of patients)

Fibromyalgia

"What Is the Most Likely Diagnosis?"

The question will describe a young woman with chronic musculoskeletal pain and tenderness with trigger points of focal tenderness at the trapezius, medial fat pad of the knee, and lateral epicondyle. The cause of fibromyalgia is unknown. Pain occurs at many sites (neck, shoulders, back, and hips) and is associated with:

- Stiffness, numbness, and fatigue
- Headaches
- Sleep disorder (nonrefreshing sleep)

There is no diagnostic testing to confirm fibromyalgia.

Sleep studies show no REM cycle. It is based on a complex of symptoms with trigger points at predictable points. All lab tests are normal such as ESR, C-reactive protein, rheumatoid factor (RF), and CPK.

Treatment is as follows:

- Tricyclic antidepressants, e.g., amitriptyline (**best initial therapy**).
- Dual reuptake inhibitors, e.g., duloxetine and venlafaxine if there is no response to tricyclics
- Milnacipran (an inhibitor of the reuptake of serotonin and norepinephrine, approved specifically for fibromyalgia)
- Pregabalin
- Trigger point injection with local anesthetic
- Aerobic exercise (very helpful)

> Fibromyalgia best initial therapy:
> - Aerobic exercise
> - TCAs

> **Steroids** are the **wrong answer** for fibromyalgia.

Carpal Tunnel Syndrome

Carpal tunnel syndrome is a peripheral neuropathy from the compression of the median nerve as it passes under the flexor retinaculum. Pressure on the nerve interferes with both sensory and motor function of the nerve.

The etiology is not often clear, but it is associated with overuse of the hand and wrist, as well as:

- Pregnancy
- Diabetes
- RA
- Acromegaly
- Amyloidosis
- Hypothyroidism

"What Is the Most Likely Diagnosis?"

Look for a person with pain in the hand affecting the palm, thumb, index finger, and the radial half of the ring finger, with muscle atrophy of the thenar eminence. The pain is worse at night and is more frequent in those whose work involves prolonged use of the hands such as typing.

- Tinel sign: reproduction of the pain and tingling with tapping or percussion of the median nerve
- Phalen sign: reproduction of symptoms with flexion of the wrists to 90°

Carpal tunnel syndrome is usually obvious from the symptoms. Diagnostic testing is as follows:

- Tinel and Phalen signs
- Simple compression of the nerve by squeezing it helps to confirm diagnosis
- Electromyography and nerve conduction testing (**most accurate tests**)

Do not do wrist MRI!

Treatment is as follows:

- Splinting of the wrist to immobilize the hand in a position to relieve pressure
- Avoid manual activity
- Steroid injection if splint and NSAIDs do not control symptoms.
- Surgery can be curative by mechanically decompressing the tunnel such as with cutting open the flexor retinaculum.

When the exam question describes muscle wasting, the answer is surgical release.

> **Sensory** symptoms happen **before motor** symptoms in the progression of carpal tunnel syndrome.

> Wrist MRI is wrong for carpal tunnel!

Dupuytren Contracture

This is the hyperplasia of the palmar fascia leading to nodule formation and contracture of the fourth and fifth fingers. There is a genetic predisposition and an association with alcoholism and cirrhosis. Patients lose the ability to extend their fingers, which is more often a cosmetic embarrassment than a functional impairment.

> Collagenase injection helps early Dupuytren contracture.

Treatment is triamcinolone, lidocaine, or collagenase injection. When function is impaired, surgical release is performed.

Vasculitis

The cause of vasculitis is unknown. Symptoms develop over weeks to months.

There are many vasculitides, including polyarteritis nodosa, granulomatosis with polyangiitis (Wegener granulomatosis), Churg-Strauss, and giant cell arteritis. All cause the following symptoms:

- Fever
- Malaise/fatigue
- Weight loss
- Arthralgia/myalgia

Polyarteritis Nodosa

Polyarteritis nodosa (PAN) is a disease of small and medium-sized arteries leading to a diffuse vasculitis that inexplicably spares the lungs. Chronic hepatitis B and C are associated with PAN.

PAN is very difficult to identify because there is no single pathognomonic feature. Common features include:

- **GI**: abdominal pain is worsened by eating from vasculitis of the mesenteric vessels; bleeding occurs; nausea/vomiting are common
- **Renal**: biopsy is required to distinguish it from other forms of glomerulonephritis, i.e., UA is not enough to diagnose
- **Neurological**: peroneal neuropathy leading to foot drop is most common, but any large peripheral nerve can be involved; look for a stroke in a young person
- **Skin**: lower extremity ulcers are most common; livedo reticularis, purpura, nodules, and rarely gangrene also occur

Mononeuritis multiplex is a confusing term. How can it be "mono" and "multi" at the same time?

Mononeuritis multiplex is multiple simultaneous peripheral neuropathies of nerves that are large enough to have a name—for example, the radial nerve and the peroneal nerve or the ulnar nerve and the lateral femoral cutaneous nerve.

> The lung is spared in PAN.

Diagnostic Tests

Angiography of the renal, mesenteric, or hepatic artery shows abnormal dilation or "beading." All PAN patients should be tested for hepatitis B and C.

The **most accurate test** is a biopsy of a symptomatic site.

Other abnormalities are anemia, leukocytosis, ESR, and C-reactive protein. P-ANCA (antimyeloperoxidase or MPO-ANCA) (<20% of cases). Urinalysis will show protein and RBCs but is nonspecific.

Treatment

Treat PAN with prednisone and cyclophosphamide. Treat hepatitis when found.

Polymyalgia Rheumatica

Polymyalgia rheumatica (PMR) is common age >50. Symptoms include:

- Pain and stiffness in shoulder and pelvic girdle muscles
- Difficulty combing hair and rising from a chair

Diagnostic testing includes:

- Elevated ESR
- Normochromic, normocytic anemia
- No lab findings of muscle destruction, in spite of muscle pain
- Normal CPK and aldolase

Treatment is steroids, which are highly effective even in low doses.

Giant Cell Arteritis

Giant cell arteritis (or temporal arteritis) is on a spectrum with PMR. The difference is the presence of:

- Visual symptoms
- Jaw claudication (pain in jaw when chewing)
- Scalp tenderness
- Headache
- Symptoms in other arteries such as decreased arm pulses, bruits near the clavicles, or aortic regurgitation

ESR and C-reactive protein are elevated. The **most accurate test** is a biopsy of the affected artery such as the temporal artery.

Treatment is prednisone. Starting high-dose prednisone quickly is more important than waiting for the biopsy. Tocilizumab, an anti-IL6 agent, gets the patient off steroids.

> Blindness is not reversible.

Granulomatosis with Polyangiitis

Granulomatosis with polyangiitis (GPA) is also known as Wegener granulomatosis.

"What Is the Most Likely Diagnosis?"

Look for a combination of upper and lower respiratory tract findings in association with renal insufficiency.

Symptoms include:

- Sinusitis
- Otitis media
- Mastoiditis
- Oral and gingival involvement

GPA is also associated with skin, joint, and eye lesions.

The **best initial test** is antineutrophil cytoplasmic antibody (ANCA). Cytoplasmic antibodies are also called "C-ANCA."

- C-ANCA = anti-proteinase-3 (PR3) antibodies
- P-ANCA = anti-myeloperoxidase (MPO) antibodies

The **most accurate test** is a biopsy:

- Lung biopsy (best)
- Renal biopsy (somewhat accurate)
- Sinus biopsy (least accurate)

Treatment is prednisone and cyclophosphamide. Rituximab is an alternative to cyclophosphamide for GPA and microscopic polyangiitis.

- GPA: C-ANCA
- Churg-Strauss and microscopic polyangiitis: P-ANCA

▶ **TIP**

The clue to answering the "most likely diagnosis" question is nonresolving pneumonia that fails to improve with antibiotics. You will not first think of Wegener when presented with the case.

Eosinophilic Granulomatosis with Polyangiitis

Eosinophilic granulomatosis with polyangiitis (or Churg-Strauss syndrome) is a pulmonary–renal syndrome. Symptoms include:

- Asthma
- Eosinophilia
- Fever, weight loss, joint pain, and skin findings (but they are nonspecific)

Eosinophilic GPA is associated with zafirlukast.

Biopsy is the **most accurate test**. Treatment is prednisone and cyclophosphamide. Interleukin inhibitors such as benralizumab or mepolizumab inhibit eosinophils without chronic steroid use in both asthma and eosinophilic GPA.

Henoch-Schönlein Purpura

Henoch-Schönlein purpura (HSP) is a vasculitis commonly seen in children. It is characterized by involvement of:

- **GI**: pain, bleeding
- **Skin**: purpura
- **Joint**: arthralgia
- **Renal**: hematuria

HSP is most often a clinical diagnosis; however, biopsy is the **most accurate test**.

- The presence of leukocytoclastic vasculitis on biopsy confirms diagnosis.
- Serum IgA level is not reliable when testing for HSP.

Most cases resolve spontaneously. Treat with steroids if there is severe abdominal pain or progressive renal insufficiency. (Steroids do not reverse renal insufficiency but may slow progression.) ACE inhibitors are used for proteinuria.

Cryoglobulinemia

Cryoglobulinemia is most commonly associated with chronic hepatitis C infection. It is also found with endocarditis and other connective tissue disorders such as Sjögren syndrome.

Do *not* confuse cryoglobulins with cold agglutinins. Both are IgM antibodies.

Cryoglobulins versus Cold Agglutinins		
	Cryoglobulins	**Cold Agglutinins**
Associated with	Hepatitis C	• EBV • *Mycoplasma* • Lymphoma
Manifestations	• Joint pain • Glomerulonephritis • Purpuric skin lesions • Neuropathy	Hemolysis
Treatment	Hepatitis C medications	• Stay warm • Rituximab, cyclophosphamide, cyclosporine

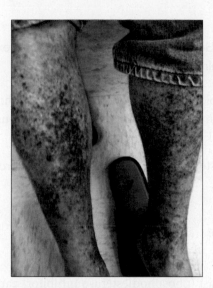

Figure 8.11 These cryoglobulinemia-induced lesions will not "blanch," or turn white, when pressed. Blood vessels are damaged and inflamed.
Source: Nitin Dhiman, MD

Lab testing includes:

- Positive rheumatoid factor
- Cold-precipitable immune complexes

Treat the underlying cause, especially hepatitis C. Steroids are not effective for cryoglobulinemia associated with hepatitis.

- **SLE** → decreased **C3** or **3** letters (SLE) = C3
- **Hep C** → decreased **C4** or **4** letters (Hep C) = C4

▶ **TIP**

Despite the rarity of the condition, the USMLE loves cryoglobulinemia questions.

Behçet Syndrome

Behçet syndrome causes widespread inflammation of blood vessels throughout the body. While rare, it is seen more often in patients who are Asian or Middle Eastern. Symptoms include painful oral and genital ulcers in association with erythema nodosum–like lesions of the skin.

Other symptoms include:

- Ocular lesions leading to uveitis and blindness
- Arthritis
- CNS lesions that mimic multiple sclerosis
- Aneurysm involving the pulmonary and coronary arteries

With Behçet, look for pathergy, in which the skin produces a sterile pustule in response to minor trauma, such as a needle scraped across the surface.

▶ **TIP**

The most common Behçet questions on the USMLE exam have to do with diagnosis and defining "pathergy."

There is no specific blood test for Behçet. The nearest thing to a specific finding is pathergy, which is the production of sterile skin pustule after a needle is scraped against the skin.

Treatment is corticosteroids. To wean patients off of steroids, use:

- Colchicine
- Azathioprine
- Cyclophosphamide
- Thalidomide

In addition, apremilast (phosphodiesterase inhibitor) can be used to alleviate the oral ulcers of Behçet syndrome.

Osteoporosis

Osteoporosis is characterized by decreased bone mass and structural deterioration of the bone. It is common in older people, especially women. The condition causes spontaneous fracture of weight-bearing bones.

Many patients are asymptomatic, and fracture is found on routine screening with bone densitometry, which is recommended for all women age >65.

Diagnostic testing includes a bone densitometry (DEXA) scan (**most accurate test**). The T-score compares the patient's bone density with normal density of a young woman.

- **Osteopenia**: bone density (T-score) 1–2.5 standard deviations below normal
- **Osteoporosis**: T-score >2.5 standard deviations below normal

All blood tests are normal in osteoporosis. Calcium, phosphate, and parathyroid hormone are normal as well.

> The HIV medication tenofovir is associated with premature osteoporosis.

Treatment is as follows:

- Vitamin D and calcium (**best initial treatment**)
- Bisphosphonates (alendronate, risedronate, ibandronate) when T-score >2.5 standard deviations below normal
  - Rarely associated with osteonecrosis of jaw
  - In prolonged contact with esophagus, can cause esophagitis (pill esophagitis)
  - Cannot be used in renal failure
  - Go on a drug holiday after 5 years of use

- Denosumab (RANKL inhibitor)
  - May be used first-line with bisphosphonates
  - Can be used renal failure
- The sclerostin inhibitor romosozumab is an alternative if bisphosphonates or denosumab are ineffective or cannot be tolerated; inhibits osteoclasts and stimulates osteoblasts
- Estrogen replacement, especially for postmenopausal women; alternatively, raloxifene is a substitute for estrogen (also reduces risk of breast cancer and decreases LDL)
- Teriparatide and abaloparatide, analogues of parathyroid hormone that stimulate new bone matrix formation
- Calcitonin used as a nasal spray, to reduce risk of vertebral fractures

> In renal failure, no bisphosphonates, but yes to denosumab.

▶ **TIP**

When multiple treatment options are presented on the exam, choose vitamin D, calcium, and bisphosphonates.

Infections

Septic Arthritis

Septic arthritis is an infection of any kind that finds its way into the joint space. Because the synovial lining has no basement membrane, it is relatively "loose" and both bacteria and antibiotics easily find their way across it.

The risk of infection is directly proportional to the degree of joint damage.

- In an undamaged joint, septic arthritis is relatively rare.
- Osteoarthritis, or degenerative joint disease (DJD), poses a slight risk; RA poses an intermediate risk (due to greater destruction); and a prosthetic joint poses the greatest risk.
- Endocarditis and injection drug use can cause septic arthritis as a result of bacteremia spreading into the joint space.

The etiology of septic arthritis is as follows:

- *Staphylococcus*: 40% of cases
- *Streptococcus*: 30% of cases
- Gram-negative rods: 20% of cases

Presentation includes a joint that is warm, red, and immobile, often with a palpable effusion. Chills and fever are common because of bacteremia.

> A joint with septic arthritis is **warm, red,** and **immobile**.

Diagnostic testing is as follows:

- Aspiration of the joint with a needle (arthrocentesis) (**best initial and most accurate test**)
- X-ray, CT, and MRI are not useful.
- Joint fluid
  - Leukocytosis: >50,000–100,000 cells, mostly neutrophils
  - Gram stain: positive (50%) gram-positive bacilli; (75%) with *Staphylococcus*
  - Synovial fluid culture: 70–90% sensitive
  - Blood cultures: 50% sensitive

Treatment

The **best initial empiric treatment** for septic arthritis is ceftriaxone and vancomycin.

Adjust antibiotics according to culture results. If the *Staphylococcus* is sensitive, switch drugs. Vancomycin is associated with a worse outcome than a beta-lactam antibiotic such as oxacillin or cefazolin.

Alternative Therapies for Septic Arthritis		
Gram-negative bacilli	**Gram-positive cocci (sensitive)**	**Gram-positive cocci (resistant)**
• Quinolones • Aztreonam • Cefotaxime • Piperacillin • Aminoglycosides	• Oxacillin, nafcillin • Cefazolin • Piperacillin with tazobactam	• Linezolid • Daptomycin • Ceftaroline • Vancomycin

Prosthetic joints are very common in the United States. An infected prosthetic joint will produce a warm, red, immobile, and tender joint. Management of an infected prosthetic joint is very specific.

- X-ray or CT scan is required to tell whether the infection is limited to the joint space or has spread into the bone around the implantation of the joint.
- MRI should not be performed, because prosthetic joints are made of metal.
- If imaging shows lucency around the implantation of joint or if the joint is physically loose, infection at the implantation site is likely.
- Treatment of an infected prosthetic joint is challenging, as it is difficult to sterilize without removing the joint; therefore, remove the joint, treat with antibiotics for 6–8 weeks, and then replace the joint.

The **most common organism** to infect recently placed artificial joints is *Staphylococcus epidermidis*.

Gonococcal Arthritis (Gonorrhea)

Look for a history of STDs or a sexually active young person. The differences in presentation from septic arthritis are:

- Polyarticular involvement
- Tenosynovitis (inflammation of the tendon sheaths, making finger movement painful)
- Petechial rash

> Gonococcal arthritis is more frequent during **menses**.

Diagnostic Tests

Detecting gonorrhea is much more difficult than detecting the *Staphylococcus*, *Streptococcus*, and gram-negative bacilli of septic arthritis.

Synovial Fluid Analysis for Infectious Arthritis		
Test sensitivity	**Septic arthritis**	**Gonococcal arthritis**
Leukocytosis	>50,000–100,000 cells/μL	30,000–50,000 cells/μL
Gram stain	50–75% sensitive	25% sensitive
Culture	90% sensitive	<50% sensitive
Blood cultures	50% sensitive	<10% sensitive

To reach maximum sensitivity, you should culture multiple diffuse sites (e.g., the pharynx, rectum, urethra, and cervix) for gonorrhea.

Additionally, if the following are present, you should culture everywhere:

- Rash
- Tenosynovitis
- Polyarticular involvement

Treatment is as follows:

- Ceftriaxone, cefotaxime, or ceftizoxime (**best empiric therapy** for disseminated gonorrhea)
- Fluoroquinolones are not the best initial treatment because >5% are resistant.
- Quinolones only if organism is confirmed to be sensitive

▶ TIP

If recurrent gonorrhea infection is described, test for terminal complement deficiency—a favorite subject of USMLE exam.

> *Salmonella* is the most commonly identified organism producing bone infection in patients with sickle cell disease.

> Bone scan is the answer *only if* you want to get an MRI and it is contraindicated (pacemaker).

Osteomyelitis

Osteomyelitis is an infection of the bone. Although *Staphylococcus aureus* is the most common cause, any organism can infect the bone.

- Children get osteomyelitis through hematogenous spread.
- Adults get osteomyelitis from a contiguous (nearby) infection, most often as a result of vascular insufficiency and diabetes.

Look for a diabetic patient with an ulcer from peripheral neuropathy or vascular disease with warmth, redness, and swelling in the area. There may also be a draining "purulent sinus tract" in the lesion. Most patients are afebrile.

Diagnostic testing includes:

- X-ray (**best initial test**); if x-ray is normal, MRI is most appropriate next step
- Biopsy (**most accurate test**); obtain biopsy before starting antibiotics
- CT scan not useful

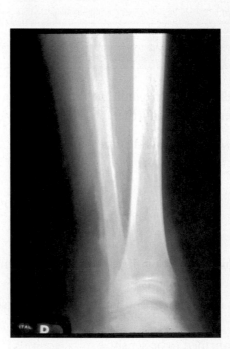 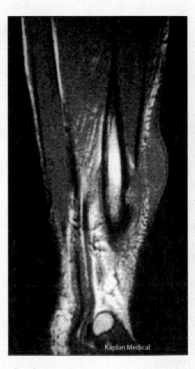

Figures 8.12, 8.13 Osteomyelitis. In the x-ray (left), look for periosteal elevation. The MRI (right) is just as sensitive as a bone scan and reveals abnormality 48 hours after onset of infection, with far greater specificity.

When is ESR the answer?

- To follow the response to therapy.

When is "culture the drainage" the answer?

- Never. You cannot reliably distinguish superficial colonization from whatever organism is inside the bone causing the bone infection.

Treatment

Osteomyelitis takes weeks to progress. Obtain a biopsy to identify what organism is present and what it is sensitive to. Then treat the organism that is found.

- Oxacillin, cefazolin, nafcillin, or ceftriaxone for sensitive staphylococci
- Vancomycin, daptomycin, dalbavancin, or oritavancin for resistant staphylococci; dalbavancin and oritavancin are long-acting versions of vancomycin (single IV dose lasts 1–2 weeks) that are ideal for the long-term treatment of osteomyelitis
- Fluoroquinolones such as ciprofloxacin for gram-negative bacilli such as *E. coli* (sensitivity of the organism must be confirmed before administering ciprofloxacin)
  - Side effects of fluoroquinolones include Achilles tendon rupture due to interference with chondrocyte growth.
  - Fluoroquinolones are contraindicated in pregnancy and in children due to interference with bone growth.

> Ciprofloxacin is the only oral therapy for osteomyelitis, but it should be used only if the organism is confirmed as a sensitive gram-negative bacillus.

> The most common wrong answer in osteomyelitis is "6 weeks of empiric treatment."

Hematology 9

Anemia

Anemia is a condition characterized by decreased RBCs (hemoglobin) in the blood. Symptoms for all types of anemia can be identical if they have the same hematocrit. In other words, you cannot diagnose simply from symptoms.

The **best initial test** for anemia is complete blood count (CBC), which establishes the presence of anemia. The first clue to etiology is mean corpuscular volume (MCV).

Symptoms of anemia are often based on the severity of disease (not the on the etiology).

- Hematocrit >**30%**: no expected symptoms
- Hematocrit **25–30%**: dyspnea (worse on exertion), fatigue
- Hematocrit **20–25%**: lightheadedness
- Hematocrit <**20%**: syncope, chest pain

Ultimately, cardiac ischemia from anemia proves fatal.
Myocytes in the heart cannot distinguish between:

- Anemia
- Hypoxia
- Coronary artery disease
- Carbon monoxide poisoning

All of these conditions will cause decreased oxygen delivery to tissues.

Microcytic Anemia

Microcytic anemia is characterized by low MCV (normal <80 fL). Most causes relate to *production*:

- **Iron deficiency**: caused by blood loss
  - The body only needs a tiny amount of iron, ~1–2 mg per day.
  - Menstruating women need ~2–3 mg per day, while pregnant women need as much as 5–6 mg per day.
  - The duodenum can absorb ~4 mg per day.
  - Thus, as little as one teaspoon (5 mL) a day of blood loss will lead to iron deficiency over time.
- **Thalassemia (very common cause)**: often asymptomatic in those with thalassemia trait alone
- **Sideroblastic anemia**: caused by an inability of iron to incorporate with heme
  - Most common cause is suppressive effect of alcohol on bone marrow
  - Less common causes are lead poisoning, isoniazid, and vitamin B6 deficiency
  - Can be macrocytic as well when associated with myelodysplasia, a preleukemic syndrome
- **Chronic disease**: any cancer or chronic infection
  - Iron is locked in storage or trapped in macrophages or in ferritin.
  - Hemoglobin synthesis will not occur because the iron just does not move forward.
  - Initially the MCV is normal, and then it decreases.
  - Inflammation gives an increase in hepcidin, which regulates iron absorption. Hepcidin will be elevated in anemia of chronic disease.

> Sideroblastic anemia can be **microcytic** or **macrocytic**.

Production problems are nearly synonymous with low reticulocyte count. (Only alpha thalassemia with 3 genes deleted has an elevated reticulocyte.)

Routine blood smear will not distinguish the types of microcytosis. All of them will be hypochromic and all of them potentially give target cells.

Normocytic Anemia

- Acute blood loss or hemolysis can cause a drop in hematocrit so rapid that there is no time for the MCV to change. Blood loss ultimately leads to iron deficiency and microcytosis.
- Eventually, hemolysis will elevate the reticulocyte count, which will elevate the MCV (since reticulocytes are slightly larger than normal cells).
- Methotrexate causes macrocytic anemia, while RA causes the anemia of chronic disease.

> Blood loss and hemolysis will elevate the reticulocyte count.

Chronic renal failure routinely produces normocytic anemia.

If the anemia is severe, treatment is transfusion of packed RBCs. Knowing when to transfuse depends on the following factors:

- **Is patient symptomatic?** Then transfuse. Symptoms include:
  - Shortness of breath, lightheadedness, confusion
  - Possible syncope
  - Hypotension and tachycardia
  - Chest pain
- **Is hematocrit very low in an elderly patient or one with heart disease?** Then transfuse.
  - "Very low" hematocrit means 25–30% in an elderly patient or one with heart disease.
- **Is patient asymptomatic and young?** Not necessary to transfuse.

Whole blood is never given. Whole blood is divided into PRBCs or FFP.

- **Packed red blood cells** (PRBCs), a concentrated form of blood, are a unit of whole blood with ~150 mL of plasma removed.
  - Hematocrit of PRBCs is 70–80% (due to plasma removal, double the normal).
  - Each unit of PRBCs should raise hematocrit by ~3 points, or 1 g/dL of Hb.
- **Fresh frozen plasma** (FFP) replaces clotting factors in those with elevated PT, aPTT, or INR + bleeding; combine FFP with plasmapheresis.
- **Cryoprecipitate** is used to replace fibrinogen and has some utility in disseminated intravascular coagulation. It provides high amounts of clotting factors in a smaller plasma volume. High levels of factor VIII and VWF are found in it.
- **Platelets** are pooled from the donations of multiple donors. Give to a bleeding patient if platelet count <50,000. Platelet infusion is contraindicated in TTP. Prothrombin complex concentrate (PCC) has all vitamin K factors used to reverse warfarin toxicity.

> - For IgA-deficient recipients, use IgA-deficient donor FFP.
> - FFP is not used for hemophilia A/B or von Willebrand disease.
> - Cryoprecipitate is not used *first* for anything.

"What Is the Most Likely Diagnosis?"

You cannot distinguish the types of anemia based on symptoms alone. The history might provide some suggestions.

| How to Answer "What Is the Most Likely Diagnosis?" for Anemia ||
Feature in the history	Most likely diagnosis
Blood loss (GI bleeding)	Iron deficiency
Menstruation	Iron deficiency
Cancer or chronic infection	Chronic disease
Rheumatoid arthritis	Chronic disease
Alcoholic	Sideroblastic
Asymptomatic	Thalassemia

Diagnostic Tests

Iron studies are the **best initial test** for anemia.

- **Low ferritin**: very specific for iron deficiency anemia
  - Because ferritin is an acute phase reactant, ~35% of patients have normal or elevated ferritin. This means that any concurrent infection or inflammation can elevate the ferritin.
  - Both iron deficiency and the anemia of chronic disease are associated with a low serum iron. However, iron deficiency is associated with an increase in the total iron-binding capacity (TIBC). This is a measure of the unbound sites on transferrin.
  - When there are a lot of open sites on transferrin, the capacity of unbound sites increases. Iron divided by TIBC equals transferrin saturation.
- **High iron** suggests sideroblastic anemia, the only form of microcytic anemia in which circulating iron is elevated.
- **Normal iron** suggests thalassemia, a genetic disease with normal iron.
- **Low iron** suggests chronic disease because iron is trapped in storage. That is why the ferritin ("stored iron") is elevated or normal. Circulating iron is decreased. However, the major point of difference is that TIBC is low.

Peripheral smear is not useful, as all of the causes of microcytic anemia can be hypochromic or associated with target cells (target cells are most common with thalassemia).

Unique laboratory features include:

- **Iron deficiency**: The RBC distribution of width (RDW) is increased because the newer cells are more iron deficient and smaller. As the body runs out of iron, the newer cells have less hemoglobin and get progressively smaller. There is an elevated platelet count. The single **most accurate test** is a bone marrow biopsy for stainable iron which is decreased.
- **Thalassemia**: Hemoglobin electrophoresis is the **most accurate test**, except in alpha thalassemia, where genetic studies are the **most accurate test**. Only 3-gene deletion alpha thalassemia is associated with hemoglobin H and elevated reticulocytes. All forms have a normal RDW.
- **Sideroblastic anemia**: Prussian blue staining for ringed sideroblasts is the **most accurate test**. Basophilic stippling can occur in any cause of sideroblastic anemia.

> Alpha thalassemia is diagnosed by DNA analysis.

> Only 3-gene deletion alpha thalassemia has high reticulocytes.

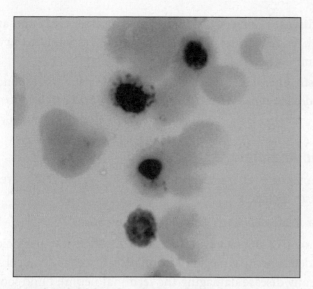

Figure 9.1 Ringed sideroblasts are detected with Prussian blue staining.
Source: Alireza Eghtedar, MD

Electrophoresis Findings	
Alpha thalassemia	**Beta thalassemia**
One gene deleted: normal	One gene defective: minor • HbA slightly decreased • HbA$_2$ increased to 5% (normal 2.5%) • HbF increased to 2% (normal 1%)
Two genes deleted: mild anemia, normal electrophoresis	Two genes defective: major • Little or no HbA • Increased HbA$_2$ and HbF
Three genes deleted: moderate anemia with hemoglobin H, which are beta-4 tetrads; increased reticulocytes	N/A
Four genes deleted: gamma-4 tetrads or hemoglobin Bart; CHF causes death in utero	N/A

Treatment

- **Iron deficiency**: Replace iron with oral ferrous sulfate. If this is insufficient, occasionally patients are treated with intravenous iron.

- **Thalassemia**: Trait is not treated. Beta thalassemia major (Cooley anemia) is managed with chronic transfusion lifelong.

  - Iron overload is managed with deferasirox or deferiprone, oral iron chelators. Deferoxamine is a parenteral version of an iron chelator.

  - Luspatercept (tissue growth factor) decreases transfusion dependence in beta thalassemia and myelodysplasia.

> Deferiprone and deferasirox are oral iron chelators used to treat hemochromatosis resulting from transfusion.

- **Chronic disease**: Correct the underlying disease. Only the anemia associated with end-stage renal failure routinely responds to erythropoietin replacement.
- **Sideroblastic anemia**: Correct the cause. Some patients respond to vitamin B6 or pyridoxine replacement. This is why isoniazid can lead to sideroblastic anemia.

Macrocytic Anemia

Macrocytic anemia is characterized by high MCV, i.e., RBCs are larger than normal. Causes include:

- B12 and/or folate deficiency (**most common causes**)
  - **Causes of B12 deficiency**: pancreatic insufficiency; pernicious anemia; dietary deficiency (e.g., vegan); Crohn disease, celiac, tropical sprue, radiation (or any disease damaging the terminal ileum); blind loop syndrome (gastrectomy or gastric bypass for weight loss); *Diphyllobothrium latum*, HIV, metformin
  - **Causes of folate deficiency**: dietary deficiency (e.g., goat's milk has no folate and provides limited iron and B12); psoriasis and skin loss or turnover; drugs (e.g., phenytoin, sulfa, methotrexate)
- Sideroblastic anemia
- Alcoholism
- Antimetabolite medication such as azathioprine, 6-MP, or hydroxyurea
- Liver disease or hypothyroidism
- Medication such as zidovudine or phenytoin
- Myelodysplastic syndrome (MDS)
- Cold agglutinins (falsely elevate MCV by clumping cells)

Macrocytic anemia will cause a low reticulocyte count. Although alcohol can cause macrocytic anemia and neurological problems, it will not lead to hypersegmented neutrophils.

> A 73-year-old man presents with increasing fatigue over several months. He is also short of breath when he walks up a flight of stairs. He drinks 4 vodka martinis a day. He has numbness and tingling in his feet. On physical examination decreased sensation of the feet is noted. Hematocrit is 28% and MCV 114 fL (elevated). What is the most appropriate next step in management?
>
> a. Vitamin B12 level
> b. Folate level
> c. Peripheral blood smear
> d. Schilling test
> e. Methylmalonic acid level
>
> Answer: **C.** Whatever the cause of the macrocytic anemia, the first step is a peripheral smear to detect hypersegmented neutrophils. Once those are seen, you would get B12 and folate levels.

> Metformin is associated with B12 deficiency.

> Celiac disease causes B12, folate, and iron deficiency.

> Megaloblastic anemia is the presence of hypersegmented neutrophils. Many factors raise the MCV, but only B12 and folate deficiency and antimetabolite medications cause hypersegmentation.

▶ **TIP**

B12 deficiency can lead to any neurological abnormality, however:

- Peripheral neuropathy (**most common**)
- Dementia (least common)
- Posterior column damage to position and vibratory sensation or "subacute combined degeneration" of the cord (**classic**)
- Look for ataxia

Diagnostic Tests

B12 deficiency and folate deficiency are identical hematologically and on blood smear. Lab abnormalities common to both B12 and folate deficiencies are:

- Megaloblastic anemia
- Elevated LDH
- Elevated indirect bilirubin level
- Decreased reticulocyte count
- Hypercellular bone marrow
- Macroovalocytes
- Increased homocysteine levels

Increased methylmalonic acid (MMA) level is associated only with B12 deficiency.

> **B12 deficiency:**
>
> High LDH + high bilirubin + low reticulocytes = **ineffective erythropoiesis**

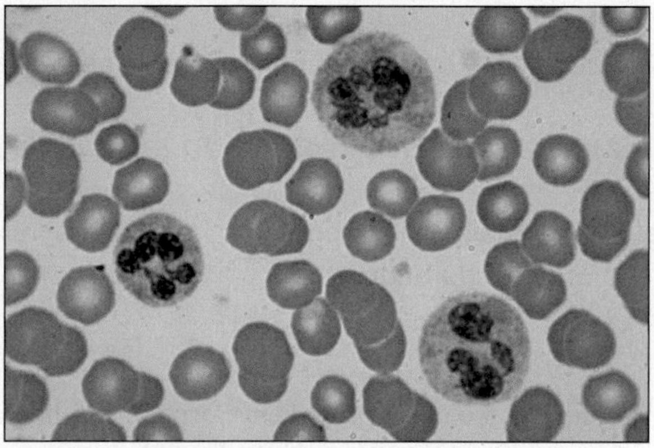

Figure 9.2 Hypersegmented Neutrophils (best initial test for determining the etiology of macrocytic anemia).
Source: Alireza Eghtedar, MD

A 73-year-old woman comes with decreased positional and vibratory sensation of the lower extremities, hematocrit 28%, MCV 114 fL, and hypersegmented neutrophils. B12 level is decreased but near the borderline of normal. What is the most appropriate next step in management?

a. Methylmalonic acid level
b. Anti-intrinsic factor antibodies
c. Anti-parietal cell antibodies
d. Schillings test
e. Folate level
f. Homocysteine level

Answer: **A.** The USMLE Step 2 exam often tests the fact that while both B12 and folate deficiency increase homocysteine levels, only B12 is associated with an increased MMA. B12 can be normal in as many as 35% of patients with B12 deficiency because the carrier protein, transcobalamin, is an acute phase reactant and can be elevated from many forms of stress such as infection, cancer, or trauma. When the vignette suggests B12 deficiency but the B12 level is equivocal, use an elevated MMA to confirm the diagnosis of vitamin B12 deficiency.

▶ **TIP**

Tested facts about macrocytic anemia:

- Schilling test is never the right answer.
- Pernicious anemia is confirmed with anti-intrinsic factor and anti-parietal cell antibodies.
- RBCs are destroyed as they leave the marrow, so the reticulocyte count is low.
- B12 and folate deficiency can cause pancytopenia as well as macrocytic anemia.
- Pancreatic enzymes are needed to absorb B12. They free it from carrier proteins.
- Neurological abnormalities will improve as long as they are minor (e.g., peripheral) and of short duration.

| B12 deficiency can produce neurological or hematological abnormalities—or both. |

Treatment

Replace what is deficient. Folate replacement corrects the hematologic problems of B12 deficiency, but not the neurological problems.

| Pancreatic enzymes are needed to remove B12 from the R-protein so it can bind with intrinsic factor. |

Which of the following is a complication of B12 or folate replacement?

a. Seizures
b. Hemolysis
c. Hypokalemia
d. Hyperkalemia
e. Diarrhea

Answer: **C.** Extremely rapid cell production in the bone marrow causes hypokalemia. There is no other condition in which cells are generated so rapidly that they use up all the potassium. Hyperkalemia from massive tissue or cellular breakdown has many causes. Hypokalemia from cell production is rare. When replacing B12 and folate, particularly if there is pancytopenia, cells in the marrow are produced so rapidly that the marrow packages up all the potassium, lowering the serum level. Observe and replace.

Hemolytic Anemia

All forms of hemolysis can lead to:

- Sudden decrease in hematocrit
- Increased LDH, indirect bilirubin, and reticulocytes
- Decreased haptoglobin
- Slight increase in MCV because reticulocytes are larger than normal cells
- Hyperkalemia from cell breakdown
- Folate deficiency from increased cell production using it up; folate stores are limited

Chronic hemolysis is associated with bilirubin gallstones.

Sickle Cell Disease

Sickle cell is a chronic, usually well-compensated hemolytic anemia with a reticulocyte count that is always high. It is commonly seen in African American patients.

Excess copper causes hemolysis.

Sickle cell is caused by a point mutation at position 6 of the beta globin chain: valine replaces glutamic acid.

Symptoms of sickle cell include:

- Bilirubin gallstones from chronically elevated bilirubin
- Increased infection from autosplenectomy, particularly encapsulated organisms
- Osteomyelitis, often from *Salmonella*
- Retinopathy
- Stroke

Children present with dactylitis (inflammation of fingers).

- Lower extremity skin ulcers
- Avascular necrosis of the femoral head (x-ray is **best initial test**, while MRI is **most accurate test**)

Acute, painful vaso-occlusive crisis presents with sudden, severe pain in the chest, back, and thighs, and possible fever. Causes of acute crisis include hypoxia, dehydration, infection/fever, and cold temperatures. It is rare for an adult to present with an acute crisis without a clear history of sickle cell.

Papillary necrosis of the kidney arises from chronic kidney damage.

Diagnostic testing includes peripheral smear (**best initial test**). Sickle cell trait (AS disease) does not produce sickled cells. Hemoglobin electrophoresis is the **most accurate test.**

Which of the following can be found on smear in sickle cell disease?

a. Basophilic stippling
b. Howell-Jolly bodies
c. Bite cells
d. Schistocytes
e. Morulae

Answer: **B.** Howell-Jolly bodies are precipitated remnants of nuclear material seen inside the RBCs of a patient who has no spleen. There is no change in management if they are present. Basophilic stippling is associated with a number of causes of sideroblastic anemia, especially lead poisoning. Bite cells are seen in glucose 6 phosphate dehydrogenase deficiency. Schistocytes are fragmented RBCs seen with intravascular hemolysis. Morulae are seen inside WBCs in *Anaplasma* and *Ehrlichia* infections.

> Nucleated RBCs are found with premature release of precursor blood cells.

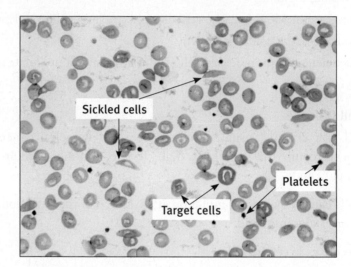

Figure 9.3 Target cells can occur with many hematological diseases, including sickle cell disease. *Source: Abhay Vakil, MD.*

Begin treatment of **acute crisis** with oxygen/hydration/analgesia.

If there is fever or high WBCs, give antibiotics (ceftriaxone, levofloxacin, or moxifloxacin). Do not wait for test results to start antibiotics if there is a fever. The absence of a functional spleen leads to overwhelming infection.

Manage **chronic disease** as follows:

- Replace folic acid as needed.
- Give pneumococcal vaccination because of autosplenectomy.
- Give hydroxyurea to prevent recurrences.
  - Increase hydroxyurea dose until hemoglobin F rises >10–15%.
  - However, if WBC count is low, do not increase the dose.

Hydroxyurea in prevention and antibiotics with fever will lower mortality in sickle cell disease. In addition, give agents to promote oxygen-carrying capacity:

- **Voxelotor** increases capacity by decreasing hemoglobin S polymerization.
- **Crizanlizumab-IgG** decreases platelet aggregation and promotes oxygen-carrying capacity by binding to p-selectin.

> **Exchange transfusion is used if there is severe vaso-occlusive crisis presenting with:**
> - Acute chest syndrome
> - Priapism
> - Stroke
> - Visual disturbance from retinal infarction

Aplastic Crisis

A 43-year-old man with sickle cell disease is admitted with an acute pain crisis. His only routine medication is folic acid. His hematocrit on admission is 34%, and on hospital day 3 it drops to 22%. What is the best initial test?

a. Reticulocyte count
b. Peripheral smear
c. Folate level
d. Parvovirus B19 IgM level
e. Bone marrow

Answer: **A.** Patients with sickle cell disease usually have very high reticulocytes because of the chronic compensated hemolysis. When reticulocyte count is normal in sickle cell disease, it is a very bad sign. Parvovirus B19 causes an aplastic crisis that freezes the growth of the marrow. Nothing will be visible on blood smear. Although the bone marrow will show giant pronormoblasts, this would not be done routinely, and certainly never as the initial test. The first clue to parvovirus is a sudden drop in reticulocyte level.

> The **most accurate test** for parvovirus B19 is a PCR for DNA. This is more accurate than the IgM level. IV immunoglobulin is the best initial treatment.

Sickle Cell Trait

Sickle cell trait means the patient is heterozygous for the sickle gene (AS). The only manifestation of sickle cell trait is a defect in the ability to concentrate the urine or "isosthenuria."

Patients are clinically asymptomatic and have both a normal CBC level and a normal smear result. Hematuria can occur.

There is no treatment for sickle cell trait.

Hereditary Spherocytosis

Hereditary spherocytosis is a defect in the cytoskeleton of the RBC leading to an abnormal round shape and loss of the normal flexibility characteristic of the biconcave disc that allows RBCs to bend in the spleen.

Symptoms include:

- Recurrent episodes of hemolysis
- Intermittent jaundice
- Splenomegaly
- Family history of anemia or hemolysis
- Bilirubin gallstones

Diagnostic testing includes:

- Low MCV
- Increased mean corpuscular hemoglobin concentration (MCHC)
- Negative Coombs test
- Eosin-5-maleimide flow cytometry (**most accurate test**) (more accurate than osmotic fragility testing, where cells are placed in a slightly hypotonic solution and the increased swelling of the cells leads to hemolysis)

Treatment is chronic folic acid replacement to support RBC production. Splenectomy will stop the hemolysis but will not eliminate the spherocytes.

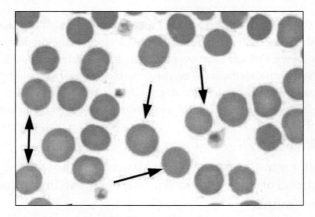

Figure 9.4 Spherocytes lose the central pallor of normal red blood cells. MCHC is elevated. *Source: Alireza Eghtedar, MD*

Autoimmune (Warm or IgG) Hemolysis

There is no identified etiology in 50% of cases. Clear causes are:

- Chronic lymphocytic leukemia (CLL)
- Lymphoma
- Systemic lupus erythematosus (SLE)
- Drugs: penicillin, alpha-methyldopa, rifampin, phenytoin

Autoimmune hemolysis is associated with microspherocytes.

- Autoantibodies remove small amounts of RBC membrane and lead to a smaller membrane, forcing the cell to become round.
- Biconcave discs need a greater surface area than a sphere.

The **most accurate test** is the Coombs test, which detects IgG antibody on the surface of the RBCs. (Direct and indirect Coombs tests tell basically the same thing, but the indirect test is associated with a greater amount of antibody.)

▶ **TIP**

The smear does not show fragmented cells in autoimmune hemolysis because the RBC destruction occurs inside the spleen or liver, not in the blood vessel.

Treatment is as follows:

- Glucocorticoids, e.g., prednisone (**best initial therapy**)
  - Intravenous immunoglobulin (IVIG) for severe, acute hemolysis when no response to prednisone
  - Cyclophosphamide, cyclosporine, azathioprine, and mycophenolate mofetil are alternative treatments to diminish the need for steroids
- Splenectomy for recurrent episodes
  - Rituximab, azathioprine, cyclophosphamide, or cyclosporine when splenectomy does not control hemolysis

Cold Agglutinin Disease

Cold agglutinins are IgM antibodies against the red blood cell developing in association with Epstein-Barr virus, Waldenström macroglobulinemia, or *Mycoplasma pneumoniae*.

Symptoms occur in colder parts of the body, for instance, numbness or mottling of the nose, ears, fingers, and toes. Symptoms resolve upon warming of the body part.

The direct Coombs test is positive only for complement. The smear is normal or may show only spherocytes. Cold agglutinin titer is the **most accurate test**.

Treatment is as follows:

- Keep patient warm
- Rituximab
- Plasmapheresis in some cases
- Cyclophosphamide, cyclosporine, or another immunosuppressive agent to stop production of the antibody
- Steroids and splenectomy are not effective

▶**TIP**

Steroids and splenectomy do not work in cold agglutinin disease. Prednisone is the most common wrong answer.

Do not mix up **cryoglobulins** with **cold agglutinins**. Although both are IgM and neither responds to steroids, only cryoglobulins are associated with:

- Hepatitis C
- Joint pain
- Glomerulonephritis

Glucose 6 Phosphate Dehydrogenase Deficiency

Glucose 6 phosphate dehydrogenase (G6PD) deficiency is an X-linked recessive disorder that leads to an inability to generate glutathione reductase and protect the RBCs from oxidant stress such as:

- Infection (**most common oxidant stress**)
- Dapsone, quinidine, primaquine, nitrofurantoin
- Fava beans

Look for sudden anemia and jaundice in an African American or Mediterranean man with a normal-sized spleen who has an infection or is using one of the drugs listed.

Testing is as follows:

- Heinz bodies and bite cells (**best initial test**)
- G6PD level (2–3 months after an acute episode of hemolysis) (**most accurate test**); the G6PD will be normal after a hemolytic event
- Heinz bodies are seen on special stain (methylene blue or crystal violet)

There is no treatment for hemolysis. Avoid oxidant stress. Use caution with rasburicase, which provokes hemolysis in G6PD.

> Because G6PD deficiency is X-linked recessive, it manifests almost exclusively in men.

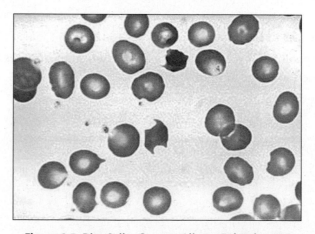

Figure 9.5 Bite Cells. *Source: Alireza Eghtedar, MD*

Thrombotic Thrombocytopenic Purpura and Hemolytic Uremic Syndrome

Thrombotic thrombocytopenic purpura (TTP) and hemolytic uremic syndrome (HUS) are variants of what is probably the same disease. TTP is associated with HIV, cancer, and drugs such as cyclosporine, ticlopidine, and clopidogrel. HUS is more common in children, and the most frequently tested association is *E. coli* 0157:H7 and *Shigella*. Both TTP and HUS are associated with:

- Intravascular hemolysis
- Renal insufficiency
- Thrombocytopenia (<30,000)

The hemolysis is visible on smear with schistocytes, helmet cells, and fragmented red blood cells.

TTP is associated with:

- Neurological symptoms
- Fever

It is not necessary to have all 5 manifestations to establish a diagnosis of TTP. In fact, the only indispensable finding to establish the diagnosis is the intravascular hemolysis. A low ADAMTS 13 level supports the diagnosis of TTP.

> PT and aPTT are normal in HUS/TTP.

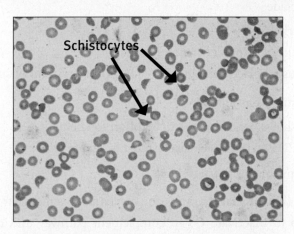

Figure 9.6 Fragmented red blood cells, or schistocytes, are characteristic of intravascular hemolysis. *Source: Abhay Vakil, MD.*

Treatment of TTP and HUS is as follows:

- Plasmapheresis is generally urgent in TTP. Severe HUS also needs urgent plasmapheresis. If plasmapheresis is not one of the choices, use infusions of fresh frozen plasma (FFP).
- Most cases of HUS from *E. coli* resolve spontaneously. Eculizumab treats severe, atypical HUS.
  - "Atypical" means HUS does not arise from infection; instead, it occurs when complement erroneously attacks red blood cells.
  - Eculizumab blocks complement (C5a). This is why vaccination for meningococcus is required with eculizumab use.

- Steroids help in TTP, but not in HUS. This is because there are antibodies to ADAMTS 13 in TTP; it is not the mechanism of HUS.
- Caplacizumab is an antibody against VWF, so it acts like ADAMTS 13. Rituximab and ocrelizumab are anti-CD20 drugs that stop the production of antibodies to ADAMTS 13.

▶ **TIP**

Platelet transfusion is never the correct choice for TTP or HUS.

Paroxysmal Nocturnal Hemoglobinuria

Paroxysmal nocturnal hemoglobinuria (PNH) is a clonal stem cell defect with increased sensitivity of RBCs to complement in acidosis.

- Mechanism is complement overactivation
- Cause is deficiency of the complement regulatory proteins CD 55 and 59 (known as decay-accelerating factor)

The gene for phosphatidylinositol class A (PIG-A) is defective. This leads to overactivation of the complement system. In an unaffected person, that would mean nothing, but in PNH it leads to hemolysis and thrombosis (**most common form of death**).

> PNH is a stem cell defect that may cause aplastic anemia, myelodysplasia, or acute leukemia.

Symptoms include:

- Episodic dark urine
- Pancytopenia and iron deficiency anemia
- Clots in unusual places (not just DVT or pulmonary embolism)

Diagnostic testing is as follows:

- CBC often shows pancytopenia in addition to anemia
- CD55 and CD59 will be decreased (**most accurate test**)

> The Ham and sucrose hemolysis tests are obsolete. **Flow cytometry** is another way of saying CD55/CD59 testing.

Treatment of PNH is as follows:

- Prednisone (**best initial therapy**); the mechanism is not clear
- Eculizumab to inactivate C5 in complement pathway and decrease RBC destruction
  - Eculizumab is essentially a "complement inhibitor." It treats hemolysis and thrombosis.
  - Give meningococcal vaccine prior to administering.
- Folic acid and replacement with transfusions as needed
- Allogeneic bone marrow transplant (only curative treatment)

> Large vessel thrombosis of the mesenteric and hepatic veins is the most common site of thrombosis.

A patient presents with increased bilirubin, LDH, and reticulocyte count and decreased platelet count of 30,000. Creatinine is elevated, and smear is positive for schistocytes. There is no history of diarrhea. What is the next step in management?

a. Steroids
b. Eculizumab
c. Platelets
d. IVIG
e. Ciprofloxacin

Answer: **B**. This patient has hemolytic uremic syndrome (HUS). Eculizumab removes complement C5 and interrupts the hemolysis of HUS. Steroids help TTP because antibodies attack ADAMTS 13. Platelets worsen both HUS and TTP. IVIG is useless (although plasma exchange helps). Antibiotics can worsen HUS.

Aplastic Anemia

Aplastic anemia is pancytopenia (low levels of all 3 blood types, i.e., RBCs, WBCs, and platelets) of unclear etiology. The condition acts as an autoimmune disorder, whereby the T cells attack the patient's own marrow.

Any infection or cancer can invade the bone marrow, causing decreased production, or hypoplasia. Other causes of pancytopenia are:

- Radiation and toxins such as toluene, insecticides (DDT), and benzene
- Drug effect: sulfa, phenytoin, carbamazepine, chloramphenicol, alcohol, chemotherapy
- SLE
- PNH
- Infection: HIV, hepatitis, CMV, EBV
- B12 and folate deficiency
- Thyroid-inhibiting medications such as propylthiouracil (PTU) and methimazole

Symptoms include the fatigue of anemia, infections from low WBC counts, and bleeding from thrombocytopenia.

Diagnosis is confirmed by excluding all the causes of pancytopenia. Bone marrow biopsy is the **most accurate test**.

Treatment starts with management of the underlying cause. Additionally, give supportive therapy such as blood transfusion for anemia, antibiotics for infection, and platelets for bleeding.

- If patient is young enough and there is a matched donor, consider allogeneic bone marrow transplantation (BMT) for true aplastic anemia.

- If patient is too old for BMT (age >50) or there is no matched donor, treatment is as follows:
  - Antithymocyte globulin
  - Cyclosporine (or tacrolimus)
  - Alemtuzumab, an anti-CD52 agent that suppresses T cells

Treatment of aplastic anemia is medication such as cyclosporine that inhibits T cells. This brings the marrow back to life.

> ABO-matched platelets last longer.

Myeloproliferative Disorders

Polycythemia Vera

Polycythemia vera (P vera) is the unregulated overproduction of all 3 cell lines, but RBC overproduction is the most prominent. There is a mutation in the JAK2 protein which regulates marrow production. The RBCs grow wildly despite a low erythropoietin level.

"What Is the Most Likely Diagnosis?"

Patients present with symptoms of hyperviscosity from the increased RBC mass:

- Headache, blurred vision, and tinnitus
- Hypertension
- Fatigue
- Splenomegaly (not in reactive polycythemia from hypoxia)
- Bleeding from engorged blood vessels
- Thrombosis from hyperviscosity (**most common cause of death**)

> Pruritus often follows warm showers because of histamine release from increased numbers of basophils.

Diagnostic testing includes:

- JAK2 mutation (95% of patients) (**most accurate test**)
- Markedly elevated hematocrit >60%
- Elevated platelets and WBCs (exclude hypoxia as a cause of the erythrocytosis)
- Elevated total RBC mass
  - Reduced iron because it has all been used up to make red blood cells
  - Reduced mean corpuscular volume
- Normal oxygen
- Reduced erythropoietin
- Elevated vitamin B12 increased transcobalamin
- Elevated basophils (as with all myeloproliferative disorders)

> Renal cell cancer is associated with an elevated hematocrit, but the erythropoietin level is elevated with kidney cancer.

Treatment is as follows:

- Phlebotomy and aspirin to prevent thrombosis
- Target hematocrit <45%

- Hydroxyurea to help lower cell count; if no response, use ruxolitinib (an inhibitor of JAK)
- Allopurinol or rasburicase to protect against uric acid rise
- Antihistamines
- Spleen removal (platelet counts will elevate temporarily)

> Ruxolitinib inhibits JAK2.

A small number of P vera patients can convert to AML.

Essential Thrombocytosis

With essential thrombocytosis (ET), a markedly elevated platelet count >1 million leads to thrombosis and bleeding. ET can be very difficult to distinguish from an elevated platelet count as a reaction to another stress such as infection, cancer, or iron deficiency.

Treatment is as follows:

- If **patient is age <60, is asymptomatic, or has platelets <1.5 million**: no treatment
- If **patient age >60, there are thromboses, or platelets >1.5 million**: begin treatment
  - Hydroxyurea (**best initial treatment**)
  - Anagrelide if hydroxyurea causes red blood cell suppression
  - Aspirin for erythromelalgia

> Mutations and ET
> - JAK2 mutation is found in 50% of ET cases.
> - CALR mutation distinguishes ET from reactive thrombocytosis.

Hypereosinophilic Syndrome

Hypereosinophilic syndrome presents with rashes (eczema, urticaria), cough, and shortness of breath >6 months. No cancer or parasitic infection is present.

Testing includes:

- Total eosinophil count >1,500
- Negative ANA
- Normal cosyntropin stimulation test
- No blasts

Treatment is steroids. If left untreated, hypereosinophilic syndrome will lead to death from cardiomyopathy or thromboembolic disease.

Systemic Mastocytosis

Systemic mastocytosis is triggered by narcotics, aspirin, and NSAIDs. Mast cells proliferate abnormally in the skin and marrow, and sometimes infiltrate the liver, spleen, and nodes.

Symptoms include:

- Itchy skin lesions (common)
- Abdominal pain
- Nausea, vomiting, diarrhea

- Urticaria pigmentosa and Darier sign (urtication at point of touch)
- Possible flushing, hypotension, and anaphylaxis

The **best initial test** is serum tryptase level, and the **most specific test** is skin and marrow biopsy.

Treatment is antihistamines, steroids, montelukast (for early disease), and cladribine, hydroxyurea (for extremely severe disease).

> JAK inhibitors increase the risk of TB reactivation.

Bone Marrow Disorders

Myelofibrosis

Myelofibrosis is a disease of older patients with a pancytopenia that is associated with bone marrow showing marked fibrosis. Blood production shifts to the spleen and liver, which become markedly enlarged.

Testing includes blood smear showing teardrop-shaped cells and nucleated red blood cells.

Treatment is as follows:

- Thalidomide and lenalidomide (TNF inhibitors) to increase bone marrow production
- Allogeneic bone marrow transplant (age <50)
- Ruxolitinib to inhibit JAK2 and suppress myelofibrosis

Myelodysplasia

Myelodysplasia, also called myelodysplastic syndrome (MDS) is a preleukemic disorder presenting in older patients (age >60) with a pancytopenia despite a hypercellular bone marrow. Most patients never develop AML because complications of infection and bleeding lead to death beforehand.

- 5q deletion is the characteristic abnormality of MDS. Patients with 5q have a better prognosis than do those without it.
- There is no single pathognomonic finding in the history or physical examination.
- Many patients present with asymptomatic pancytopenia on routine CBC.
- If symptoms do occur, they include:
  - Fatigue and weight loss
  - Infection
  - Bleeding
  - Possible splenomegaly

Diagnostic testing includes:

- CBC: anemia with increased MCV, nucleated RBCs, and a small number of blasts (severity is based on percentage of blasts)
- Marrow: hypercellular
- Prussian blue stain shows ringed sideroblasts
- Pelger-Huet cells (**most distinct lab abnormality**)

> Pelger-Huet cells are the most distinct lab abnormality in MDS.

Treatment is as follows:

- Transfusion
- Erythropoietin (20% success rate)
- Azacitidine or decitabine
- Lenalidomide for those with the 5q deletion can decrease transfusion dependence.
- Luspatercept (growth factor) decreases transfusion dependence in MDS.
- Bone marrow transplant age <50

> Hyperparathyroidism and ACE inhibitors cause erythropoietin resistance.

> **Azacitidine** decreases transfusion dependence and increases survival in MDS.

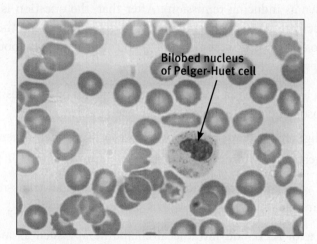

Bilobed nucleus of Pelger-Huet cell

Figure 9.7 Pelger-Huet cells are seen in MDS.
Source: Alireza Eghtedar, MD

Leukemia

Acute Leukemia

Symptoms include:

- Signs of pancytopenia (fatigue, infection, bleeding) even though WBCs are normal or increased (common)
- Infection (despite increased WBCs) is common, because leukemic cells (blasts) do not function normally in controlling infection

> Look for a history of myelodysplastic syndrome to suggest acute leukemia.

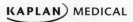

> ▶ **TIP**
>
> There is no distinct clinical presentation between the 3 subtypes of ALL, so for the exam, there is no point in learning the differences between them.

> ▶ **TIP**
>
> The acute leukemia **most frequently seen on the USMLE exam** is M3, or acute promyelocytic leukemia. This is because promyelocytic leukemia is associated with DIC.

M3 is associated with translocation between chromosomes 15 and 17.

Testing includes:

- Blood smear showing blasts (**best initial test**)
- Flow cytometry (**most accurate test**) will distinguish the CD subtypes of acute leukemia (myeloperoxidase is characteristic of AML)

Treatment for both acute myelocytic leukemia (AML) and acute lymphocytic leukemia (ALL) is chemotherapy to remove blasts from the peripheral blood smear (known as inducing remission). After that, the question is whether to proceed directly to BMT after remission or to give more chemotherapy alone. If the prognosis is poor, go straight to BMT. If the prognosis is good, give more chemotherapy.

Rasburicase prevents tumor lysis–related rise in uric acid.

Prognosis in acute leukemia is done with cytogenetics or by assessing the specific chromosomal characteristics found in each patient.

- Good cytogenetics = Less chance of relapse = More chemotherapy
- Bad cytogenetics = More chance of relapse = Immediate BMT

In **patients with M3** (promyelocytic leukemia), add all-trans-retinoic acid (ATRA) or arsenicals.

Auer rods: - Eosinophilic inclusions associated with AML - Most commonly associated with M3

In **patients with ALL**, add intrathecal chemotherapy such as methotrexate. This prevents relapse of ALL in the CNS.

> ▶ **TIP**
>
> The most-tested facts for acute leukemia are:
>
> - M3 (promyelocytic leukemia) gives DIC
> - Add ATRA to M3
> - Auer rods = AML
> - Add intrathecal methotrexate to ALL

Leukostasis Reaction

A 54-year-old man comes to the ED for shortness of breath, blurry vision, confusion, and priapism. WBC count is 225,000/μL. The cells are predominantly neutrophils, with about 4% blasts. What is the most appropriate next step in management?

a. Leukapheresis
b. BCR-ABL testing
c. Bone marrow biopsy
d. Bone marrow transplant
e. Consult hematology/oncology
f. Hydroxyurea

Answer: **A.** In acute leukostasis reaction, it is more important to remove the excessive WBCs from the blood than to establish a specific diagnosis. In other words, specific testing is not as important as treatment. No matter what the etiology, you still have to take the cells off. The symptoms are caused by blocking the delivery of oxygen to tissues because the RBCs simply cannot get to the tissues. Afterward, you can establish a specific diagnosis. Hydroxyurea will lower the cell count, but not as rapidly as leukapheresis.

Chronic Myelogenous Leukemia

Chronic myelogenous leukemia (CML) has the greatest likelihood of all myeloproliferative disorders to transform into acute leukemia (blast crisis). If CML is untreated, this will happen in 20% of patients a year.

"What Is the Most Likely Diagnosis?"

Look for a patient with a persistently high WBC count that is all neutrophils.

- Pruritus (common after hot baths/showers from histamine release from basophils)
- Splenomegaly presents with early satiety, abdominal fullness, and LUQ pain
- Vague symptoms of fatigue, night sweats, and fever due to hypermetabolic syndrome
- High WBC sometimes on routine exam

Diagnostic testing starts with neutrophils.

- High neutrophils (**best initial test**)
- Small numbers of blasts (<5%)
- Increased basophils
- BCR-ABL (**most accurate test**)
  - Do after high neutrophils are confirmed to determine if it truly is leukemia or is a reaction to another infection or stress (leukemoid reaction)
  - Use PCR or FISH (fluorescent in-situ hybridization) on peripheral blood

> "BCR-ABL" = 9:22 translocation = Philadelphia chromosome (95% of cases)

Treatment:

- Tyrosine kinase inhibitors, i.e., imatinib, dasatinib, nilotinib (**best initial therapy**)
- Bone marrow transplant is curative (but is never initial therapy)

Chronic Lymphocytic Leukemia

Chronic lymphocytic leukemia (CLL) is a clonal proliferation of normal, mature-appearing B lymphocytes that function abnormally.

The great majority of those with CLL are age >50. Many are asymptomatic at presentation, with only a markedly elevated WBCs. There are no unique physical findings.

Symptoms include:

- Fatigue (**most common**)
- Lymphadenopathy (80%)
- Spleen or liver enlargement (50%)
- Infection from poor lymphocyte function
- Hemolysis sometimes

CLL is paradoxical. When the body needs a useful antibody for an infection, it is often not made; on the other hand, the CLL cells attack normal RBCs and platelets.

Diagnostic testing:

- WBCs ≥20,000/μL with 80–98% lymphocytes
- Hypogammaglobulinemia (50% of patients)
- Anemia and thrombocytopenia (from marrow infiltration or autoimmune warm IgG antibodies)

Treatment is as follows:

- **Stage 0** (elevated WBC): no treatment
- **Stage I** (lymphadenopathy): no treatment
- **Stage II** (hepatosplenomegaly): no treatment
- **Stage III** (anemia): fludarabine, cyclophosphamide, and rituximab
- **Stage IV** (thrombocytopenia): fludarabine, cyclophosphamide, and rituximab
  - On the exam, if an answer choice lists fludarabine, cyclophosphamide, and rituximab, then that is the **best initial treatment** for advanced-stage disease or anyone who is symptomatic (severe fatigue, painful nodes).
  - Alemtuzumab (anti-CD-52) is used when fludarabine fails.

Although fludarabine and rituximab are used in combination for most symptomatic CLL patients age <70, there is no clear first-line treatment among the agents just described. You will not be asked to choose between them.

Richter phenomenon (the conversion of CLL into high-grade lymphoma) is seen in 5% of patients.

A smudge cell is a lab artifact in which the fragile nucleus is crushed by the cover slip.

Step 2 will not ask you to choose between fludarabine and rituximab for CLL.

Ibrutinib is an inhibitor of Bruton tyrosine kinase. It can be combined with cyclophosphamide.

Which is less dangerous: thrombocytopenia and anemia from autoimmune effect or from marrow infiltration with CLL cells?

- Thrombocytopenia and anemia caused by autoimmune effect is less dangerous. Treatment is prednisone, and is not the same as stage III and IV disease.

> **To get a score of 250 on the USMLE Step 2 CK exam, know the following treatments:**
> - Refractory cases: cyclophosphamide (more efficacy, but more toxic)
> - Mild cases: bendamustine (elderly)
> - Severe infection: intravenous immunoglobulins
> - Autoimmune thrombocytopenia or hemolysis: prednisone
> - Bendamustine with rituximab = fludarabine

	PCP prophylaxis is indicated in CLL.

Hairy Cell Leukemia

Hairy cell leukemia (HCL) is seen in middle-aged men with:

- Pancytopenia
- Massive splenomegaly
- Monocytopenia
- Inaspirable "dry" tap despite hypercellularity of the marrow

Smear showing hairy cells is the **best initial test**. Immunotyping by flow cytometry (e.g., CD11c) is the **most accurate test**.

Treatment is cladribine or pentostatin.

	In hairy cell leukemia, B cells with filamentous projections are seen on smear.

Lymphoma

Non-Hodgkin Lymphoma

Non-Hodgkin lymphoma (NHL) is a proliferation of lymphocytes in the lymph nodes and spleen. Typically, it is widespread at presentation and can affect any lymph node or organ that has lymphoid tissue.

	NHL and CLL are extremely similar, but NHL is a solid mass and CLL is "liquid" or circulating.

"What Is the Most Likely Diagnosis?"

In the majority of cases, symptoms present at an advanced stage.

- Painless lymphadenopathy
- May involve pelvic, retroperitoneal, or mesenteric structures
- Nodes not warm, red, or tender
- "B" symptoms: fever, weight loss, drenching night sweats

	Infection, not NHL, will produce nodes that are warm, red, and tender.

Testing includes:

- Excisional biopsy (**best initial test**)
- CBC is normal in most cases
- High lactate dehydrogenase (LDH) correlates with worse severity

Staging NHL will determine the intensity of treatment, but the treatment itself does not often change because disease is usually widespread.

- **Stage I**: 1 lymph node group
- **Stage II**: 2 or more lymph node groups on same side of the diaphragm
- **Stage III**: both sides of the diaphragm
- **Stage IV**: widespread disease

Typical staging procedures are CT scan of the chest/abdomen/pelvis and bone marrow biopsy.

▶ **TIP**

The **most common wrong answer** is needle aspiration of the lymph node. Aspiration is not enough, because the individual lymphocytes appear normal.

Treatment is as follows:

- **Local disease (stages Ia and IIa)**: local radiation and small dose/course of chemotherapy
- **Advanced disease (stages III and IV, any "B" symptoms)**: combination chemotherapy with CHOP and rituximab, an antibody against CD20
  - **C**: cyclophosphamide
  - **H**: adriamycin (doxorubicin or "hydroxydaunorubicin")
  - **O**: vincristine (Oncovin)
  - **P**: prednisone

One type of NHL is mucosa-associated lymphoid tissue (MALT), a lymphoma of the stomach that is associated with *Helicobacter pylori*. Treatment is clarithromycin and amoxicillin.

Waldenström Macroglobulinemia

Waldenström macroglobulinemia is the overproduction of IgM from malignant B cells leading to hyperviscosity. It presents with:

- Lethargy
- Blurry vision and vertigo
- Engorged blood vessels in the eye
- Mucosal bleeding
- Raynaud phenomenon

Anemia is common, but an IgM spike on SPEP results in hyperviscosity. There are no bone lesions. Plasmapheresis is the best initial therapy to remove the IgM and decrease viscosity. Long-term treatment is with rituximab or prednisone cyclophosphamide. Control the cells that make the abnormal immunoglobulins. Decrease the means of production. Use bortezomib or lenalidomide as in myeloma.

Hodgkin Disease

The definition, presentation, testing, "B" symptoms, and staging of Hodgkin disease (HD) are the same as NHL. However, HD shows Reed-Sternberg cells on pathology.

HD versus NHL	
Hodgkin disease	**Non-Hodgkin lymphoma**
Local, stage I, and stage II in 80–90%	Stage III and stage IV in 80–90%
Centers around cervical area	Disseminated
Reed-Sternberg cells on pathology	No Reed-Sternberg cells
Pathologic classification: • Lymphocyte predominant has the best prognosis. • Lymphocyte depleted has the worst prognosis.	Pathologic classification: • Burkitt and immunoblastic have the worst prognosis.

Treatment is as follows:

- **Stage Ia and IIa**: local radiation with small course of chemotherapy
- **Stage III and IV, or anyone with "B" symptoms**: ABVD
    - **A**: adriamycin (doxorubicin)
    - **B**: bleomycin
    - **V**: vinblastine
    - **D**: dacarbazine

Relapses after radiation therapy are treated with chemotherapy. Relapses after chemotherapy are treated with extra high dose chemotherapy and bone marrow transplantation.

> Note the complications of radiation and chemotherapy:
>
> - Radiation increases the risk of solid tumors such as breast, thyroid, or lung cancer.
> - Radiation increases the risk of premature CAD.
> - Chemotherapy increases the risk of acute leukemia, MDS, and NHL very slightly.
> - Screening for breast cancer is recommended 8 years or more after treatment.

Which of the following is the most useful to determine dosing of chemotherapy in HD?

a. Echocardiogram
b. Bone marrow biopsy
c. Gender
d. MUGA or nuclear ventriculogram
e. Hematocrit
f. Symptoms

> Radiation alone is never right for lymphoma.

Answer: D. Adriamycin (or doxorubicin) is cardiotoxic. The nuclear ventriculogram is the most accurate way to assess left ventricular ejection fraction. Use the MUGA scan to determine whether cardiac toxicity has occurred prior to the development of symptoms. You cannot use adriamycin if ejection fraction <50%.

Adverse Effects of Chemotherapy	
Chemotherapeutic agent	**Toxicity**
Doxorubicin	Cardiomyopathy
Vincristine	Neuropathy
Bleomycin	Lung fibrosis
Cyclophosphamide	Hemorrhagic cystitis
Cisplatin	Renal toxicity, ototoxicity, neurotoxicity

Myeloma

Multiple Myeloma

Myeloma is an abnormal proliferation of plasma cells. These plasma cells are unregulated in their production of useless immunoglobulin that is usually IgG or IgA. These immunoglobulins do not fight infection but do clog up the kidney.

IgM is a separate disease called *Waldenström macroglobulinemia*.

"What Is the Most Likely Diagnosis?"

Symptoms include:

- Bone pain from pathologic fractures (**most common**)
  - *Pathologic fracture* means the bone breaks under "normal use"; this is from osteoclast activating factor (OAF), which attacks the bone and causes lytic lesions.
  - OAF is also the reason for hypercalcemia.
  - Infection is common because the abnormal plasma cells do not make immunoglobulins that are effective against infections.

- Hyperuricemia from increased turnover of the nuclear material of plasma cells
- Anemia from infiltration of the marrow with massive numbers of plasma cells
- Renal failure from accumulation of immunoglobulins and Bence-Jones protein in the kidney; hypercalcemia and hyperuricemia also damage the kidney

> Renal failure and infection are the most common causes of death in myeloma.

Diagnostic testing:

- X-ray of affected bone will show lytic ("punched out") lesions (**initial diagnostic test**)
- Serum protein electrophoresis shows an IgG (60%) or IgA (25%) spike of a single type or "clone" (this one clone is called a monoclonal spike or "M-spike"); 15% have light chains or Bence-Jones protein only
- Hypercalcemia
- Bence-Jones protein on urine immunoelectrophoresis
- Beta$_2$ microglobulin (levels correspond to severity of disease)
- Smear on rouleaux
- Elevated BUN and creatinine
- Bone marrow biopsy: >10% plasma cells defines myeloma
- Elevated total protein with normal albumin

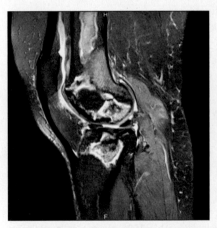
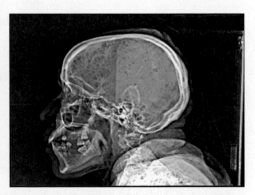

> Serum free light chains (FLC) ratio of 100:1 is highly consistent with myeloma.

Figures 9.8, 9.9 Myeloma: MRIs showing bone infarcts (left) and lytic lesions in the skull (right). Bone lesions in myeloma are exclusively lytic. Nuclear bone scan will show nothing, because there is no blastic activity. The bone can pick up the nuclear isotope only where there is blastic activity.
Source: Pramod Theetha Kariyanna, MD

> Myeloma has a decreased anion gap. IgG is cationic. Increased cationic substances will increase chloride and bicarbonate levels. This decreases the anion gap.

Rouleaux form when the IgG paraprotein sticks to the RBCs, causing them to adhere to each other in a stack or "roll."

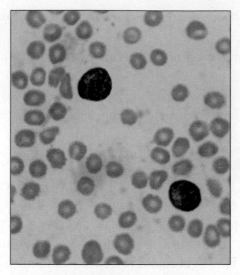

Figure 9.10 Plasma cell in myeloma. The lucency, or light area, near the nucleus is the "Hof," which is the Golgi apparatus.
Source: Vlad Gottlieb, MD.

What is the explanation for the difference between the urinary level of protein on urinalysis and the 24-hour urine?

a. False positive 24-hour urine is common in myeloma.
b. Calcium in urine creates a false negative urinalysis.
c. Uric acid creates a false positive 24-hour urine.
d. Bence-Jones protein is not detected by dipstick.
e. IgG in urine inactivates the urine dipstick.

Answer: **D**. Bence-Jones protein is detected by urine immunoelectrophoresis. The urine dipstick will detect only albumin.

What is the single most accurate test for myeloma?

a. Skull x-ray
b. Bone marrow biopsy
c. 24-hour urine
d. SPEP
e. Urine immunoelectrophoresis (Bence-Jones protein)

Answer: **B**. Nothing besides myeloma is associated with >10% plasma cells on bone marrow biopsy. The most common wrong answer is SPEP. Of those with an "M-spike" of immunoglobulins, 99% do not have myeloma. Most IgG spikes are from monoclonal gammopathy of unknown significance that does not progress or need treatment. Skull x-ray shows lytic lesions, but this is not as specific as massive plasma cell levels in the marrow.

Treatment is needed if plasma cells >60% in marrow or FLC ratio >100.

- Dexamethasone + lenalidomide or bortezomib (or both) (**best initial therapy**)
- Melphalan for older, fragile patients who cannot tolerate side effects

- Autologous bone marrow transplant with stem cell support for those age <70 (**most effective therapy**)
  - Do after induction chemotherapy with lenalidomide and steroids
  - Daratumumab is an anti-CD38 drug used in relapse
- Bortezomib (often causes neurologic complications)
- Thalidomide and lenalidomide (can cause increased clotting); give prophylaxis against clotting beforehand

> Myeloma therapy is in a state of rapid flux due to numerous advances.

Monoclonal Gammopathy of Unknown Significance

IgG or IgA spikes on an SPEP are common in older patients. The main issue is to evaluate with bone marrow biopsy to exclude myeloma. Monoclonal gammopathy of unknown significance (MGUS) has small numbers of plasma cells.

There is no treatment for MGUS, but know that 1% of cases per year transform into myeloma. The quantity or amount of immunoglobulin in the spike is the main correlate of risk for myeloma: More MGUS means more myeloma.

> More MGUS = More myeloma

Smoldering Myeloma

Smoldering myeloma is characterized by 10–60% plasma cells with an M-spike on SPEP. There is elevated urine monoclonal protein and elevated FLC ratio but no hypercalcemia, renal failure, anemia, or bone lesions.

There is no specific treatment.

Coagulation Disorders

Bleeding Disorders

Bleeding in the brain or GI system can be caused by platelet or clotting factor deficiency. The first step in evaluation is to determine if the bleeding seems related to platelets or clotting factors.

Types of Bleeding	
Platelet bleeding	**Factor bleeding**
Superficial	Deep
Epistaxis, gingival, petechiae, purpura, mucosal surfaces such as the gums, vaginal bleeding	Joints and muscles

Immune Thrombocytopenia

Idiopathic thrombocytopenia (ITP) is a diagnosis of exclusion. Look for isolated thrombocytopenia (normal hematocrit, normal WBC count) and normal-sized spleen.

Occasional diagnostic tests are:

- Megakaryocytes are elevated
- Antiplatelet antibodies lack specificity, so of limited benefit
- U/S or CT scan to exclude hypersplenism
- Bone marrow not routine; indicated only before splenectomy
- Mean platelet volume is elevated

> Platelets are large in ITP.

Treatment is as follows:

- **No bleeding, count >30,000**: no treatment
- **Mild bleeding, count <30,000**: glucocorticoids
- **Severe bleeding (GI/CNS), count <10,000**: IVIG, anti-Rho (anti-D)
- **Recurrent episodes, steroid-dependent**: splenectomy (before splenectomy, vaccinate for *N. meningitidis*, *H. influenzae*, and Pneumococcus)
- **Splenectomy or steroids not effective**: romiplostim, eltrombopag, avatrombopag, rituximab, azathioprine, cyclosporine, mycophenolate

> Romiplostim, avatrombopag, and eltrombopag are synthetic thrombopoietin for ITP.

A 23-year-old woman comes to the ED with markedly increased menstrual bleeding, gum bleeding when she brushes her teeth, and petechiae on physical examination. Physical examination is otherwise normal. Platelet count is 17,000/μL. What is the most appropriate next step in therapy?

a. Bone marrow biopsy
b. Intravenous immunoglobulins
c. Prednisone
d. Antiplatelet antibodies
e. Platelet transfusion

Answer: **C.** The bleeding in this case is mild, meaning there is no intracranial bleeding or major GI bleeding, and platelets are not profoundly low. Prednisone is the best initial therapy. Initiating prednisone is more important than checking for increased megakaryocytes or the presence of antiplatelet antibodies, which is characteristic of ITP. Bone marrow is rarely needed.

Von Willebrand Disease

Von Willebrand disease (VWD) (**most common inherited bleeding disorder**) is decreased level or functioning of von Willebrand factor (VWF). It is autosomal dominant.

Look for bleeding related to platelets (epistaxis, gingival, gums) with a normal platelet count. VWD is markedly worsened after the use of aspirin.

Diagnostic testing is as follows:

- Decreased VWF (antigen)
- Ristocetin cofactor assay: detects VWF dysfunction (also called VWF activity)
- Factor VIII activity
- Normal platelets

- Elevated aPTT (50% of patients)
- Bleeding time: increased duration of bleeding (rarely done)

Treatment is DDAVP (desmopressin), which releases subendothelial stores of VWF. If there is no response, use factor VIII replacement or VWF concentrate.

Glanzmann Thrombasthenia and Bernard-Soulier Syndrome

Both disorders present with platelet-type bleeding (e.g., epistaxis and petechiae) with normal platelet count. Both have a normal VWF level. Both are diagnosed with platelet studies.

The distinguishing feature is Bernard-Soulier has giant platelets, while Glanzmann does not.

Treatment of both disorders is the same.

> Glanzmann: IIb/IIIa defect
>
> Bernard-Soulier: Ib/IX defect

- Desmopressin to release subendothelial stores of VWF and factor VIIIa
- Tranexamic acid and epsilon-aminocaproic acid to inhibit fibrinolysis and plasminogen
- Recombinant factor VIIa
- Estrogen upregulates VWF

Hemophilia

Look for delayed joint or muscle bleeding in a male child, since the condition is X-linked recessive. Bleeding is delayed because the primary hemostatic plug is with platelets.

- Normal prothrombin time (PT)
- Prolonged aPTT

The **most accurate test** is a specific assay for factor VIII or IX.

Treatment is as follows:

- Mild bleeding: DDAVP
- Severe bleeding
  - Very low levels of factor VIII or IX: replace the specific factor
  - Exception: for severe bleeding from factor VIII antibodies, replace with factor VII (bypasses the usual pathway and directly activates factor X)
- Mixing studies with normal plasma to correct the aPTT to normal

Factor XII Deficiency

Patients have elevated aPTT but there is no bleeding. No treatment is needed.

> Treatment of clotting-factor deficiencies includes **recombinant versions of factors VII, VIII, IX, and X:**
>
> - DDAVP to counteract factor VIII deficiency and von Willebrand disease (VWD)
> - Recombinant VWF to treat VWD
> - Prothrombin complex concentrate (PCC) to reverse warfarin toxicity
>   - Has all the vitamin K–dependent factors and works faster than giving vitamin K or FFP
>   - Has factors II, VII, IX, and X and proteins C and S

Factor XI Deficiency

Most of the time, there is no increase in bleeding with factor XI deficiency. With trauma or surgery, there is increased bleeding. Look for a normal PT with a prolonged aPTT. Mixing study will correct the aPTT to normal, as occurs whenever there is a deficiency of clotting factors. Use fresh frozen plasma (FFP) to stop the bleeding.

Disseminated Intravascular Coagulation

Disseminated intravascular coagulation (DIC) does not occur in otherwise healthy people. Look for a definite risk such as:

- Sepsis
- Burns
- Abruptio placentae or amniotic fluid embolus
- Snake bites
- Trauma resulting in tissue factor release
- Cancer

There is bleeding related to both clotting factor deficiency as well as thrombocytopenia.

Look for:

- Elevation in both the PT and aPTT
- Low platelet count
- Elevated d-dimer and fibrin split products
- Decreased fibrinogen level (it has been consumed)

Treatment is as follows:

- If platelets <50,000/μL and patient has serious bleeding, replace platelets as well as clotting factors by using FFP.
- If bleeding is not controlled with FFP, cryoprecipitate may be effective to replace fibrinogen.
- Heparin has no definite benefit.

Hypercoagulable States/Thrombophilia

The most common cause of thrombophilia is factor V Leiden mutation. There is no difference in the intensity of anticoagulation. Use warfarin for 6 months to INR 2–3.

Heparin-Induced Thrombocytopenia

Heparin-induced thrombocytopenia (HIT) is more common with the use of unfractionated heparin, but can still occur with low-molecular-weight (LMW) heparin. HIT presents 5–10 days after the start of heparin with a marked drop in platelet count (>30%). Both venous and arterial thromboses can occur, although venous clots are more common. HIT rarely leads to bleeding. The platelets just precipitate out.

HIT is confirmed with an ELISA for platelet factor 4 (PF4) antibodies or the serotonin release assay.

Treatment is as follows:

- Stop all heparin-containing products immediately. You cannot just switch unfractionated heparin to LMW heparin.
- Give fondaparinux or direct thrombin inhibitors (argatroban, bivalirudin); fondaparinux is easiest to use.

Antiphospholipid Syndromes

The 2 main antiphospholipid (APL) syndromes are the lupus anticoagulant and anticardiolipin antibody. Both cause thrombosis.

- APL syndromes are the only cause of thrombophilia with an abnormality in the aPTT.
- Anticardiolipin antibodies are associated with multiple spontaneous abortions.

The **best initial test** is the mixing study. Because it is a circulating inhibitor, the aPTT will remain elevated even after the mix. The **most accurate test** for the lupus anticoagulant is the Russell viper venom test.

Treatment is heparin and warfarin. APL syndrome requires lifelong anticoagulation. Warfarin is superior to a NOAC only for APL syndrome, metal valves, and mitral stenosis with atrial fibrillation.

> Warfarin is superior to a NOAC in patients with APL, metal valves, or mitral stenosis.

> Do not transfuse platelets into those with HIT, because it may worsen the thrombosis.

> The only thrombophilia important to test for with first clot is APL syndrome. APL requires lifelong warfarin with only one clot.

Stroke

Stroke (**third most common cause of death in United States**) is the sudden onset of a neurological deficit from the death of brain tissue. In a stroke, a cerebral vessel is blocked by a thrombosis occurring in the vessel or by an embolus to the vessel. Causes include:

- Sudden blockage in the flow of blood to the brain (85% of cases)
- Bleeding (15% of cases)

Emboli originate from carotid stenosis or from the heart (A-fib, valvular heart disease, or a DVT paradoxically getting into the brain through a patent foramen ovale [PFO]).

Risk factors for stroke are the same as those for myocardial infarction: hypertension, diabetes, hyperlipidemia, and tobacco smoking. Control risk factors as follows:

- Control diabetes to hemoglobin A1C <7% mg/dL
- Control hypertension
- Reduce LDL to at least <70 mg/dL
- Stop tobacco smoking

Presentation includes:

- **Middle cerebral artery (MCA)** stroke (90% of cases)
  - Weakness or sensory loss on opposite (contralateral) side of the lesions causing stroke
  - Homonymous hemianopsia: loss of visual field on opposite side of the stroke
    - Left-sided MCA stroke will cause loss of right visual fields
    - For instance, the eyes cannot see the right side, so the eyes deviate to the left (toward the side of the lesion)
  - Aphasia (if stroke occurs on same side as the speech center, i.e., for most people on the left side)

> Speech is controlled by the same side as "handedness." Right-handed people (left-brain dominant) have a speech center on the left-hand side of the brain.

- **Anterior cerebral artery (ACA)** stroke
  - Personality/cognitive defects such as confusion
  - Urinary incontinence
  - Leg (more than arm) weakness

- **Posterior cerebral artery (PCA)** stroke
  - Ipsilateral sensory loss of the face, 9th and 10th cranial nerves
  - Contralateral sensory loss of the limbs
  - Limb ataxia

Diagnostic testing is as follows:

- For any kind of stroke, the **best initial test** is a CT scan of the head without contrast. MRI is the **most accurate test**.
- CT scan is done first only so that hemorrhage can be excluded as a cause of the stroke prior to initiating treatment.
- CT scan needs 4–5 days to reach >95% sensitivity, while MRI needs only 24–48 hours to reach >95% sensitivity.

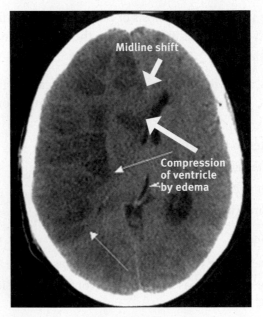

Figure 10.1 Nonhemorrhagic stroke is characterized by edema without blood.
Source: Mohammad Maruf, MD

Beyond that, testing to determine the cause of a stroke—and treatment—is as follows:

- **Echocardiogram**
  - Surgical replacement or repair of certain damaged valves
  - Patent foramen ovale (PFO)
  - Thrombi: anticoagulation

- **EKG**
  - A-fib or A-flutter is treated with a NOAC (or warfarin) as long as the arrhythmia persists
  - Stroke or TIA means CHADS-VASc score ≥2
- **Holter monitor**
  - 24–48 hr ambulatory EKG to detect atrial arrhythmias with greater sensitivity if EKG is normal
  - If negative, long-term monitoring (1–6 months) with a loop recorder is needed to find atrial arrhythmias

  > 24–48 hours of Holter monitoring is not enough to label a stroke "cryptogenic" for PFO closure.

- **Carotid duplex ultrasound**
  - Carotid stenosis is a frequent cause of emboli to the brain. If a patient has symptomatic cerebrovascular disease and severe stenosis (71–99% occlusion) is detected, perform surgical correction of the narrowing.
  - Endarterectomy is superior to carotid angioplasty (but it has no value for mild stenosis [<50%] and unclear value for moderate stenosis [50–70%]).
  - If the stenosis is 100%, however, no intervention is needed since there is no point in opening a passage that is 100% occluded.

Treatment is as follows:

- **Hemorrhagic stroke**: no treatment; surgical drainage will not help the outside posterior fossa
- **Nonhemorrhagic stroke**:
  - If <**3 hours** since onset of stroke: thrombolytics
  - If >**3 hours** since onset of stroke: aspirin (if patient already taking aspirin at time of stroke, add dipyridamole or clopidogrel)
    - Some patients still get thrombolytics
    - Aspirin
    - Dipyridamole or clopidogrel (added for a few weeks if patient is already taking aspirin at time of stroke)

> The major difference in management of TIA vs. stroke: No tPA or mechanical clot retrieval for TIA.

If patient is age <80, NIH stroke scale <25 (i.e., not maximally severe, leading to more bleeding), and not a diabetic with a previous stroke, use the following treatment guidelines:

- If <**4.5 hours** since onset of stroke: thrombolytics
- If >**4.5 hours** since onset: clot removal via catheter (pulls clot out like a corkscrew); useful 24 hours after stroke

> **Catheter retrieval of clot** is useful up to 24 hours after stroke.

Additional treatment guidelines are as follows:

- Give all stroke and TIA patients a statin, regardless of LDL; although target-based therapy for lipid management is unclear at this time, LDL should be lowered to at least <70 mg/dL.

Carotid stenosis is considered an equivalent of coronary artery disease, so control LDL to <70 mg/dL.

When aspirin and clopidogrel are combined, the clopidogrel is stopped after several weeks.

- Patent foramen ovale (PFO) occurs in 30% of the population. Do closure of PFO (in addition to antiplatelet treatment) under the following conditions:
  - Patient has right-to-left shunt detected by bubble study
  - Patient has embolic-appearing cryptogenic ischemic stroke

Prevention of a stroke is done with aspirin, clopidogrel, and sometimes the combination of aspirin and clopidogrel. You can combine dipyridamole with aspirin as an equivalent of clopidogrel.

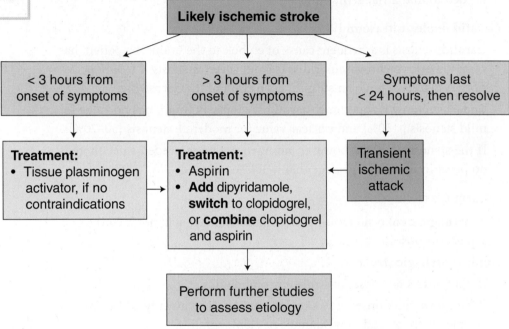

Figure 10.2 Initial Treatment for Nonhemorrhagic Stroke

On the exam, you will be shown an image of a stroke and asked what to add.

Stroke patients should be placed on telemetry to detect A-fib/A-flutter.

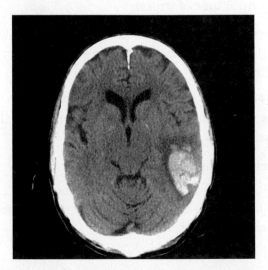

Figure 10.3 Acute blood appears white on CT scan.
(Contrast is not needed to detect blood.)
Source: Saba Ansari, MD

▶ **TIP**

The Step 2 CK exam will avoid controversial or unclear topics such as the management of moderate carotid stenosis (50–70%). Your exam question will be clear: **Definitely operate** with >70% stenosis, but **do not operate** with <50% stenosis.

Subarachnoid Hemorrhage

Subarachnoid hemorrhage (SAH) is caused by the rupture of an aneurysm that is usually located in the anterior portion of the circle of Willis.

Aneurysms are found in 2% of routine autopsies. The vast majority never rupture. They are more frequent in those with:

- Polycystic kidney disease
- Tobacco smoking
- Hypertension
- Hyperlipidemia
- High alcohol consumption

What provokes a rupture is not clear in the majority of cases.

"What Is the Most Likely Diagnosis?"

Look for the sudden onset of an extremely severe headache with meningeal irritation (stiff neck, photophobia) and fever. Fever is secondary to blood irritating the meninges. Loss of consciousness occurs in 50% from the sudden increase in intracranial pressure. Focal neurological complications occur in as many as 30%.

Unlike meningitis, **SAH** has very sudden onset and loss of consciousness.

Diagnostic testing includes:

- CT without contrast (**best initial test**) (95% sensitive)
- LP (**most accurate test**) showing blood (needed only for the 5% of patients with a falsely negative CT)
  - Xanthochromia is a yellow discoloration of CSF from the breakdown of RBCs in the CSF
  - The CSF in SAH will have an increased number of WBCs, which can mimic meningitis. However, the ratio of WBCs to RBCs will be normal in SAH. When the WBC count exceeds the normal ratio, you should suspect meningitis.

Normal ratio is **1 WBC** for every **500–1,000 RBCs**

- Angiogram is used to determine the site of the aneurysm in order to guide repair of the lesion. The diagnosis of SAH is based on CT and sometimes LP. The only way to tell precisely which vessel ruptured is with CT angiogram, standard angiogram with catheter, or MRA.
- EKG may show large or inverted T waves suggestive of myocardial ischemia (cerebral T waves). This is thought to be from excessive sympathetic activity.

> Contrast on CT or MRI improves detection of mass lesions such as cancer or abscess. **Do not use contrast when looking for blood.**

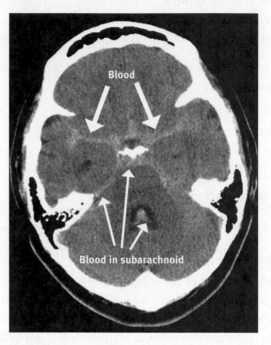

Figure 10.4 Head CT without contrast is 95% sensitive in the detection of SAH. Lumbar puncture is 100% sensitive. *Source: Saba Ansari, MD.*

Treatment is as follows. There is nothing that can reverse the hemorrhage.

- Nimodipine (CCB) to prevent subsequent ischemic stroke
- Embolization (coiling) using a catheter to "clog up" the site of bleeding and prevent a repeat hemorrhage

> 50–70% of those who rebleed will die.

  - An interventional neuroradiologist places platinum wire into the site of hemorrhage.
  - Embolization is superior to surgical clipping in terms of survival and complications.
- Ventriculoperitoneal shunt: SAH is associated with hydrocephalus. Place a shunt only if hydrocephalus develops.
- Seizure prophylaxis: Medication is generally given to prevent seizures. If the question asks "Which of the following is indicated?" antiepileptic therapy is the answer, although controversial.

A woman comes to the ED with a severe headache that started the previous day. On physical examination she has a temperature of 39.4 C (103 F), nuchal rigidity, and photophobia. Head CT is normal. LP shows CSF with 1,250 white blood cells and 50,000 red blood cells. What is the most appropriate next step in management?

a. Angiogram
b. Ceftriaxone and vancomycin
c. Nimodipine
d. Embolization
e. Surgical clipping
f. Repeat the CT scan with contrast
g. Neurosurgical consultation

Answer: **B.** The number of WBCs in the CSF in this patient far exceeds the normal ratio of 1 WBC to each 500–1,000 RBCs. With 50,000 RBCs, there should be no more than 50–100 WBCs, so 1,250 WBCs indicates an infection. Ceftriaxone and vancomycin are the best initial therapy for bacterial meningitis. Contrast is not useful when looking for blood. Try never to answer "consultation" for anything.

▶ **TIP**

On the USMLE exam, "consultation" is the right answer only when you want to do a particular procedure and the procedure is not included as an answer choice. If the right answer is "embolization" and it is not listed, but "interventional neuroradiology consultation" is one of the choices, then the right answer in that case is "consultation."

Cerebral Vein Thrombosis

Cerebral vein thrombosis mimics subarachnoid hemorrhage. It presents with:

- Clotting in cerebral veins
- Headache over several days
- Possible weakness and speech difficulty like a stroke
- Normal LP

The most accurate test is magnetic resonance venography (MRV).

Treat with LMW heparin followed by warfarin.

Headache

Tension headache is, by far, the most common cause of headache. It is a diagnosis of exclusion.

"What Is the Most Likely Diagnosis?"

Diagnosis of tension headache starts with exclusion of more serious conditions:

- **Migraine**: visual disturbance (flashes, sparks, stars, luminous hallucinations), photophobia, aura, relationship to menses, association with food (chocolate, red wine, cheese). May be precipitated by emotions. Associated with nausea and vomiting.
- **Cluster headache**: frequent, short duration, high-intensity headaches (with men affected 10× more than women)
- **Giant cell (temporal) arteritis**: visual disturbance; systemic symptoms such as muscle pain, fatigue, and weakness; jaw claudication
- **Pseudotumor cerebri**: associated with obesity, venous sinus thrombosis, oral contraceptives, and vitamin A toxicity. Mimics a brain tumor with nausea, vomiting, and visual disturbance.

Physical Examination

- **Tension headache**: no physical findings
- **Migraine**: no physical findings usually, but rare cases have aphasia, numbness, dysarthria, or weakness
- **Cluster headache**: red, tearing eye with rhinorrhea; Horner syndrome occasionally
- **Giant cell (temporal) arteritis**: visual loss, tenderness of the temporal area
- **Pseudotumor cerebri**: papilledema with diplopia from sixth cranial nerve (abducens) palsy

> Pseudotumor cerebri is also known as idiopathic intracranial hypertension.

> Evaluate for glaucoma with headache and a red eye.

There are no specific diagnostic tests for tension headache, migraine, and cluster headache. If there is a clear history of a particular type of headache, imaging is not needed.

- Head CT or MRI can exclude intracranial mass lesions if diagnosis is unclear or syndrome has recently started.
- To diagnose pseudotumor cerebri, CT or MRI must first exclude an intracranial mass lesion and LP must show increased pressure. (In pseudotumor cerebri, the pressure is abnormal but the CSF itself is normal.)
- To diagnose giant cell arteritis, the most accurate test is a biopsy. ESR is markedly elevated.

> It is critical to start steroids without waiting for biopsy in giant cell arteritis.

Treatment

- NSAIDs and other analgesics: tension headache
- Triptans, ergotamine, lasmiditan, or ubrogepant as abortive therapy: migraine

- Triptans, ergotamine, or 100% oxygen as abortive therapy: cluster headache
- Prednisone: giant cell (temporal) arteritis
- Acetazolamide to decrease production of CSF: pseudotumor cerebri
  - Weight loss, steroids
  - Repeat LP will rapidly lower intracranial pressure
  - If no response to treatment, place a ventriculoperitoneal shunt or fenestrate (cut into) the optic nerve

Abortive treatment for migraine and cluster headache is as follows:

- Both migraine and cluster: ergotamine or a triptan (e.g., sumatriptan, eletriptan, almotriptan, zolmitriptan)
- Cluster only: 100% oxygen
- Migraine only:
  - Lasmiditan (5-HT1 inhibitor that does not cause vasoconstriction) is used when there is a contraindication to triptans (hypertension, coronary disease)
  - Ubrogepant (calcitonin gene-related peptide [CGRP] antagonist)

> CGRP antagonists can be prophylactic or abortive. Use these ones for prophylaxis when beta blockers are ineffective:
> - Erenumab
> - Fremanezumab
> - Galcanezumab

Prophylactic (preventive) treatment for migraine and cluster headache is as follows:

- Migraine: propranolol, CGRPs (erenumab, fremanezumab, galcanezumab), CCBs; tricyclic antidepressants (amitriptyline), SSRIs; topiramate; and botulinum toxin injections)
- Cluster: verapamil, prednisone, lithium

Headache Management			
Presentation	• Bilateral "bandlike" pressure • Lasts 4–6 hours • Normal physical exam	• +/− aura, photophobia • Related to food/emotions/menses • Rare: aphasia, numbness, dysarthria	• Episodic pain • Unilateral periorbital intense pain • Lacrimation • Eye reddening • Nasal stuffiness • Lid ptosis
Type	Tension headache	Migraine	Cluster headache
Treatment	• NSAIDs • Acetaminophen	• Avoid triggers • NSAIDs • 5-HT1 agonists (triptans)	• Sumatriptan • Octreotide • Oxygen
Prophylaxis		If 3 attacks/month: • Propranolol • CGRP antagonists	• Verapamil • Prednisone • CGRP antagonists

Neuralgia

Trigeminal Neuralgia

Trigeminal neuralgia is an idiopathic disorder of the fifth cranial nerve resulting in severe, overwhelming pain in the face. Attacks of pain can be precipitated by chewing, touching the face, or pronouncing certain words in which the tongue strikes the back of the front teeth. Patients describe the pain as feeling as if a "knife is being stuck into the face." There is no specific diagnostic test.

Treatment is oxcarbazepine or carbamazepine. Baclofen and lamotrigine may also help. If medications do not control the pain, gamma knife surgery or surgical decompression can be curative.

Postherpetic Neuralgia

Herpes zoster reactivation (or shingles) is associated with a pain syndrome after resolution of the vesicular lesions in ~15% of cases. Treatment with antiherpetic medications such as acyclovir, famciclovir, and valganciclovir seems to reduce the incidence of postherpetic neuralgia, but steroids do not.

The pain is treated with tricyclic antidepressants, gabapentin, pregabalin, carbamazepine, or phenytoin until an effective therapy is found. Topical capsaicin is helpful. Most antiepileptic medications have some beneficial effect in neuropathic pain such as postherpetic neuralgia or peripheral neuropathy. However, none work in $\geq$50$\square$70% of patients.

Zoster vaccine is indicated in **all persons age >50** to prevent herpes zoster (shingles). The vaccine is similar to the varicella vaccine routinely administered to children to prevent chicken pox or varicella, except that the dose is much higher.

> Topical lidocaine effectively treats postherpetic neuralgia.

> There is no clear routinely effective treatment for peripheral neuropathy.

Seizures

Seizure disorders can be classified as follows:

- **Partial seizure**: a seizure that is focal to one part of the body, e.g., an arm or a leg; can be simple (intact consciousness) or complex (loss or alteration of consciousness)
- **Tonic-clonic seizure**: a generalized seizure with varying phases of muscular rigidity (tonic) followed by jerking of the muscles of the body for several minutes (clonic)
- **Absence (petit-mal) seizure** (common in children): a seizure where consciousness is impaired only briefly; patient often remains upright and gives a normal appearance (or seems to stare into space)

Generalized tonic-clonic seizures are caused by:

- Hyponatremia or hypernatremia
- Hypoxia

- Hypoglycemia
- Any CNS infection (encephalitis, meningitis, abscess)
- Any CNS anatomic abnormality (trauma, stroke, tumor)
- Hypocalcemia
- Uremia (elevated creatinine)
- Hepatic failure
- Alcohol, barbiturate, and benzodiazepine withdrawal
- Cocaine toxicity
- Hypomagnesemia (rare)

An EEG would not be the right answer unless all of these tests were done and were normal including a CT or MRI of the head. There is no point in doing an EEG to identify the cause of a seizure if there is a clear metabolic, toxic, or anatomic defect causing the seizure.

In other words, what would be the point of doing an EEG if the patient had hyponatremia or a brain lesion? You have already found the cause of the seizure.

> - Seizures of unclear etiology are called **epilepsy**.
> - If there is a clear cause, it is not epilepsy.

Delirium, Stupor, and Coma

These terms represent variations on a spectrum of abnormalities of altered consciousness or unresponsiveness to stimuli. All of the metabolic, toxic, and CNS anatomic problems previously listed can cause confusion or difficulty with arousal described as delirium, stupor, obtundation, or coma. When the condition is severe enough, a seizure occurs. Confusion is to coma and seizure as angina is to myocardial infarction.

Treatment

Treatment for **status epilepticus** is the only seizure treatment that is truly clear.

- For a persistent seizure: benzodiazepine such as lorazepam or diazepam intravenously (**best initial therapy**)
- If seizure persists: levetiracetam, valproic acid, phenytoin, or fosphenytoin.
  - Fosphenytoin (preferred) and phenytoin are equally effective.
  - Fosphenytoin has fewer side effects and can be given more rapidly.
  - Like lidocaine, phenytoin is a class 1b antiarrhythmic medication; given intravenously, it is associated with hypotension and AV block.
- If no response after benzodiazepines and fosphenytoin, give phenobarbital.
- The final option for unresolving seizure is a neuromuscular blocking agent such as succinylcholine, vecuronium, or pancuronium.
  - A neuromuscular blocking agent will just stop muscular contraction or the external manifestations of the seizure.
  - This will allow you to intubate the patient and give general anesthesia such as midazolam or propofol. If propofol is used, place the patient on a ventilator beforehand, since it can stop breathing.

> **Treatment of Status Epilepticus**
> 1. Benzodiazepine
> 2. Fosphenytoin
> 3. Levetiracetam, valproic acid, or phenobarbital
> 4. General anesthesia

Other treatment guidelines for seizure are as follows:

- Antiepileptic drugs (AED) are not needed after a single seizure, with the following exceptions:
  - Presentation in status epilepticus or with focal neurological signs
  - Abnormal EEG or lesion on CT
  - Family history of seizures
  - Uncorrectable cause such as stroke, tumor, or anatomical brain defect
- In **pregnancy**, the best AEDs are levetiracetam and lamotrigine.
- For **epilepsy**, the best treatment is not clear. A number of medications are effective, but none is clearly superior. In other words, levetiracetam, phenytoin, valproic acid, and carbamazepine all have nearly equal efficacy. You cannot be asked to choose between them based on efficacy. Levetiracetam has the fewest side effects. Alternative treatment is gabapentin, topiramate, lamotrigine, oxcarbazepine, or levetiracetam.
- For **absence seizures**, the best treatment is ethosuximide. If seizures are not controlled with a single agent, an alternate medication should be tried. If seizures are still not controlled, adding a second drug may help. If multiple medications do not control the seizure, surgical correction of a seizure focus may slow recurrence.

Regarding duration of treatment, the standard of care is to wait until the patient has been seizure-free for 2 years. A sleep deprivation EEG is the best way to tell if there is the possibility of recurrence. Sleep deprivation can elicit abnormal activity on an EEG, but the test lacks high sensitivity.

> Alcohol withdrawal seizures are not treated with long-term antiepileptic drugs.

Pregnancy	Levetiracetam, lamotrigine
Highest risk of hyponatremia	Carbamazepine
Estrogens (OCPs)	Increase metabolism of lamotrigine to ineffective levels
HLA B*1502 testing	Predicts Stevens-Johnson syndrome: carbamazepine and phenytoin

A 38-year-old man is evaluated for seizures. He achieves partial control with the addition of a second antiepileptic medication. He drives to work each day. What do you do about his ability to drive?

a. Confiscate his license.

b. Allow him to drive if he is seizure-free for 1 year.

c. Allow him to drive as long as his seizure history is noted on his license.

d. Recommend that he find an alternate means of transportation.

e. Do not let him leave the office unless he is picked up by someone; no further driving.

f. Allow him to drive as long as he is accompanied.

Answer: **D.** As a physician, you do not have the right to confiscate a patient's driver's license. The rules on seizure disorder and motor vehicles vary from state to state. Reporting his condition to the department of motor vehicles does not have the same clarity as, for instance, reporting child abuse, in which the doctor is legally protected for all reports made in good faith. You cannot hold a patient (incarcerate) for seizures in the way that you can for TB. Being accompanied in a car does not prevent seizures.

Spine Disorders

Anterior Spinal Artery Infarction

Anterior spinal artery infarction presents with:

- Loss of all function except for the posterior column (position and vibratory sensation intact)
- Flaccid paralysis below the level of the infarction
- Loss of deep tendon reflexes (DTRs) at the level of the infarction
- Transition into spastic paraplegia several weeks later
- Loss of pain and temperature
- Extensor plantar response

There is no specific treatment.

Subacute Combined Degeneration of the Cord

- From B12 deficiency or neurosyphilis.
- Position and vibratory sensation are lost.

Spinal Trauma

Acute onset of limb weakness and/or sensory disturbance below the level of the injury with the severity in proportion to the degree of injury. Sphincter function impaired. Loss of DTRs at the level of the injury followed by hyperreflexia below the level of the trauma. Glucocorticoids are not clearly beneficial.

Brown-Sequard Syndrome

After unilateral hemisection of spinal cord from an injury such as a knife wound cutting half the cord or compression from a mass lesion, patients lose pain and temperature sensation on the contralateral side from the injury, and lose motor function as well as position and vibratory sense on the ipsilateral side of the injury. For a mass, surgically decompress.

Syringomyelia

Syringomyelia is a fluid-filled, dilated central canal in the spinal cord. This widening bubble or cavitation first damages neural fibers passing near the center of the spine. It is caused by tumor or severe trauma to the spine or is congenital.

"What Is the Most Likely Diagnosis?"

Look for the loss of pain and temperature bilaterally across the upper back and both arms. Look for the phrase *capelike distribution of deficits*. Syringomyelia (literally a "bubble in the cord") also causes loss of reflexes and muscle atrophy in the same bilateral distribution.

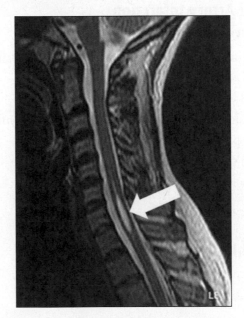

Figure 10.5 Syringomyelia is a fluid-filled lesion inside the center of the cord resulting in a capelike distribution of sensory loss across the neck and upper extremities. *Source: Mohammad Maruf, MD*

MRI is the **most accurate test**.

Treatment is surgical removal of tumor if present and drainage of fluid from the cavity.

Parkinsonism

Parkinsonism is the loss of cells in the substantia nigra resulting in a decrease in dopamine, which leads to a significant movement disorder presenting with tremor, gait disturbance, and rigidity.

There are many causes of parkinsonism. However, for the USMLE exam it is important to remember only the ones that will help you answer the "What is the most likely diagnosis?" question.

For instance, gait disturbance with a history of repeated head trauma from boxing or the use of antipsychotic medications such as chlorpromazine will help you establish the diagnosis. Other causes are encephalitis, reserpine, or metoclopramide.

> The most common cause of parkinsonism is idiopathic.

▶ **TIP**

There is no test for parkinsonism. The diagnosis is based entirely on the clinical presentation.

Presentation is as follows:

- Look for a patient age ≥50–60 who presents with a tremor, muscular rigidity, bradykinesia (slow movements), and a shuffling gait with unsteadiness on turning and a tendency to fall. Cogwheel rigidity is the slowing of movement on passive flexion or extension of an extremity. Facial expression is limited (hypomimia) and writing is small (micrographia). Postural instability is orthostatic hypotension. This happens because the same slowness that results in bradykinesia results in the inability of the pulse and blood pressure to reset appropriately. When an unaffected person stands up, the pulse speeds up within seconds. This response is impaired in parkinsonism, leading to lightheadedness when getting up from a seated position.
- Painful, contracted muscles from damage to the CNS (called spasticity). Spasticity is often associated with MS.

▶ **TIP**

The most frequent parkinsonism question is treatment. Know the drugs.

Treatment
Mild disease:

- Anticholinergic medications (benztropine and trihexyphenidyl) relieve tremor and rigidity. It is unclear why blocking acetylcholine improves symptoms of insufficient dopamine. Adverse effects of dry mouth, worsening prostate hypertrophy, and constipation occur more frequently in older patients.
- Amantadine may work by increasing the release of dopamine from the substantia nigra. It is definitely the answer in older patients (age >60) intolerant of anticholinergic medications.

> Which migraine drugs worsen Parkinson disease?
> - Prochlorperazine
> - Metoclopramide
> - Chlorpromazine
>
> All of these therapies are **antidopaminergic**.

Severe disease (inability to care for themselves, orthostatic):

- Dopamine agonists:
  - Pramipexole and ropinirole (**best initial therapy**)
  - Apomorphine or rotigotine (a patch)
- Levodopa/carbidopa (**most effective medication**)
  - Associated with "on/off" episodes: "off" is insufficient dopamine characterized by bradykinesia, while "on" is excessive dopamine characterized by dyskinesia
- COMT inhibitor (tolcapone, entacapone): extends the duration of levodopa/carbidopa by blocking the metabolism of dopamine (evens out dopamine level during "on/off" or when no response to treatment)
- Istradefylline (adenosine A2 antagonist): decreases the "off" phenomenon
- MAO inhibitors (rasagiline, selegiline, safinamide) as a single agent or in addition to levodopa/carbidopa; blocks metabolism of dopamine
- Deep brain stimulation: highly effective for tremors and rigidity

Pimavanserin is an antipsychotic medication that does not worsen Parkinson disease. It works by inhibiting 5HT, not through dopamine inhibition.

> Avoid tyramine-containing foods (e.g., cheese) with MAO inhibitors; they precipitate hypertension.

For spasticity, no single treatment is universally effective. Baclofen, dantrolene, and the central acting alpha agonist tizanidine may work.

> A 70-year-old man with extremely severe parkinsonism comes by ambulance to the ED secondary to psychosis and confusion developing at home. He is maintained on levodopa/carbidopa, ropinirole, and tolcapone. What is the most appropriate next step in management?
>
> a. Stop levodopa/carbidopa
> b. Start quetiapine
> c. Stop ropinirole
> d. Stop tolcapone
> e. Start haloperidol
>
> **Answer: B.** When a patient has very severe parkinsonism, you cannot stop medications, because the patient will become "locked in" with severe bradykinesia. Psychosis and confusion are a known adverse effect of antiparkinsonian treatment. Use antipsychotic medications with the fewest extrapyramidal (antidopaminergic) effects.

> Lewy body dementia = parkinsonism with dementia

> Shy-Drager syndrome = parkinsonism predominantly with orthostasis

Essential Tremor

Essential tremor is an action tremor that is activated by voluntary movement or when the arms are held in a fixed posture against gravity. It may affect some manual skills such as handwriting or the use of a computer keyboard. Caffeine makes the tremor worse.

Treatment is as follows:

- Propranolol (**best initial treatment**)
- If tremor persists, add primidone (an antiepileptic medication that controls tremor)

- If tremor still persists, switch treatment to topiramate or gabapentin
- If tremor remains severe despite these interventions and interferes with functioning, consider thalamotomy, which ablates the thalamus with magnetic resonance focused U/S or unilateral thalamotomy by delivering local heat (very effective at improving tremor severity)

▶ TIP

Tremor at rest and exertion improved with a drink of alcohol is the key to the diagnosis.

Restless Leg Syndrome

With restless leg syndrome (RLS), patients report an uncomfortable sensation in the legs that is "creepy and crawly" at night. The discomfort is worsened by caffeine and relieved by moving the legs. This can happen during sleep; a patient is sometimes brought in by a bed partner who is being kicked at night.

RLS is associated with iron deficiency.

Treatment is gabapentin, pregabalin, or dopamine agonists such as pramipexole. Iron replacement can improve symptoms.

Huntington Disease

Huntington disease (HD) is a hereditary disease characterized by CAG trinucleotide repeat sequences on chromosome 4.

"What Is the Most Likely Diagnosis?"

HD is the answer when you see:

- Choreiform movement disorder (dyskinesia)
- Dementia
- Behavior changes (irritability, moodiness, antisocial behavior)
- Onset age 30–50 with a family history of HD

The movement disorder of HD starts with "fidgetiness" or restlessness progressing to dystonic posturing, rigidity, and akathisia.

There is a specific genetic test in HD; it is 99% sensitive. CAG trinucleotide repeat sequences are found on genetic analysis. The symptom triad (movement/memory/mood) is confirmed with the test.

No treatment reverses HD.

- Psychosis is treated with haloperidol, quetiapine, or a trial of different antipsychotics.
- Movement disorders such as tardive dyskinesia and Huntington disease are treated with vesicular monoamine transporter 2 (VMAT2) inhibitors such as deutetrabenazine and tetrabenazine. They alter levels of monoamine (e.g., dopamine, serotonin, norepinephrine).

> Movement disorder may be troubling in HD, but it is far worse to progress to no movement at all (rigidity).

Tourette Syndrome

Tourette is an idiopathic disorder of:

- Vocal tics, grunts, and coprolalia
- Motor tics (sniffing, blinking, frowning)
- Obsessive-compulsive behavior

There are no specific diagnostic tests.

Treatment is fluphenazine, clonazepam, pimozide, or other neuroleptic medications. Methylphenidate and ADHD treatment are intrinsic to Tourette management.

Multiple Sclerosis

Multiple sclerosis (MS) is an idiopathic disorder exclusively of CNS (brain and cord) white matter. MS is more common in white women who live in colder climates.

"What Is the Most Likely Diagnosis?"

Look for multiple neurological deficits of the CNS affecting any aspect of CNS functioning.

- Focal sensory symptoms (most common), especially with gait and balance
- Optic neuritis (blurry vision/visual disturbance from optic neuritis is no longer the most common symptom)
- Motor problems
- Fatigue
- Spasticity and hyperreflexia
- Cerebellar deficits
- Trigeminal neuralgia (30%)

The least common abnormalities are cognitive defects and dementia. Sexual function remains relatively intact.

Diagnostic testing:

- MRI (**best initial and most accurate test**)
- Lumbar puncture shows CSF with a mild elevation in protein and <50–100 WBCs
- Oligoclonal bands (85% of patients) but these not specific to MS

> Internuclear ophthalmoplegia (INO) is the inability to adduct one eye with nystagmus in the other eye. INO is characteristic of MS.

> Visual and auditory evoked potentials are always the wrong answer.

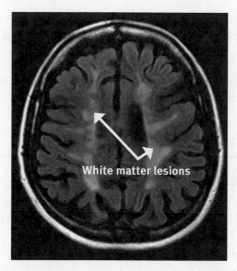

Figure 10.6 MS plaques appear white and are exclusively in the white matter of the CNS. *Source: Saba Ansari, MD*

▶ **TIP**

Oligoclonal bands are the answer in the 3–5% of patients with an equivocal or nondiagnostic MRI.

Treatment:

- For acute exacerbations, high-dose steroids will shorten the duration.
- To prevent relapse and progression:
  - Ocrelizumab (anti-CD20), siponimod, and cladribine (**the preferred agents**)
  - Glatiramer (copolymer 1)
  - Beta-interferon
  - Fingolimod, dimethyl fumarate, and teriflunomide (oral)
  - Natalizumab (an inhibitor of alpha-4 integrin; can be associated with PML)
  - Mitoxantrone
  - Azathioprine
  - Cyclophosphamide
  - Alemtuzumab (anti-CD52 also for CLL)

> Dalfampridine increases walking distance.

> Neurogenic (weak) bladder is treated with bethanechol, which is acetylcholine.

Allergic reactions to MRI gadolinium contrast are less common than allergic reactions or renal injury to CT iodine contrast. However, a systemic overreaction to gadolinium can occur, whereby increased collagen deposits in soft tissues and hardened fibrotic nodules develop in the skin, heart, lung, and liver. This condition, called "nephrogenic systemic fibrosis," occurs only in renal insufficiency. There is no specific treatment.

If neurologic deficits worsen with a chronic suppressive medication, and MRI shows multiple white matter hypodense lesions, what medication is likely the cause?

- Natalizumab, an inhibitor of alpha-4 integrin, has been associated with progressive multifocal leukoencephalopathy (PML).

Neuromuscular Disorders

Amyotrophic Lateral Sclerosis

Amyotrophic lateral sclerosis (ALS) (or motor neuron disease) is a loss exclusively of upper and lower motor neurons. The cause is unknown.

"What Is the Most Likely Diagnosis?"

Look for weakness of unclear etiology starting age 20s–40s with a unique combination of upper and lower motor neuron loss. The most serious symptom is difficulty in chewing and swallowing and a decrease in gag reflex. This leads to pooling of saliva in the pharynx and frequent episodes of aspiration. A weak cough and loss of swallowing offer poor prognosis.

| Presentation of Amyotrophic Lateral Sclerosis ||
Upper motor neurons	Lower motor neurons
Weakness	Weakness
Spasticity	Wasting
Hyperreflexia	Fasciculations
Extensor plantar responses	

> In ALS, there is no sensory loss and the sphincters are spared.

Diagnostic testing:

- Electromyography shows loss of neural innervation in multiple muscle groups
- Elevated CPK

Treatment:

- Riluzole to reduce glutamate buildup in neurons
- Edaravone, an antioxidant, to help the oxidative stress thought to play a role in killing neurons in those with ALS
- Baclofen to help spasticity
- CPAP and BiPAP to help with respiratory difficulties secondary to muscle weakness

> Both riluzole and edaravone delay progression of ALS. On the USMLE exam, you will not be asked to choose between them.

Tracheostomy and maintenance on a ventilator are often necessary when the disease advances. The most common cause of death in ALS is respiratory failure.

Pseudobulbar Affect

This is a condition of emotional lability, or emotional incontinence, with intermittent episodes of inappropriate laughter or crying. Half of patients with ALS have pseudobulbar affect. Stroke and MS also cause it.

Treat with dextromethorphan combined with quinidine. SSRIs are also effective in some patients.

Charcot-Marie-Tooth Disease

Charcot-Marie-Tooth (CMT) is a genetic disorder with loss of both motor and sensory innervation leading to:

- Distal weakness and sensory loss
- Wasting in the legs
- Decreased deep tendon reflexes
- Tremor

Foot deformity with a high arch is common (pes cavus). The legs look like inverted champagne bottles. The **most accurate test** is electromyography.

There is no treatment.

Peripheral Neuropathy

The most common cause of peripheral neuropathy is diabetes mellitus. Other causes include uremia, alcoholism, and paraproteinemias like monoclonal gammopathy of unknown significance.

Specific Peripheral Nerve Neuropathies		
Nerve	**Precipitating event described in the stem**	**Manifestations/Presentation**
Ulnar	Biker, pressure on palms of hands, trauma to the medial side of elbow	Wasting of hypothenar eminence, pain in 4th and 5th fingers
Radial	Pressure of inner, upper arm; falling asleep with arm over back of chair ("Saturday night palsy"); using crutches and pressure in the axilla	Wrist drop
Lateral cutaneous nerve of thigh	Obesity, pregnancy, sitting with crossed legs	Pain/numbness of outer aspect of one thigh
Tarsal tunnel (tibial nerve)	Worsens with walking	Pain/numbness in ankle and sole of foot
Peroneal	High boots, pressure on back of knee	Weak foot with decreased dorsiflexion and eversion
Median	Typists, carpenters, working with hands	Thenar wasting, pain/numbness in first 3 fingers

Treatment is pregabalin or gabapentin. Tricyclic antidepressants and most seizure medications (phenytoin, carbamazepine, lamotrigine) may be effective.

Complex Regional Pain Syndrome

Complex regional pain syndrome (or reflex sympathetic dystrophy) is characterized by severe, excruciating pain in a limb (arms, legs) with allodynia (pain elicited by normal stimuli). There are vasomotor symptoms as well as intermittent edema and skin color changes.

There is always a history of trauma damaging the myelin of the peripheral nerves.

The cause is unknown, and there is no precise testing; however, nuclear bone scan/MRI is abnormal in affected persons.

Treatment is similar to peripheral neuropathy: NSAIDs, TCAs, gabapentin or pregabalin.

Facial (Seventh Cranial) Nerve Palsy or Bell Palsy

Most cases of facial palsy are idiopathic. Some identified causes are Lyme disease, sarcoidosis, herpes zoster, and tumors.

Paralysis of the entire side of the face is classic. Stroke will paralyze only the lower half of the face because the upper half of the face receives innervation from both cerebral hemispheres. There is difficulty with closing the eye. If the patient can wrinkle her forehead on the affected side, worry about stroke. The inability to wrinkle the forehead on the affected side indicates Bell palsy.

Two additional features are:

- Hyperacusis: Sounds are extra loud because the seventh cranial nerve normally supplies the stapedius muscle, which acts as a "shock absorber" on the ossicles of the middle ear.
- Taste disturbances: The seventh cranial nerve supplies the sensation of taste to the anterior two-thirds of the tongue.

> Eating is "sloppy" because of difficulty closing the lips.

▶ TIP

Look for statements that "the face feels stiff" or "pulled to one side" to answer "What is the most likely diagnosis?"

Testing is not typically done because of the characteristic presentation of paralysis of half of the face. The **most accurate test** (if asked on the exam) is electromyography and nerve conduction study.

Treatment is prednisone, but even without treatment 60% of patients fully recover.

A 38-year-old carpenter comes with pain near his ear that is quickly followed by weakness of one side of his face. Both the upper and lower parts of his face are weak, but sensation is intact. What is the most common complication of his disorder?

a. Corneal ulceration
b. Aspiration pneumonia
c. Sinusitis
d. Otitis media
e. Deafness
f. Dental caries

Answer: **A**. Corneal ulceration occurs with seventh cranial nerve palsy because of difficulty in closing the eye, especially at night. This leads to dryness of the eye and ulceration. Prevent eye dryness and ulceration by taping the eye shut and using lubricants in the eye. Dental caries don't happen; although there is drooling from difficulty closing the mouth, saliva production is normal. Rather than deafness, sounds are extra loud. Aspiration does not occur, because gag reflex and cough are normal.

Guillain-Barré Syndrome

Guillain-Barré Syndrome (GBS) (or acute inflammatory polyneuropathy) is an autoimmune damage of multiple peripheral nerves.

There is no CNS involvement. A circulating antibody attacks the myelin sheaths of the peripheral nerves, removing their insulation.

GBS is associated with *Campylobacter jejuni* infection.

"What Is the Most Likely Diagnosis?"

Look for weakness in the legs that ascends from the feet and moves toward the chest, associated with a loss of DTRs. A few patients have a mild sensory disturbance. The main problem is that when GBS hits the diaphragm, it is associated with respiratory muscle weakness. Autonomic dysfunction with hypotension, hypertension, or tachycardia can occur.

> Ascending weakness + Loss of reflexes = GBS

Diagnostic testing:

- Nerve conduction study/electromyography (**most specific test**) will show a decrease in the propagation of electrical impulses along the nerves, but it takes 1–2 weeks to become abnormal.
- CSF shows increased protein with a normal cell count.
- Tests of respiratory muscle involvement: When diaphragm is involved, there is a decrease in forced vital capacity and peak inspiratory pressure; inspiration is the "active" part of breathing, and patient loses the strength to inhale.
  - PFTs tell who might die from GBS.
  - Death, although rare, is caused by dysautonomia and respiratory failure.

Treatment is intravenous immunoglobulin (IVIG) or plasmapheresis (equal in efficacy). Do not combine them.

Prednisone does not help.

A woman comes to the ED with bilateral leg weakness over the last few days. She has lost her knee jerk and ankle jerk reflexes. The weakness started in her feet and progressed up to her calves and then her thighs. She is otherwise asymptomatic. Which of the following is the most urgent next step?

a. Pulmonary function testing
b. Arterial blood gas
c. Nerve conduction study
d. Lumbar puncture
e. Peak flow meter

Answer: **A.** The most dangerous thing that can happen with GBS is dysautonomia or involvement of the respiratory muscles. Peak **inspiratory** pressure or a decrease in forced vital capacity (FVC) is the earliest way to detect impending respiratory failure. If you wait until there is CO_2 accumulation on an ABG, it is too late. Nerve conduction studies are the most accurate test, but their results are not as important as answering the question "Do you know who is going to die from respiratory failure?" Peak flow assesses **expiratory** function, which is not greatly impaired in GBS; peak flow is best used to assess obstructive disease such as COPD or asthma.

Miller Fisher is a variant of GBS, with weakness descending, from top down. A key physical finding is oculomotor nerve involvement. Perform GQ1b antibody testing. Treat like GBS, with IVIG or plasmapheresis.

Myasthenia Gravis

Myasthenia gravis (MG) is a disorder of muscular weakness from the production of antibodies against acetylcholine receptors at the neuromuscular junction.

"What Is the Most Likely Diagnosis?"

Look for a question describing "double vision and difficulty chewing," "dysphonia," or "weakness of limb muscles worse at the end of the day."

This is because the extraocular muscles and mastication (masseter) are often the only 2 muscular activities universally done by people (i.e., watching TV and eating).

Physical examination reveals ptosis, weakness with sustained activity, and **normal pupillary responses.**

| Severe myasthenia affects respiratory muscles. |

Diagnostic testing includes:

- Acetylcholine receptor antibodies (**best initial test**)
  - 80–90% sensitive
  - Better first test than edrophonium testing
  - For patients without those antibodies, get anti-MUSK antibodies (muscle-specific kinase)
- Edrophonium: short-acting inhibitor of acetylcholinesterase. The temporary bump up in acetylcholine levels is associated with a clear improvement in motor function that lasts for a few minutes.
- Electromyography (**most accurate test**) shows decreased strength with repetitive stimulation

► **TIP**

Exam questions often ask, "What imaging test should be done?" For MG, answer: chest something. Chest x-ray, CT, or MRI is done to look for thymoma or thymic hyperplasia. CT with contrast is best.

Treatment is as follows:

- Neostigmine or pyridostigmine (**best initial treatment**), a long-acting version of edrophonium
  - Glycopyrrolate, an anticholinergic drug that blocks muscarinic receptors, can minimize the drooling and diarrhea that are side effects of neostigmine and pyridostigmine; can help with COPD; and can reduce oral secretions during intubation.
  - It blocks adverse effects at the muscarinic receptors of the salivary gland without blocking the nicotinic receptors at the neuromuscular junction.
- If there is no response to neostigmine or pyridostigmine, do the following:
  - If patient age <60: thymectomy
  - If patient age >60: prednisone
  - Azathioprine, tacrolimus, cyclophosphamide, or mycophenolate to get patient off of steroids before serious side effects occur
  - The main point is to suppress T cell function in order to control antibodies made against acetylcholine receptors.
- Refractory and recurrent disease
  - Rituximab to eliminate CD20 cells (source of the antibodies that attack Ach receptors)
  - Eculizumab to remove complement, which destroys receptors

> Thymectomy in myasthenia is like splenectomy in idiopathic thrombocytopenic purpura. It markedly improves recurrent, hard-to-control disease.

Acute myasthenic crisis presents with severe, overwhelming disease with profound weakness or respiratory involvement. Treatment is IVIG or plasmapheresis.

Lambert-Eaton Myasthenic Syndrome

Lambert-Eaton myasthenic syndrome (LEMS) presents with muscle weakness in those with small-cell lung cancer. There is decreased release of acetylcholine at the neuromuscular junction.

Unlike MG or the muscle weakness of any paraneoplastic syndrome, **with LEMS there is increased strength with increased use.** Deep tendon reflexes increase after exercise.

- **Best initial test**: anti-P/Q-type voltage-gated calcium channel (VGCC) antibody
- **Best initial treatment**: pyridostigmine
- **Best treatment for acute, severe disease**: IVIG, amifampridine (K^+ channel blocker)

Dementia

Alzheimer disease is by far the most common cause of dementia. Since there is no specific test for Alzheimer disease, your challenge is to know how far to go in testing to diagnose it and what the other dementia syndromes are.

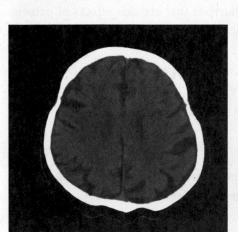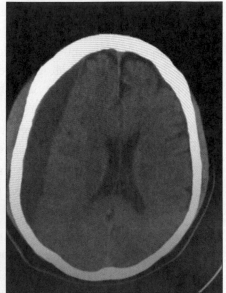

Figures 10.7, 10.8 Alzheimer disease, chronic alcoholism, and untreated HIV can all give diffuse symmetrical atrophy (left). Draining a chronic subdural hematoma (right) may improve memory. This is a key reason why an MRI of the head is done in dementia.
Source: left: Pramod Theetha Kariyanna, MD
Source: right: Naveen Paddhu, MD

Diagnostic testing includes:

- MRI of brain
- VDRL or RPR to exclude syphilis
- B12 with possible methylmalonic acid level
- Thyroid function test

Treatment is as follows:

- Donepezil, rivastigmine, and galantamine (all equal in efficacy) to increase acetylcholine level
- Memantine

Lewy Body Dementia

- Associated with Parkinson disease
- Treat Parkinson disease with dopamine agonists and replacement (as previously described) and Alzheimer disease with acetylcholinesterase inhibitors

Frontotemporal Dementia (Pick Disease)

- Emotional and social appropriateness are lost first
- Memory deteriorates later
- No special therapy beyond acetylcholine medications

Creutzfeldt-Jakob Disease (CJD)

- Rapidly progressive dementia
- Myoclonic jerks
- Normal head MRI or CT
- CSF with 14-3-3 protein
- Biopsy is most accurate
- No specific therapy

Normal Pressure Hydrocephalus

- Dementia with gait ataxia and urinary incontinence
- Diagnose with head scan
- Treat with shunt

Neurocutaneous Diseases

Neurocutaneous disorders are neurologic conditions that affect the brain, spine, and peripheral nerves but have manifestations on the skin.

Tuberous Sclerosis

- Neurological abnormalities: seizures, progressive psychomotor retardation, slowly progressive mental deterioration
- Skin:
  - Adenoma sebaceum (reddened facial nodules)
  - Shagreen patches (leathery plaques on the trunk)
  - Ash leaf (hypopigmented) patches
- Retinal lesions
- Cardiac rhabdomyomas

There is no specific treatment. Control seizures.

Neurofibromatosis (von Recklinghausen Disease)

- Neurofibromas: soft, flesh-colored lesions attached to peripheral nerves
- Eighth cranial nerve tumors
- Cutaneous hyperpigmented lesions (café au lait spots)
- Meningioma and gliomas

There is no specific treatment. Eighth cranial nerve lesions may need surgical decompression to help preserve hearing.

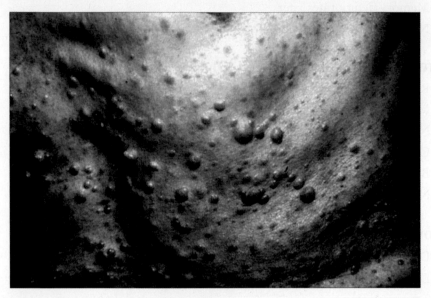

Figure 10.9 The lesions of neurofibromatosis are flesh-colored, soft, and nontender.
Source: Mohammad Maruf, MD

Sturge-Weber Syndrome

Presents with:

- Port-wine stain of the face
- Seizures
- CNS: homonymous hemianopsia, hemiparesis, mental subnormality

Skull x-ray shows calcification of angiomas. There is no treatment beyond controlling seizures.

Nephrology 11

Diagnostic Tests in Nephrology

In nephrology, the **best initial tests** are urinalysis, blood urea nitrogen (BUN), and creatinine.

Urinalysis

The urinalysis (urine analysis or UA) measures chemical reactions associated with:

- Protein
- WBCs (direct microscopic examination) or leukocyte esterase (dipstick)
- RBCs
- Specific gravity and pH
- Nitrites (indicates presence of gram-negative bacteria on dipstick)

The dipstick gives some quantitative values as well. This means it is not just positive or negative but can give an approximation of the quantity of the protein, WBCs, and RBCs. This can be described as a direct number (e.g., 300 mg protein) or a scale: 0, 1+, 2+, 3+, or 4+.

> Urinalysis is two parts:
> 1. dipstick if positive
> 2. microscopic analysis

▶ TIP

Every USMLE Step 2 CK administration will have a range of normal values available for you to reference.

Protein

It is normal to excrete a very tiny amount of protein. The tubules secrete slight amounts of protein normally known as Tamm-Horsfall protein. This should be <150 mg per 24 hours. Greater amounts of protein can be associated with either tubular disease or glomerular disease. Very large amounts of protein can only be excreted with glomerular disease.

> Severe proteinuria means
> **glomerular damage**.

In terms of proteinuria, the problem with using the scale of "trace" through 4+ is that UA measures only the amount of protein excreted at a particular moment in the day. It does not give an average or total amount of protein excreted over 24 hours, because renal function itself varies during the day based on bodily position and physical activity. It is like the difference between

Standing and physical activity increase urinary protein excretion.	an EKG and a Holter monitor. Transient proteinuria is present in 2–10% of the population, with most of this being benign, without representing pathology. If proteinuria persists and is not related to prolonged standing (orthostatic proteinuria), a kidney biopsy should be performed.

Assuming constant protein excretion throughout the day, 1+ protein is about 1 gram excreted per 24 hours, 2+ protein is about 2 grams per 24 hours, and so on. The methods used to assess the total amount of protein in a day are:

Urine dipstick for protein detects only albumin. Bence-Jones protein in myeloma is **not detectable** on a dipstick. Use immunoelectrophoresis.

- Single protein-to-creatinine ratio
- 24-hour urine collection

These tests are considered equal in accuracy. Since the 24-hour urine is much harder to collect, however, it is rarely performed. Normal protein is less than 150 mg per 24 hours.

Normal urinary protein excretion is <150 mg/24 hr.

▶ TIP

To assess proteinuria, UA is the **initial test**. Protein-to-creatinine ratio is **more accurate** at determining the amount.

Protein-to-Creatinine Ratio

The P:Cr ratio can be superior in accuracy to a 24-hour urine because of technical difficulties in collecting a full day's worth of urine. If you collect a little less, it will *underestimate* the true excretion. If you add a single extra urination, you might overestimate the protein excretion.

- P:Cr ratio of 1 is equivalent to 1 gram of protein on a 24-hour urine.
- P:Cr ratio of 2.5 is equivalent to 2.5 grams of protein found on a 24-hour urine.

Biopsy determines the cause of proteinuria.

▶ TIP

If both P:Cr ratio and 24-hour urine are in the choices, choose the P:Cr ratio. It is faster and technically easier to perform.

Microalbuminuria

The presence of tiny amounts of protein that are too small to detect on the UA is called microalbuminuria. This is very important to detect in diabetic patients. Long-term microalbuminuria leads to worsening renal function in a diabetic patient and should be treated. Be aware that <30 mg on spot urine is normal.

Microalbuminuria = 30–300 mg/24 hr

A diabetic patient is evaluated with a UA that shows no protein. Microalbuminuria is detected (30–300 mg/24 hr). What is the next best step in management?

a. Enalapril
b. Kidney biopsy
c. Hydralazine
d. Renal consultation
e. Low-protein diet
f. Repeat UA annually and treat when trace protein is detected

Answer: **A.** An ACE inhibitor or angiotensin receptor blocker (e.g., losartan, valsartan) is the **best initial therapy** for any degree of proteinuria in a diabetic patient. They decrease the progression of proteinuria and delay the development of renal insufficiency in diabetic patients. Hydralazine is not as effective and has more adverse effects. Low-protein diets are less effective than ACE inhibitors. Do not consult for initiating medications like ACE inhibitors.

White Blood Cells

WBCs detect inflammation, infection, or allergic interstitial nephritis. You cannot distinguish neutrophils from eosinophils on a UA. Neutrophils indicate infection. Eosinophils indicate allergic or acute interstitial nephritis. It is very useful if eosinophils are found because of their specificity. It is less important if they are absent, because the sensitivity of the test is limited. Microscopic examination gives a precise numerical count of the number of white blood cells present. Persistent WBC on UA with negative culture can be TB.

No nitrites or WBCs on UA means there is no infection.

> No nitrites or WBCs on UA = **No infection**

> NSAID-induced renal disease does not show eosinophils.

▶ TIP

Wright and Hansel stains detect eosinophils in the urine. They are the answer for allergic interstitial nephritis.

Hematuria

Normal urinalysis has <5 RBCs per high power field. Hematuria is indicative of:

- Stones in bladder, ureter, or kidney
- Hematologic disorders that cause bleeding (coagulopathy)
- Infection (cystitis, pyelonephritis)
- Cancer of bladder, ureters, or kidney (however, do not use urinalysis to screen for bladder cancer)
- Treatments (cyclophosphamide gives hemorrhagic cystitis)
- Trauma; simply "banging" the kidney or bladder makes it shed red blood cells
- Glomerulonephritis

False-positive tests for hematuria on dipstick are caused by hemoglobin or myoglobin. Ascorbic acid (vitamin C) causes a false-negative test.

> IgA nephropathy is common for mild recurrent hematuria.

A woman is admitted to the hospital with trauma and dark urine. The dipstick is markedly positive for blood. What is the best initial test to confirm the etiology?

a. Microscopic examination of the urine
b. Cystoscopy
c. Renal ultrasound
d. Renal/bladder CT scan
e. Abdominal x-ray
f. Intravenous pyelogram

Answer: **A.** Hemoglobin and myoglobin make the dipstick positive for blood, but no red blood cells are seen on microscopic examination of the urine. Abdominal x-ray detects small bowel obstruction (ileus) but is very poor at detecting stones or cancer. Renal CT is the most accurate test for stones, but would not be done until the etiology of the positive dipstick had been confirmed as blood.

The **best initial test** of the bladder is microscopic examination of the urine. The **most accurate test** is cystoscopy.

> Cystoscopy is the most accurate test of the bladder.

▶ **TIP**

Intravenous pyelogram (IVP) is always wrong. It is slower and the contrast is renal toxic.

▶ **TIP**

When "dysmorphic" red blood cells are described, the correct answer is glomerulonephritis.

When is cystoscopy the answer?

- When there is hematuria without infection or prior trauma; renal U/S/CT shows no etiology; and bladder sonography shows a mass for possible biopsy.

Casts

These are microscopic collections of material clogging up the tubules and being excreted in the urine.

> Casts are very useful if found, but they are often absent.

Urinary Casts and Their Significance	
Type of cast	**Association**
Red blood cell	Glomerulonephritis
White blood cell	Pyelonephritis
Eosinophil	Acute (allergic) interstitial nephritis
Hyaline	Dehydration concentrates the urine and the normal Tamm-Horsfall protein precipitates or concentrates into a cast.
Broad, waxy	Chronic renal disease
Granular, "muddy-brown"	Acute tubular necrosis; these are collections of dead tubular cells

▶ **TIP**

The presence of urinary casts helps answer the "most likely diagnosis" question because they are specific.

Acute Kidney Injury

Acute kidney injury (AKI), formerly called acute renal failure (ARF), is a decrease in creatinine clearance which causes a sudden rise in BUN and creatinine. AKI is categorized into 3 types:

- Prerenal azotemia (decreased perfusion)
- Postrenal azotemia (obstruction)
- Intrinsic renal disease (ischemia and toxins)

Prerenal Azotemia

Prerenal azotemia is caused by inadequate perfusion of the kidney; the kidney itself is normal. Any cause of hypoperfusion or hypovolemia will raise the BUN and creatinine, with the BUN rising more than the creatinine. Causes include the following:

- Hypotension (systolic <90 mm Hg) from sepsis, anaphylaxis, bleeding, dehydration
- Hypovolemia: diuretics, burns, pancreatitis
- Renal artery stenosis: even though the blood pressure may be high, the kidney is underperfused
- Relative hypovolemia from decreased pump function: CHF, constrictive pericarditis, tamponade
- Hypoalbuminemia
- Cirrhosis
- NSAIDs constricting the afferent arteriole

Postrenal Azotemia

Obstruction of any cause damages the kidney by blocking filtration at the glomerulus. As in prerenal azotemia, the kidney itself is normal. Causes of postrenal azotemia include:

- Prostate hypertrophy or cancer
- Stone in the ureter
- Cervical cancer
- Urethral stricture
- Neurogenic (atonic) bladder
- Retroperitoneal fibrosis (look for bleomycin, or radiation in the history)

> The kidney in prerenal and postrenal disease would function normally if transplanted into another person.

> **Both** kidneys must be obstructed to cause a rise in creatinine.

> CT angiogram is dangerous in a patient with borderline renal function.

Management of prerenal and postrenal azotemia is based on correcting the underlying cause. The majority are reversible.

The major force favoring filtration is the hydrostatic pressure in the glomerular capillary. If hydrostatic pressure in Bowman space rises, fluid cannot filter through. Unilateral obstruction causes renal failure if the person has only one kidney.

Intrinsic Renal Disease

The most common cause of intrinsic renal disease is acute tubular necrosis (ATN) from toxins or ischemia of the kidney. Glomerulonephritis is rarely acute, but when the kidney is injured from any cause, there is always a greater risk of AKI. For example, a few hours of hypotension might result in no damage at all to a normal kidney but cause AKI in a kidney with underlying renal damage. Other causes are:

- Acute (allergic) interstitial nephritis (commonly from medications such as penicillin)
- Rhabdomyolysis and hemoglobinuria
- Contrast agents, aminoglycosides, cisplatin, amphotericin, cyclosporine, and NSAIDs (the **most common toxins** causing AKI from ATN)
- Crystals such as hyperuricemia, hypercalcemia, or hyperoxaluria
- Proteins such as Bence-Jones protein from myeloma
- Poststreptococcal infection

Acute Kidney Injury Etiologies		
Prerenal	**Intrinsic renal**	**Postrenal**
Hypotension	Acute tubular necrosis	BPH/prostate cancer
• Sepsis	• Toxins	Ureteral stone
• Anaphylaxis	– NSAIDs	Cervical cancer
• Bleeding	– Aminoglycoside antibiotics, amphotericin	Urethral stone
• Dehydration	– Cisplatin, cyclosporine	Neurogenic bladder
Hypovolemia	• Prolonged ischemia	Retroperitoneal fibrosis (chemotherapy or external-beam therapy)
• Diuretics	AIN	
• Burns	• Penicillin, sulfa drugs	
• Pancreatitis	Rhabdomyolysis/hemoglobinuria	
• ↓ pump function	Contrast	
• Low albumin	Crystals	
• Cirrhosis	Bence-Jones proteins	
Renal artery stenosis	Poststreptococcal infection	
• Congestive heart failure		

Presentation of AKI

AKI may present with only an asymptomatic rise in BUN and creatinine. When AKI is symptomatic, symptoms include:

- Nausea and vomiting
- Fatigue/malaise
- Weakness
- Shortness of breath and edema from fluid overload

Very severe disease presents with:

- Confusion
- Arrhythmia from hyperkalemia and acidosis
- Sharp, pleuritic chest pain from pericarditis

▶ **TIP**

No symptoms are specific enough to answer the "most likely diagnosis" question without lab testing.

> There is no pathognomonic physical finding of AKI.

Presentation of Postrenal Azotemia

Bladder distention and massive diuresis after Foley catheter placement are events specific to urinary obstruction. This is the closest you will get to a specific presentation for any form of AKI.

Diagnostic Tests

The **best initial test** for AKI is the BUN and creatinine. With completely dead kidneys, the creatinine will rise about one point (1 mg/dL) per day. If the BUN:creatinine ratio is above 20:1, the etiology is either prerenal or postrenal damage of the kidney. Intrinsic renal disease has a ratio closer to 10:1. Renal sonogram is the **best initial imaging test**. Sonography does not require contrast, and contrast should be avoided in renal insufficiency.

Prerenal azotemia is usually a clear diagnosis. Look for a question describing *all of the following*:

- BUN:creatinine ratio above 20:1
- Clear history of **hypoperfusion or hypotension**

Postrenal azotemia is usually a clear diagnosis. Look for a question involving *all of the following*:

- BUN:creatinine ratio above 20:1
- **Distended bladder or massive release of urine** with catheter placement
- Bilateral **hydronephrosis** on sonogram (ultrasound)

▶ **TIP**

Some medications give the false impression of renal injury by elevating creatinine. These drugs inhibit creatinine secretion in the proximal tubule:

- Trimethoprim
- Febuxostat
- Cimetidine
- Cobicistat

Tests for AKI of Unclear Etiology

When the cause of AKI is not clear, the "best next diagnostic step" is:

- Urinalysis
- Urine sodium (UNa)
- Fractional excretion of sodium (FENa) or urea
- Urine osmolality

▶ **TIP**

If all of these are choices, always go with urinalysis first.

Urine Sodium and Fractional Excretion of Sodium

> **Prerenal** azotemia:
> **low UNa** (<20) =
> **low FENa** (<1%)

Decreased blood pressure (or decreased intravascular volume) normally will increase aldosterone. Increased aldosterone increases sodium resorption. It is normal for urine sodium to decrease when there is decreased renal perfusion because aldosterone levels rise.

> Urine sodium and FENa give you the same information.

▶ **TIP**

You can answer all the questions on USMLE Step 2 CK without knowing the mathematical formula for FENa.

Urine Osmolality

When intravascular volume is low, normally ADH levels should rise. A healthy kidney will resorb more water to fill the vasculature and increase renal perfusion.

When more water is resorbed from the urine, will the urine become more concentrated, or more dilute?

- Increased resorption leads to an increase in urine osmolality: more concentrated urine.

Normal tubule cells resorb water. In ATN, the urine cannot be concentrated because the tubule cells are damaged. The urine produced in ATN is similar in osmolality to the blood (about 300 mOsm/L). This is called isosthenuria. Urine osmolality in ATN is inappropriately low. Isosthenuria is especially problematic when the patient is dehydrated.

Isosthenuria means the urine is the same (*iso*) strength (*sthenos*) as the blood. The term *isosthenuria* is used interchangeably with the phrase *renal tubular concentrating defect*.

Dehydration should normally increase urine concentration (osmolality). If there is damage to the tubular cells from ischemia or toxins, however, the kidney loses the ability to absorb sodium and water. In ATN, the body inappropriately loses sodium (UNa above 20) and water (UOsm below 300) into the urine.

Normal osmolality changes in a healthy person:
- Fluid overload → **low** urine osmolality (dilute urine)
- Dehydration → **high** urine osmolality (concentrated urine)

A 20-year-old African American man comes for a screening test for sickle cell. He is found to be heterozygous (trait or AS) for sickle cell. What is the best advice for him?

a. Nothing needed until he has a painful crisis
b. Avoid dehydration
c. Hydroxyurea
d. Folic acid supplementation
e. Pneumococcal vaccination

Answer: **B.** The only significant manifestation of sickle cell trait is a defect in renal concentrating ability or isosthenuria. These patients will continue to produce inappropriately dilute, high-volume urine despite dehydration. Hydroxyurea is used to prevent painful crises when they occur more than 4×/year. Painful crises rarely occur in sickle cell trait. Patients with sickle cell trait do not have hemolysis, so there is no need for additional folic acid supplementation. Splenic function is abnormal only in those who are homozygous, so pneumococcal vaccination is not routinely indicated.

Classification of Acute Renal Failure by Laboratory Testing		
Test	**Prerenal azotemia**	**Acute tubular necrosis**
BUN:creatinine	>20:1	<20:1
Urine sodium (UNa)	<20 mEq/L	>20 mEq/L
Fractional excretion of sodium (FENa)	<1%	>1%
Urine osmolality (UOsm)	>500 mOsm/kg	<300 mOsm/kg

Urine specific gravity correlates to urine osmolality.

High UOsm = High specific gravity

Specific Gravity on UA Correlated with Urine Osmolarity	
UA specific gravity	**Urine osmolarity**
1.010	300
1.020	600
1.040	1,200

To correlate the specific gravity with the osmolarity, multiply the last two numbers by 30.

Acute Tubular Necrosis (ATN)

ATN is an injury to the kidneys from ischemia and/or toxins that causes tubular cells to slough off into the urine. The mechanisms for resorbing sodium and water are lost with the tubular cells. Proteinuria is not significant in ATN since protein spills into the urine when glomeruli (not tubules) are damaged.

Knowing the causes of ATN is critical, since there is no specific diagnostic test to prove the etiology. You cannot do a blood level of a drug or a biopsy to prove that a particular toxin caused the renal failure.

▶ TIP

Acute renal failure and a toxin in the history are your clues to the "What is the most likely diagnosis?" question for ATN.

Specific Causes of ATN

A patient comes with fever and acute left lower quadrant abdominal pain. Blood cultures on admission grow *E. coli* and *Candida albicans*. She is started on vancomycin, metronidazole and gentamicin, and amphotericin. She has a CT scan that identifies diverticulitis. After 36 hours, her creatinine rises dramatically. Which of the following is most likely the cause of the patient's renal insufficiency?

a. Vancomycin
b. Gentamicin
c. Contrast media
d. Metronidazole
e. Amphotericin

Answer: **C.** Radiographic contrast media has a very rapid onset of injury. Creatinine rises the next day. Vancomycin, gentamicin, and amphotericin are all potentially nephrotoxic, but they would not cause renal failure with just 2 or 3 doses. They need 5–10 days to result in nephrotoxicity. Metronidazole is hepatically excreted and does not cause renal failure.

A 74-year-old blind man is admitted with obstructive uropathy and chest pain. He has a history of hypertension and diabetes. His creatinine drops from 10 mg/dL to 1.2 mg/dL 3 days after catheter placement. The stress test shows reversible ischemia. What is the most appropriate next step in management?

a. Coronary artery calcium score on CT scan
b. One to two liters of normal saline hydration prior and during angiography
c. N-acetylcysteine prior to angiography
d. Mannitol during angiography
e. Furosemide during angiography
f. Intravenous sodium bicarbonate before and during angiography

Answer: **B.** Saline hydration has the **most proven benefit** at preventing contrast-induced nephrotoxicity. Mannitol and furosemide may or may not prevent nephrotoxicity. There is minimal data to support their use. N-acetylcysteine and sodium bicarbonate have some benefit, but the evidence is not as clear as that with saline. Calcium scoring on CT scan is still considered experimental. It does not provide sufficient information to eliminate angiography.

Extra-Difficult Question—How to Get a 280 on Step 2 CK

A patient with mild renal insufficiency undergoes angiography and develops a 2 mg/dL rise in creatinine from ATN despite the use of saline hydration before and after the procedure. What do you expect to find on laboratory testing?

a. Urine sodium 8 (low), FENa >1%, urine specific gravity 1.035 (high)
b. Urine sodium 58 (high), FENa >1%, urine specific gravity 1.005 (low)
c. Urine sodium 5 (very low), FENa <1%, urine specific gravity 1.040 (very high)
d. Urine sodium 45 (high), FENa >1% urine specific gravity 1.005 (low)

Answer: **C.** Although contrast-induced renal failure is a form of ATN, the urinary lab values are an exception from the other forms of ATN. Contrast causes spasm of the afferent arteriole that leads to renal tubular dysfunction. There is tremendous resorption of sodium and water, leading the specific gravity of the urine to become very high. This results in profoundly low urine sodium. The usual finding in ATN from nephrotoxins would be UNa >20, FENa >1%, and a *low* specific gravity. Specific gravity correlates with urine osmolality.

A patient with extremely severe myeloma with a plasmacytoma is admitted for combination chemotherapy. Two days later, the creatinine rises. What is the most likely cause?

a. Cisplatin
b. Hyperuricemia
c. Bence-Jones proteinuria
d. Hypercalcemia
e. Hyperoxaluria

Answer: **B.** Two days after chemotherapy, the creatinine rises in a person with a hematologic malignancy; this is most likely from tumor lysis syndrome leading to hyperuricemia. Cisplatin, as with most drug toxicities, would not produce a rise in creatinine for 5–10 days. Bence-Jones protein and hypercalcemia both cause renal insufficiency, but it would not be rapid and it would not happen as a result of treatment. Treatment for myeloma would end up decreasing both the calcium and Bence-Jones protein levels because they are produced from the leukemic cells. Cancer cells do not release oxalate.

What would have prevented the creatinine rise described in the preceding vignette?

• Allopurinol, hydration, and rasburicase should be given prior to chemotherapy to prevent renal failure from tumor lysis syndrome.

> Rasburicase causes hemolysis in those with G6PD deficiency.

A patient who is suicidal ingests an unknown substance and develops renal failure 3 days later. Her calcium level is also low, and the urinalysis shows an abnormality. What did she take?

a. Aspirin
b. Acetaminophen
c. Ethylene glycol
d. Ibuprofen
e. Opiates
f. Methanol

Answer: C. Ethylene glycol is associated with acute kidney injury based on oxalic acid and oxalate precipitating within the kidney tubules, causing ATN. Oxalate appears as envelope-shaped crystals. The calcium level is low because ethylene glycol precipitates as calcium oxalate. Aspirin is renally toxic but does not lower calcium levels and has no abnormality on urinalysis. Acetaminophen is hepatotoxic. Ibuprofen and all NSAIDs are renally toxic; they constrict the afferent arteriole and cause allergic interstitial nephritis and papillary necrosis. They have no impact on calcium levels, and the only time something would be found in the urine is in the case of papillary necrosis (which causes sudden flank pain and fever). Methanol causes inflammation of the retina; it has no renal toxicity. Opiates do not cause AKI.

Toxins Producing ATN

> The body loses 1% of renal function for every year past the age of 40.

Toxins have an increased likelihood of producing ATN if there is hypoperfusion of the kidney and if there is underlying renal insufficiency such as from hypertension or diabetes. The risk of ATN is directly proportional to increasing age of the patient.

Summary of Causes of ATN

- Nonoliguric renal injury: caused by aminoglycoside antibiotics, amphotericin, cisplatin, vancomycin, acyclovir, and cyclosporine
  - Slower onset (usually 5–10 days)
  - Dose dependent (the more administered, the sicker the patient becomes)
  - Aminoglycoside and cisplatin: low magnesium level may increase the risk of toxicity
- Contrast media
  - Cause immediate renal toxicity
  - Best prevented with saline hydration
  - N-acetylcysteine and sodium bicarbonate do not help
- Hemoglobin and myoglobin (rhabdomyolysis)
- Hyperuricemia from tumor lysis syndrome (acute) or from gout (if long-standing, can cause chronic renal failure)
- Precipitation of calcium oxalate in the renal cortex from ethylene glycol overdose
- Bence-Jones protein (directly toxic to renal tubules)
- NSAIDs

Rhabdomyolysis

Rhabdomyolysis is caused by trauma, prolonged immobility, snake bites, seizures, and crushing injuries. Additional etiologies:

- Cocaine (constricts vessels)
- Low K^+ (constricts vessels)
- Low PO_4 (breaks cells)
- Statins
- Viral infections

Creatine phosphokinase (CPK) levels are markedly elevated, and myoglobin spills into the urine. Hyperkalemia occurs from the release of potassium from damaged cells because 95% of the potassium in the body is intracellular. Hyperuricemia occurs for the same reason it does in tumor lysis syndrome. When cells break down, nucleic acids are released from the cell's nuclei and are rapidly metabolized to uric acid. Damaged muscle releases phosphate. Hypocalcemia occurs from increased calcium binding to damaged muscle.

Diagnostic testing begins with urinalysis (**best initial test**) to confirm the diagnosis. The UA will be positive only on dipstick for large amounts of blood, but no cells will be seen on microscopic examination. The **most specific diagnostic test** is a urine test for myoglobin.

Urine dipstick cannot tell the difference between:
- Hemoglobin
- Myoglobin
- Red blood cells

Why doesn't **hemolysis** cause **hyperuricemia**? RBCs have no nuclei.

Treat rhabdomyolysis with:

- Saline hydration
- Mannitol as an osmotic diuretic

Myoglobin is a severe oxidant stress on the tubular cells. Saline and mannitol increase urine flow rates, decreasing the contact time between the myoglobin and the tubular cells.

A man comes to the ED after participating in a triathlon, then undergoing status epilepticus. He takes simvastatin at triple the recommended dose. The patient's muscles are tender, and the urine is dark. Intravenous fluids are started. What is the best next step in management?

a. CPK level
b. EKG
c. Potassium replacement
d. Urine dipstick
e. Urine myoglobin

Answer: **B**. EKG is done to detect life-threatening hyperkalemia. Your question may have "potassium level" as the answer. CPK level, urine dipstick for blood, and urine myoglobin must all be done, but the EKG will show if the patient is about to die of a fatal arrhythmia from hyperkalemia. Potassium replacement in a person with rhabdomyolysis would be fatal.

Treatment

No therapy is proven to benefit ATN. Diuretics increase urine output but do not change overall outcome. Dopamine, mannitol, and steroids are likewise ineffective in reversing ATN.

> More urine output with diuretics does not mean renal failure is reversing.

Manage patients with hydration, if they are volume-depleted, and correct any electrolyte abnormalities.

▶ **TIP**

Answer treatment questions for ATN correctly by recognizing the most common wrong answers:

- **Low-dose dopamine**
- **Diuretics**
- **Mannitol**
- **Steroids**

> Correct the underlying cause in ATN.

Initiating dialysis is not based on a specific level of BUN or creatinine. It is based on the development of life-threatening conditions that cannot be corrected another way. Hypocalcemia, for example, is life-threatening (seizures, prolonged QT interval leading to arrhythmia), but it can be corrected by giving vitamin D and calcium. You do not dialyze a patient with hypocalcemia.

When is dialysis the answer?

- Fluid overload
- Encephalopathy
- Pericarditis
- Metabolic acidosis
- Hyperkalemia

A patient develops ATN from gentamicin. She is vigorously hydrated and treated with high doses of diuretic, low-dose dopamine, and calcium acetate as a phosphate binder. Urine output increases, but the patient still progresses to end-stage renal failure. She also becomes deaf. What caused the hearing loss?

a. Hydrochlorothiazide
b. Dopamine
c. Furosemide
d. Chlorthalidone
e. Calcium acetate

Answer: **C.** Furosemide causes ototoxicity by damaging the hair cells of the cochlea, resulting in sensorineural hearing loss. This is related not only to the total dose, but how fast it is injected. It essentially "burns" the inner ear. Aminoglycoside antibiotics also cause hearing loss. Furosemide in ATN *adds no proven overall benefit*. It does add ototoxicity to the gentamicin.

Hepatorenal Syndrome

Hepatorenal syndrome is renal failure developing secondary to liver disease. The kidneys are intrinsically normal. Look for:

- Severe liver disease (cirrhosis)
- New-onset renal failure with no other explanation
- Very low urine sodium (<10–15 mEq/dL)
- FENa <1%
- Elevated BUN:creatinine ratio (>20:1)

Treatment is with:

- Midodrine
- Octreotide
- Albumin (benefit is less clear)

> Lab values in hepatorenal syndrome fit in with prerenal azotemia.

Atheroemboli

Cholesterol plaques in the aorta or near the coronary arteries are sometimes large and fragile enough that they can be "broken off" when these vessels are manipulated during catheter procedures. Cholesterol emboli lodge in the kidney, leading to AKI. Look for blue/purplish skin lesions in fingers and toes, livedo reticularis, and ocular lesions.

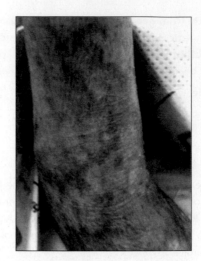

Figure 11.1 Livedo Reticularis. *Source: Farshad Bagheri, MD.*

Test for the following:

- Eosinophilia
- Low complement levels
- Eosinophiluria
- Elevated ESR

To diagnose atheroembolism, biopsy of one of the purplish skin lesions (**most accurate diagnostic test**). Biopsy will show cholesterol crystals.

There is no specific therapy to reverse atheroembolic disease.

> Peripheral **pulses are normal** in atheroembolism. The emboli are too small to occlude large vessels such as the radial or brachial artery.

Acute (Allergic) Interstitial Nephritis

Acute (allergic) interstitial nephritis (AIN) is a form of acute renal failure that damages the tubules occurring on an idiosyncratic (idiopathic) basis. Antibodies and eosinophils attack the cells lining the tubules as a reaction to drugs (70% of cases), infection, and autoimmune disorders (20%).

Although any medication can cause AIN, certain medications are more allergenic (allergy-inducing) than others.

- Penicillins and cephalosporins (**common**)
- Sulfa drugs (**common**)
- Phenytoin
- Rifampin
- Quinolones
- Allopurinol
- Proton pump inhibitors

> Some medications are just not allergenic—i.e., it is extremely rare for them to cause a rash:
> - CCBs
> - SSRIs
> - Beta blockers
>
> These drugs are also almost never associated with AIN, toxic epidermal necrolysis, or hemolysis.

The medications that cause AIN are the same as those that cause drug allergy and rash, Stevens-Johnson, toxic epidermal necrolysis, and hemolysis. These are outcomes of the same process, with different target organs affected.

Allergenic substances affect:

- Skin
- Kidney
- Red blood cells

In addition to drugs, AIN is caused by infections and autoimmune disease like systemic lupus erythematosus (SLE), Sjögren, and sarcoidosis.

"What Is the Most Likely Diagnosis?"

Look for acute renal failure (rising BUN and creatinine) with the following symptoms (occur simultaneously in 10% of patients):

- Fever
- Rash
- Arthralgias
- Eosinophilia and eosinophiluria

Diagnostic Tests

- Elevated BUN and creatinine (ratio below 20:1)
- White and red blood cells in the urine

The Hansel or Wright stain (**most accurate test**) shows whether eosinophils are present (unlike the UA, which detects only WBCs, RBCs, and protein).

Treatment

AIN usually resolves spontaneously upon stopping the drug or controlling the infection. Severe disease is managed with dialysis, which may be temporary. When the creatinine continues to rise after stopping the drug, the answer is to give glucocorticoids (prednisone, hydrocortisone, methylprednisolone).

> Eosinophils are not found in the urine with AKI from NSAIDs.

> Urine sodium and osmolality are not uniformly up or down in AIN. They cannot establish the diagnosis.

Analgesic Nephropathy

Analgesic nephropathy presents with:

- ATN from direct toxicity to the tubules
- AIN
- Membranous glomerulonephritis
- Vascular insufficiency of the kidney from inhibiting prostaglandins. Prostaglandins dilate the afferent arteriole. NSAIDs constrict the afferent arteriole and decrease renal perfusion. This is asymptomatic in healthy patients. When patients are older and have underlying renal insufficiency from diabetes and/or hypertension, then NSAIDs can tip them over into clinically apparent renal insufficiency.
- Papillary necrosis

There is no specific diagnostic test to determine NSAIDs caused the disease previously described. Exclude other causes and look for NSAIDs in the history.

Papillary Necrosis

Papillary necrosis is a sloughing off of the renal papillae. It is caused by toxins such as NSAIDs or by sudden vascular insufficiency leading to death of the papillary cells, which drop off the internal structure of the kidney.

Papillary necrosis does not occur in people who are otherwise healthy. There must be some underlying renal damage—even if baseline BUN and creatinine levels are normal. Remember that a patient must lose at least 60–70% of renal function before creatinine even begins to rise. Look for extra NSAID use with a history of:

- Sickle cell disease
- Diabetes
- Urinary obstruction
- Chronic pyelonephritis

> Papillary necrosis can give grossly visible **necrotic material** passed **in the urine**. These are the renal papillae.

Presentation

Papillary necrosis can be very hard to distinguish from pyelonephritis. Look for the sudden onset of flank pain, fever, and hematuria in a patient with one of the diseases previously listed.

Diagnostic Tests

Urinalysis (**best initial test**) shows red and white blood cells and may show necrotic kidney tissue. The urine culture will be normal (no growth). CT scan (**most accurate test**) shows the abnormal internal structures of the kidney from the loss of the papillae.

Treatment

There is no specific treatment. You cannot reattach the sloughed-off part of the kidney.

Pyelonephritis versus Papillary Necrosis		
	Pyelonephritis	**Papillary necrosis**
Onset	Few days	Few hours
Symptoms	Dysuria	Necrotic material in urine
Urine culture	Positive	Negative
CT scan	Diffusely swollen kidney	"Bumpy" contour of interior where papillae were lost
Treatment	Antibiotics such as ampicillin/gentamicin or fluoroquinolones	No treatment

Tubular Disease

Tubular diseases are caused by toxins (drugs, myoglobin, hemoglobin, oxalate, urate, NSAIDs, contrast). These conditions are generally acute.

- Never cause nephrotic syndrome or give massive proteinuria
- Biopsy not needed to establish a diagnosis

Treatment of tubular diseases is correction of the hypoperfusion and removal of the toxin. They are not treated with steroids or additional immunosuppressive medications (cyclophosphamide, mycophenolate). Like all drug allergies, AIN usually resolves spontaneously.

> Acute = Tubular = Toxin

Tubular Diseases

- Acute
- Toxins
- None nephrotic
- No biopsy usually
- No steroids
- Never additional immunosuppressive agents

Glomerular Diseases

Glomerular diseases are generally chronic. They can all cause nephrotic syndrome.

The causes of glomerular disease are generally not toxins or hypoperfusion.

- Biopsy (**most accurate test**) is not always needed.
- Several diseases resolve spontaneously, but for those that do not steroids are used. Also consider immunosuppressive medications (cyclophosphamide, mycophenolate).

> Any form of glomerular disease can produce nephrotic syndrome.

> Glomerular = Slow = Sample = Steroids = Immuno**suppressives**

Glomerular Diseases

- Chronic
- Not from toxins/drugs
- All potentially nephrotic
- Biopsy sample
- Steroids often

Diagnostic Tests

All types of glomerulonephritis cause proteinuria, red blood cells and red blood cell casts in urine, hypertension, and edema.

- UA with hematuria
- "Dysmorphic" red blood cells (deformed as they "squeeze" through an abnormal glomerulus)

- Red blood cell casts
- Urine sodium and FENa are low
- Proteinuria

So how do they all differ?

The main difference between **glomerulonephritis** and **nephrotic syndrome** is the degree/amount of proteinuria.

Complement Levels and Renal Disease	
Low complement	**Normal complement**
• SLE	• Vasculitis (GPA, EoGPA)
• Endocarditis	• Goodpasture syndrome
• Cryoglobulinemia	• IgA
• Post-streptococcal glomerular disease	• HIV

Goodpasture Syndrome

Goodpasture also presents with lung and kidney involvement, but unlike granulomatosis with polyangiitis (GPA) (Wegener granulomatosis), there is no upper respiratory tract involvement. Goodpasture is also limited to just the lung and kidney, so signs of systemic vasculitis are absent. There is no skin, joint, GI, eye, or neurological involvement.

Diagnostic Tests/Treatment

> Kidney biopsy in Goodpasture syndrome shows "**linear deposits.**"

The antiglomerular basement membrane test is the **best initial test**, while a lung or kidney biopsy is the **most accurate test**. Anemia is often present from chronic blood loss from hemoptysis. Chest x-ray will be abnormal but is insufficient to confirm the diagnosis.

Treat with plasmapheresis and steroids. Cyclophosphamide can be helpful.

IgA Nephropathy (Berger Disease)

> IgA levels don't help in IgA nephropathy.

IgA nephropathy is the most common cause of acute glomerulonephritis in the United States. Look for IgA nephropathy with recurrent episodes of gross hematuria 12 days after an upper respiratory tract infection (synpharyngitic). All the other causes have some specific physical findings.

Poststreptococcal glomerulonephritis follows pharyngitis by 1–2 weeks.

▶ **TIP**

There are **no unique physical findings or blood tests** in IgA nephropathy to allow you to answer the "most likely diagnosis" question.

Diagnostic Tests

IgA levels are increased in only 50%. The **only accurate test** is a kidney biopsy.

> Proteinuria levels correspond to severity of disease and likelihood of progression.
>
> More proteinuria = Worse progression

Treatment

There is no treatment proven to reverse the disease: 30% of cases will completely resolve, while up to 50% of cases will progress to end-stage renal disease.

Severe proteinuria is treated with ACE inhibitors and steroids. Fish oil is of uncertain benefit.

> IgA nephropathy
> - ACE for everybody
> - High protein gets steroids
> - BP goal <130/80 mm Hg

Postinfectious Glomerulonephritis

The most common organism leading to postinfectious glomerulonephritis (PIGN) is *Streptococcus*, but almost any infection can lead to abnormal activation of the immune system and PIGN. Poststreptococcal glomerulonephritis (PSGN) follows throat infection or skin infection (impetigo) by 1–3 weeks.

Patients present with:

- Dark (cola-colored) urine
- Edema that is often periorbital
- Hypertension
- Oliguria

Diagnostic Tests

A UA with proteinuria, red blood cells, and red blood cell casts tells you that glomerulonephritis is present. PSGN from group A beta hemolytic streptococci (*pyogenes*) is confirmed by antistreptolysin O (ASO) titers and anti-DNase antibody titers (**best initial test**). Biopsy is the **most accurate test**, but you should not routinely do a kidney biopsy because the blood test is sufficiently accurate and the disorder usually resolves spontaneously.

> Complement levels are low in PSGN.

Treatment

Management of PSGN does not reverse the glomerulonephritis. Use supportive therapies such as:

- Antibiotics
- Diuretics to control fluid overload

> Less than 5% of those with PSGN will progress.

Alport Syndrome

Alport syndrome is a congenital defect of collagen that results in glomerular disease combined with:

- Sensorineural hearing loss
- Visual disturbance from loss of the collagen fibers that hold the lens of the eye in place

There is no specific therapy to reverse this defect of type IV collagen. Thin basement membrane disease is a variant of Alport syndrome.

Polyarteritis Nodosa

Polyarteritis nodosa (PAN) is a systemic vasculitis of small and medium-sized arteries that most commonly affects the kidney. Virtually every organ in the body can be affected, but it tends to spare the lung.

PAN can be associated with hepatitis B or C.

PAN presents with glomerulonephritis and nonspecific symptoms of fever, malaise, weight loss, myalgia/arthralgia over weeks to months (as with almost every type of vasculitis). Common organ systems involved are:

- **GI**: abdominal pain, bleeding, nausea, and vomiting; pain can be worsened by eating because of mesenteric vasculitis
- **Neurological**: vasculitis damages the blood vessels surrounding larger peripheral nerves such as the peroneal, ulnar, radial, and brachial nerves.
  - Damage to small blood vessels around nerves starves them into neuropathy.
  - When more than one large peripheral nerve is involved, it is called "mononeuritis multiplex." When that presents with stroke in a young person, look for vasculitis.
- **Skin**: vasculitis of any cause leads to purpura (large) and petechiae (small). PAN also gives ulcers, digital gangrene, and livedo reticularis.
- **Cardiac disease** (30% of patients)

▶TIP

PAN is nonspecific. There is no single finding that allows you to answer the "most likely diagnosis" question.

Diagnostic Tests

There is no blood test to confirm PAN. However, blood tests will show:

- Anemia and leukocytosis
- Elevated ESR and C-reactive protein
- **ANCA not present in most cases**
- ANA and rheumatoid factor: sometimes present in low titer

Stroke or MI in a young person suggests PAN.

Angiography of the renal, mesenteric, or hepatic artery showing aneurysmal dilation in association with new-onset hypertension and characteristic symptoms is the **best initial test** that has specificity for PAN. (Angiography is the best diagnostic test whenever the most involved organ is not easily accessible for a biopsy, such as the kidney.)

The **most accurate test** is a biopsy of a symptomatic site such as skin, nerves, or muscles.

Treatment

Prednisone and cyclophosphamide are the standard of care and they lower mortality.

Treat hepatitis B or C when it is found.

Lupus Nephritis

SLE can give any degree of renal involvement. The kidneys in SLE can be normal or present with mild, asymptomatic proteinuria. Severe disease presents with membranous glomerulonephritis. Longstanding SLE may simply "scar" the kidneys, and biopsy will show glomerulosclerosis, which has no active inflammatory component but may lead to such damage as to require dialysis.

Biopsy is the **most accurate test** of lupus nephritis—not to diagnose but rather to determine treatment based on the stage. Mild inflammatory changes may respond to glucocorticoids. Severe, proliferative disease such as membranous nephropathy is treated with glucocorticoids combined with either cyclophosphamide or mycophenolate.

Use steroids + cyclophosphamide to treat:

- SLE
- PAN
- Granulomatosis with polyangiitis
- Eosinophilic granulomatosis with polyangiitis
- Microscopic polyangiitis

Amyloidosis

Amyloid is an abnormal protein produced in association with:

- Myeloma
- Chronic inflammatory disease
- Rheumatoid arthritis
- Inflammatory bowel disease
- Chronic infections

Amyloid, HIV nephropathy, polycystic kidneys, and diabetes give **large kidneys** on sonogram and CT scan.

There is also a primary form of amyloidosis in which the protein is produced for unknown reasons. The kidney is the primary target of the protein.

Biopsy (**most accurate test**) will show green birefringence with Congo red staining.

Treatment is control of the underlying disease. When that is unsuccessful or there is no primary disease to control, use melphalan, prednisone, bortezomib (or whatever you would use for myeloma). Patisiran and tafamidis treat amyloidosis.

Nephrotic Syndrome

Nephrotic syndrome is a measure of the severity of proteinuria in association with any form of glomerular disease; diagnosis of nephrotic syndrome is not based on etiology. It occurs when proteinuria is so massive that the liver can no longer increase the production of albumin to compensate for urinary losses. The cause is not definitively known.

Nephrotic syndrome is most commonly seen with diabetes and hypertension, which can cause massive protein loss. Other conditions (limited to the kidney) that have an association with nephrotic syndrome include:

The major difference between "nephritic" and "nephrotic" is the amount of proteinuria.

- Cancer (solid organ): membranous
- Minimal change disease (in children)
- Injection drug use and AIDS (focal-segmental)
- NSAIDs
- SLE (any)

Presentation

Massive proteinuria can lead to the following:

CHF: edema in dependent areas (legs)

Nephrotic syndrome: edema everywhere

- Edema (periorbital edema is characteristic of nephrotic syndrome)
- Hyperlipidemia
- Thrombosis/clots (from urinary loss of the natural anticoagulants protein C, protein S, and antithrombin)
- Infections (from urinary loss of immunoglobulins and complement)

Diagnostic Tests

The **best initial test** is the urine albumin/creatinine spot urine ratio. It is equal in accuracy to a 24-hour urine but is much easier to obtain. It gives a measure of the average protein produced over 24 hours.

- Ratio 2:1 means 2 grams of protein excreted over 24 hours
- Ratio 5.4:1 means 5.4 grams excreted over 24 hours

Although UA protein level corresponds to the amount of protein excreted over 24 hours, UA is not sufficient to diagnose nephrotic syndrome:

- UA only detects albumin as a protein.
- Variations in renal function mean significant differences in results (trace proteinuria on one UA and 2+ protein on another) with the time of day and posture (flat or upright).

Renal biopsy is the **most accurate test** to identify the cause of nephrotic syndrome. Although each type of nephrotic syndrome has certain associations, only a biopsy can distinguish between the forms:

- Focal-segmental
- Membranous
- Membranoproliferative
- Minimal change
- Mesangial

By definition, nephrotic syndrome is:

- Hyperproteinuria (>3.5 grams per 24 hours)
- Hypoproteinemia
- Hyperlipidemia
- Edema

Lipid levels rise because the lipoprotein signals that turn off the production of circulating lipid are now lost in the urine. With loss of these lipoproteins that surround chylomicrons and VLDLs, all lipid levels in the blood will rise. Iron, copper, and zinc are low because their carrier protein is lost in the urine. UA shows Maltese crosses, which are lipid deposits in sloughed-off tubular cells.

UA shows Maltese crosses.

Anything with a carrier protein can be lost in urine.

Treatment

- Glucocorticoids; if no response after several weeks, try another immunosuppressive medication such as cyclophosphamide
- ACE inhibitors or ARBs to control proteinuria
- Salt restriction and diuretics to manage the edema
- Statins to manage the hyperlipidemia

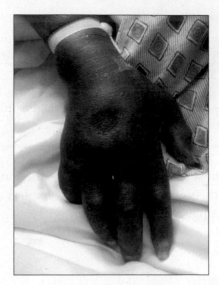

Figure 11.2 Pitting Edema.
Source: Pramod Theetha Kariyanna, MD

End-Stage Renal Disease

End-stage renal disease (ESRD), or chronic renal failure, is a general term for kidney failure so severe that it needs dialysis or renal transplantation. There is a massive loss of renal function leading to characteristic symptoms and lab abnormalities ("uremia").

Causes of ESRD include:

- Diabetes and hypertension (**by far most common**)
- Any other form of tubular or glomerular damage

Uremia (a term interchangeable with the conditions for which dialysis is the treatment) is defined as the presence of:

- Metabolic acidosis
- Fluid overload
- Encephalopathy
- Hyperkalemia
- Pericarditis (uncommon)

Each of these conditions is an indication for dialysis; they are usually seen at the same time that creatinine clearance drops below the level at which acids, fluid, and potassium can be excreted.

> Peritoneal dialysis and hemodialysis are equally effective at removing wastes from the body.

▶ TIP

ESRD usually implies disease that has been present for years; however, rapidly progressive glomerulonephritis is so named because it can lead to ESRD over weeks.

Manifestations of Renal Failure

- **Anemia**: Loss of erythropoietin leads to normochromic, normocytic anemia.
- **Hypocalcemia**: The kidney transforms the less active 25-hydroxy-vitamin D into the much more active 1,25-dihydroxy-vitamin D. Without the 1,25 dihydroxy form of vitamin D, the body will not absorb enough calcium from the gut.
- **Osteodystrophy**: Low calcium leads to secondary hyperparathyroidism. High parathyroid hormone level will remove calcium from bones, making them soft and weak.
- **Bleeding**: platelets do not work normally in a uremic environment; they do not degranulate. If a platelet does not release the contents of its granules, it will not work.
- **Infection**: The same defect occurs with neutrophils. Without degranulation, neutrophils will not effectively combat infection.
- **Pruritus**: Urea accumulating in skin causes itching (unclear reasoning).
- **Hyperphosphatemia**: Phosphate is normally excreted through kidneys. High parathyroid hormone levels release phosphate from bones but the body cannot excrete it.
- **Hypermagnesemia**: from loss of excretory ability
- **Accelerated atherosclerosis and hypertension**: The immune system (lymphocytes) helps keep arteries clear of lipid accumulation. White blood cells don't work normally in a uremic environment. This is the most common cause of death in those on dialysis.
- **Endocrinopathy**: Women are anovulatory, and men have low testosterone. Erectile dysfunction is common. Insulin tends to elevate because it is excreted renally. However, insulin resistance also increases. Glucose, therefore, can be up or down.

> Patiromer and zirconium bind potassium, allowing longer use of ACEIs to decrease progression.

> Hyperparathyroidism and ACE inhibitors block the effect of erythropoietin.

> Cardiac disease kills triple the number that infection does in ESRD.

Treatment of the Manifestations of ESRD	
Manifestation	**Treatment**
Anemia	Erythropoietin replacement and iron supplementation
Hypocalcemia and osteomalacia	Replace vitamin D and calcium
Bleeding	DDAVP increases platelet function; use only when bleeding
Pruritus	Dialysis and ultraviolet light
Hyperphosphatemia	Oral binders: see "Treatment of Hyperphosphatemia"
Hypermagnesemia	Restriction of high-magnesium foods, laxatives, and antacids
Atherosclerosis	Dialysis
Endocrinopathy	Dialysis, estrogen and testosterone replacement

> Anemia from ESRD is the only time erythropoietin is always used.

> Use sevelamer and lanthanum to bind phosphate when the calcium level is high.

Treatment of Hyperphosphatemia

Oral phosphate binders will prevent phosphate absorption from the bowel. Treatment of hypocalcemia will also help because it is the hyperparathyroidism that causes increased phosphate release from bone. When vitamin D is replaced to control hypocalcemia, it is critical to also give phosphate binders; otherwise vitamin D will increase GI absorption of phosphate. Use:

- Sevelamer
- Lanthanum
- Calcium acetate
- Calcium carbonate
- Cinacalcet and etelcalcetide (inhibitors of PTH that mimic the effect of calcium on the parathyroid gland)

> Cinacalcet and etelcalcetide stimulate the calcium-sensing receptor on the parathyroid gland.

Complications of ESRD

Calciphylaxis is calcification of blood vessels with skin vessel clotting and necrosis.

- It can also be caused by hypercalcemia with milk-alkali syndrome or hyperparathyroidism.
- Normalize calcium and phosphate levels and increase the amount of dialysis. Thiosulfate and cinacalcet work.

> **Never use** aluminum-containing phosphate binders. Aluminum causes dementia.

Nephrogenic systemic fibrosis is a proliferation of dermal fibrocytes leading to hardened areas of fibrotic nodules skin.

- This form of fibrosis occurs following administration of the MRI contrast agent gadolinium in a person with ESRD or a severely low GFR (<30 mL).
- Joint and skin contractures occur.
- There is no therapy.

Kidney Transplantation

Only 50% of ESRD patients will be suitable for transplantation. The donor does not have to be alive or related, although these are both better.

Survival by Method			
	1 year	**3 years**	**5 years**
Living, related donor	95%	88%	72%
Deceased donor	90%	78%	58%
Dialysis alone	Variable	Variable	30–40%
Diabetics on dialysis	Variable	Variable	20%

> HLA-identical, related-donor kidneys last 24 years on average.

Cystic Disease

The single most important point in cystic disease is how to recognize a cyst that is potentially malignant and needs to be aspirated. If any of the qualities of a complex cyst are found, it should be aspirated to exclude malignancy.

Benign (Simple) Cysts Versus Potentially Malignant Cysts		
	Simple cyst	Complex cyst (potential malignancy)
Echogenicity	Echo free	Mixed echogenicity
Walls	Smooth, thin	Irregular, thick
Demarcation	Sharp	Lower density on back wall
Transmission	Good through to back	Debris in cyst

Polycystic Kidney Disease

Polycystic kidney disease (PCKD) presents with:

- Pain
- Hematuria
- Stones
- Infection
- Hypertension

What is the most common cause of death from PCKD?

a. Intracerebral hemorrhage
b. Stones
c. Infection
d. Malignancy
e. Renal failure

Answer: **E**. Renal failure occurs in PCKD from recurrent episodes of pyelonephritis and nephrolithiasis causing progressive scarring and loss of renal function. PCKD does not have malignant potential. Only 10–15% of affected people have cerebral aneurysms, most of which do not rupture. Connective tissue is weak throughout the body. These patients may have:

- Liver cysts (most common site outside the kidney)
- Ovarian cysts
- Mitral valve prolapse
- Diverticulosis

No treatment exists to prevent or reverse cysts of any type.

Sodium Disorders

Hypernatremia

Hypernatremia occurs when there is loss of free water. Examples are:

- Sweating
- Burns
- Fever
- Pneumonia: from insensible losses from hyperventilation
- Diarrhea
- Diuretics

Diabetes insipidus (DI) leads to high-volume water loss from insufficient or ineffective antidiuretic hormone (ADH). Any CNS disorder (stroke, tumor, trauma, hypoxia, infection) can damage the production of ADH in the hypothalamus or storage in the posterior pituitary, leading to central diabetes insipidus (CDI).

Nephrogenic DI is a loss of ADH effect on the collecting duct of the kidney. This is much less common. Nephrogenic diabetes insipidus (NDI) is caused by lithium or demeclocycline, chronic kidney disease, hypokalemia, or hypercalcemia. They make ADH ineffective at the tubule.

DI and hypernatremia of any cause present with neurological symptoms such as confusion, disorientation, lethargy, and seizures. If uncorrected, severe hypernatremia causes coma and irreversible brain damage.

> High-volume **nocturia** is the first clue to the **presence of DI**.

▶ TIP

Polyuria is high urine volume. Frequency just means increased attempts at voiding. The volume in urinary frequency might be very small (such as in urethritis or cystitis).

High serum sodium is nearly equivalent to hyperosmolality since the majority of osmolality is sodium. Fluid losses from the skin, kidneys, or stool generally lead to:

- Decreased urine volume (high urine volume in DI)
- Increased urine osmolality (decreased urine osmolality in DI)
- Decreased urine sodium

> Increased urine volume despite dehydration and hyperosmolality of the blood suggests DI.

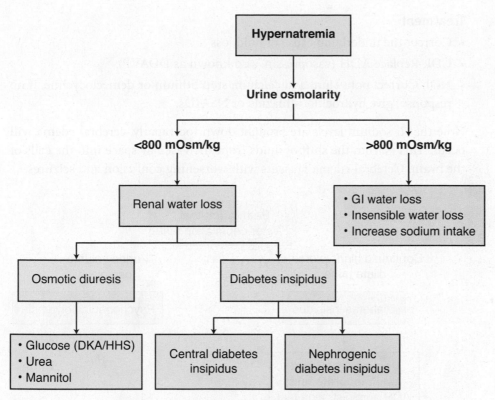

Figure 11.3 Hypernatremia Algorithm. ©Kaplan

The **best initial test** for DI is the water deprivation test: Prevent the patient from drinking water, then observe urine output and urine osmolality. With DI, urine volume stays high and urine osmolality stays low despite vigorous urine production and despite developing dehydration.

ADH further distinguishes DI. The ADH level is **low in CDI**, and markedly **elevated in NDI**. Response to ADH administration is as follows:

- CDI: **sharp decrease** in urine volume, increase in osmolality
- NDI: **no change** in urine volume or osmolality

Comparison of Central versus Nephrogenic Diabetes Insipidus		
	CDI	**NDI**
Polyuria and nocturia	Yes	Yes
Urine osmolality and sodium	Low	Low
Positive water deprivation test	Yes	Yes
Response to ADH	Yes	No
ADH level	Low	High

A "positive" water deprivation test means **urine volume stays high** despite withholding water.

Treatment

- Correct the underlying cause of fluid loss
- CDI: Replace ADH (vasopressin, also known as DDAVP).
- NDI: Correct potassium and calcium; stop lithium or demeclocycline; if no response, give hydrochlorothiazide or NSAIDs.

Note that if sodium levels are brought down too rapidly, cerebral edema will occur. This is from the shift of fluids from the vascular space into the cells of the brain. Cerebral edema presents with worsening confusion and seizures.

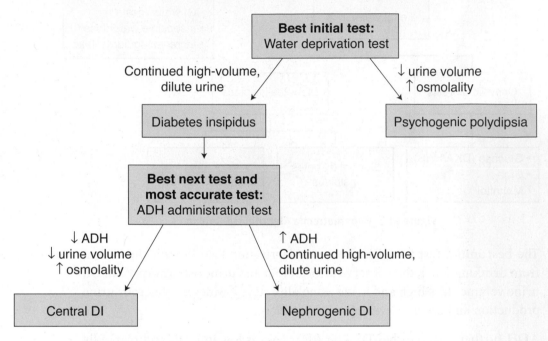

Figure 11.4 Diagnosing Diabetes Insipidus

Hyponatremia

Hyponatremia is characterized according to overall volume status of the body.

Hypervolemia

The **most common causes** of hyponatremia with a hypervolemic state are:

- CHF
- Nephrotic syndrome
- Cirrhosis

These are cases in which intravascular volume depletion leads to increased ADH levels. Pressure receptors in the atria and carotids sense the decrease in volume and stimulate ADH production and release. Although the sodium level drops, it is more important to maintain vascular volume and organ perfusion.

> Perfusion is more important than normal sodium.

Hypovolemia

The **most common causes** of hyponatremia with a hypovolemic state are:

- Sweating
- Burns
- Fever
- Pneumonia (due to insensible losses from hyperventilation)
- Diarrhea
- Diuretics

All of these are also causes of hypernatremia; however, they cause hyponatremia instead if there is chronic replacement with free water. A little sodium and a lot of water are lost in urine, which is then replaced with free water that has no sodium. Over time, this process depletes the body of sodium and the serum sodium level drops.

Another cause of hyponatremia is Addison disease (loss of adrenal function), because of loss of aldosterone. Aldosterone causes sodium resorption. If the body loses aldosterone, it loses sodium.

> Loss of aldosterone means loss of sodium.

Euvolemia

The **most common causes** of hyponatremia with euvolemia (normal volume status) are:

- Pseudohyponatremia (hyperglycemia)
- Psychogenic polydipsia
- Hypothyroidism
- Syndrome of inappropriate ADH release (SIADH)

Hyperglycemia: Very high glucose levels lead to a decrease in sodium levels. Hyperglycemia acts as an osmotic draw on fluid inside the cells. Free water leaves the cells to correct the hyperosmolar serum; this drops the sodium level. For every 100 mg/dL of glucose above normal, there is a 1.6 mEq/L decrease in sodium. Manage by correcting the glucose level.

Psychogenic polydipsia: Massive ingestion of free water above 12–24 liters a day will overwhelm the kidney's ability to excrete water. The minimum urine osmolality is 50 mOsm/kg. The body can produce 12–24 liters of urine a day, depending on whether you can get the urine osmolality down to 50–100 mOsm/kg.

▶ **TIP**

Look for a history of bipolar disorder to suggest psychogenic polydipsia.

Hypothyroidism: Thyroid hormone is needed to excrete water. If the thyroid hormone level is low, free water excretion is decreased.

SIADH: Any lung or brain disease can cause SIADH for unclear reasons. Certain drugs such as SSRIs, sulfonylureas, vincristine, cyclophosphamide, or tricyclic antidepressants can cause SIADH. Certain cancers, especially small-cell cancer of the lung, produce ADH. Pain causes SIADH.

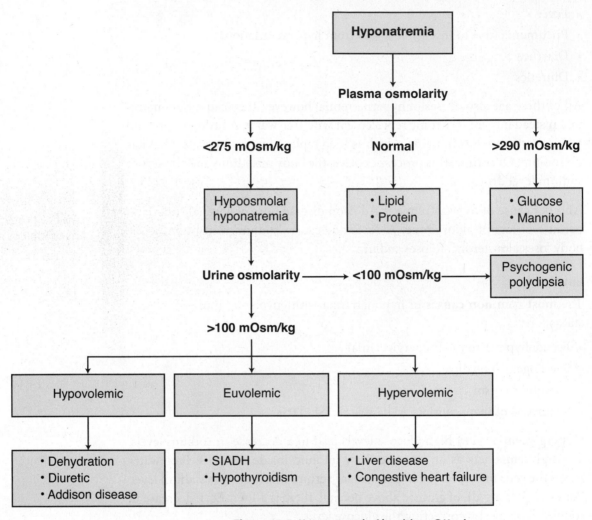

Figure 11.5 Hyponatremia Algorithm. ©Kaplan

Presentation

Hyponatremia presents entirely with CNS symptoms:

- Confusion
- Lethargy
- Disorientation
- Seizures
- Coma

> Symptoms of hyponatremia depend on how quickly sodium is lost.

> Sodium loss means **CNS symptoms**.

If the sodium levels drop very fast, the patient can immediately seize. Slow drops may be entirely asymptomatic even if the level is very low.

Response to Hyponatremia		
	Expected levels	**SIADH**
Urine osmolality	Low (<100 mOsm/kg)	High
Urine sodium	Low (<20 mEq/L)	High (>40 mEq/L)

Diagnostic Tests

In SIADH, the urine is inappropriately concentrated (high urine osmolality), making urine sodium is inappropriately high. Meanwhile, uric acid level and BUN are low.

Treatment

Clinical Manifestations of Hyponatremia by Severity		
Degree of hyponatremia	**Specific manifestation**	**Management**
Mild hyponatremia	No symptoms	Restrict fluids
Moderate	Minimal confusion	Saline and loop diuretic
Severe	Lethargy, seizures, coma	Hypertonic saline, conivaptan, tolvaptan

▶ **TIP**

The treatment answer is not based on the sodium level; it is based on the symptoms.

> In SIADH, saline without a diuretic makes it worse.

Additional agents in the treatment of SIADH include the following:

- **ADH antagonists**: Tolvaptan and conivaptan are antagonists of ADH. They are the answer as part of urgent therapy for severe, symptomatic SIADH. Use only for urgent treatment in hospital.
- **Demeclocycline**: SIADH can be from an underlying disorder that cannot be corrected, such as metastatic cancer. Demeclocycline treats chronic SIADH by blocking the action of ADH at the collecting duct of the kidney tubule.

Complications of Treatment

Correction of sodium must occur slowly. "Slowly" is defined as <0.5–1 mEq per hour or <12–24 mEq per day. If the sodium level is brought up to normal too rapidly, the neurological disorder known as central pontine myelinolysis or osmotic demyelination occurs.

Potassium Disorders

Hyperkalemia

High potassium levels (hyperkalemia) are an absolutely indispensable portion of your knowledge because of the life-threatening nature of potassium disorders. Severe hyperkalemia can stop the heart in seconds if the level is high enough.

Etiology

Pseudohyperkalemia (falsely elevated levels) arises from:

- Hemolysis
- Repeated fist clenching with tourniquet in place
- Thrombocytosis or leukocytosis will leak out of cells in the lab specimen

None of these causes of hyperkalemia needs further treatment or investigation. Simply repeat the sample.

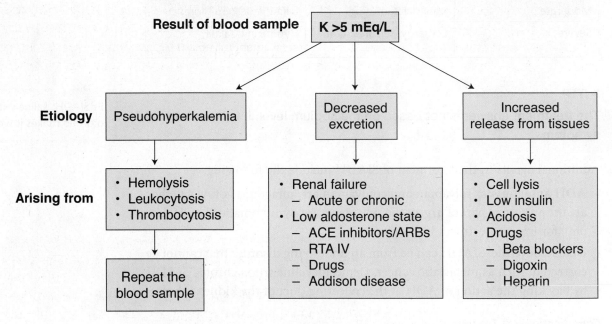

Figure 11.6 Hyperkalemia Etiology

Decreased excretion results from:

- Renal failure
- Aldosterone decrease:
    - ACE inhibitors/ARBs
    - Type IV renal tubular acidosis (hyporeninemic, hypoaldosteronism)
    - Spironolactone and eplerenone (aldosterone inhibitors)
    - Triamterene and amiloride (potassium-sparing diuretics)
    - Addison disease

Release of potassium from tissues has several causes:

- Any tissue destruction, such as hemolysis, rhabdomyolysis, or tumor lysis syndrome, can release potassium.
- Decreased insulin: Insulin normally drives potassium into cells.
- Acidosis: Cells will pick up hydrogen ions (acid) and release potassium in exchange.
- Beta blockers and digoxin: These drugs inhibit the sodium/potassium ATPase that normally brings potassium into the cells.
- Heparin increases potassium levels, presumably through increased tissue release.

> Since 95% of potassium in the body is intracellular, shifting potassium out of cells can easily be fatal.

Presentation

Potassium disorders interfere with muscle contraction and cardiac conductance. Look for:

- Weakness
- Paralysis when severe
- Ileus (paralyzes gut muscles)
- Cardiac rhythm disorders

> Hyperkalemia does not cause seizures.

Diagnostic Tests

Besides a potassium level, testing is aimed at finding the causes previously described. The **most urgent test in severe hyperkalemia** is an EKG.

The EKG in severe hyperkalemia shows:

- Peaked T waves
- Wide QRS
- PR interval prolongation

> Sodium = CNS symptoms
>
> Hyperkalemia = Muscular and cardiac symptoms

Treatment

Hyperkalemia treatments lower potassium levels by either moving it into cells or removing it from the body.

In life-threatening hyperkalemia (abnormal EKG), give the following:

1. Calcium chloride or calcium gluconate
2. Insulin and glucose to drive potassium back into cells
3. Bicarbonate: drives potassium into cells (most important when acidosis causes hyperkalemia)

> Calcium is only used if the EKG is abnormal to protect the heart. It does not lower the potassium level.

Sodium polystyrene sulfonate (Kayexalate) removes potassium from the body through the bowel. The patient ingests Kayexalate orally and over several hours it will bind potassium in the gut and remove it from the body. Patiromer and zirconium are long-term, oral potassium-lowering agents that can be used chronically.

> Insulin does not remove potassium from the body.

> Patiromer and zirconium allow use of ACEI/ARB despite rising potassium levels.

Insulin and bicarbonate lower the potassium level through redistribution into the cells.

Other methods to lower potassium are:

- Inhaled beta agonists (albuterol)
- Loop diuretics
- Dialysis
- Oral potassium binder (patiromer or zirconium)

▶ TIP

When there is hyperkalemia and an abnormal EKG, the "most appropriate next step" is clearly calcium chloride or gluconate.

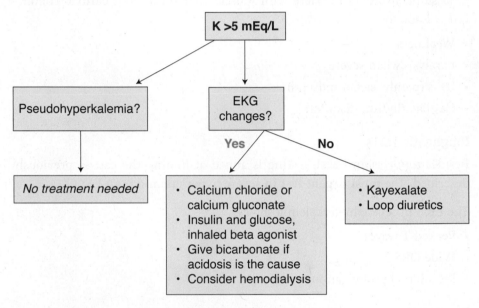

Figure 11.7 Hyperkalemia Treatment

Hypokalemia

Potassium is essential for proper neuromuscular contraction. Hypokalemia leads to problems with muscular contraction and cardiac conduction. Muscular abnormalities may be so severe as to cause rhabdomyolysis.

Etiology

Decreased intake: This is unusual because the kidney can decrease potassium excretion to extremely small amounts.

Shift into cells:

- Alkalosis (hydrogen ions come out of the cell in exchange for potassium entering)
- Increased insulin
- Beta adrenergic stimulation (accelerates sodium/potassium ATPase)

Renal loss:

- Loop diuretics
- Increased aldosterone
  - Primary hyperaldosteronism (Conn syndrome)
  - Volume depletion raises aldosterone
  - Cushing syndrome
  - Bartter syndrome (genetic disease causing salt loss in loop of Henle)
  - Licorice
- Hypomagnesemia: When magnesium is low, magnesium-dependent potassium channels in the body open and spill potassium into the urine.
- Renal tubular acidosis (RTA), both proximal and distal

Gastrointestinal loss:

- Vomiting
- Diarrhea
- Laxative abuse

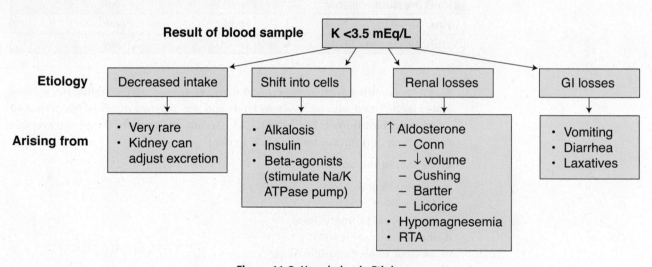

Figure 11.8 Hypokalemia Etiology

Presentation

- Weakness
- Paralysis
- Loss of reflexes

EKG Findings

U waves are the **most characteristic EKG finding** of hypokalemia.

Other findings are ventricular ectopy (PVCs), flattened T waves, and ST depression.

> Muscular abnormalities in hypokalemia may be severe enough to cause rhabdomyolysis.

> Hypokalemia does **not** cause seizures.

Treatment

Restore potassium level and manage the cause of the hypokalemia.

- For **oral** replacement of potassium, there is **no maximum rate**. The gastrointestinal system cannot absorb potassium faster than the kidneys can excrete it, so you cannot go too far too fast.

- **Intravenous** replacement of potassium, however, **can cause a fatal arrhythmia** if done too fast. You must allow time for potassium to equilibrate into the cells.

> Intravenous potassium replacement must be very slow.

> Bartter acts like a furosemide-secreting tumor.

Diseases That Cause Hypokalemia			
	Bartter syndrome	**Gitelman syndrome**	**Liddle syndrome**
Drug analogy	Like furosemide	Like thiazide	Like excess aldosterone
Site of defect	Ascending loop	Distal tubule	Distal tubule
Precise defect	Loss of Na absorption	Loss of Na absorption	Excess ENaC channel activity
Blood pressure	Low	Low	High
Urine chloride	High	High	Low
Serum potassium	Low	Low	Low

A man is admitted with vomiting and diarrhea from gastroenteritis. His volume status is corrected with intravenous fluids and the diarrhea resolves. His pH is 7.40 and serum bicarbonate has normalized. Despite vigorous oral and intravenous replacement, his potassium level fails to rise.

What should you do?

a. Consult nephrology
b. Magnesium level
c. Parathyroid hormone level
d. Intracellular pH level
e. 24-hour urine potassium level

Answer: **B**. Hypomagnesemia can lead to increased urinary loss of potassium. If magnesium is replaced, it will close up the magnesium-dependent potassium channels and stop urinary loss. Although magnesium is necessary for parathyroid hormone release, this would have nothing to do with potassium levels. There will be increased potassium on a 24-hour urine with hypomagnesemia, but there is no point in performing this test because you still have to detect and treat hypomagnesemia.

A woman with ESRD and glucose 6-phosphate dehydrogenase deficiency skips dialysis for a few weeks and then is crushed in a motor vehicle accident. She is taking dapsone and has recently eaten fava beans. What is the most urgent step?

a. Initiate dialysis

b. EKG

c. Bicarbonate administration

d. Insulin administration

e. Kayexalate

f. Urine dipstick

g. CPK levels

h. Urine myoglobin

Answer: **B.** All of these interventions may be helpful in a person with life-threatening hyperkalemia. The most important step is to determine if there are EKG changes from hyperkalemia. If the EKG is abnormal, she needs calcium chloride or gluconate in order to protect her heart while the other interventions are performed. Kayexalate and dialysis take hours to remove potassium from the body. Bicarbonate and insulin work in 15–20 minutes, but their effect is not as instantaneous as giving calcium.

▶ **TIP**

Protect the heart first in potassium disorders.

Phosphate Disturbances

Phosphate balance follows diet:

Feed more = More tissues produced = Low phosphate

Starve more = Tissues break down = High phosphate

Low blood phosphate	High blood phosphate
• Vitamin D deficiency	• Vitamin D toxicity
• Refeeding starved people	• Starving people
• **Hyper**parathyroid	• **Hypo**parathyroid
• Respiratory alkalosis	• Acute acidosis
• Insulin	• DKA
• Tenofovir	

Acid-Base Disturbances

Renal Tubular Acidosis

Renal tubular acidosis (RTA) is a metabolic acidosis with a normal anion gap. The anion gap is defined as sodium minus chloride plus bicarbonate.

$$(Na^+) \text{ minus } (Cl^- \text{ and } HCO_3^-)$$

A normal anion gap is 6–12. The difference between the cations and the anions is predominantly from negative charges that are on albumin.

The most important causes of a metabolic acidosis with a normal anion gap are:

- RTA
- Diarrhea

The anion gap is normal in both of these because the chloride level rises. Hence, they are also referred to as hyperchloremic metabolic acidosis.

The anion gap increases from ingested substances such as ethylene glycol or methanol, or organic acids such as lactate that are anionic and drive down the chloride level.

Distal RTA (Type I)

The distal tubule is responsible for generating new bicarbonate under the influence of aldosterone. Drugs such as amphotericin and autoimmune diseases such as SLE or Sjögren syndrome can damage the distal tubule. If new bicarbonate cannot be generated at the distal tubule, then acid cannot be excreted into the tubule, raising the pH of the urine.

The USMLE urgently wants examinees to know that topiramate causes distal RTA.

In an alkaline urine, there is increased formation of kidney stones from calcium oxalate.

The **best initial diagnostic test** is a UA looking for an abnormally high pH >5.5. The **most accurate test** is to infuse acid into the blood with ammonium chloride. A healthy person will be able to excrete the acid and thus decrease the urine pH. Those with distal RTA cannot excrete the acid, and the urine pH will remain basic (>5.5) despite an increasingly acidic serum.

Treat distal RTA by replacing bicarbonate, which will be absorbed at the proximal tubule. Since the majority of bicarbonate is absorbed at the proximal tubule, distal RTA is relatively easy to correct. Just give more bicarbonate and the proximal tubule will absorb it and correct the acidosis.

Proximal RTA (Type II)

Normally 85–90% of filtered bicarbonate is resorbed at the proximal tubule. However, damage to the proximal tubule (from amyloidosis, myeloma, Fanconi syndrome, acetazolamide, or heavy metals) decreases the kidney's ability to resorb most of filtered bicarbonate, phosphate, glucose, or citrate. Bicarbonate is lost in the urine until the body is so depleted of bicarbonate that the distal tubule can absorb the rest. When this happens, the urine pH will become low (≤5.5). Chronic metabolic acidosis leaches calcium out of the bones and they become soft (osteomalacia).

No acid into the tubule makes the urine basic.

Distal RTA calcifies the kidney parenchyma (nephrocalcinosis).

Distal = Stones

RTA does not mean the tubule is always acidic.

In proximal RTA, tenofovir kills tubules.

The **most accurate test** is to evaluate bicarbonate malabsorption in the kidney by giving bicarbonate and testing the urine pH.

- The urine pH is variable in proximal RTA. First it is basic (>5.5) until most bicarbonate is lost from the body, then it is low (<5.5).
- Because the kidney cannot absorb bicarbonate, the urine pH will rise when bicarbonate is administered.

Treat with vigorous bicarbonate replacement and thiazide diuretics.

- Because bicarbonate is not absorbed well in proximal RTA, it is difficult to treat, and massive doses of bicarbonate are necessary.
- Thiazide diuretics cause volume depletion, which enhances bicarbonate resorption.

Type IV RTA

Type IV RTA occurs most often in diabetes. Either the amount or the effect of aldosterone at the kidney tubule is abnormally low, leading to loss of sodium and retention of potassium and hydrogen ions.

Test for type IV RTA by finding a persistently high urine sodium despite a sodium-depleted diet. In addition, hyperkalemia is a main clue to answering "What is the most likely diagnosis?"

▶ TIP

Just because RTA is difficult does not mean it isn't tested. RTA is tested. Learn it.

> - Both proximal and distal RTA are **hypo**kalemic. Potassium is lost in the urine.
> - Type IV RTA is **hyper**kalemic.

Types of Renal Tubular Acidosis (RTA)			
	Proximal (Type II)	**Distal (Type I)**	**Type IV**
Urine pH	Variable	High >5.5	<5.5
Blood potassium level	Low	Low	High
Nephrolithiasis	No	Yes	No
Diagnostic test	Administer bicarbonate	Administer acid	Urine salt loss
Treatment	Thiazides	Bicarbonate	Fludrocortisone

> Fludrocortisone is the steroid with the highest mineralocorticoid or "aldosteronelike" effect.

Urine Anion Gap

The urine anion gap (UAG) is a way to distinguish between diarrhea and RTA as causes of normal anion gap metabolic acidosis.

$$UAG = sodium\ minus\ chloride$$
$$or$$
$$Na^+\ minus\ Cl^-$$

Acid excreted by the kidney is buffered off as NH_4Cl or ammonium chloride. The more acid excreted, the greater the amount of chloride found in the urine.

> RTA has a positive UAG. Diarrhea has a negative UAG.

In RTA there is a defect in acid excretion into the urine, so the amount of chloride in the urine is diminished. This gives a positive number when calculating Na^+ minus Cl^-.

In diarrhea, the ability to excrete acid through the kidney remains intact. Because diarrhea is associated with metabolic acidosis, the kidney tries to compensate by increasing acid excretion. Hence, in diarrhea there is more acid in the urine. Acid (H^+) is excreted with chloride. So, in diarrhea, more acid in the urine means more chloride in the urine. Na^+ minus Cl^- will become a negative number in diarrhea.

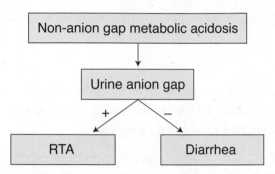

Figure 11.9 Urine Anion Gap: Definition

Metabolic Acidosis

Metabolic disturbances kill patients through cardiac arrhythmias. They also alter potassium levels.

An increase in metabolic acidity occurs with or without anion gap elevation. The compensation for metabolic acidosis is respiratory alkalosis through hyperventilation.

> Respiratory alkalosis from hyperventilation compensates for all forms of metabolic acidosis.

- **Normal anion gap (6–12):** RTA and diarrhea
- **Elevated anion gap (>12):** The anion gap is increased if there are unmeasured anions driving the bicarbonate level down. Examples are found in the table.

Causes of Metabolic Acidosis with an Increased Anion Gap			
	Cause	**Test**	**Treatment**
Lactate	Hypotension or hypoperfusion	Blood lactate level	Correct hypoperfusion
Ketoacids	DKA, starvation	Acetone level	Insulin and fluids
Oxalic acid	Ethylene glycol overdose	Crystals on UA	Fomepizole, dialysis
Formic acid	Methanol overdose	Inflamed retina	Fomepizole, dialysis
Uremia	Renal failure	BUN, creatinine	Dialysis
Salicylates	Aspirin overdose	Aspirin level	Alkalinize urine

▶ **TIP**

You cannot determine the etiology of metabolic acidosis from the ABG.

Metabolic Alkalosis

By definition, metabolic alkalosis has an elevated serum bicarbonate level. The compensation for metabolic alkalosis is **respiratory acidosis**. There will be a relative hypoventilation that will increase the pCO_2 to compensate for metabolic alkalosis.

Metabolic problems always show compensation.	

Etiology

- GI loss: vomiting or nasogastric suction
- Increased aldosterone: primary hyperaldosteronism, Cushing syndrome, ectopic ACTH, volume contraction, licorice
- Diuretics
- Milk-alkali syndrome: high-volume liquid antacids
- Hypokalemia: hydrogen ions move into cells so potassium can be released

Arterial Blood Gas in Metabolic Alkalosis

The ABG in metabolic alkalosis will always have:

- Increased pH >7.40
- Increased pCO_2 indicating respiratory acidosis as compensation
- Increased bicarbonate

Metabolic derangements kill patients with cardiac arrhythmia.	

▶ TIP

You cannot determine the etiology of metabolic alkalosis from the ABG.

Respiratory Acidosis and Alkalosis

Respiratory acid/base disturbances are easy to understand because they come down to the single pathway of the effect on minute ventilation.

$$\text{Minute ventilation} = \text{Respiratory rate} \times \text{Tidal volume}$$

Minute ventilation is more precise than respiratory rate. Hyperventilation may occur with a tiny tidal volume. This does not increase minute ventilation.

Minute ventilation is more precise than respiratory rate.	

Causes of Respiratory Acidosis and Alkalosis	
Respiratory alkalosis	**Respiratory acidosis**
Decreased pCO_2	Increased pCO_2
Increased minute ventilation	Decreased minute ventilation
Metabolic acidosis as compensation	Metabolic alkalosis as compensation
• Anemia • Anxiety • Pain • Fever • Interstitial lung disease • Pulmonary emboli	• COPD/emphysema • Drowning • Opiate overdose • Alpha 1-antitrypsin deficiency • Kyphoscoliosis • Sleep apnea/morbid obesity

Nephrolithiasis

The most common cause of kidney stones (nephrolithiasis) is calcium oxalate, which forms more frequently in an alkaline urine. The **most common risk factor** is the overexcretion of calcium in the urine. Fat malabsorption also increases stone formation.

> Crohn disease causes kidney stones because of increased oxalate absorption.

A 46-year-old man comes to the ED with excruciating pain in his left flank radiating to the groin. He has some blood in his urine. What is the most appropriate next step in management?

a. Ketorolac
b. X-ray
c. Sonography
d. Urinalysis
e. Serum calcium level

Answer: **A.** Ketorolac is an NSAID that is available orally and intravenously. It provides a level of analgesia similar to opiate medications. When the presentation of nephrolithiasis is clear, it is more important to provide relief for this excruciating form of pain than to obtain specific diagnostic tests.

What is the most accurate diagnostic test for nephrolithiasis?

a. CT scan
b. X-ray
c. Sonography
d. Urinalysis
e. Intravenous pyelogram

Answer: **A.** The CT scan for nephrolithiasis does not need contrast and is more accurate (sensitive) than an x-ray or sonogram. Intravenous pyelogram (IVP) needs intravenous contrast and takes several hours to perform. Urinalysis and straining the urine may show blood or the passage of a stone, but will not help manage acute renal colic. X-ray has a false negative rate of 10–20%. X-rays of the abdomen are useful only in detecting an ileus.

▶ **TIP**

IVP is always a wrong answer for nephrolithiasis.

The **best initial therapy** for acute renal colic is analgesics and hydration.

Use CT and sonography to detect obstruction such as hydronephrosis.

- Stones <5 mm pass spontaneously
- Stones 5–7 mm get nifedipine and tamsulosin to help them pass

Cystine stones are managed with surgical removal, alkalinizing the urine. Urinary tract infection gives struvite stones (magnesium/ammonium/phosphate). Remove them surgically.

> **Uric acid stones** are not detectable on x-ray but are **visualized on CT.**

> Stones 5–7 mm get nifedipine + tamsulosin to help them pass.

The etiology of the stone is determined with:

- Stone analysis
- Serum calcium, sodium, uric acid, PTH, magnesium, and phosphate levels
- 24-hour urine for volume, calcium, oxalate, citrate, cystine, pH, uric acid, phosphate, and magnesium

A woman with her first episode of renal colic is found to have a 1.8 cm stone in the left renal pelvis. She has no obstruction and her renal function is normal (normal BUN and creatinine). What is the most appropriate next step in management?

a. Wait for it to pass; hydrate and observe
b. Lithotripsy
c. Surgical removal
d. Hydrochlorothiazide
e. Stent placement

Answer: **B.** Lithotripsy is used to manage stones 0.5–2 cm. Small stones (<5 mm) will spontaneously pass. Stones larger than 2 cm are not well-managed with lithotripsy because the fragments will get caught in the ureters. These large stones are best managed surgically. *Stent placement relieves hydronephrosis* from stones caught in the distal ureters. Stones halfway up the ureters are treated with lithotripsy. Those halfway down the ureter are removed from below with a basket.

Long-Term Management of Nephrolithiasis

Fifty percent of those with kidney stones will have a recurrence over the next 5 years.

A man with a calcium oxalate stone is managed with lithotripsy and the stone is destroyed and passes. His urinary calcium level is increased. Besides increasing hydration, which of the following is most likely to benefit this patient?

a. Calcium restriction
b. Hydrochlorothiazide
c. Furosemide
d. Stent placement
e. Increased dietary oxalate

Answer: **B.** Hydrochlorothiazide removes calcium from the urine by increasing distal tubular resorption of calcium. Furosemide increases calcium excretion into the urine and can make it worse. Calcium restriction actually does not help decrease overexcretion of calcium into the urine. In fact, it can make it more likely to form a stone. This is because calcium binds oxalate in the bowel. When calcium ingestion is low, there is increased oxalate absorption in the gut because there is no calcium to bind it in the gut. Stent placement is done when there is an obstruction in the ureters, especially at the ureteropelvic junction. Hydrochlorothiazide desaturates the urine of calcium. The risk of stone formation is increased if there is a dietary decrease in calcium, increase in oxalate, or decrease in citrate.

Metabolic Acidosis and Stone Formation

Metabolic acidosis removes calcium from bones and increases stone formation. In addition, metabolic acidosis decreases citrate levels. Citrate binds calcium, making it unavailable for stone formation.

Urinary Incontinence

Urinary Incontinence		
	Stress incontinence	**Urge incontinence**
Symptoms	Older woman with painless urinary leakage with coughing, laughing, or lifting heavy objects	Sudden pain in the bladder followed immediately by the overwhelming urge to urinate
Test	Have patient stand and cough; observe for leakage	Pressure measurement in half-full bladder; manometry
Treatment	1. Kegel exercises 2. Local estrogen cream 3. Surgical tightening of urethra	1. Bladder training exercises 2. Anticholinergic therapy • Oxybutynin or tolterodine • Solifenacin, darifenacin, or trospium 3. Beta-3 agonist: mirabegron 4. Botulinum toxin 5. Surgical tightening of urethra

Hypertension

Hypertension is defined as:

- Systolic pressure >140 mm Hg
- Diastolic pressure >90 mm Hg

JNC 8 says:

- In diabetes, blood pressure goal is 140/90 mm Hg.
- Thiazides are not better than CCBs, ACEIs, or ARBs.
- BP 150/90 mm Hg age >60.

In order to establish the diagnosis of hypertension, blood pressure measurements must be repeated in a calm state over time. The precise interval between measurements over what period of time is not clear.

Hypertension is:

- The **most common disease** in the United States
- The **most common risk factor** for the most common cause of death: myocardial infarction

> A **diabetic** patient with BP >140/90 mm Hg is **hypertensive**.

Etiology

Ninety-five percent of hypertension has no clear etiology and can be called "essential hypertension." Known causes of hypertension are:

- Renal artery stenosis
- Glomerulonephritis
- Coarctation of the aorta
- Acromegaly
- Obstructive sleep apnea
- Pheochromocytoma
- Hyperaldosteronism
- Cushing syndrome or any cause of hypercortisolism including therapeutic use of glucocorticoids
- Congenital adrenal hyperplasia

Presentation

The vast majority of cases are found on routine screening of asymptomatic patients. When hypertension does have symptoms, they are from end-organ damage from atherosclerosis such as:

- Coronary artery disease
- Cerebrovascular disease
- CHF
- Visual disturbance
- Renal insufficiency
- Peripheral artery disease

Presentation of Secondary Hypertension

- Renal artery stenosis: Bruit is auscultated at the flank. The bruit is continuous throughout systole and diastole.
- Glomerulonephritis
- Coarctation of the aorta: upper extremity > lower extremity blood pressure
- Acromegaly
- Pheochromocytoma: episodic hypertension with flushing
- Hyperaldosteronism: weakness from hypokalemia

Diagnostic Tests

Repeated in-office measurement or home ambulatory measurements carry equal significance.

Those with hypertension are also tested with:

- EKG
- Urinalysis
- Glucose measurements to exclude concomitant diabetes
- Cholesterol screening

> **Hypertension is rarely symptomatic** at first presentation.

For renal artery stenosis, the **most accurate test** is MRA.

Treatment

The **best initial therapy** is with lifestyle management such as:

- Weight loss (**most effective**)
- Sodium restriction
- Dietary modification (less fat and red meat, more fish and vegetables)
- Exercise
- Tobacco cessation does not stop hypertension but becomes especially important to prevent cardiovascular disease.

Treat renal artery stenosis by dilating fibromuscular dysplasia and using a stent. If the stenosis is from atherosclerosis and cannot be dilated, use an ACE inhibitor or ARB (the most effective medications).

Summary of JNC 8 Management of Hypertension

- Blood pressure goal in diabetes is 140/90 mm Hg.
- Initial management is with either thiazides or calcium blockers or ACE inhibitor or angiotensin receptor blocker. Diuretics are not considered specifically better as the initial therapy.
- The main point is to control the blood pressure. The specific agent is not as important.
- With age >60, the goal of BP is 150/90 mm Hg.
- With diabetes and CKD, the goal is BP <140/90 mm Hg.

Drug Therapy

The **best initial therapy** is a thiazide diuretic, calcium blocker, ACE inhibitor, or angiotensin receptor blocker.

A single medication controls hypertension in 60–70% of patients. If blood pressure is very high on presentation (>160/100 mm Hg), 2 medications should be used at the outset.

If diuretics do not control blood pressure, the most appropriate next step in management is:

- ACE inhibitor
- Angiotensin receptor blocker (ARB)
- Beta blocker (BB)
- Calcium channel blocker (CCB)

Medications that are not considered first-line or second-line therapy are:

- Central-acting alpha agonists (alpha methyldopa, clonidine)
- Peripheral-acting alpha antagonists (prazosin, terazosin, doxazosin)
- Direct-acting vasodilators (hydralazine, minoxidil)

Lifestyle modifications are tried for 3–6 months before medications are started.

In renal artery stenosis, the most effective BP medications are ACE inhibitors or ARBs.

Hypertension will be controlled by 2–3 medications in 90% of patients.

Pregnancy-safe hypertension drugs:
- BB—use first
- CCB
- Hydralazine
- Alpha methyldopa

Compelling Indications for Specific Drugs

If there is another significant disease in the history, you should add a specific drug to lifestyle modifications. In these circumstances you should not start with a thiazide.

Compelling Indications	
If this is in the history...	**This is the best initial therapy...**
Coronary artery disease	BB, ACE, ARB
Diabetes mellitus	ACE, ARB (goal <140/90 mm Hg)
Benign prostatic hypertrophy	Alpha blockers
Depression and asthma	Avoid BBs
Hyperthyroidism	BB first
Osteoporosis	Thiazides
Proteinuria	ACE, ARB

Hypertensive Crisis

Hypertensive crisis is defined as high blood pressure in association with:

- Confusion
- Blurry vision
- Dyspnea
- Chest pain

Treatment is aimed at reducing blood pressure. However, do not lower blood pressure to normal in hypertensive crisis or you may provoke a stroke.

The **best initial therapy** for hypertensive crisis is labetalol or nitroprusside. Because nitroprusside needs monitoring with an arterial line, it is not usually the first choice.

Equally acceptable forms of therapy for acute hypertensive crises are:

- Enalapril
- CCBs: diltiazem, verapamil
- Esmolol
- Hydralazine
- Peripheral dopamine receptor agonist: fenoldopam

Any intravenous medication is acceptable. The specific drug available is not as important as giving enough of it to control the blood pressure.

> Hypertensive crisis is not defined as a specific level of blood pressure. It is defined as **hypertension associated with end-organ damage**.

Breast Cancer

Breast cancer is found in asymptomatic women on screening mammography or by the palpation of a mass by the patient or a physician. When breast cancer presents as a palpable mass, it is hard to the touch. It may also be associated with retraction of the nipple because ligaments in the breast will withdraw and pull the nipple inward.

> Breast cancer is usually painless.

Diagnostic Tests

Biopsy is the best initial test. The different methods of biopsy are:

- **Fine needle aspiration** (FNA) (**best initial biopsy**): false-positive rate <2%, but because FNA is a small sample, the disadvantages are a false-negative rate 10%
- **Core needle biopsy**: larger sample of the breast; can test for estrogen receptors (ER), progesterone receptors (PR), and HER 2/neu; disadvantages are greater deformity of the breast and the possibility that the needle will miss the lesion
- **Open biopsy** (**most accurate diagnostic test**): allows for frozen section to be done while the patient is in the operating room, followed by immediate resection of cancer, followed by sentinel node biopsy

> An FNA cannot test for ER, PR, HER 2/neu.

Mammography

Mammography is indicated to screen for breast cancer in the general population starting at age 50.

A woman finds a hard, nontender breast mass on self-examination. There is no alteration of the mass with menstruation. She is scheduled to undergo a FNA biopsy. Which of the following is most likely to benefit the patient?

a. Mammography
b. BRCA testing
c. Ultrasound
d. Bone scan
e. PET scan

The precise utility of MRI for breast cancer is not yet clear.

Answer: **A.** If breast biopsy is going to be performed, why do a screening test like mammography? The answer is that 5–10% of patients have bilateral disease. In addition, there is a huge difference in management if there is a single lesion or multiple lesions within the same breast. BRCA testing confirms an extra risk of cancer compared to the general population, but will add nothing to a patient who must already undergo biopsy. Ultrasound is useful in evaluating whether masses that are equivocal by clinical examination are cystic or solid. Bone scan is used after a diagnosis of breast cancer is made to exclude occult metastases. PET scan helps determine the content of abnormal masses within the body or enlarged nodes without biopsy, but it does not eliminate the need to establish an initial diagnosis with biopsy. MRI is used in young women with dense breasts.

When Is Ultrasound the Answer?

To evaluate clinically indeterminant mass lesions. It tells cysts versus solid lesions. Answer ultrasound if the lesion:

- Is painful
- Varies in size or pain with menstruation

When Is PET Scan the Answer?

To determine the content of abnormal lymph nodes that are not easily accessible to biopsy. Cancer increases uptake on PET scan.

Suppose an 80-year-old woman with biopsy-proven breast cancer has no nodes with cancer in the axilla. The primary lesion is small and the woman may not need adjuvant chemotherapy. Chest CT shows an abnormal hilar lymph node.

In this case, PET scan is useful to exclude a metastasis and the need for additional chemotherapy.

How do you tell the content of an abnormal, inaccessible lesion without biopsy? Try PET scan.

When Is BRCA Testing the Answer?

- BRCA is definitely associated with an increased risk of breast cancer, particularly within families.
- BRCA is associated with ovarian cancer and pancreatic cancer.

What is not clear is what to do when BRCA is positive. BRCA has not yet been shown to add mortality benefit to usual management. However, some patients opt for bilateral mastectomy.

We do not know what to do about BRCA when it is positive.

With so many methods to lower mortality in breast cancer, the Step 2 exam will not engage in speculation about who should get BRCA testing. It is just not clear.

When Is Sentinel Lymph Node Biopsy the Answer?

The first node identified near the operative field of a definitively identified breast cancer is the sentinel node. Contrast or dye is placed into the operative field and the first node identified that it travels to is the sentinel node.

- Sentinel node biopsy is done routinely in all patients at the time of lumpectomy or mastectomy.
- A negative sentinel node eliminates the need for axillary lymph node dissection.

When Are Estrogen- and Progesterone-Receptors Tested?

Always. These are routine for all patients. If either test is positive, hormone manipulation therapy is done.

Treatment

Surgery

Lumpectomy plus radiation is equal in efficacy to modified radical mastectomy but much less deforming. The addition of radiation to lumpectomy is not a small issue.

- Radiation at the site of the cancer is indispensable in preventing recurrences in the breast.
- Lumpectomy is contraindicated if the cancer is multifocal or if radiation is contraindicated.
- Radical mastectomy is always the wrong answer.

Hormonal Manipulation

All ER- or PR-positive patients should receive tamoxifen, raloxifene, or one of the aromatase inhibitors (anastrozole, letrozole, exemestane). Aromatase inhibitors seem to have a slight superiority in efficacy. If both are among the answer choices, aromatase inhibitors are the answer to the "most likely to benefit the patient" question. Aromatase inhibitors are generally for postmenopausal women, while tamoxifen is better for premenopausal patients.

▶ **TIP**

If 2 treatments are very close in efficacy, how can you be tested on them? You will need to understand the differences in their adverse effects.

When is trastuzumab the answer?

- All breast cancers should be tested for HER-2/neu. This is an abnormal ER.
- Those who are positive should receive anti-HER-2/neu antibodies known as trastuzumab.
- Trastuzumab decreases the risk of recurrent disease and increases survival.

When is adjuvant chemotherapy the answer?

- When lesion size >1 cm or when positive axillary lymph nodes are found.

Adjuvant chemotherapy is not prophylactic, since patients already have the disease. It is not *treatment*, since the term implies there are no clearly identified metastases. *Adjuvant* means an additional therapy to clean up presumed microscopic cancer cells too small in amount to be detected.

Side effects:

- **Tamoxifen** (selective estrogen receptor modifier): endometrial cancer and clots
- **Aromatase inhibitors** (inhibit estrogen effect everywhere, including good effects like bone density): **osteoporosis**

Trastuzumab is cardiotoxic.

When all 3 receptors are negative, the chemo to give is atezolizumab.

Use SERMs or aromatase inhibitors when multiple first-degree relatives have breast cancer. It lowers the risk of breast cancer.

All of the following definitely lower mortality:

- Mammography
- ER/PR testing, then tamoxifen/raloxifene
- Aromatase inhibitors
- Adjuvant chemotherapy
- Lumpectomy and radiation
- Modified radical mastectomy
- Trastuzumab (anti-Her 2/neu)
- Prophylaxis with tamoxifen (or raloxifene)
- Atezolizumab

Prostate Cancer

Prostate cancer presents with obstructive symptoms on voiding similar to benign prostatic hypertrophy or a palpable lesion on examination. Biopsy is the best initial test and the most accurate test. Most prostate cancers are asymptomatic.

Gleason grading is a measure of the aggressiveness or malignant potential of prostate cancer. A high Gleason grade suggests a greater benefit of surgical removal of the prostate. If the Gleason grade is high, get it out before it metastasizes.

Treatment

- Prostatectomy may have a slight benefit over radiation in terms of survival, but it has some common complications:
  - Erectile dysfunction
  - Urinary incontinence

- In localized prostate cancer, it is not known whether prostatectomy, external beam radiation, implantable radioactive pellets, or watchful waiting is superior.

- Hormonal manipulation (not like tamoxifen in breast cancer; they do not prevent recurrence but rather shrink lesions that are already present)

  - Flutamide, GNRH agonists, ketoconazole, and orchiectomy help control the size and progression of metastases once they have occurred.

  - Abiraterone is an inhibitor of 17-hydroxylase that stops production of all androgens in the body, including adrenal production of androgens; it decreases the progression of metastatic prostate cancer and reduces risk of death by 30%

> Exam questions about *adverse effects* are always clear. You will be expected to know that surgery is more likely to give erectile dysfunction compared to radiation. Radiation also leads to diarrhea.

> Hormone manipulators such as abiraterone, enzalutamide, and apalutamide lower mortality in metastatic prostate cancer.

Management That Is Definitely Not Beneficial in Prostate Cancer

These answers are always wrong:

- **"Screening" imaging study**. Prostate ultrasound is not a screening test. It is used to localize lesions to biopsy when PSA is high.
- **Lumpectomy**.
- **Chemotherapy**. It is used only if hormonal therapy does not work.
- **Hormonal manipulation to prevent recurrences**. It is used only to shrink existing tumors.

Prostate Specific Antigen (PSA)

PSA corresponds to the volume of cancer. The higher the PSA, the greater the risk of cancer. However, PSA is a controversial subject for the following reasons:

- A normal PSA does not exclude the possibility of prostate cancer.
- There is no clear mortality benefit with PSA.
- PSA is not to be routinely offered to patients; if patient is age >75, do not do the test, even if asked.

▶ **TIP**

If the exam question specifically says, "The patient is requesting PSA to screen for cancer," then the answer is do the test.

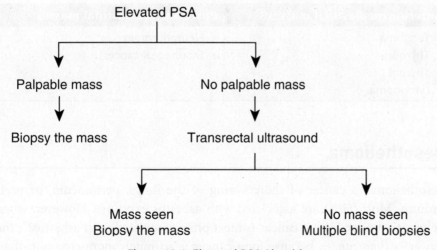

Figure 12.1 Elevated PSA Algorithm

Lung Cancer

The most important question for lung cancer is, "Who should be treated with surgery?"

The size of the lesion is not the most important factor in whether the lesion is resectable. If the lesion is large, but is surrounded by normal lung and there is enough remaining lung function post-resection, then surgery is still possible.

Surgery is not possible in these cases:

- Bilateral disease or lymph nodes involved on opposite side
- Malignant pleural effusion
- Heart, carina, aorta, or vena cava is involved

Small cell cancer is considered unresectable in 95% of cases because it is metastatic or spread outside one lung.

When the question describes lung cancer that tests positive for the programmed death (PD) biomarker (not the specific histology), the answer is pembrolizumab and nivolumab. These PD inhibitors are more effective and better tolerated than platinum therapy for non–small cell lung cancer.

> Screen for lung cancer annually with low-dose chest CT in those with:
> - 20 pack-year smoking history
> - Age 50–80

Mediastinal Masses

Anterior mediastinal masses	Posterior mediastinal masses
• Teratoma • Thymoma • Thyroid • Lymphoma	• Neurofibromas • Esophageal cancer

Mesothelioma

Mesothelioma is cancer of the covering of the lungs, peritoneum, or pericardium. Most (80%) are associated with asbestos exposure. However, when the question asks, "What cancer is most often associated with asbestos?", the answer is *lung cancer*, because lung cancer is so much more common than mesothelioma.

Patients with mesothelioma typically present with the symptoms of pleural inflammation and effusion such as chest pain, dyspnea, and cough.

- **Best initial test**: chest x-ray, then chest CT
- **Most accurate test**: pleural or peritoneal biopsy
- Management: surgical removal of the cancerous tissue and, in some, both radiation and chemotherapy

Pleurodesis is a procedure to seal shut the pleural space in those with recurring large pleural effusions. In pleurodesis, the pleura is purposely inflamed with minocycline, bleomycin, or talc to obliterate the pleural space.

Ovarian Cancer

There is no screening test for ovarian cancer.

Look for a woman age >50 with increasing abdominal girth who is still losing weight. BRCA is associated with ovarian cancer.

The **best initial test** is an ultrasound or CT scan. The **most accurate diagnostic test** is a biopsy. CA-125 is not for screening; it is used only for follow-up of treatment.

Ovarian cancer is the only cancer in which removing large amounts of locally metastatic disease will benefit the patient. Remove all visible tumor and pelvic organs and give chemotherapy. PARP inhibitors are especially effective in ovarian cancer.

Cervical Cancer

(See the Gynecology section for evaluation and management of cervical cancer.)

Testicular Cancer

Testicular cancer presents with a painless lump in the scrotum that does not transilluminate. Risk is increased with history of cryptorchidism.

> Cryptorchid → cancer

Treatment is to remove the whole testicle with inguinal orchiectomy. Do not cut the scrotum, which can spread the disease. Needle biopsy of the testicle is always a wrong answer.

Alpha fetoprotein is secreted only by nonseminomatous cancers. HCG is elevated in all of them.

> Seminoma: sensitive to chemotherapy **and** radiation
>
> **Non**-seminoma: sensitive to chemotherapy

Staging is performed with CT scan of the abdomen, pelvis, and chest. Testicular cancer metastasizes up through the lymphatic channels in the retroperitoneum and moves up into the chest.

After orchiectomy, **radiation** is used for **local** disease and **chemotherapy** is used for **widespread** disease. This refers to seminomas. Testicular cancer is one of the only malignancies in which chemotherapy can cure widely metastatic disease, including when it has spread into the brain.

Chemotherapy-Induced Nausea

The 3 main classes of medications used to treat chemotherapy-induced nausea are 5-hydroxytryptamine (5HT) inhibitors, neurokinin-1 (NK) receptor antagonists, and glucocorticoids. All 3 types of drugs can be combined in severe nausea and vomiting from chemotherapy.

- **5HT inhibitors** (ondansetron, granisetron, palonosetron, dolasetron)
  - The answer to "**best initial therapy**" question
  - *Exception*: Do not give if QT prolongation on EKG (good exam question)

- **Glucocorticoids**
  - Dexamethasone used first
  - Steroids have major antinausea effect
  - Combination with steroids effective *only with 5HT inhibitors*

- **NK receptor antagonists** (aprepitant, rolapitant, netupitant)

  - The answer if 5HT inhibitors do not work or cannot be given because of QT prolongation on EKG

The phenothiazines prochlorperazine and chlorpromazine are antiemetics that are less effective than 5HT and NK antagonists; they will be the wrong answer choice in questions about chemotherapy-induced nausea. Metoclopramide is useful for the nausea of diabetic gastroparesis. These medications have no utility in combination, because they are all dopamine receptor antagonists.

> Do not give 5HT inhibitors with QT prolongation on EKG.

> A question about antiemetics that work through dopamine receptors will describe a patient whose **parkinsonism gets worse**.

PART 2

Preventive Medicine

In terms of preventive medicine, the hardest thing for a medical student to know is which guidelines will be tested. The answer is that the most reliable preventive medicine guidelines, and the standard of care, is the recommendations of the United States Preventive Services Task Force (USPSTF). These guidelines are as objective a source as we have. They are not based on the financial incentives of a particular specialty, and they are created by those who simply interpret the best available objective data without regard for personal or professional gain. A specialized nonprofit organization like the American Cancer Society or a private professional group like the American Urological Association has a vested interest in increasing detection of certain diseases, even if a given screening test has not clearly been shown to decrease mortality.

▶ **TIP**

Let mortality benefit be your guide in choosing which test to do, or "Which of the following is most likely to benefit the patient?"

Cancer Screening

The single most important preventive medicine question is:

Which cancer screening method lowers mortality the most? In other words, which of the following is most likely to benefit the patient?

a. Pap smear
b. Colonoscopy
c. Prostate-specific antigen (PSA)
d. Mammography age >40
e. Mammography age >50

Answer: **E.** Controversy may surround the question of how early to begin mammography. Recommendations have recently changed to start mammography at age 50, instead of 40. What is not controversial, however, is that screening those age >50 has a greater mortality benefit. That is because the incidence of breast cancer is greater age >50. So if you screen 1,000 women age >50, you will detect more cancer than if you screen 1,000 women age >40.

> Age to start mammography can be controversial (40–50). Age of maximum benefit (>50) is clear.

Breast Cancer

Mammography should be done starting at age 50 every 2 years. The reduction in mortality is greatest age >50. Screening can end at age 74.

▶ **TIP**

Breast self-examination is a wrong answer. Although it may seem to benefit, there is no proof.

On average, you will detect 10 cases of breast cancer by screening 1,000 women age >50, but you will detect only 2 cancers by screening 1,000 women age 40–49. The MRI, CT, and ultrasound do not yet have a clear place in terms of screening for breast cancer.

> As a screening test, only mammography is proven to lower mortality.

Which of the following prevents cancer in patients with multiple first-degree relatives with breast cancer?

a. BRCA testing
b. Aromatase inhibitors (anastrozole, letrozole)
c. Dietary modification (low fat, soy diet)
d. HER2/neu testing
e. Estrogen and/or progesterone receptor testing

Answer: B. Selective estrogen receptor modulators (SERMs), tamoxifen, raloxifene, and aromatase inhibitors result in a 50–66% reduction in breast cancer when compared with placebo. The benefit is greatest in those with 2 first-degree relatives with breast cancer (mother or sister). Dietary modification is unproven. HER2/neu testing is useful to guide the use of trastuzumab, which will block this receptor in those with proven cancer, but not as prophylaxis. Estrogen and progesterone receptor testing has no place in managing asymptomatic women. These tests are used in those proven to have cancer.

> Start these breast cancer prevention drugs at age 35–40 and use for 5 years:
> • SERMs
> • Aromatase inhibitors

BRCA Testing

BRCA is associated with increased risk of breast and ovarian cancer. However, this does not mean it is a clearly beneficial screening test. The missing piece is: What to do when the patient is positive for BRCA? *It is not clear.* The only truly unambiguous statement about BRCA testing is that a positive test means an increased risk of cancer. Management remains undetermined.

▶ **TIP**

When BRCA is positive, "offer prophylactic bilateral mastectomy" is a wrong answer.

Cervical Cancer Screening

(See the Gynecology section for more details.)

There are 7,000–10,000 cases of cervical cancer a year in the United States. For these, Pap smear definitely lowers mortality. Recommendations are as follows:

- Papillomavirus vaccine should be routine for all women age 11–45.
- First Pap smear should be done for all women at age 21.
- If one combines Pap smear + HPV testing, testing can be done every 5 years in women age 30–65.

HPV testing is rarely done age <30.

> Adding HPV testing to Pap increases interval to 5 years.

> Chlamydia screen women 15–25 years old.

▶ **TIP**

USMLE Step 2 CK will not engage in controversy. The answer must be clear.

Colon Cancer Screening

The lifetime risk of colon cancer for an American is 6–8%. Each year, 50,000 people die of colon cancer in the United States. With screening, 95% of these deaths are preventable.

Which of the following is most likely to benefit the patient?

a. Colonoscopy every 10 years after age 40
b. Colonoscopy every 10 years after age 45
c. Sigmoidoscopy every 3–5 years after age 45
d. Barium enema after age 50
e. Fecal occult blood testing
f. Virtual colonoscopy with CT scanning
g. Capsule endoscopy
h. Digital rectal examination after age 50

Answer: **B**. Colonoscopy is unquestionably the **best colon cancer screening method**. Sigmoidoscopy will miss the 40% of cancers occurring proximal to the sigmoid colon. Barium enema does not allow for biopsy or removal of polyps. Virtual colonoscopy misses cancers in polyps smaller than 0.5 cm. It is inferior to endoscopic colon cancer detection methods. Fecal occult blood testing will detect cancer. If positive, however, it must be followed by colonoscopy. The age cutoff for screening is 45.

> Capsule endoscopy detects small bowel bleeding. It is not a cancer screening method.

> Standard colon screening is colonoscopy every 10 years after age 50.

▶ **TIP**

Digital rectal exam is not proven to lower mortality in any disease. It is always a wrong choice.

Prostate Cancer Screening

Unfortunately, there is no clearly beneficial test to lower mortality in prostate cancer screening. Neither the prostate-specific antigen nor the digital rectal exam has proven sufficiently sensitive or specific to lower mortality. Although PSA does detect prostate cancer, the lesions detected are most often not ones that need treatment. Of patients with prostate cancer, 25% have a normal PSA, and 25% of those with an elevated PSA do not have cancer.

The mortality benefit question for PSA is clear: There is no benefit. Whether to do the test is controversial.

▶ **TIP**

If the question asks mortality benefit for PSA, say "No."

If the question says, "The patient wants/requests a PSA," say "Yes."

Lung Cancer Screening

Long-term smokers with 20 pack-years of smoking should be screened by chest CT at age 50. Chest x-ray detects many lesions that turn out to be insignificant and misses many small cancers. High-resolution CT scanning lowers lung cancer mortality in those with a long history of smoking. Screen annually.

However: If the patient quit >15 years ago, lung cancer screening is not needed.

▶ **TIP**

Smoking cessation is always the single **most beneficial** disease-preventive method of any type.

Lipid Screening

Cholesterol and LDL measurement is recommended for healthy patients when:

- Men are age >35
- Women are age >45

Lipid screening is recommended for all patients with diabetes, hypertension, coronary artery disease, or the equivalents of coronary disease such as:

- Carotid disease
- Peripheral vascular disease
- Aortic disease

> Lung cancer screening is not needed if the patient quit >15 years ago.

Hypertension

Blood pressure testing is indicated for all patients age >18 at every visit.

Hypertension screening has never been prospectively evaluated in a meaningful way and probably never will. In order to do the study correctly, you would have to withhold BP measurement and observe for years to detect a mortality difference, which would be unethical.

Screen adults for hypertension every 2 years.

Diabetes Mellitus

Screening for diabetes with fasting blood glucose levels (2 measurements over 125 or HbA1c >6.5%) is done when the patient has:

- Obesity
- Hypertension
- Hyperlipidemia

There is no clear recommendation for diabetes mellitus screening in the general asymptomatic public.

Vaccinations

For adults, the 2 most beneficial vaccines are:

- Influenza
- Pneumococcus

Influenza and Pneumococcal Vaccines

Live attenuated vaccine should not be used in patients age >50 or with additional medical conditions, as listed. Both influenza and pneumococcal vaccine are recommended for all patients with:

- Chronic heart, lung, liver, and kidney disease including asthma
- HIV/AIDS
- Steroid users
- Immunocompromised patients in general such as cancer or functional or anatomic asplenia
- Diabetes mellitus

Egg allergy is not a contraindication to flu vaccine.

> Age ≥50 or with chronic medical illness: Use only inactivated flu vaccine.

> Egg allergy is not a contraindication to flu vaccine.

> Give both the 13 and 23 polyvalent pneumococcal vaccines in immunocompromised patients.

Differences in Indications between Influenza and Pneumococcal Vaccination

The differences in indications for these 2 vaccines are small.

Indications for Influenza and Pneumococcal Vaccination	
Influenza vaccine	**Pneumococcal vaccine**
• Everyone yearly • Healthcare workers • Pregnant patients	• Everyone age >65 • Cochlear implant • CSF leaks • Alcoholics • Tobacco smokers • One vaccine age >65 only • Single revaccination after 5 years if the patient is immunocompromised or the first injection was prior to age 65

Herpes (Varicella) Zoster Vaccine

> Zoster vaccine prevents shingles in adults. Start at age 50.

Although varicella vaccination is routinely indicated in all children, there is a higher-dose version of the varicella vaccine that is indicated in all patients age >50. This prevents postherpetic neuralgia.

Hepatitis A and B Vaccines

> Hepatitis A and B vaccines are **most beneficial** in those with chronic liver disease.

Both hepatitis A and B vaccines are routinely indicated in children. They are both indicated in adults if any of the following is true:

- Chronic liver disease
- Men who have sex with men or multiple sexual partners
- Household contacts with hepatitis A or B
- Injection drug users

Differences in Indication for Hepatitis A and B Vaccine	
Hepatitis A	**Hepatitis B**
• Travelers to countries of high endemicity • Homeless patients	• Patients with end-stage renal disease (dialysis) • Healthcare workers • Diabetics

Postexposure Prophylaxis: Hepatitis A

Hepatitis A vaccine for postexposure prophylaxis is enough for healthy people. In those younger than 12 months, give immune globulin. If the exposed patient is immunocompromised or has chronic liver disease, the answer is also immune globulin.

Meaningful exposures to hepatitis A are household and sexual contacts.

Postexposure Prophylaxis: Hepatitis B

Needle-stick and sexual exposures to those positive for hepatitis B surface antigen get hepatitis B immune globulin and hepatitis B vaccine. If the person exposed already has protective surface antibody, however, no therapy is needed.

Postexposure Prophylaxis: Hepatitis C

There is no postexposure prophylaxis for hepatitis C.

Tetanus Vaccine

- Td (toxoid) every 10 years
- One Tdap (tetanus with acellular pertussis) as one of the boosters
- Tetanus immune globulin in those never vaccinated
- Give Tdap with *every* pregnancy.

> **Tetanus**
>
> Never vaccinated: Immune globulin
>
> Dirty wound: Booster after 5 years
>
> Clean wound: Booster after 10 years

Meningococcal Vaccine

Meningococcal vaccine is routinely indicated at the age 11 visit. The vaccine is also indicated for adults with the following circumstances:

- Asplenia
- Terminal complement deficiency and those getting eculizumab
- Military recruits
- Residents of college dormitories
- Travelers to Mecca or Medina in Saudi Arabia for the Hajj (pilgrimage)
- HIV

> Eculizumab increases the risk of meningococcus 1,000-fold

Which of the following is the strongest indication for meningococcal vaccination (i.e., who will benefit the most)?

a. Asplenia
b. Military recruits
c. Residents of college dormitories
d. Travelers to Mecca or Medina
e. 11-year-old child

Answer: **A.** Asplenia represents a person at high risk for disseminated meningococcal infection. If exposed to the organism, an asplenic person has the highest risk of dissemination. The other choices represent increased exposure, but not an increased risk of immune compromise leading to dissemination.

Osteoporosis

Every woman should be screened with bone densitometry at the age of 65 with a DEXA scan. Hip fracture in an elderly patient carries an extremely high risk of mortality. Preventing fracture with bisphosphonates to increase bone density is potentially more life-saving than beta blockers in coronary disease. In an older woman, a hip fracture is more deadly than a myocardial infarction. Screening for men is much less clear.

Abdominal Aortic Aneurysm

All men age >65 with a smoking history should be screened once with an ultrasound to exclude an aneurysm. Also screen age 65–75 with family history of AAA.

Abdominal aortic aneurysm (AAA) should be repaired if it is wider than 5 centimeters.

Smoking Cessation

All patients should:

- Be **asked**, "Do you smoke?"
- Be **advised** to stop smoking.
- Receive an **attempt:** Find out who really wants to stop.
- Be **assisted:** Prescribe a method of aiding nicotine dependence.
- **Arrange** to meet with the patient again to find out if they have set a quit date and have really managed to stop.

Varenicline is the most effective medical means of stopping smoking. Both varenicline and bupropion are more effective than nicotine patches and gum.

Intimate Partner Violence (Domestic Violence)

All patients should be asked about the possibility of intimate partner violence. Patients will most often not volunteer this information. You cannot report this form of injury without the consent of the patient.

Alcoholism (Alcohol Dependence)

Alcoholism is a "self-diagnosed" disease. Alcoholism is not defined as an amount of alcohol used. It is not defined as alcohol use leading to loss of employment. Many alcoholics still maintain their jobs.

Ask:

- **C**: Do they feel the need to **cut down** the amount they are drinking?
- **A**: Do they feel **angry** when asked about their drinking?
- **G**: Do they feel **guilty** about the amount they drink?
- **E**: Do they feel the need for a morning **eye-opener**?

The **CAGE** questions are excellent at helping patients recognize they are alcohol dependent.

Routine Screening Methods That Are Always Incorrect

Chest x-ray, EKG, and stress testing are never correct as screening methods in the otherwise healthy general population.

PART 3

Dermatology

Cutaneous Malignancies

Dermal malignancies occur more frequently in those with pale skin on more sun-exposed areas. Diagnose with biopsy. Treat with surgical removal.

Skin Cancer

- More sun, more cancer
- Biopsy
- Remove

Malignant Melanoma

Although melanoma occurs more frequently in sun-exposed areas, it is not exclusive to those areas. Since there are many benign skin lesions, the main question is one of diagnosis. Melanoma is best diagnosed clinically by ABCDE:

- **A**: asymmetry
- **B**: border irregularity
- **C**: color irregularity
- **D**: diameter >6 mm
- **E**: evolution (changing in appearance over time)

For any suspicious lesion, biopsy should be done, including the entire lesion if possible.

| Benign versus Malignant Lesions ||
Benign	**Malignant**
Round	Asymmetric
Even borders	Borders uneven
Color evenly spread	Color uneven
Diameter constant	Diameter increases

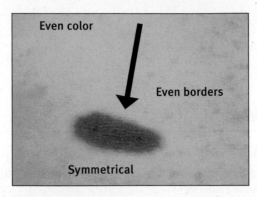

Figure 3.1 Benign lesions are characterized by even coloring, with smooth borders and no asymmetry. *Source: Andrew Peredo, MD*

> Sentinel node biopsy is essential to determining the stage of melanoma. A positive sentinel node also changes therapy.

Diagnostic testing is:

- Full thickness biopsy (indispensable in diagnosis)
- Sentinel lymph node biopsy
- Do not do a shave biopsy.

Treatment is surgical removal, and it must include a significant removal of normal skin surrounding the lesion. Melanoma has a strong tendency to metastasize to the brain.

- PD1 blockade: nivolumab or pembrolizumab
- CTLA4 blockade: ipilimumab
- Dabrafenib + trametinib or vemurafenib + cobimetinib if BRAF mutation is present
- Imatinib if C-kit mutation is present
- Talimogene (modified HSV injected into lesions)
- Interferon injection: helpful in widespread disease

Growing lesions have the worst prognostic significance.

Squamous Cell Cancer

Besides sunlight, SCC is greatly increased by organ transplant secondary to the long-term use of immunosuppressive drugs.

All forms of SCC start out by looking like an ulcer that does not heal or continues to grow.

Biopsy and remove.

Basal Cell Carcinoma

In BCC (**most common form of skin cancer**), lesions appear waxy and shiny like a pearl.

Shave biopsy is a fine way to make the diagnosis, as unlike melanoma, wide margins are not necessary.

Basal cell and squamous cell carcinomas are good uses of Mohs micrographic surgery, removal of skin cancer under a dissecting microscope with immediate frozen section.

- One of the most precise methods for treating skin cancer
- Allows removal of the skin cancer with the loss of only the smallest amount of normal tissue.
- Under microscopy, very thin slices of skin are removed and examined for cancer by frozen section.
- You can stop resecting as soon as the margin is cancer-free. In other words, there is no need to remove a wide margin routinely.

Recurrence rate of BCC is <5%.

> Use imiquimod or topical 5-fluorouracil in addition to resection for basal cell carcinoma.

> Mohs is best for delicate areas like the eyelid or ear.

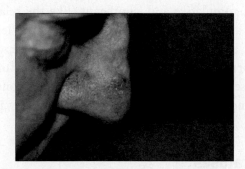

Figure 3.2 Basal cell carcinoma is very slow to grow and is not hyperpigmented. *Source: Andrew Peredo, MD*

Kaposi Sarcoma

In the past, Kaposi sarcoma (KS) was seen in older men of Mediterranean origin. The most common cause now is AIDS. KS is from human herpes virus 8, which is oncogenic. The lesion is reddish/purplish in color because it is more vascular than other forms of skin cancer. KS is also found in the GI tract and in the lung. Only AIDS acquired through sexual contact is associated with KS; AIDS from injection drug use is rarely associated with KS.

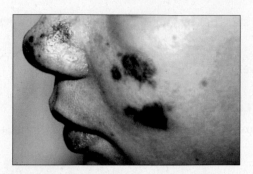

Figure 3.3 Kaposi sarcoma occurs in patients with AIDS and <100 CD4 cells per µL. *Source: Andrew Peredo, MD*

Treatment

Unlike other skin cancers, KS is not routinely treated with surgical removal.

1. Treat the AIDS with antiretrovirals and the majority of KS will disappear as the CD4 count improves.

2. Intralesional injections of vincristine or interferon are very successful.

3. For extensive disease, use chemotherapy with liposomal doxorubicin.

Actinic Keratoses

Actinic keratoses are premalignant skin lesions from high-intensity sun exposure in fair-skinned people. Each individual lesion has a very small risk of squamous cell cancer. Since many actinic keratoses can occur in a single person, the risk is cumulative and significant (like the relationship between cervical dysplasia and the risk of cervical cancer). The lesions are slow to progress but must be removed with curettage, cryotherapy, laser, or topical 5-fluorouracil before they transform. The local immunostimulant imiquimod is also effective (used for molluscum contagiosum and condyloma acuminatum as well). Ingenol mebutate clears actinic keratoses by inducing death in fast-growing cells.

> Ingenol mebutate:
> - Programmed death inducer
> - Milkweed derivative
> - Clears actinic keratoses

Seborrheic Keratoses

Seborrheic keratoses are hyperpigmented lesions commonly referred to as liver spots. They are very common in the elderly. They have a "stuck on" appearance.

Although they may look like melanoma to some people, seborrheic keratoses have no premalignant potential. They do not transform into melanoma.

Treatment is removal with cryotherapy, surgery, or laser for cosmetic reasons.

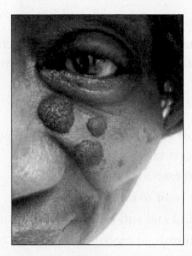

Figure 3.4 Seborrheic Keratoses. *Source: Pramod Theetha Kariyanna, MD*

Scaling Disorders

Psoriasis

Psoriasis is very common, with nearly 2 million patients in the United States.

- Silvery, scaly plaques that are not itchy most of the time (classic symptom)
- Arthritis (<10% of cases)
- Extensive disease is associated with depression.

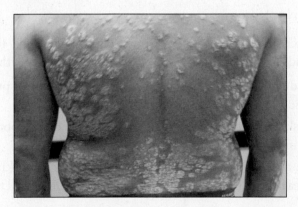

Figure 3.5 Psoriasis is characterized by silvery, scaly plaques.
Source: Andrew Peredo, MD

Treatment

For local disease, treatment is as follows:

1. Topical high-potency steroids: fluocinonide, triamcinolone, betamethasone, clobetasol; **no oral steroids for psoriasis**

2. Vitamin A (acitretin) and vitamin D ointment (calcipotriene) help get the patient off steroids, which cause skin atrophy

> Steroids cause atrophy because they inhibit collagen formation and growth. Steroids try to convert all amino acids into glucose for gluconeogenesis.

3. Coal tar preparation

4. Pimecrolimus and tacrolimus for delicate areas such as the face and penis; these agents are an alternative to steroids and are less potentially deforming

For extensive disease, treatment is as follows:

- Ultraviolet light
- Tumor necrosis factor (TNF) inhibitors (etanercept, adalimumab, infliximab) (very high success rate)
  - TNF inhibitors can reactivate tuberculosis
  - Screen with a PPD prior to using
- Ustekinumab: anti-IL12 and anti-IL23
- Secukinumab, ixekizumab, or brodalumab: anti-IL17
- Methotrexate (last resort except for psoriatic arthritis) due to adverse effects on liver and lung

> Apremilast is an oral phosphodiesterase inhibitor for psoriasis.

Atopic Dermatitis (Eczema)

Atopic dermatitis is a common skin disorder associated with overactivity of mast cells and the immune system. Onset is in early childhood; it is very rare to start after age 30. Look for a history of:

- Asthma
- Allergic rhinitis
- Family history of atopic disorders

IgE levels are elevated.

Symptoms include long-lasting, severe itching, which leads to scratching. Scratching leads to more itching. Atopic dermatitis presents with:

- Pruritus and scratching (most common presentation) due to premature and idiosyncratic release of transmitters such as histamine
- Superficial skin infections from *Staphylococcus* due to microorganisms that are driven under the epidermis from scratching.
- Scaly rough areas of thickened skin on the face, neck, and skin folds of the popliteal area behind the knee (called *lichenified skin*) due to all the scratching

Food allergies do not exacerbate atopic dermatitis.

Treatment

- **Skin care**
  - Frequent moisturizer use: dry skin is more itchy
  - Room humidifier, especially in the winter
  - Avoid brushes, soap, washcloths, and even hot water; the skin in atopic dermatitis is hyperirritable
  - Cotton clothing, which is less irritating to skin than wool

- Medical therapy
  - Topical corticosteroids for flares of disease (oral steroids for only the most severe, acute flares)
  - Topical crisaborole (phosphodiesterase inhibitor) for mild eczema
  - Tacrolimus and pimecrolimus, T cell–inhibiting agents, to provide longer-term control and help patient get off steroids; used topically for atopic dermatitis because it is a form of immune system hyperactivity but also used systemically in organ transplantation to prevent organ rejection and keep patients off steroids
  - Antihistamines: nonsedating drugs (cetirizine, fexofenadine, loratadine) (for mild disease); hydroxyzine, diphenhydramine, doxepin (for severe disease)
  - Antibiotics such as cephalexin, mupirocin, retapamulin for possible impetigo
  - Ultraviolet light (phototherapy) or cyclosporine for severe, recalcitrant disease

> Tacrolimus and pimecrolimus are rarely associated with developing lymphoma.

Seborrheic Dermatitis

Seborrheic dermatitis (dandruff) is a hypersensitivity reaction to a dermal infection with noninvasive dermatophyte organisms. This is why both topical steroids (hydrocortisone, alclometasone) and antifungal agents (ketoconazole or ciclopirox) are useful. Topical calcineurin inhibitors (tacrolimus & pimecrolimus) are useful as well.

It is increased in those with AIDS and Parkinson disease.

▶ TIP

The term **seborrheic** is synonymous with **benign**.

Pityriasis Rosea

Pityriasis rosea is an idiopathic, transient dermatitis that starts out with a single lesion (herald patch) and then disseminates. It can look like secondary syphilis, but it spares the palms and soles. It is transient, but if it is symptomatic, it is treated with steroids or ultraviolet light.

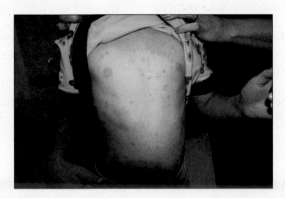

Figure 3.6 Note the diffuse erythematous, largely macular lesions.
Source: Andrew Peredo, MD

Blistering Diseases

Pemphigus Vulgaris

Pemphigus vulgaris has both an idiopathic autoimmune form and a drug-induced form.

Pemphigus, although idiopathic, is associated with:

- ACE inhibitors
- Penicillamine
- Phenobarbital
- Penicillin

Autoantibodies split the epidermis, resulting in:

- Bullae that easily rupture because they are thin walled
- Involvement of the mouth
- Fluid loss and infection if widespread; they act like a burn

The **most characteristic finding** is the Nikolsky sign, the loss or "denuding" of skin (e.g., the removal of the superficial layer of skin in a single sheet) while pulling on it with just mild pressure.

Biopsy is the **most accurate test**, showing autoantibodies on immunofluorescent studies.

Treatment is as follows:

1. Systemic steroids (prednisone)
2. Azathioprine or mycophenolate to wean the patient off steroids
3. Rituximab (anti-CD20 antibodies) or IVIG in refractory cases

Without treatment, pemphigus is a fatal disease.

Bullous Pemphigoid

This is a much milder disease than pemphigus vulgaris because:

- Bullae stay intact and there is less loss of fluid and infection.
- Mouth involvement is uncommon.

The **most accurate test** is biopsy with immunofluorescent stains, and the **best initial therapy** is prednisone. To get patients off steroids, use azathioprine, cyclophosphamide, or mycophenolate.

Mild bullous pemphigoid responds to erythromycin, dapsone, and nicotinamide (not niacin).

> Nikolsky sign is absent in bullous pemphigoid.

Porphyria Cutanea Tarda

Porphyria cutanea tarda (PCT) is a hypersensitivity of the skin to abnormal porphyrins when they are exposed to light. In other words, it is a blistering skin disease of sun-exposed areas in those with a history of:

- Liver disease (hepatitis C [**most common**], alcoholism)
- Estrogen use
- Iron overload (hemochromatosis)

Look for involvement of the back of the hands and face.

▶ **TIP**

Hepatitis C is the most frequently tested association with PCT.

Because this is a deficiency of uroporphyrin decarboxylase activity, the **most accurate test** is increased uroporphyrins in a plasma or urine collection.

Treatment is correction of the underlying cause: Stop alcohol, stop estrogens, and remove iron with phlebotomy.

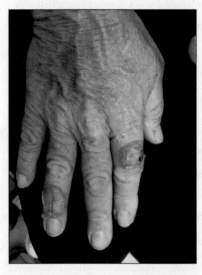

Figure 3.7 Skin Lesions of Porphyria Cutanea Tarda.
Source: Pramod Theetha Kariyanna, MD

Skin Infections

On the Step 2 CK exam, you will be expected to know the best route of administration (oral versus IV). However, you will not be expected to know the exact dosing of antibiotics.

Bacterial Infections

Impetigo

Impetigo is the most superficial of the bacterial skin infections. *Staphylococcus* and *Streptococcus* invade the epidermis, resulting in weeping, crusting, oozing, and draining of the skin. Treat topically with mupirocin.

Erysipelas

Erysipelas is a much more severe disease than impetigo because it occurs at a deeper level in the skin.

- More often the result of *Streptococcus* than *Staphylococcus*
- Invades dermal lymphatics
- Causes bacteremia, leukocytosis, fever, and chills
- Untreated disease can be fatal

Look for a bright red, hot, swollen lesion on the face. Leukocytosis can occur because it is more often a systemic disease.

Cellulitis

Cellulitis is an infection of the soft tissue of the skin. It extends from the dermis into the subcutaneous tissue. The skin is warm, red, swollen, and tender.

- Involves legs more often than arms
- Does not have collections of walled-off infection (that is an abscess)
- Is not only at hair follicle (that is folliculitis, furuncles, and carbuncles)

No diagnostic testing is needed to establish a diagnosis of cellulitis. The **most accurate test** is injection of sterile saline into the skin with aspiration for culture (20% yield). *Staphylococcus* is much more common than *Streptococcus*.

Folliculitis, Furuncles, Carbuncles

These infections originate around hair follicles. The different terms do not have precise definitions, and there is no cutoff point in size that distinguishes them from one another.

Folliculitis < Furuncle < Carbuncle

- Folliculitis: earliest and mildest
- Furuncle: small abscess or collection of infected material
- Carbuncle: collection of furuncles

> Skin infections with group A beta hemolytic *Streptococcus* can cause glomerulonephritis, but not rheumatic fever.

> Skin infection is caused by *Staphylococcus aureus*, **not *S. epidermidis*.** *S. epidermidis* lives on the skin as part of normal flora.

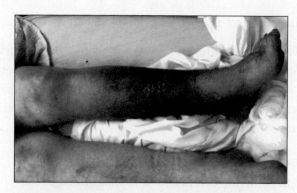

Figure 3.8 Cellulitis is often bright red, warm, and tender.
There is no weeping of purulent material as in impetigo.
Source: Farshad Bagheri, MD

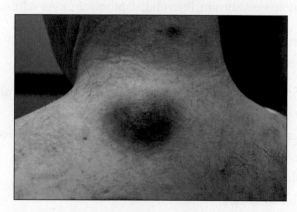

Figure 3.9 A furuncle is a small skin abscess
(note the small area of folliculitis above it on the neck).
Source: Andrew Peredo, MD

Treatment of Bacterial Skin Infections

The treatment of all skin infections is similar.

- **Mild disease**: oral medication
  - Dicloxacillin, cephalexin, cefadroxil
  - Penicillin allergic: erythromycin, clarithromycin, clindamycin
  - MRSA: doxycycline, clindamycin, TMP/SMX, delafloxacin
- **Severe disease** (fever present): IV medication
  - Oxacillin, nafcillin, cefazolin
  - Penicillin-allergic: clindamycin, vancomycin
  - MRSA: vancomycin, linezolid, daptomycin, dalbavancin, oritavancin, ceftaroline

Cross-reaction between penicillins and cephalosporins is very rare.

Antistaphylococcal penicillins
OX*CLOX*DICLOX*NAF

Severe disease = Fever, chills, bacteremia

Ceftaroline = Only cephalosporin covering MRSA

Disease-specific treatment is given additionally as follows:

- **Cellulitis**: Topical antibiotics will not cover cellulitis. The infection is below the dermal/epidermal junction and topical antibiotics will not reach it.
- **Erysipelas**: Although it is often caused by streptococci, you must treat for *Staphylococcus* as well unless you have a definitive diagnostic test such as blood cultures.

Penicillin Allergy

If the reaction to penicillin is a rash, use cephalosporins.

If the reaction is anaphylaxis:

- Mild infection: macrolides, clindamycin, doxycycline, or TMP/SMX
- Severe infection: vancomycin, linezolid, daptomycin, tigecycline, or ceftaroline

Other Antistaphylococcal Medications

See the list of drugs described in the section on erysipelas.

Medications that cover *Staphylococcus* but are not specific for skin infections are:

- Second-generation cephalosporins (cefoxitin, cefotetan, cefuroxime)
- Beta-lactam/beta-lactamase combinations
  - Amoxicillin/clavulanate
  - Ticarcillin/clavulanate
  - Ampicillin/sulbactam
  - Piperacillin/tazobactam
- Carbapenems (imipenem, meropenem)

These agents cover additional gram-negative organisms.

These medications *would not* be used as first-line agents for skin infections because they would be considered excessive in terms of spectrum. They all cover more than is necessary. However, if the patient is already on one of these medications, you do not need to add anything to cover skin infection.

Fungal Infections

Dermatophytes are superficial fungal infections. The proper term for superficial fungal infections is *tinea*, followed by the name of the body part in Latin.

- **Tinea corporis** = body
- **Tinea manus** = hand
- **Tinea pedis** = foot
- **Tinea cruris** = groin ("jock itch")

To prepare for the Step 2 CK exam, we extract the questions from each disease, "What is the best initial test?" "What is the most accurate test?" "What is the best initial treatment?" The answer to these questions is the same for all forms of tinea, so we do not learn them separately.

Diagnostic tests for tinea are as follows:

- KOH (potassium hydroxide) preparation (**best initial test**). KOH will dissolve epidermal skin cells and leave the fungi intact so they can be visualized.
- Fungal culture (**most accurate test**)

▶ **TIP**

Remember that "What is the most accurate test?" and "What will you do?" are often not the same answer. Fungal culture may be "the most accurate test" for tinea cruris, but it is not what you will do next. In most cases, tinea cruris is treated without a specific diagnostic test. A KOH-aided scraping is often useful for immediate diagnosis, and if positive, no culture is necessary.

Treatment of tinea depends on the location of the infection.

- The **best initial therapy** is a topical antifungal agent **if no hair or nails** are involved.
- The **best initial therapy for hair** (tinea capitis) **and nail** (tinea unguium) infections is terbinafine. Itraconazole is close in efficacy.

Topical antifungal agents:

- Clotrimazole
- Ketoconazole
- Econazole
- Miconazole
- Nystatin (effective only in yeast infections, not other common fungal infections)
- Ciclopirox

> Ketoconazole is antiandrogenic. **Oral** ketoconazole causes gynecomastia.

> Griseofulvin has less efficacy compared to terbinafine or itraconazole.

Oral and Vaginal Candidiasis

For the purpose of preparing for the exam, these 2 infections are the same disease. KOH is the best initial test and fungal culture the most accurate test. However, with a clear presentation of the disease, what you will do next is treat with a topical antifungal from the previous list.

Drug Reactions

Hypersensitivity reactions to medications vary in severity. When the severity of the reaction changes, the name of the reaction changes.

The drugs that cause hypersensitivity reactions of the skin are the same that cause hemolysis, interstitial nephritis, and often drug-induced thrombocytopenia (except heparin).

The drugs that commonly cause hypersensitivity reactions are:

- Penicillins
- Sulfa drugs (including thiazides, furosemide, and sulfonylureas)
- Allopurinol
- Phenytoin
- Lamotrigine
- NSAIDs

Morbilliform Rash

Morbilliform rash is a mild skin reaction, oftentimes to a drug. The skin stays intact, without mucous membrane involvement. There is no specific treatment.

Erythema Multiforme

Erythema multiforme is widespread, small "target" lesions, mostly seen on the trunk. There is no mucous membrane involvement.

This condition may also result from herpes or mycoplasma. Treatment is prednisone, but it is not helpful in all cases.

Stevens-Johnson Syndrome and Toxic Epidermal Necrolysis

Stevens-Johnson syndrome (SJS) is a very severe condition. There is mucous membrane involvement and may lead to respiratory failure. The skin sloughs off respiratory epithelium. Treatment is intravenous immunoglobulins (IVIG). Steroids are not clearly beneficial.

Toxic epidermal necrolysis (TEN) is a rash with mucous membrane involvement. Nikolsky sign is characteristic. Treatment is intravenous immunoglobulins (IVIG). Steroids are of no benefit.

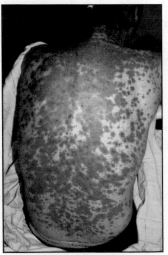

Figure 3.10 Erythema multiforme is characterized by multiple small target-shaped lesions that can be confluent.
Source: Andrew Peredo, MD

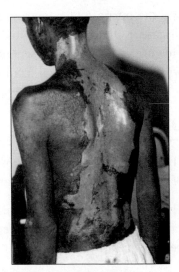

Figure 3.11 In TEN, the skin comes off in a sheet, simulating a burn.
Source: Conrad Fischer, MD

Toxin-Mediated Diseases

Staphylococcal scalded skin syndrome (SSSS) and **toxic shock syndrome** (TSS) are different severities of the same event: a reaction to a toxin in the surface of *Staphylococcus*.

SSSS looks similar to TEN, including Nikolsky sign. TSS has the same skin involvement as well as life-threatening multiorgan involvement such as:

- Hypotension
- Renal dysfunction (elevated BUN and creatinine)
- Liver dysfunction
- CNS involvement (delirium)

Treatment for both is supportive care and antistaphylococcal medication. In the absence of penicillin allergy and with a sensitive organism, use oxacillin or nafcillin (**most effective medications**). Cefazolin is interchangeable to treat *Staphylococcus*. Antibiotics do not reverse the disease, but they kill the *Staphylococcus* that is producing the toxin.

Acne

Treatment

- **Mild acne**: topical antibacterials such as benzoyl peroxide; if no response, add a topical antibiotic, e.g., clindamycin or erythromycin
- **Moderate acne**: add a topical vitamin A derivative, e.g., tretinoin, adapalene, or tazarotene, to a topical antibiotic; if no response, use an oral antibiotic, e.g., minocycline or doxycycline
- **Severe acne**: add oral vitamin A (isotretinoin) to an oral antibiotic; note that isotretinoin causes hyperlipidemia

Vitamin A derivatives are extremely teratogenic. They must not be used in patients who are pregnant or might become pregnant during treatment. Do a pregnancy test. Use only in patients on suitable hormonal and barrier birth control.

Hidradenitis Suppurativa (HS)

HS is a chronic inflammatory condition involving occluded apocrine glands and hair follicles that is characterized by painful cutaneous draining lesions, abscesses, and sinuses. The exact pathogenesis is not fully known, but multiple risk factors play a role, including obesity, smoking, and family history. HS can affect the axillae (most common site), inguinal area, inner thighs, and perianal and perineal areas.

A diagnosis of HS is straightforward in patients who demonstrate the constellation of recurrent inflammatory nodules, sinus tracts, and hypertrophic scarring in intertriginous areas.

Management is as follows:

- Tobacco cessation, weight loss, topical antibiotics, and measures to keep the skin clean and friction-free
- Short course of antibiotics, e.g., tetracycline, if no response to conservative therapy
- For antibiotic-refractory or worsening disease, consider TNF alpha inhibitors or surgery

PART 4

Surgery

by Niket Sonpal, MD

Preoperative Evaluation

Patients undergoing surgery must be risk stratified prior to surgery in order to decrease perioperative and postoperative complications. The number 1 limiting factor prior to surgery is history of cardiovascular disease.

- **Ejection fraction** <**35%:** increased risk for noncardiovascular surgery
- **Recent myocardial infarction:** must defer surgery 6 months and stress patient at that time
- **CHF (JVD, lower extremity edema):** medically optimize patient with ACE inhibitors, beta blockers, and spironolactone to decrease mortality

The Revised Cardiac Risk Index (RCRI) is a tool used to estimate a patient's risk of perioperative cardiac complications based on the following risk factors:

- History of ischemic heart disease
- History of CHF
- History of cerebrovascular disease (stroke or transient ischemic attack)
- History of diabetes requiring preoperative insulin use
- Chronic kidney disease (creatinine >2 mg/dL)
- Undergoing suprainguinal vascular, intraperitoneal, or intrathoracic surgery

RCRI score >2 indicates increased risk for cardiac death, nonfatal myocardial infarction, and nonfatal cardiac arrest. Patients require perioperative cardioselective beta blockade to reduce cardiac mortality.

The **best next step in management** for patients with scores ≥2 on the RCRI is perioperative beta blockade to reduce cardiac mortality. Higher scores mean the patient requires preoperative medical optimization.

The USMLE may require you to classify preoperative patients according to the Physical Status Classification System created by the American Society of Anesthesiologists (ASA). The ASA system assesses the fitness of patients before surgery, giving 1 point for each of the following aspects of physical status:

1. Healthy person
2. Mild systemic disease
3. Severe systemic disease
4. Severe systemic disease that is a constant threat to life
5. A moribund person who is not expected to survive without the operation
6. A declared brain-dead person whose organs are being removed for donor purposes

On the USMLE, ASA classification scores >3 require preoperative assessment and testing for elective conditions and optimization before surgical emergencies.

Cardiovascular Disease Assessment

An obese 57-year-old man presents for preoperative evaluation after he decides to have an elective inguinal hernia repair. His medical history is significant for hypertension, diabetes mellitus type 2, and elevated cholesterol. Physical examination reveals a grade 3/6 systolic ejection murmur. How many risk factors does this patient have?

a. 3
b. 4
c. 5
d. 6
e. 7
f. 8

> Being male age >45 is a risk factor.

Answer: **B.** Diabetes is equivalent to having coronary artery disease. In addition, the patient is a man age >45, is a known hypertensive, and has high cholesterol. Choices (C) through (F) are testing to see whether you can risk-stratify a patient. Systolic ejection murmur is not considered a risk factor. This patient needs his blood pressure medications adjusted, daily finger sticks monitored, and insulin regimen adjusted. He would also need a stress test with EKG, and possibly an echo to assess his murmur.

If the patient is age <35 with no history of cardiac disease, EKG is the only test needed. However, if the patient has a history of cardiac disease, the following tests are required regardless of age:

- EKG
- Stress testing to evaluate for ischemic coronary lesions
- Echocardiogram only if there is a history of structural disease and to assess ejection fraction (not part of routine testing)

A 61-year-old man is due to undergo his first screening colonoscopy. His medical history is significant for hypertension. Current medications are lisinopril and amlodipine. The patient denies headache and chest pain. Blood pressure today is 160/100 mm Hg. What is the next step in management?

a. Schedule a colonoscopy.
b. Retake patient's blood pressure.
c. Improve blood pressure control.
d. Refer for cardiology consultation.
e. Cancel the colonoscopy and get a CT colonoscopy.

Answer: **C.** Controlling hypertension to under 140/90 mmHg reduces perioperative cardiac complications, and systolic hypertension should be controlled prior to any elective surgery. There is no need to repeat the blood pressure reading. The patient cannot have the colonoscopy yet due to his uncontrolled blood pressure. CT colonoscopy has no role in the prevention of colorectal cancer on the USMLE.

> Consultations of any kind are always wrong on the USMLE exam.

Pulmonary Disease Risk Assessment

Patients with known lung disease or a smoking history require pulmonary function testing is necessary to evaluate for vital capacities. Have the patient quit smoking for 6–8 weeks prior to surgery and use nicotine replacement therapy (bupropion or varenicline).

Renal Disease Risk Assessment

Patients with known renal disease require adequate hydration; otherwise, hypoperfusion of the kidneys can lead to increased mortality. If there is a pre-existing renal disease, volume loss during surgery will adversely and acutely affect renal function. Subsequent renin-angiotensin system activation will lead to further constriction of renal vasculature and make the creatinine clearance even lower.

To ensure adequate kidney perfusion:

- Give fluids before and during surgery.
- If the patient is on dialysis, dialyze the patient 24 hours prior to surgery.

A 71-year old man is undergoing femoropopliteal bypass for severe claudication of the left leg, which causes unbearable pain with exercise. His medical history is significant for insulin-dependent DM type 2 and a remote appendectomy. What preoperative testing is recommended?

a. Basic metabolic panel (BMP) only
b. BMP + EKG
c. BMP + EKG + PFTs
d. BMP + EKG + exercise stress test
e. BMP + EKG + thallium stress test

Answer: **E.** Vascular surgery is very high-risk surgery. This patient has 2 significant risk factors for a cardiac event: diabetes (coronary disease equivalent) and age >70. Therefore, he needs a thorough workup, including a stress test. Since his claudication prevents him from exercising, it must be nonexercise stress testing.

Trauma

ABC Assessment

The mainstay of trauma has always been the ABCs.

By itself, "ABC" is not enough to answer exam questions. You must answer specifically what you want to do.

- **Airway:** in any trauma, the primary step is to assess and secure the airway
  - Patients with facial trauma require a cricothyroidotomy.
  - Patients with cervical spine injury also require an orotracheal tube intubation; perform with flexible bronchoscopy to reduce risk of further injury to cervical spine
- **Breathing:** proper ventilation is necessary to maintain oxygen saturation; routine goal is to keep oxygen saturation >90%
- **Circulation:** insert 2 large-bore IVs into the patient and begin aggressive fluid resuscitation to prevent hypovolemic shock

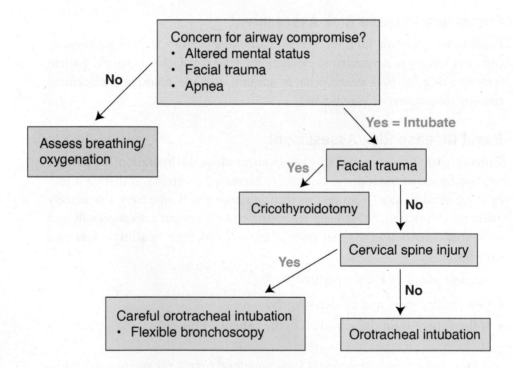

Figure 4.1 Trauma/ABC Assessment Algorithm

A 43-year-old woman loses control of her car and runs into a tree. At the ED, physical examination reveals pallor, cool extremities, heart rate 120 bpm, JVD, and blood pressure 80/40 mm Hg. The patient has chest pain, and chest x-ray reveals 3 broken ribs over the left side of the chest. This patient is in which of the following types of shock?

a. Hypovolemic shock
b. Cardiogenic shock
c. Neurogenic shock
d. Septic shock

Answer: **B.** Cardiogenic shock is most likely secondary to pericardial tamponade. The patient's car injury caused blood to collect in the pericardial sac, leading to right ventricular diastolic collapse and impaired filling. The broken ribs are the source of injury to the pericardium. Hypovolemic shock is unlikely, as the patient cannot lose that much volume into her pericardium. Neurogenic shock would have hyperreflexia and upgoing toes. Septic shock is unlikely as there is no fever and chills.

Systemic Inflammatory Response Syndrome

Systemic inflammatory response syndrome (SIRS) is a global inflammatory state that yields a particular set of symptoms and objective findings before sepsis and shock set in. There are 4 SIRS criteria. The presence of ≥2 indicates SIRS.

1. Body temperature <36 C (96.8 F) or >38 C (100.4 F)
2. Heart rate >90 BPM
3. Tachypnea >20 breaths/min or PCO_2 <32 mm Hg
4. WBC <4,000 cells/mm^3 or >12,000 cells/mm^3

Interpretation of SIRS criteria:

- 2 criteria = **SIRS**
- 2 criteria + source of infection = **sepsis**
- 2 criteria + source of infection + organ dysfunction = **severe sepsis**
- 2 criteria + source of infection + organ dysfunction + hypotension = **septic shock**

Shock

Shock occurs when the tissues in the body do not receive enough oxygen and nutrients to allow the cells to function. Shock is more than just tachycardia and hypotension. You will see:

- Brain: confusion
- Kidney: increased BUN:creatinine ratio
- Liver: elevated AST and ALT
- Heart: chest pain and shortness of breath
- Blood: increased lactic acid

Four Kinds of Shock								
	Signs and symptoms	**CVP**	**SVR**	**Heart Rate**	**CO**	**PCWP**	**Treatment**	**Most common cause**
Hypovolemic	Pale and cool	↓	↑	↑	↓	↓	Fluids and pressors	Massive hemorrhage
Cardiogenic	Pale and cool	↑	↑	↑	↓	↑	Treat cardiac problem	Myocardial infarction
Neurogenic	Warm	↓	↓	↑	↓	↓	Fluids and pressors	Spinal cord injury (cervical or thoracic)
Septic	Warm and faint	↓	↓	↑	↑	No change	Fluids, antibiotics, and pressors	*E. coli* and *S. aureus*
CVP = central venous pressure, PCWP = pulmonary capillary wedge pressure, SVR = systemic vascular resistance								

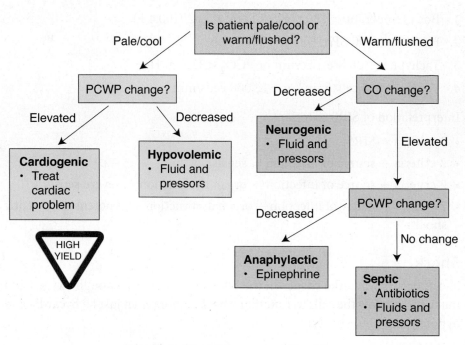

Figure 4.2 Shock Management Algorithm

"Shocking" Reminder

Cardiac output = Stroke volume × Heart rate

and

Stroke volume = End-diastolic volume − End-systolic volume

Thus:

Cardiac output = (End-diastolic volume − End-systolic volume) × Heart rate

and

Total peripheral resistance = Mean arterial pressure − Mean venous pressure

Therefore:

Blood pressure = Cardiac output × Total peripheral resistance

A 74-year-old woman is brought in for respiratory distress and altered mental status. Her medical history records right-sided hemiplegia from a stroke several years ago. She has blood pressure 86/52 mm Hg, heart rate 123 BPM, breathing rate 33/min, temperature 39 C (102.3 F), and O2 sat 84%. Exam reveals rhonchi bilaterally with "E to A" changes and warm extremities with faint pulses. Chest x-ray shows bilateral infiltrates. What is the likely etiology of this patient's hypotension?

a. Neurogenic shock
b. Septic shock
c. Hemorrhagic shock
d. Hypovolemic shock
e. Cardiogenic shock

Answer: **B.** This patient is presenting with 3 SIRS criteria: hypotension, altered mental status, and a source of infection (pneumonia). The physical exam is also consistent with septic shock: Massive vasodilation has yielded warm extremities and faint pulses. Both hypovolemic shock and cardiogenic shock would have pale and cool extremities. There is no mention of bleeding, ruling out hemorrhagic shock.

An 85-year-old woman presents with nausea, vomiting, and profuse, watery diarrhea of 4 days' duration. She was recently on a cruise ship where many people fell ill due to norovirus. Today she lost consciousness in the ED while talking to the nurse. Her blood pressure is 70/40 mm Hg, and heart rate is 140 bpm. Bladder scan shows an empty bladder. Which of the following is the most likely diagnosis?

a. Septic shock
b. Anaphylactic shock
c. Hemorrhagic shock
d. Hypovolemic shock
e. Cardiogenic shock

Answer: **D.** This patient is in hypovolemic shock caused by intravascular volume loss. Common findings in a patient with hypovolemic shock and systolic BP <90 mmHg are organ dysfunction such as low urine output; cold, clammy extremities; and lightheadedness. The low volume decreases the cardiac output (CO) because of lack of preload. Meanwhile, systemic vascular resistance (SVR) increases in an effort to compensate for the diminished cardiac output and maintain perfusion to the vital organs.

An 11-year-old boy who was given a suspension of amoxicillin for acute otitis media a few hours ago is now in severe respiratory distress. His eyes and lips are swollen, and he is having difficulty swallowing. His blood pressure is 70/40 mm Hg, and heart rate 130 bpm. The child is unable to speak. Exam reveals bilateral wheezing and tachycardia. What is the most likely diagnosis?

a. Anaphylactic shock
b. Cardiogenic shock
c. Sepsis
d. Pulmonary embolus
e. Pneumonia

Answer: **A.** This acute-onset illness involving the skin and mucosa, combined with respiratory compromise, reduced blood pressure, and subsequent end-organ dysfunction, is anaphylactic shock. The trigger for this child is most likely severe allergy to penicillin. It cannot be sepsis because there is no fever and onset was sudden rather than gradual. Pulmonary embolism would have a normal lung exam, and it is not plausible that a child this young would have pneumonia without a fever or cough.

Perioperative Management

Perioperative Medical Management		
Drug class	**What to do?**	**Additional information**
Analgesia	• NSAIDs and COX-2 inhibitors stopped 7 days before surgery • Narcotics should be tapered on a case-by-case basis if possible.	
Anticoagulant	Discontinue before major surgery	Very high-risk patients may require heparin bridge
Antiplatelet	Noncardiac patients: discontinue before major surgery	• Discontinuation in patients with cardiac stents is controversial. • Aspirin should be started before CABG.
Cardiovascular	• Continue beta blockers and CCBs • Discontinue diuretics on day of surgery	
Estrogen	Discontinue several weeks before surgery due to increased risk of DVT	
GI medications	Continue H2 and PPI meds	
Glucocorticoids	Continue steroids	Stress dose steroids for patients on chronic steroids >3 weeks
Herbal medications	Stop 1 week before surgery	
Hypoglycemic agents	• Oral hypoglycemics: stop 3 days before surgery • Short-acting insulin: withhold on the morning of surgery • Long-acting insulin: continue at half-dose	Hypoglycemia is more dangerous than hyperglycemia.
Immunomodulators	• Nontransplant: discontinue 2 weeks before surgery • Transplant: continue all except sirolimus	Sirolimus may lead to poor wound healing or dehiscence and should be discontinued before surgery.
Lipid-lowering medications	Withhold on the day of the surgery	
Neurologic	• Continue antiepileptic medication • Discontinue dementia drugs before surgery	
Pulmonary	Continue all inhalers and glucocorticoids	
Thyroid medications	Continue thyroid medications	

Thoracic Trauma

A 29-year-old woman presents to the ED with a sudden onset of left-sided chest pain and difficulty breathing. She states her only medication is birth control pills. She has smoked 1 pack of cigarettes per day for 10 years. She is tachypneic (24 BrPM) and heart rate is 120 bpm. Physical examination reveals diminished breath sounds on the left and the trachea deviated to the right. What is the most likely diagnosis?

a. Pericardial tamponade
b. Pulmonary embolus (PE)
c. Tension pneumothorax
d. Hemothorax

Answer: **C.** Tension pneumothorax presents with decreased breath sound on one side and tracheal deviation. PE does not give tracheal deviation, although it does have chest pain and tachycardia. Muffled heart sounds are seen typically in pericardial tamponade. This patient's risk for pneumothorax is that she is a smoker. It is likely she has a pleural bleb that burst due to her smoking history.

Thoracic Abnormalities Secondary to Trauma				
Abnormality	**Etiology**	**Signs and symptoms**	**Diagnostic tests**	**Treatment**
Pericardial tamponade	Trauma with penetration to the pericardium; secondary to broken ribs, knives, or bullet wounds	JVD, hypotension, muffled heart sounds, and electrical alternans on EKG	Cardiac echocardiogram	Pericardiocentesis is the most effective therapy.
Pneumothorax	Air in the pleural space	Chest pain, hyperresonance, and decreased breath sounds	Chest x-ray	Chest tube placement
Tension pneumothorax	Air in the pleural space through a one-way leak	Chest pain, hyperresonance and decreased breath sounds, and tracheal deviation away from the involved lung	Chest x-ray	Immediate needle decompression followed by chest tube placement
Hemothorax	Blood in the pleural space	Absent breath sounds and dull to percussion	Blunting of costophrenic angle on chest x-ray and CT scan	Chest tube drainage and possible thoracotomy

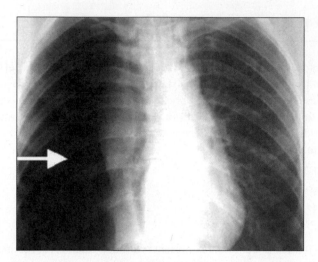

Figure 4.3 Pneumothorax on chest x-ray is characterized by absent vascular patterns and lack of x-ray absorption leading to a "blackout" of the affected lung.
Source: Niket Sonpal, MD

Lung trauma and the trachea:

- Tension pneumothorax pushes it **away from** the involved lung.
- Atelectasis pulls it **toward** the involved lung.

The Abdomen

Abdominal Trauma

Blunt abdominal trauma (BAT) is the most common cause of abdominal injury, and motor vehicle–related trauma is the most common cause.

Patient presentation ranges from stable and communicative to hemorrhagic shock. An absence of abdominal pain or tenderness on physical exam does not rule out the presence of significant intra-abdominal injury. The seatbelt sign—bruising in the location where a seatbelt lies—is highly correlative to abdominal trauma.

A 27-year-old man presents with severe abdominal pain radiating to his back after another car struck his while he was driving home. He says his abdomen hurts from colliding with the steering wheel. He is admitted, and after 2 days in the hospital a large ecchymosis is seen on the right flank. What is the most likely diagnosis?

a. Hemorrhagic pancreatitis
b. Pseudocyst
c. Renal trauma
d. Aortic dissection

Answer: **A.** The patient's history of blunt abdominal trauma leads to the diagnosis of pancreatitis. The bruising and its flank location suggest a retroperitoneal hemorrhage. This is where blood collects in pancreatitis. Pseudocyst develops much later, 6–8 weeks postpancreatitis. Renal trauma does not present with ecchymosis. Aortic dissection presents with extremely elevated BP and tearing midepigastric pain that radiates sharply into the back; it does not cause bruising.

The goal of initial management is to assess for intraperitoneal bleeding. Follow the ABCDE pattern:

- Airway
- Breathing
- Circulation
- Disability (neurologic status)
- Exposure

After that, look for free fluid in the abdomen and pelvis using the Focused Assessment with Sonography for Trauma (FAST).

The **most accurate test** is CT scan of the retroperitoneum. Exploratory laparotomy is the answer for hemodynamically unstable patients.

Splenic Rupture

Rupture of the spleen can result from BAT or abdominal procedures such as surgery and colonoscopy. Diagnosis is with FAST or abdominal CT.

CT allows for grading of the injury:

- **Grade I**: subcapsular hematoma <10% of surface area
- **Grade II**: subcapsular hematoma 10–50% of surface area
- **Grade III**: subcapsular hematoma >50% of surface area or expanding
- **Grade IV**: laceration involving segmental or hilar vessels
- **Grade V**: shattered spleen

Treatment is as follows:

- **Hemodynamically stable with low-grade injury** (grades I–III): supportive care and monitoring of hemoglobin; if patient worsens, do angiographic embolization or surgical exploration
- **Hemodynamically unstable with positive FAST exam showing splenic rupture**: surgical exploration
- **High-grade injury** (grades IV–V): exploratory laparotomy for more precise staging, repair, or removal of the spleen

> **Removal of spleen =** Vaccination against encapsulated organisms

Splenic Infarction

Splenic infarction occurs in patients with A-fib and hypercoagulable states when the splenic artery becomes occluded by an embolus. It can also occur in sickle cell disease and mononucleosis.

On physical exam, look for acute LUQ pain that radiates to the left shoulder along with tenderness with splenomegaly. Labs reveal elevated LDH.

Treatment is aimed at the underlying cause and providing pain relief. Splenectomy is required only if there are complications such as abscess formation.

Splenic Abscess

Splenic abscess is an infection that is seeded by endocarditis. It presents with LUQ pain, and splenomegaly is seen on physical exam.

CT scan is the **most accurate test**.

Treatment is antibiotics and splenectomy.

Signs Associated with Abdominal Trauma		
Sign	**What is it?**	**Cause(s)**
Cullen sign	Bruising around the umbilicus	Hemorrhagic pancreatitis, ruptured abdominal aortic aneurysm
Grey Turner sign	Bruising in the flank	Retroperitoneal hemorrhage
Kehr sign	Pain in the left shoulder	Splenic rupture
Balance sign	Dull percussion on the left and shifting dullness on the right	Splenic rupture
Seatbelt sign	Bruising where a seatbelt was	Deceleration injury

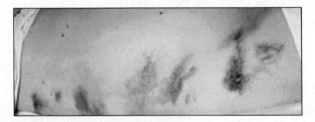

Figure 4.4 Bruising in the flanks is seen in acute pancreatitis (up to 50% of patients). *Source: Niket Sonpal, MD*

Abdominal Pain

A 75-year-old man with a history of atrial fibrillation, coronary artery disease, and dyslipidemia presents with severe abdominal pain that is worsened with eating. He states the pain is 10/10 but no peritoneal signs are present. Lab analysis shows white blood cell count 15×10^3/uL with increased neutrophils and decreased bicarbonate. What is the most appropriate next step in management?

a. CT scan of the abdomen
b. Angiography
c. Liver function tests
d. Colonoscopy
e. Oral antibiotics

Answer: **B.** Angiography is the most appropriate next step in a patient suffering from acute mesenteric ischemia. The patient will present with complaints of abdominal pain that is severe and out of proportion to physical findings. This patient could also be a surgical candidate, but that was not an answer choice. Angiography is done prior to surgery as quickly as possible to avoid perforation; colonoscopy may lead to perforation.

Ischemic Colitis

Ischemic colitis is caused by a lack of blood flow to the mesentery of the bowel. Ischemia of the bowel is most damaging to the mucosa.

The most common symptoms are:

- Abdominal pain that is described as cramping
- Bloody diarrhea

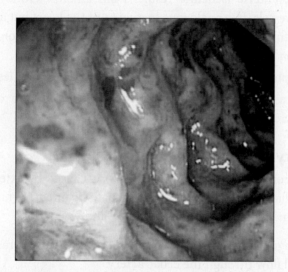

Figure 4.5 A lack of blood flow causes ischemia to the bowel wall and sloughing of the mucosa. *Source: Niket Sonpal, MD*

Testing includes:

- CT of the abdomen (**best initial test**)
- Angiogram (**most accurate test**)
- Colonoscopy with biopsy can show ischemic mucosa, but it takes time for pathology to come back

Treatment is IV normal saline and antibiotics if fever is present.

Severe abdominal pain that is "out of proportion to physical findings" is:

- 10/10 pain
- Soft abdomen
- No guarding
- No rebound tenderness

Causes of abdominal pain that do not require surgery include MI, GERD, lower lobe pneumonia, and acute porphyria.

Mesenteric Ischemia

- **Acute mesenteric ischemia** is the acute occlusion of mesenteric arteries (most commonly the superior mesenteric artery).
  - A-fib is number 1 risk factor (causes emboli to occlude the vessel).
  - Symptoms include excruciating pain that is out of proportion to the physical exam.
  - Labs may show increased lactic acid and leukocytosis.
  - Abdominal x-ray showing air in the bowel wall (**best initial test**). The **most accurate test** is angiography.
  - Treatment is emergent laparotomy with resection of necrotic bowel; if there is a clear reason to avoid surgery, use endovascular therapy.
- **Chronic mesenteric ischemia** results from atherosclerotic disease of ≥2 mesenteric vessels. It is analogous to angina of the heart but affects only the gut. In intestinal ischemia, eating is the equivalent of exertion in "chest pain with exertion."
  - Angiography (**best initial test**) is done first to locate the lesions.
  - Then, stenting or bypass reestablishes blood flow to allow surgical correction.

> The most common locations for infarction are watershed areas.

Celiac Artery Compression Syndrome

Celiac artery compression syndrome (CACS) is caused by external compression of the celiac trunk by the median arcuate ligament. Symptoms include severe postprandial abdominal pain, nausea, and weight loss.

CACS is a diagnosis of exclusion. Confirm with duplex ultrasonography to measure blood flow through the celiac artery.

Treatment is surgical decompression of the celiac artery.

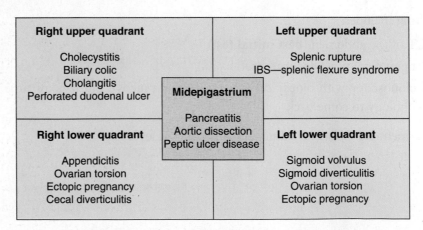

Right upper quadrant	Left upper quadrant
Cholecystitis Biliary colic Cholangitis Perforated duodenal ulcer	Splenic rupture IBS—splenic flexure syndrome
Midepigastrium Pancreatitis Aortic dissection Peptic ulcer disease	
Right lower quadrant	Left lower quadrant
Appendicitis Ovarian torsion Ectopic pregnancy Cecal diverticulitis	Sigmoid volvulus Sigmoid diverticulitis Ovarian torsion Ectopic pregnancy

Figure 4.6 Causes of Abdominal Pain by Location

Referred Pain

Pain in one part of the body are often referred to another part of the body. It is key to remember these associations, as they are a favorite on the USMLE.

> Referred pain associations are a **USMLE favorite**.

Cause	Site of Referred Pain
Myocardial ischemia	Left chest, jaw, and left arm
Cold foods such as ice cream	"Brain freeze" secondary to rapid temperature change of the sinuses
Gall bladder	Right shoulder/scapula
Pancreas	Back pain
Pharynx	Ears
Prostate	Tip of penis/perineum
Appendix	Right lower abdominal quadrant
Esophagus	Substernal chest pain
Pyelonephritis, nephrolithiasis	Costovertebral angle

A 65-year-old woman presents to the ED with substernal chest pain that began shortly after vomiting. The patient has a history of alcoholism and has just finished a 3-day binge. Physical examination reveals a "snap, crackle, and pop" upon palpation around the clavicles. What is the most likely diagnosis?

a. Boerhaave syndrome
b. Pancreatitis
c. Biliary colic
d. Volvulus
e. Myocardial infarction

Answer: **A.** Boerhaave syndrome is a full-thickness tear of the esophagus secondary to retching. The patient will have a history of severe incessant vomiting, often due to alcoholism. MI is unlikely in this patient given the subcutaneous emphysema. The other choices do not have substernal chest pain. Pancreatitis presents with abdominal pain that radiates to the back upon alcohol intake, not air in the subcutaneous space. Biliary colic has postprandial RUQ pain. Volvulus is malrotation of the colon.

Esophageal Perforation

The most common cause of esophageal perforation is iatrogenic. The most common procedure that causes an esophageal perforation is upper endoscopy. It can also occur due to the rapid increase in intraesophageal pressure combined with negative intrathoracic pressure caused by vomiting.

Symptoms include:

- Severe and acute onset of excruciating retrosternal chest pain
- Odynophagia
- Positive Hamman sign, a crunching heard upon palpation of the thorax due to subcutaneous emphysema
- Pain that can radiate to the left shoulder

Boerhaave syndrome is a full-thickness tear secondary to extreme retching and vomiting. USMLE most commonly tests it in the setting of an alcoholic. The most common location is the left posterolateral aspect of the distal esophagus. Boerhaave syndrome carries 25% mortality, even with surgery.

Mallory-Weiss syndrome is a mucosal tear, also due to vomiting. It is not a perforation. The most common location is at the gastroesophageal junction.

Esophagram (**most accurate test**) uses diatrizoate meglumine and diatrizoate sodium solution to show leakage of contrast outside of the esophagus. Barium cannot be used because it is caustic to the tissues.

Treatment is an absolute emergency, requiring surgical exploration with debridement of the mediastinum and closure of the perforation. Mediastinitis is a complication that carries a very high mortality rate.

	Mucosal tear: "Mallory-Weiss syndrome"	Esophageal perforation: "Boerhaave syndrome"
Cause	Vomiting/retching in alcoholics	Iatrogenic is #1 (endoscopy) Vomiting/retching in alcoholics
Symptoms	Hematemesis Odynophagia	Retrosternal chest pain • Severe, acute onset • Radiates to L shoulder • Subcutaneous emphysema
Location	Gastroesophageal junction	Distal esophagus • Left posterolateral aspect
Diagnosis	Gastrografin esophagogram • No leakage	Gastrografin esophagogram • Leakage
Treatment	Supportive Cauterization if necessary	Emergent surgery • High mortality (25%)
Complications	Rare	Acute mediastinitis • Very high mortality

A 53-year-old obese man presents with sudden onset of abdominal pain that radiates to his right shoulder. The patient also says he has vomited blood earlier in the day. He pulls a full bottle of esomeprazole from his pocket, saying he uses them sometimes for heartburn. Physical examination reveals rebound tenderness in the midepigastrum. Upright chest x-ray shows air under the diaphragm. What is the most likely diagnosis?

a. Gastric perforation
b. Hemorrhagic ulcer
c. Cholecystitis
d. Ischemic colitis

Answer: A. This is gastric perforation in the setting of peptic ulcer disease. The patient's bottle filled with PPIs is due to his history of ulcers. The fact that it is a full bottle implies the patient is noncompliant with his medication. Hemorrhagic ulcers will present with hematemesis, specifically coffee-ground emesis. Cholecystitis would have right upper quadrant pain that is colicky in nature. Ischemic colitis would have an abdominal pain that is out of proportion to physical findings.

Gastric Perforation

Gastric perforation is most commonly seen secondary to ulcer disease.

- Risk factors are conditions that either diminish the stomach's barrier against acid or elevate gastric acid: *Helicobacter pylori* infection, NSAID abuse, burns, head injury, trauma, and cancer.
- Alcohol and smoking prevent ulcer healing.
- The ulcer, once it erodes deep enough into the stomach, allows for the leakage of gastric acid into the abdominal cavity and causes peritonitis.
- Gastric acid has also been shown to cause pancreatitis if the ulcer is in the posterior part of the stomach. (The acid leaks out the back of the stomach and effectively "fries" the pancreas.)

Symptoms include:

- Acute abdominal pain that is progressively worsening and radiates to the right shoulder as a result of acid irritation of the phrenic nerve
- Guarding, rebound tenderness, and abdominal rigidity (likely signs of peritonitis) by the time the patient comes to the ED

> Upright chest x-ray is the best initial test to evaluate free air under the diaphragm. Free air under the diaphragm indicates a perforation of the bowel.

Upright chest x-ray (**best initial test**) shows free air under the diaphragm. CT scan is the **most accurate test**.

Treatment is as follows:

- Make patient NPO: prevents further extrusion of gastric contents into peritoneal cavity
- Place NG tube: suctions gastric contents and mitigates risk from newly formed acid
- Medical management: IV antibiotics to combat infection and IV fluids to prepare for surgery. Abdominal antibiotics are:
  - Piperacillin-tazobactam
  - Ampicillin-sulbactam
  - Carbapenems
  - Ciprofloxacin and metronidazole
- Emergent surgery: exploratory laparotomy and repair of the perforation

A 9-year-old boy comes to school with decreased appetite and abdominal pain around his umbilicus. His parents thought he simply didn't want to go to school. While in class he begins to have sharp pain in his right lower abdomen. He is rushed to the ED and laboratory analysis shows WBC 12,500/mm^3. What is the most likely diagnosis?

a. Acute appendicitis
b. Acute diverticulitis
c. Cholecystitis
d. Acute pancreatitis

Answer: **A.** Acute appendicitis presents with pain that originates in the umbilical region and later begins to localize to the right lower quadrant. The patient will then develop signs of peritonitis. This patient is too young for diverticulitis. Diverticulitis also gives pain in the left lower quadrant. Cholecystitis would present with right upper quadrant pain. Pancreatitis would have midepigastric pain that radiates to the back with high amylase and lipase levels. The number one consideration is the location of the pain. It gives away 95% of the diagnosis.

If the RLQ pain presents in a female patient of childbearing age, **ectopic pregnancy, cysts**, and **torsion** must be considered.

- Get a beta-hCG and pelvic sonogram.
- *Avoid radiation* imaging tests (CT and x-rays) in a patient who may be pregnant.
- If the sonogram shows an ectopic pregnancy, emergent surgery must be performed.

A 76-year-old woman with no significant medical history presents with severe left lower quadrant pain, fever, and anorexia of 1 day's duration. The patient's daughter says her only medical history is frequent constipation, for which she takes daily stool softeners. Physical exam shows guarding and rigidity. What is the most likely diagnosis?

a. Acute appendicitis
b. Acute diverticulitis
c. Ectopic pregnancy
d. Cholecystitis
e. Acute pancreatitis

Answer: **B.** Acute diverticulitis has an acute onset of severe abdominal pain, most likely in the lower left quadrant. Diverticulitis is highly associated with constipation. Appendicitis produces pain in the right lower quadrant. Pregnancy is implausible in this age group. Cholecystitis would produce right upper quadrant pain, and pancreatitis would produce pain that radiates to the back.

Barium enema and colonoscopy are **contraindicated** in diverticulitis due to an increased incidence of perforation.

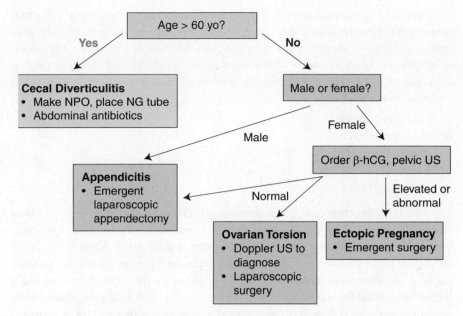

Figure 4.7 Right Lower Quadrant Pain Algorithm

Abdominal Abscess

Abscesses occur after invasive procedures, inflammatory conditions, and traumatic events. They are diagnosed by CT scan and incision and drainage is the only therapy. Percutaneous drainage can be done by CT or ultrasound guidance. Antibiotics must also be given to prevent bacteremia.

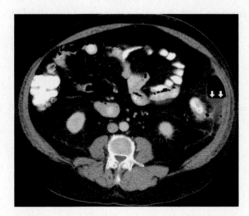

Figure 4.8 Abdominal Abscess. *Source: Joel McFarland, Medpix 28716.*

A 40-year-old obese woman with 5 children presents with a "gnawing" pain that recently has become severe. She explains that the pain starts immediately after eating and that it radiates to her right shoulder. Physical exam reveals a cessation of inspiration upon palpation of the right upper quadrant and rebound tenderness. Lab analysis shows white blood cell count of 15,000 and a left shift. What is the most likely diagnosis?

a. Acute appendicitis
b. Acute diverticulitis
c. Ectopic pregnancy
d. Cholecystitis
e. Acute pancreatitis

Answer: **D.** Acute cholecystitis is a common inflammatory condition seen in obese women in their 40s. A gallstone occludes the lumen of the cystic duct. Symptoms include peritoneal signs and a positive Murphy sign. A sonographic Murphy sign is the ultrasound probe causing a cessation of breathing when it presses against the abdominal wall. On ultrasound, cholecystitis is characterized by pericholecystic fluid and a thickened gallbladder wall. Appendicitis would present with RLQ pain. Diverticulitis would present with LLQ or RLQ pain in an elderly person with a history of constipation. Ectopic pregnancy would present with LLQ or RLQ pain. Pancreatitis would have deep epigastric pain radiating to the back.

> Abdominal pain that radiates to the back has 2 emergent conditions: pancreatitis and aortic dissection.

> HIDA scan will show delayed emptying of the gallbladder in acute cholecystitis by failure to visualize the gallbladder from isotope accumulation.

Signs of Appendicitis

- **Rovsing sign:** palpation of the left lower quadrant causes pain in the right lower quadrant
- **Psoas sign:** pain with extension of the hip
- **Obturator sign:** pain with internal rotation of the right thigh

Pancreatitis

There are many causes of pancreatitis, as recorded in the mnemonic **"I get smashed"**:

- Idiopathic
- Gallstones (most common cause)
- Ethanol
- Trauma
- Steroids
- Mumps, malignancy (pancreatic cancer)
- Autoimmune
- Scorpion sting
- Hypercalcemia, hypertrigliceridemia (usually >1,000 mg/dL)
- ERCP
- Drugs

Inflammatory Abdominal Conditions					
	Etiology	**Signs and symptoms**	**Diagnostic tests**	**Treatment**	**Complications**
Cholecystitis	Gallstones occluding the lumen of the cystic duct, causing inflammation of the gallbladder	Fever, severe RUQ tenderness, Murphy sign; pain on inspiration causing a cessation of breathing, nausea, and vomiting	Ultrasound will reveal pericholecystic fluid, gallbladder wall thickening, and stones in the gallbladder. HIDA scan is the most accurate test.	Laparoscopic surgery, or open surgery if there is perforation of the gallbladder	Perforation of the gallbladder
Acute pancreatitis	Alcohol or gallstone obstruction of the duct, causing inflammation	Fever, severe midabdominal pain radiating to the back, nausea and vomiting	CT scan is the best test. Amylase is sensitive and lipase is specific.	Aggressive IV fluids and NPO until symptoms resolve	Hemorrhagic pancreatitis and pseudocyst formation
Appendicitis	Fecalith obstructing the appendiceal orifice, causing inflammation	Anorexia, fever, periumbilical pain with RLQ tenderness. Elevated white count with left shift.	CT scan is most accurate test.	Laparoscopic surgery	Abscess formation and gangrenous perforation
Diverticulitis	Fecal impaction into pseudodiverticula, causing inflammation	Fever, nausea, most commonly LLQ pain, and peritonitis	CT scan is the best and most accurate test.	Antibiotics for the first attack; surgical resection if it recurs or perforates	Abscess formation. No endoscopy due to risk of perforation.

Bowel Obstruction

Bowel obstruction is a mechanical or functional obstruction of the intestines. The most common cause of small bowel obstruction is previous abdominal surgery.

- Upon occlusion of the lumen, gas and fluid build up, severely increasing pressure within the lumen.
- This leads to decreased perfusion of the bowel and necrosis.

In **partial obstruction**, a small amount of GI contents can pass. In **complete obstruction**, no GI contents can pass.

Symptoms include:

- Severe waves of intermittent crampy abdominal pain
- Nausea and vomiting
- Fever
- Hyperactive bowel sounds
- High-pitched "tinkling" sounds indicate that the intestinal fluid and air are under high pressure in the bowel.
- Hypovolemia due to third spacing

Methylnaltrexone has been shown to alleviate obstruction from stool impaction in patients on chronic opioids.

The etiology of bowel obstruction includes:

- Adhesions from previous abdominal surgery (MCC)
- Hernias
- Crohn disease
- Neoplasms
- Intussusception
- Volvulus
- Foreign bodies
- Intestinal atresia
- Carcinoid

Diagnostic testing is as follows:

- Elevated WBC count is sensitive but not specific
- Elevated lactate with marked acidosis (**hallmark sign**)
- Abdominal x-ray (**best initial test**) will show multiple air-fluid levels with dilated loops of small bowel
- CT scan of the abdomen (**most accurate test**) will show a transition zone from dilated loops of bowel with contrast to an area of bowel with no contrast

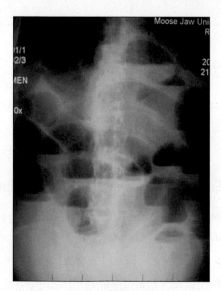

Figure 4.9 X-ray of Bowel Obstruction.
Source: James Heilman, MD, commons.wikimedia.org

Treatment is as follows:

- Make patient NPO: prevents further increase in bowel pressure
- Place NG tube with suction: lowers bowel pressure proximal to obstruction
- IV fluids to replace volume lost via third spacing
- Surgical decompression if there is no response or complete obstruction (emergent)

A 63-year-old woman presents to the ED with nausea, vomiting, and severe abdominal pain of increasing intensity. She has not had a bowel movement in 3 days and cannot remember the last time she passed gas. Her medical history is significant for an abdominal hysterectomy. The resident performs a physical exam and hears hyperactive bowel sounds plus a possible tinkling sound. Lab results show WBC count 15,000/mm^3. Her temperature is 38.6 C (101.5 F). What is the most likely diagnosis?

a. Acute appendicitis
b. Acute diverticulitis
c. Small bowel obstruction
d. Cholecystitis
e. Acute pancreatitis

Answer: **C**. Small bowel obstruction is characterized by failure to pass stool and flatus and hyperactive bowel sounds. Nausea, vomiting, and abdominal pain with hyperactive bowel sounds are hallmark signs. Past abdominal surgery is a very significant risk factor, as adhesions can form from surgery. The other answer choices have abdominal pain localized to one quadrant, whereas with obstruction, diffuse unlocalized pain is seen.

Hepatobiliary Diseases

Cholelithiasis

Asymptomatic gallstones should be monitored and observed.

Biliary Colic

The classic presentation of biliary colic is as follows:

- Abdominal pain in the right upper quadrant, radiating to the right shoulder and back
- Often triggered by fatty food due to gallstones

The etiology of the pain is a temporary "ball valving" of the gallstone in the cystic duct with contraction and falling out again with gallbladder relaxation.

Sonogram (**best initial test**) will show acoustic shadowing, i.e., no sound waves seen below the stone or posterior to it.

Treatment is elective cholecystectomy.

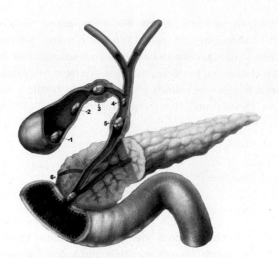

Figure 4.10 Obstruction of the Common Bile Duct.
Source: Oleg Reznik

Acute Ascending Cholangitis

Cholangitis is a life-threatening emergency caused by obstruction of the common bile duct (CBD) with a gallstone that has escaped the gallbladder. Symptoms include:

- Jaundice
- Fever
- RUQ pain
- Altered mental status
- Hypotension or shock

Abdominal U/S (**best initial test**) is taken once patient is stable; obstruction is confirmed by identification of dilated intra- and extrahepatic ducts plus dilated CBD. MRCP of the abdomen is the **most accurate test**.

Treatment is IV antibiotics followed by ERCP to decompress the CBD and remove the stone. If the patient is unstable, the best next step is decompression of the CBD through the liver by percutaneous transhepatic cholangiogram (PTC). Eventually the patient must undergo an elective cholecystectomy.

Bile Leak

Biliary leakage should be suspected in a patient who presents after cholecystectomy with fever, abdominal pain, and/or bilious ascites. The **most accurate test** for bile leak is HIDA scan. Large loculated collections should be percutaneously drained with radiologic guidance. ERCP finds the leak and a stent closes it.

> A Klatskin tumor (or hilar cholangiocarcinoma) is a cholangiocarcinoma occurring at the confluence of the right and left hepatic bile ducts.

Sphincter of Oddi Dysfunction

The sphincter of Oddi is the muscle that combines the distal common bile duct and the pancreatic duct as they enter the wall of the duodenum. Sphincter of Oddi dysfunction (SOD) is a clinical syndrome of biliary or pancreatic obstruction related to mechanical or functional abnormalities of the sphincter of Oddi.

Suspect SOD in patients who have biliary-type pain without other apparent causes. All of the following conditions must be present for a diagnosis of SOD to be made:

- Pain located in the epigastrium and/or RUQ
- Episodes lasting ≥30 minutes
- Recurrent symptoms occurring at different intervals (not daily)
- Pain that builds up to a steady level
- Pain severe enough to interrupt the patient's daily activities or lead to an emergency department visit
- Pain not significantly related to bowel movements
- Pain not significantly relieved by postural change or acid suppression

Sphincter of Oddi manometry (SOM) is the **most accurate test** for diagnosing of SOD.

The goal of treatment with symptomatic SOD is to eliminate pain and/or recurrent pancreatitis by improving the flow of biliary and pancreatic secretions. Management is based on the type of SOD.

Type of SOD	Characteristics	Management
Type I	Biliary-type pain, abnormal liver tests, dilated common bile duct	Endoscopic sphincterotomy *without* preprocedure SOM (offers greatest relief for the patient)
Type II	Biliary-type pain *plus* abnormal liver tests *OR* dilated common bile duct	SOM followed by endoscopic sphincterotomy (most common cause: sphincter of Oddi stenosis)
Type III	Biliary-type pain, **normal** liver tests, dilated common bile duct	Medical management *without* endoscopic sphincterotomy

Pancreatic Cancer

The table compares 3 cancers involving the pancreas.

	Pancreatic cancer	**Cholangiocarcinoma**	**Gallbladder cancer**
Presentation	• Painless jaundice with weight loss • +/− depressive symptoms • History of smoking	• Painless jaundice with weight loss in patient with history of PSC • Most common cancer of the bile duct • Elevated alkaline phosphatase	• Constant RUQ pain and jaundice when metastasis occurs • Palpable "porcelain gallbladder"
Etiology	90% adenocarcinoma of the pancreatic head with common bile duct dilatation	• Most commonly PSC • Southeast Asians at risk due to *Clonorchis sinensis* and *Opisthorchis viverrini*	• 90% from adenocarcinoma • More common in women • Associated with chronic typhoid infection of gallbladder
Diagnosis & workup	• Most accurate test: CT scan of the chest, abdomen, and pelvis (also used for staging) • CA 19-9 used to measure response to therapy	• Most accurate imaging test (to localize mass): MRCP • ERCP with brushings or FNA allows for biopsy • CA 19-9 used to measure response to therapy	• Best initial test: ultrasound • Most accurate imaging test: CT scan
Treatment	• Pancreaticoduodenectomy (Whipple procedure) • Palliative CBD duct stent (for metastatic disease)	Surgical resection if possible and chemotherapy	• Surgical resection if possible and chemotherapy • Extremely poor prognosis at one year

Pyogenic Liver Abscess

Liver abscess (**most common type of visceral abscess**) is commonly caused by a recent abdominal inflammatory process (e.g., diverticulitis, cholangitis) that seeds an infection to the liver.

- Typically involves right lobe of the liver because it is larger and has greater blood supply than the left and caudate lobes
- Symptoms include fever and abdominal pain
- WBC and AST/ALT levels are elevated in a nonspecific pattern

Antibiotics to cover gram-negative bacteria and anaerobes should be the next step in management. Ultrasound is the best test to diagnose pyogenic liver abscesses. Concurrent percutaneous aspiration is therapeutic.

Most pyogenic liver abscesses are polymicrobial. Following are common associations:

- Enteric gram-negative bacilli—the most common finding
- *Klebsiella pneumoniae*—associated with colorectal cancer; do a colonoscopy
- *Staphylococcus aureus*—seen after transarterial embolization for HCC
- *Candida*—seen during recovery of neutrophil counts after a neutropenic episode
- *Burkholderia pseudomallei*—associated with recent travel to Southeast Asia
- *E. histolytica*—associated with recent travel to Central and South America and with diarrhea

Abdominal antibiotics:
- Piperacillin-tazobactam
- Ampicillin-sulbactam
- Carbapenems
- Ciprofloxacin and metronidazole

Gallbladder Polyp

Gallbladder polyps are outgrowths of the gallbladder mucosal wall. They are usually found incidentally on ultrasonogram or after cholecystectomy.

Treatment of **asymptomatic polyps** depends on their size:

- **≤5 mm**: usually benign (commonly cholesterolosis); repeat U/S at 1 year to confirm size stability
- **6–9 mm**: monitor with yearly U/S; if polyp enlarges, remove surgically
- **10–20 mm**: possibly malignant; remove by laparoscopic cholecystectomy
- **>20 mm**: treated as malignant; resect surgically

Treatment of **symptomatic polyps** is cholecystectomy, regardless of polyp size.

Mirizzi Syndrome

In this rare complication, a gallstone lodges in the cystic duct of the gallbladder, and the resulting compression of the common bile duct (CBD) or common hepatic duct causes obstruction and jaundice. Labs show elevated bilirubin and alkaline phosphatase.

U/S is the **best initial test**, while MRCP is the **most accurate test**.

Treatment for simple cases is surgical resection of the gallbladder (mainstay of therapy). If a fistula has developed, cholecystectomy and bilioenteric anastomosis may be required.

Acalculous Cholecystitis

Acalculous cholecystitis is an inflammatory disease of the gallbladder caused by bile stasis, ischemia, and bile salt concentration; there is no evidence of gallstones or cystic duct obstruction.

Critically ill patients (especially those with sepsis or those receiving TPN) are more susceptible to this condition because cholecystokinin-induced gallbladder contraction is suspended in patients who do not eat.

Once the disease is established, secondary infection with enteric pathogens is common (e.g., *Escherichia coli, Enterococcus faecalis*, Klebsiella, Pseudomonas, Proteus, and *Bacteroides fragilis*).

Diagnosis is made through a combination of clinical presentation and history. While imaging is not specific enough to confirm acalculous cholecystitis, it is used to exclude other conditions.

Treatment is cholecystostomy. Surgery is reserved for patients who have necrosis/perforation of the gallbladder or emphysematous cholecystitis.

Colorectal Disease

Fecal Incontinence

Fecal incontinence is the continuous/recurrent uncontrolled passage of fecal material (>10 mL) for at least 1 month in a patient age >3.

Diagnosis is made by clinical history, plus:

- Flexible sigmoidoscopy or anoscopy (**best initial test**)
- Anorectal manometry (**most accurate test**)
- Endorectal manometry (best test if there is a history of anatomic injury)

Treatment is as follows:

- Medical therapy: bulking agents such as fiber
- Biofeedback: control exercises and muscle strengthening exercises
- Dextranomer/hyaluronic acid injection (reduces incontinence by 50%)
- If there is no response, colorectal surgery

Pilonidal Cyst

Pilonidal cyst is an abscess of the sacrococcygeal region arising from an infection of the skin and subcutaneous tissue. Risk factors include poor hygiene, obesity, and the presence of a deep natal cleft.

- As the natal cleft stretches, it damages or breaks hair follicles and opens a pore that collects hair and skin debris.
- The movement of the skin taut over the natal cleft creates negative pressure in the subcutaneous space and draws more debris into the pore.
- The friction generates a sinus.

Symptoms include sudden onset of mild to severe pain in the intergluteal region when sitting or doing activities that stretch the skin overlying the natal cleft (e.g., bending, sit-ups).

Other symptoms may include intermittent swelling as well as mucoid, purulent, and/or bloody drainage in the area.

Treatment is incision and drainage. Recurrence is treated with sinus tract excision.

Anal Fissure

Anal fissure is a tear in the anoderm distal to the dentate line. The tear triggers cycles of recurring anal pain and bleeding, which lead to a chronic anal fissure.

- Most cases are longitudinal and occur at posterior midline; not typically past dentate line
- Most cases are primary and caused by local trauma, e.g., constipation, diarrhea, vaginal delivery, anal sex
- Acute anal fissure presents with anal pain that is present at rest but is even worse with defecation

Diagnosis can be confirmed on physical exam by directly visualizing a fissure or reproducing the patient's presenting complaints by gentle digital palpation of the posterior (or anterior) midline anal verge.

Treatment is as follows:

- Sitz baths, increased fiber intake or stool softeners, and topical vasodilators such as nitroglycerin
- If no response after 8 weeks, lateral internal sphincterotomy
- Botulinum toxin for older patients or multiparous women who are at high risk for developing fecal incontinence

> The posterior midline is the most common location for primary anal fissure.

> **Anal Fissure Pain**
> - Acute: <8 weeks
> - Chronic: >8 weeks

Rectal Procidentia

Rectal procidentia (or rectal prolapse) is the protrusion of all layers of the rectum through the anus, manifesting as concentric rings of rectal mucosa. Risk factors include advanced age, chronic constipation, multiparity, and dementia.

Symptoms include pain in the anal area, bleeding, and a palpable rectal "mass." Clinical history of exam is enough to make the diagnosis.

Treatment is surgical repair. Indications for surgical repair include the direct observation of a prolapse, sensation of a rectal prolapse, and fecal incontinence and/or constipation associated with the prolapse.

Anal Abscess

Anal abscess presents with severe, constant pain around the rectum or perineum, with or without fever. The infection usually originates from an obstructed anal crypt gland and generates pus that collects in the subcutaneous tissue, intersphincteric plane, or other tissue planes.

The patient may have a history of Crohn disease.

Physical exam will show an erythematous, indurated area of skin or a fluctuant mass over the perianal space.

Treatment is surgical drainage and antibiotics.

Hemorrhoids

Hemorrhoidal veins are normal anatomic structures located in the submucosal layer of the lower rectum which enlarge. Multiple factors can cause the enlargement, e.g., constipation, advancing age, prolonged sitting, and straining during defecation.

- 40% of patients are asymptomatic
- Of those who do experience symptoms, the most common symptom is bleeding
- Other symptoms include itching, burning, and pain

Diagnosis is made clinically but the **most accurate test** is anoscopy.

Treatment is as follows:

- Dietary management (oral hydration, stool softener, increased fiber)
- Sitz baths
- Topical steroids
- If conservative measures fail, rubber band ligation of internal hemorrhoids
- If ligation fails, surgical hemorrhoidectomy

If the patient presents with the first 3 days of symptoms, acutely thrombosed external hemorrhoids can be treated by excision. Otherwise, supportive care is indicated.

Hemorrhoid Location
- **External:** distal to the dentate line
- **Internal:** proximal to the dentate line

Acute Colonic Pseudo-Obstruction

Acute colonic pseudo-obstruction (or Ogilvie syndrome) is the acute dilatation of the colon in the absence of an anatomic lesion obstructing the flow of intestinal contents. The cause is unknown, but potential causes include:

- Trauma, such as long bone fractures
- Neurologic conditions
- Chemotherapy
- Obstetric surgery, especially involving spinal anesthesia
- Pelvic, abdominal, or cardiothoracic surgery
- Major orthopedic surgery
- Severe illness (e.g., pneumonia, myocardial infarction)
- Retroperitoneal malignancy or hemorrhage
- Metabolic imbalance of electrolytes
- Medications: narcotics, CCBs, alpha-2 agonists, epidural analgesics

Symptoms include severe abdominal distension and pain, with nausea and vomiting. On physical examination the abdomen is tympanitic, but bowel sounds are present.

Diagnosis is made clinically, but CT scan (**most accurate test**) will rule out other causes of intestinal obstruction.

Treatment is aimed at the underlying cause and patient comfort:

- Nasogastric and rectal tubes to decompress the GI tract
- If there is no relief after 24–48 hours, neostigmine administration
- If there is no response with neostigmine, colonoscopy-aided decompression, followed by surgical decompression (cecostomy or colectomy)

A 19-year-old video game champion presents with lower back pain. He reports worsening pain when he sits or bends forward. On physical exam there is a tender and fluctuant erythematous mass. There is also purulent discharge from a sinus tract. What is the most likely diagnosis?

a. Hidradenitis suppurativa
b. Anorectal fistula
c. Pilonidal cyst
d. Folliculitis
e. Perianal furuncle and carbuncle

Answer: **C.** This patient has classic symptoms of a pilonidal cyst.

Orthopedics

Fractures are always diagnosed with an x-ray. In terms of therapy, general rules are:

- **Closed reduction**: mild fractures without displacement
- **Open reduction and internal fixation**: severe fractures with displacement or misalignment of bone pieces
- **Open fractures**: skin must be closed, devitalized tissue must be debrided, and the bone must be set in the operating room

Fracture

There are 5 types of fracture, all of which present with pain, swelling, and deformity.

- **Comminuted fracture**: fracture in which the bone gets broken into multiple pieces; most commonly caused by crush injury
- **Stress fracture**: complete fracture from repetitive insults to the bone in question; most commonly located in the metatarsal bones
  - On the USMLE Step 2 CK, vignettes may describe an athlete with persistent pain.
  - X-ray does not show evidence of fracture, so CT or MRI is required for diagnosis.
  - Treatment is rehabilitation, reduced physical activity, and casting. If persistent, surgery is indicated.

- **Compression fracture**: specific fracture of the vertebra in the setting of osteoporosis; most commonly lumbar; thoracolumbar; or thoracic
- **Pathologic fracture**: fracture that occurs from minimal trauma to bone that is weakened by disease, e.g., metastatic carcinoma, multiple myeloma, and Paget disease
  - On the USMLE Step 2 CK, look for a vignette in which an older person fractures a rib from coughing.
  - Treatment is surgical realignment of the bone and treatment of the underlying disease.
- **Open fracture**: fracture that occurs when injury causes a broken bone to pierce the skin
  - Associated with high rates of bacterial infection to the surrounding tissue
  - Surgery is always the right answer.

> Surgery is always the right answer for an open fracture.

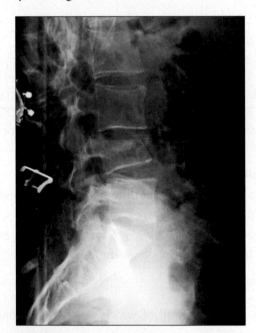

Figure 4.11 Compression Fracture of L4.
Source: James Heilman, MD, commons.wikimedia.org

Shoulder Injury

	Etiology	Signs and symptoms	Diagnosis	Treatment
Anterior shoulder dislocation	• Any injury that causes strain on the glenohumeral ligaments • **Most common type (>95%)**	Arm held to the side with externally rotated forearm with severe pain	• Best initial test: x-ray • Most accurate test: MRI • Must rule out axillary artery or nerve injury	Shoulder relocation and immobilization
Posterior shoulder dislocation	Seizure or electrical burn	Arm is medially rotated and held to the side	• Best initial test: x-ray • Most accurate test: MRI	Traction and surgery if pulses or sensation are diminished during physical exam

Finger Pain

A 39-year-old woman awakes from a nap with her index finger in severe pain and flexed, while all other fingers are extended. When she tries to pull it free, she hears a loud popping sound and the pain subsides. The next day she presents to the doctor concerned about the sound and pain. What is the most appropriate next step in management?

a. Amputate the finger

b. Steroid injection

c. Rehabilitation

d. Admit to the hospital

e. NSAID therapy

Answer: B. Trigger finger is an acutely flexed and painful finger. The cause is stenosis of the tendon sheath leading to the finger in question. Steroid injection will decrease pain and recurrence. If steroids fail, surgery to cut the sheath that is restricting the tendon is the definitive treatment.

> For clavicular fracture, a figure 8 sling is no longer used, as it is no more effective than a simple arm sling.

> Do not confuse trigger finger with **Dupuytren contracture** (common in men age >40), where the palmar fascia becomes constricted and the hand cannot properly extend open. Surgery is the only effective treatment.

Achilles Tendon Rupture

Rupture of the Achilles tendon presents as a sudden snap in the lower calf associated with acute, severe pain and inability to walk. It usually occurs after trauma or a fall. MRI is the **most accurate test**.

Treatment is surgical repair of the Achilles tendon. In elderly patients, however, casting and pain management are also considered.

A 19-year-old woman broke her femur 3 days ago during a college soccer tryout. This morning her mother brought her to the ED because she was short of breath. Physical examination reveals a confused patient who is awake but not alert or oriented and a splotchy magenta rash around the base of the neck and back. ABG reveals PO_2 under 60 mm Hg. What is the most likely diagnosis?

a. Fat embolism
b. Myocardial infarction
c. Pancreatitis
d. Rhabdomyolysis

Answer: **A.** Fat embolism syndrome is characterized by a combination of confusion, petechial rash, and dyspnea. It is caused by fracture of long bones. Myocardial infarction may have shortness of breath, but is unlikely in a 19-year-old woman. Pancreatitis would present with severe abdominal pain. Rhabdomyolysis has high CPK from muscle breakdown with a urine analysis and dipstick that shows positive blood with fewer than 5 RBCs.

Fat Embolism

Fracture of the long bone allows fat to escape as "little vesicles" and cause occlusion of vasculature throughout the body. The most common bone is the femur.

Onset of symptoms is within 5 days of the fracture:

- Confusion
- Petechial rash on the upper extremity and trunk
- Shortness of breath and tachypnea with dyspnea

Diagnostic testing includes:

- ABG will show PO_2 <60 mm Hg
- Chest x-ray will show infiltrates
- Urine analysis may show fat droplets

Treatment for fat embolism requires oxygen to keep PO_2 >95%. If the patient becomes severely hypoxic, intubation followed by mechanical ventilation is necessary.

Compartment Syndrome

Compartment syndrome is due to the compression of nerves, blood vessels, and muscle inside a closed space. This can also be within a cast after setting a fracture. The 6 signs of compartment syndrome are:

1. Pain: most commonly the first symptom
2. Pallor: lack of blood flow causes pale skin
3. Paresthesia: "pins and needles" sensation
4. Paralysis: inability to move the limb
5. Pulselessness: lack of distal pulses
6. Poikilothermia: cold to the touch

Compartment syndrome is a medical emergency, and immediate fasciotomy must be completed in order to relieve pressure before necrosis occurs.

Compartment syndrome is a medical emergency.

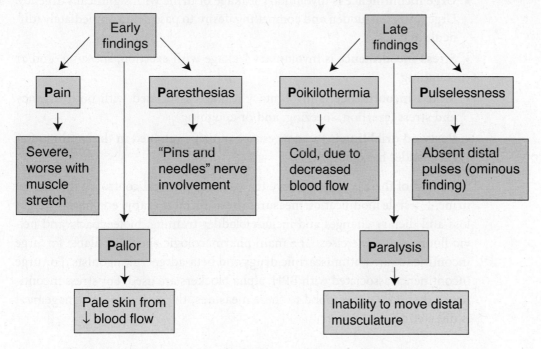

Figure 4.12 Compartment Syndrome Signs and Symptoms: The 6 P's

Urology

Hydronephrosis

Obstruction to the flow of urine from the kidney at the ureteropelvic junction causes hydronephrosis. Common obstructions include:

- Kidney stones
- Prostate hyperplasia
- Cervical cancer
- Retroperitoneal fibrosis
- Congenital malformation (e.g., bladder obstruction)
- Ureter injury during surgery (less common)

The **best test** is an ultrasound demonstrating dilatation of the renal pelvis and upper ureter.

Treat by relieving the obstruction, wherever it is. It may be necessary to place a percutaneous nephrostomy tube to allow temporary drainage of the urinary tract. After relief of the obstruction, observe the patient for post-obstructive diuresis and correct the resulting electrolyte abnormalities.

Male Incontinence

There are 4 types of male incontinence:

- **Urge incontinence** is involuntary leakage of urine with significant urgency. Urgency is the sudden and compelling desire to pass urine immediately (difficult to defer).
- **Stress incontinence** is involuntary leakage with exertion, sneezing, and/or coughing.
- **Mixed incontinence** is involuntary leakage associated with both urgency and stress (exertion, sneezing, and/or coughing).
- **Postvoid dribbling** is the slow escape of urine retained in the urethra after the bladder has emptied.

The focus of therapy is to improve the patient's physical control of the flow of urine. Lifestyle modification measures (**best initial therapy**) emphasize weight loss and dietary changes and include bladder training, biofeedback, and pelvic floor muscle exercises. The main pharmacologic agents available for urge incontinence are antimuscarinic drugs and beta-adrenergic agonists. For urge incontinence associated with BPH, alpha blockers are used. For stress incontinence that does not respond to these measures, the next step in management is duloxetine.

Benign Prostatic Hyperplasia (BPH)

BPH is a noncancerous increase in size of the prostate associated with 2 categories of symptoms:

- Storage symptoms: increased daytime urinary frequency, nocturia, urgency, and urinary incontinence
- Voiding symptoms: slow urinary stream, splitting or spraying of the urinary stream, intermittent urinary stream, hesitancy, straining to void, and terminal dribbling

These symptoms occur because the prostate is pressing on the urethra, narrowing the passage by which urine exits the bladder.

Diagnosis is made through clinical history of symptoms and a prostate that is diffusely enlarged, firm, and nontender on physical examination. Obtain a urinalysis to check for urinary tract infection or blood (which could indicate bladder calculi or cancer).

Treatment is as follows:

- Alpha-1-adrenergic antagonist (tamsulosin, terazosin, doxazosin) (**best initial therapy**) provides immediate therapeutic benefits; most common side effect is hypotension
- 5-alpha-reductase inhibitors (finasteride, dutasteride) reduce the size of the prostate gland, but patients must be counseled that significant reduction of symptoms can take 6–12 months.

> Medications like pseudoephedrine, anticholinergics, and CCBs may worsen symptoms of BPH.

> In severe BPH (i.e., requiring Foley), use 5-alpha reductase in combination with an alpha-1 antagonist.

- Surgery for persistent or progressive symptoms despite combination therapy for 12–24 months

An 18-year-old man is hit by a car while riding his bicycle. He presents to the ED with severe groin pain after falling on the central bar of the bike. Physical examination reveals blood at the urethral meatus and a high-riding prostate. What is the most appropriate next step in management?

a. Foley catheter
b. Get a retrograde urethrogram
c. Empiric antibiotics
d. CBC and electrolytes
e. Discharge the patient with reassurance

Answer: **B**. The patient has a urethral disruption that needs to be evaluated. A kidney, ureters, and bladder (KUB) x-ray followed by a retrograde urethrogram must be conducted prior to any other tests. Placing a Foley catheter without such an imaging modality can lead to further urethral damage. The step after urethrogram is a Foley catheter placement to aid in urination. There is no role for antibiotics for trauma without evidence of infection.

Erectile Dysfunction (ED)

ED is the recurrent inability to maintain an erection for the duration of sexual intercourse. Obesity, diabetes, and depression are common risk factors. History includes absence of spontaneous or nocturnal erections. The diagnosis of ED is made through history and clinical exam.

Phosphodiesterase-5 (PDE5) inhibitors such as sildenafil, vardenafil, tadalafil, and avanafil are the next step in management. They are equal in efficacy, but tadalafil has a longer duration of action and avanafil has a more rapid onset.

PDE5 inhibitors are contraindicated in men taking nitrates and should be used cautiously in men receiving an alpha-adrenergic blocker, due to an increased risk of hypotension.

If PDE5 inhibitors fail, second-line therapies are penile injections with vasodilating agents or intraurethral alprostadil. In medication-refractory ED, surgical placement of a penile prosthesis is the next step in management.

> Premature ejaculation is the most common of the ejaculatory disorders.

Urethral Abnormalities

In **hypospadias**, the urethral opening is ectopically located on the ventral side of the penis, proximal to the tip of the glans penis. Surgical correction is treatment of choice. Do not circumcise; circumcision can add to the difficulties of surgically correcting the hypospadias.

In **epispadias**, the opening to the urethra is found on the dorsal surface. Epispadias is highly associated with urinary incontinence and concomitant bladder exstrophy. Surgical correction is required.

Priapism

Priapism is a prolonged penile erection (more than 4–6 hours) in the absence of sexual stimulation. **It is a urologic emergency.** There are 2 types:

- **Ischemic** (low-flow) priapism, the more common type, is caused by decreased venous flow.
- **Nonischemic** (high-flow) priapism is caused by a fistula between cavernosal artery and corporal tissue and is often associated with trauma to the perineum.

Priapism is diagnosed with clinical exam. To determine ischemic versus nonischemic, blood should be aspirated from the corpora cavernosum for blood gas analysis:

- Ischemic: sample is black, and analysis shows hypoxemia, hypercarbia, and acidemia
- Nonischemic: sample is red, and analysis shows normal levels of oxygen, carbon dioxide, and pH

Treat ischemic priapism with intracavernosal injection of a vasoconstrictor (e.g., phenylephrine) and cavernosal blood aspiration. Nonischemic priapism can be monitored conservatively.

Hydrocele

Hydrocele is a painless, swollen, fluid-filled sac along the spermatic cords within the scrotum that transilluminates upon inspection. It is a remnant of tunica vaginalis and usually resolves within the first 12 months of life, and it does not need to be reassessed unless present after one year. For most hydroceles, watchful waiting is the appropriate management. If the hydrocele does persist beyond 12 months, surgery is recommended in order to decrease the future risk of inguinal hernias.

Varicocele

> Varicocele is the most common cause of scrotal enlargement in adult men.

Varicocele is a varicose vein in the scrotal veins causing swelling and increased pressure of the pampiniform plexus. The most common complaint is dull ache and heaviness in the scrotum.

The **best initial test** is a proper physical exam coinciding with a "bag of worms" sensation. The **most accurate test** is U/S of the scrotal sac, which will show dilatation of the vessels of the pampiniform plexus to >2 mm. Always ultrasound the other testicle as well. Varicocele is a bilateral disease. If you see it on one side, it is likely indolent on the other side.

Asymptomatic patients are monitored with yearly examination. Surgical ligation or embolization is reserved for those with pain, infertility, or delayed growth of the testes.

Cryptorchidism

Cryptorchidism is the congenital absence of one testicle in the scrotal sac. The "missing" testicle is usually found within the inguinal canal; in 90% of cases it can be palpated there. After 4 months of age, orchiopexy of congenitally undescended testes is recommended as soon as possible, and the surgery should definitely be completed before age 2 years.

> Cryptorchidism is associated with an increased risk of malignancy regardless of surgical intervention.

Testicular Torsion

Testicular torsion occurs when the spermatic cord twists, cutting off the testicle's blood supply. The most common symptom is rapid onset of severe pain and tenderness in the testicles, groin, and lower abdomen.

Physical examination will show an asymmetrically high-riding testis with its long axis oriented transversely instead of longitudinally (because the torsion shortens the spermatic cord), along with an absent cremasteric reflex. Cremasteric reflex is assessed by stroking or gently pinching the skin of the upper thigh; the normal response is elevation of the ipsilateral testis.

- **Best initial test**: physical examination
- **Most accurate test**: U/S confirming the absence of blood flow in the twisted testicle

> The testis suffers irreversible damage after 12 hours of ischemia from testicular torsion.

Treatment for suspected testicular torsion is urgent surgical exploration with intraoperative detorsion and fixation of the testes. Manual detorsion should be performed if surgical intervention is not immediately available.

Fournier Gangrene

Fournier gangrene is a necrotizing fasciitis of the perineum and scrotum from a mixed aerobic/anaerobic infection. Symptoms include severe pain that generally starts on the anterior abdominal wall and migrates into the gluteal muscles, scrotum, and penis.

Physical exam will show blisters/bullae, crepitus, and subcutaneous gas, as well as systemic findings such as fever, tachycardia, and hypotension. CT scan (**most accurate test**) will show air along the fascial planes or deeper tissue involvement.

Treatment is the same as for any other necrotizing fasciitis: surgical exploration, debridement of necrotic tissue, and antibiotic therapy.

Bariatric Surgery

Candidates for a bariatric surgical procedure are adults with a morbidly high body mass index (BMI), specifically:

- BMI ≥40 kg/m² without comorbid illness
- BMI 35.0–39.9 kg/m² with at least one serious comorbid illness (type 2 diabetes, fatty liver disease, hypertension)

The most common contraindication to bariatric surgery is major depression, psychosis, or an eating disorder that is untreated/uncontrolled.

The following are operations to promote weight loss by restricting food volume, nutrient absorption, or both.

- **Sleeve gastrectomy (most common)** is a partial gastrectomy in which the majority of the greater curvature of the stomach is removed and a tubular stomach is created. Common side effects are narrowing or stenosis of the remnant stomach, leaks, and severe GERD due to a change in the angulation of the esophagus in relation to the stomach.

- In **Roux-en-Y gastric bypass**, a small gastric pouch is created and connected to a limb of small bowel. The volume of food intake is decreased because the stomach is smaller, and absorption is decreased because the total small bowel area is reduced. Common side effects are marginal ulcer formation, cholelithiasis, dumping syndrome, and weight regain.

- **Gastric band** surgery is a purely volume-decreasing procedure in which an adjustable silicone device squeezes the gastric cardia near the gastro-esophageal junction, limiting the amount of food that it can contain. Volume restriction can be increased by slowly tightening the band over time. Common side effects are band erosion into the stomach and slippage of the band off the stomach.

Vascular

Abdominal Aortic Aneurysm (AAA)

An AAA occurs when the portion of the aorta in the abdomen grows to 1.5× its normal size or exceeds the normal diameter by >50% through dilation. It is a true aneurysm, since it involves all layers of the arterial wall.

Former or current smokers age >65 should have an abdominal ultrasound to screen for AAA, based on USPSTF recommendation. This test has >95% sensitivity and specificity.

A third-year medical student is examining a patient who has acute onset of abdominal pain. The patient is a 65-year-old smoker with HTN and DM who has had dull abdominal pain gradually building for 12 hours. It is not related to food and not relieved with famotidine. On physical examination, auscultation reveals a bruit and palpation shows a pulsatile mass. While the epigastrium is being lightly palpated, the patient suddenly becomes hypotensive and passes out. What is the most likely diagnosis?

a. Ruptured abdominal aortic aneurysm
b. Ruptured peptic ulcer
c. Hemorrhagic gastritis
d. Narcolepsy

Answer: **A.** A bruit and pulsatile abdominal mass are hallmark signs of an abdominal aortic aneurysm (AAA). The fact that the medical student was palpating the area and the patient passed out was a coincidence; however, syncope in the setting of the AAA is rupture until proven otherwise. Ruptured peptic ulcer would have more severe and sharp abdominal pain. Hemorrhagic gastritis could cause syncope, but the bleeding would cause emesis, and the patient is supine, so orthostasis is not of concern. Narcolepsy would not have hypotension. This patient's abdominal pain was from the AAA beginning to rupture and was dull and gradual in onset.

A 69-year-old man with a 50 pack-year smoking history is brought to the ED by his wife, who reports he seems "confused." He feels weak and has mid-abdominal pain. He is a pale, elderly male in moderate distress. BP is 84/55 mm Hg and pulse 120 bpm. There is a palpable, pulsatile mass in the patient's abdomen. What is the most likely diagnosis?

a. Ruptured peptic ulcer
b. Hemorrhagic gastritis
c. Hemorrhagic pancreatitis
d. Ruptured abdominal aortic aneurysm

Answer: **D.** The key to the diagnosis of this patient is a painful, pulsatile mass in the abdomen with signs of hypovolemia (hypotension and tachycardia). The ruptured aorta is pouring blood into the retroperitoneal space, and it bulges with every heartbeat. Smoking and age are 2 risk factors for AAA.

Diagnostic Tests

- CT or MRI will give information regarding the relationship of the AAA to the surrounding vessels.
- Ultrasound must be done because it gives information on size and can be used as a cost-effective and safe means to monitor the AAA over time.
- Surgery is indicated when the AAA reaches 5 cm.

Which of the following is the most appropriate screening for aortic aneurysm?

a. Everyone age >50 with CT angiography
b. Men who ever smoked age >65 with ultrasound
c. Everyone age >50 with ultrasound
d. Everyone age >65 with ultrasound
e. Men age >65 with ultrasound

Answer: **B.** When the width of the AAA is >5 cm in diameter, surgical or catheter-directed repair of the lesion is indicated. The incidence of AAA is lower in both non-smokers and in women, so there is no recommendation for screening in those groups. New-onset back pain in elderly patients (age >65) should have ultrasound of aorta to rule out AAA.

Treatment

Management of AAA is based on size of the lesion:

- 3.0–4.0 cm: ultrasound every 2–3 years
- 4.0–5.4 cm: ultrasound or CT every 6–12 months
- ≥ 5.5 cm, asymptomatic: surgical repair

Aortic Dissection

Aortic dissection occurs when a tear in the intima of the aorta creates a false lumen. This weak spot extends with each beat, extending the tear.

Risk factors include:

- Hypertension (**main risk factor**)
- Age >40
- Marfan syndrome

> Key points for presence of aortic dissection:
> - Pain in between the scapulae
> - Difference in BP between the arms.

The patient will present with sudden onset of tearing chest pain that radiates to the back, and the patient may be found to have asymmetric blood pressures in the right and left arms.

Diagnostic testing:

- Chest x-ray (**best initial test**) may show widened mediastinum
- Computed tomography angiography (CTA) is easiest to get
- MRA, TEE, and CTA are all equal in sensitivity and specificity

In treatment of aortic dissection, the most important step is to control BP.

- Beta blockers: beta blockade will decrease the "shearing forces" that are worsening the dissection
- Nitroprusside: only after beta blockers are given (to protect against reflex tachycardia of nitroprusside, which will worsen shearing forces)
- Surgical correction

A 67-year-old man comes to the ED with a sudden onset of chest pain. He also has pain between his scapulae. He has a history of hypertension and tobacco smoking. Blood pressure is 169/108 mm Hg. What is the best initial test?

a. Chest x-ray
b. Chest CT
c. MRA
d. Transesophageal echocardiogram
e. Transthoracic echocardiogram
f. CT angiogram
g. Angiography

Answer: **A.** Although not as sensitive as the other tests, chest x-ray might show widening of the mediastinum, which is an excellent clue to the presence of aortic dissection.

A 67-year-old man comes to the ED with a sudden onset of chest pain. He also has pain between his scapulae. He has a history of hypertension and tobacco smoking. Blood pressure is 169/108 mm Hg. What is the most accurate test?

a. MRA

b. Transesophageal echocardiogram

c. Transthoracic echocardiogram

d. CT angiogram

e. Angiogram

Answer: **E.** Angiography is more accurate than the other choices. It is the most invasive, as well, with potential complications of allergy to contrast and renal failure, but it is the most sensitive and specific. The diagnostic quality from TEE, MRA, and CT angiogram are comparable to those from angiogram with a catheter. CT angiogram is used most often only because it is the easiest to obtain.

> MRA, CT angiogram, and TEE are equally accurate. In other words, **MRA = CTA = TEE.**

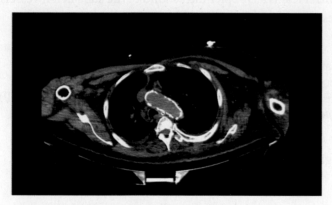

Figure 4.13 Aortic Calcification.
Source: Pramod Theetha Karivanna, MD

Varicose Veins

Varicose veins are veins that are enlarged and twisted because the leaflets of the valves have become incompetent. The condition is most common in the superficial veins of the legs, which are subject to high pressure when standing. Look for a patient whose job involves standing for extended hours daily.

Symptoms of varicose veins include an aching, swelling, heavy-feeling leg with large, swollen veins visible on the affected leg. Diagnose based on clinical history and exam.

Treatment is usually done only for aesthetic reasons. Veins that cause ulcerations or clotting require surgical stripping or sclerotherapy.

Thoracic Outlet Syndrome

Thoracic outlet syndrome (TOS) is a condition in which there is compression of the nerves, arteries, or veins in the passageway from the lower neck to the armpit. The most common cause is a congenital cervical rib—an extra rib that arises from the seventh cervical vertebra.

There are 3 main types of TOS:

- Neurogenic TOS (**most common**) presents with pain, weakness, and thenar atrophy.
- Venous type results in swelling, pain, and cyanosis of the arm.
- Arterial type causes pain, coldness, and pallor of the arm.

Some patients may have Adson sign, the loss of the radial pulse in the arm upon rotating the head to the ipsilateral side, with neck extended, and taking a deep inspiration.

The **best initial test** is a Doppler ultrasound of the subclavian vessels. The **most accurate test** is MRA.

Treatment is indicated only for symptomatic patients; incidentally found asymptomatic cervical ribs should be observed.

Neurogenic TOS should initially be managed with physical therapy. Thoracic outlet decompression is indicated for symptomatic patients with:

- Vascular symptoms of TOS
- Neurologic weakness or disabling pain and paresthesia

Hernias

A hernia is a protrusion, bulge, or projection of an organ (or part of an organ) through the body wall that normally contains it, such as the abdominal wall. Although an abdominal wall hernia can go unnoticed, the patient will usually report a bulge that may or may not be associated with symptoms of heaviness and localized pain.

Hernias can present with complications related to incarceration and strangulation of contents in the hernia sac, leading to sepsis. Large ventral hernias may present with skin ulceration due to pressure necrosis.

Type	Characteristics
Indirect inguinal hernia (**most common** hernia type in both men and women)	Protrudes via the internal inguinal ring, lateral to the inferior epigastric vessels
Direct inguinal hernia	Protrudes medial to the inferior epigastric vessels within the Hasselbalch triangle
Femoral hernia	Hernia protrudes through the femoral ring, which is inferior to the inguinal ligament, medial to the femoral vein, and lateral to the lacunar ligament
Umbilical hernia	Results from failure of the umbilical ring to close spontaneously
Epigastric hernias	Results from defects in the abdominal midline between the umbilicus and the xiphoid process

For any type of hernia, the **best initial test** is a thorough history and physical examination. When the diagnosis is not clear or the **most accurate test** is needed, choose CT scan or MRI.

The **definitive treatment** for any type of hernia is surgical repair. If there is bowel or strangulation obstruction, surgical repair should be done urgently within 4–6 hours of presentation, with antibiotics given to prevent bowel loss.

> The Hasselbalch triangle consists of:
> - Inferior inguinal ligament (Poupart ligament)
> - Lateral inferior epigastric artery
> - Medial conjoint tendon

Transplantation

	Indications	Complications
Liver	• Acute hepatic failure • Chronic liver disease (e.g., cirrhosis, PBC, PSC)	Bleeding, biliary tract strictures, reperfusion injury
Kidney	• End-stage renal disease on hemodialysis • Impending renal failure • Polycystic kidney disease, etc.	Urine leak caused by poor blood supply to the distal ureter
Pancreas	Type I diabetes	Rejection and loss of graft function
Small bowel	• Short gut syndrome • Crohn disease • Trauma • Congenital small bowel disorders	Graft failure and rejection (common)

Postoperative Care

A 57-year-old woman who underwent emergent cholecystectomy for a perforated gallbladder 3 days ago now has a fever of 38 C (>100.4 F) and is complaining of chills. The patient has not been ambulating and says she is in a great deal of pain at her incision. What is the most likely cause of her fever?

a. Atelectasis
b. UTI
c. Wound infection
d. DVT
e. Abscess

Answer: **B.** UTI is most likely, but all of the choices are possible. In this patient with a complicated surgery and obvious risk factors, the timing and presentation given in the vignette help indicate which complication is most likely to be causing the fever.

Postoperative Fever Assessment				
	Mnemonic	**Possible cause**	**Diagnostic test**	**Therapy**
POD 1–2	Wind	Atelectasis or postoperative pneumonia	Chest x-ray followed by sputum cultures	Prevention by incentive spirometry; vancomycin and tazobactam-piperacillin for hospital-acquired pneumonia
POD 3–5	Water	Urinary tract infection	Urine analysis showing positive nitrates and leukocyte esterase. Urine culture for species and sensitivity.	Antibiotics appropriate for the organism
POD 5–7	Walking	Deep vein thrombosis or thrombophlebitis of the IV access lines. Must also consider pulmonary embolism for new-onset tachycardia and chest pain.	Doppler ultrasound of the extremities. Changing of IV access lines and culture of the IV tips.	Heparin for 5 days as a bridge to warfarin for 3–6 months
POD 7	Wound	Wound infections and cellulitis	Physical exam of the wound for erythema, purulent discharge, and/or swelling	Incision and drainage if abscess or fluid followed by antibiotics
POD 8–15	Wonder	Drug fever or deep abscess	CT scan for examination of a deep fluid collection	CT guided percutaneous drainage of the abscess; otherwise surgery
POD = Postoperative Day				

Postoperative Complications

Postoperative Confusion

It is likely that a confused patient is hypoxic or septic. You must get an ABG, chest x-ray, blood cultures, urine culture, and CBC, and then treat the appropriate organism. If the patient is hypoxic, consider pulmonary embolism, atelectasis, or pneumonia as a cause.

Acute Respiratory Distress Syndrome (ARDS)

This will be seen postoperatively with severe hypoxia, tachypnea, accessory muscle use for ventilation, and hypercapnia. Diagnose with a chest x-ray that will show bilateral pulmonary infiltrates without JVD (rule out CHF) and treat with positive end expiratory pressure.

Pulmonary Embolism

PE presents as an acute onset of chest pain with clear lung exam. The **best initial diagnostic test** is an EKG, which will show sinus tachycardia without evidence of ST segment changes. You can confirm noncardiac chest pain with troponins and cardiac enzymes. Then follow with a CT angiogram of the chest. (See pulmonary section for treatment.).

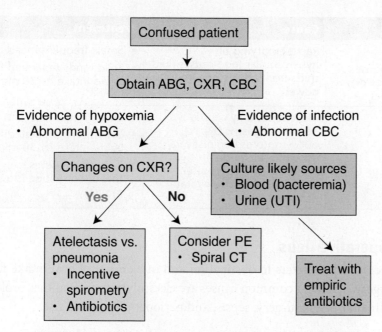

Figure 4.14 Postoperative Confusion and Complications

> The most common finding on EKG for pulmonary embolism is **nonspecific ST segment changes**. S1-Q3-T3 is not the most common; it is seen in less than 10% of patients.

A 62-year-old woman with no significant PMH underwent right total hip replacement 3 days ago. Recovery was uncomplicated until 30 minutes ago, when she reported moderate SOB and chest pain with deep inspiration. What is the best next step in management?

a. EKG only
b. EKG + V/Q scan
c. EKG + spiral CT scan
d. EKG + d-dimer
e. EKG + heparin injection

Answer: **C.** A presentation of pleuritic chest pain and shortness of breath after recent trauma and a period of immobility is a high risk for PE. The best next step is spiral CT scan (V/Q scan for those with allergy to IV contrast) and an EKG, because chest pain may indicate ischemia, and that must be ruled out. D-dimer is sensitive but not specific, and should be used to rule out PE in low-risk patients. Injection of low-molecular-weight heparin or a NOAC (oral agent) is an appropriate treatment for PE, but PE must first be diagnosed; thus, this is not the next best step here.

Dumping Syndrome

Dumping syndrome is a complication of both gastric bypass and sleeve gastrectomy. There are 2 forms of dumping syndrome.

Name	Symptoms	Cause	Treatment
Early dumping syndrome	• Hypotension • Autonomic response (flushing, tachycardia, possible syncope)	Rapid emptying of hyperosmolar food causes fluid shifts from the plasma into the bowel	• Small, frequent meals • Solid foods separated from liquid intake by 30 minutes
Late-onset dumping syndrome, or postprandial hyperinsulinemic hypoglycemia (PHH)	• Hypoglycemia • Dizziness • Fatigue • Diaphoresis • Weakness	Most commonly caused by Roux-en-Y gastric bypass, but symptoms begin several months after surgery, occurring 1–3 hours after ingestion of a carbohydrate-rich meal	• Small, frequent meals • Solid foods separated from liquid intake by 30 minutes • If these measures fail, trial of octreotide (slows motility)

Postoperative Ileus

Postoperative ileus refers to obstipation and intolerance of oral intake following surgery. The most common causes are electrolyte abnormalities, prolonged abdominal or pelvic surgery, sepsis, and perioperative opioid use.

Symptoms include oral intolerance, nausea and vomiting, obstipation, and lack of flatus. Physical exam will show decreased or absent bowel sounds.

The **best initial test** is an abdominal x-ray showing air-fluid levels, and the **most accurate test** is a CT scan demonstrating a lack of a transition zone as seen in SBO.

Treatment is supportive care, electrolyte replacement, and stopping the offending medications. Alvimopan (μ-opioid receptor antagonist) is indicated to treat postoperative ileus following partial large or small bowel resection with primary anastomosis.

Abdominal x-ray is used to evaluate ileus, which is a nonmechanical etiology for lack of peristalsis in the GI tract.

Postcardiac Surgery Syndrome

Anytime the pericardium is opened, the patient can develop postcardiac surgery syndrome. Pericarditis with or without a pericardial effusion resulting from injury to the pericardium is postcardiac injury syndrome. It begins because of damage to mesothelial pericardial cells, which releases cardiac antigens and stimulates an immune response that causes an inflammatory cascade in the local tissues.

The patient will present with tachycardia, tachypnea, and distant, muffled heart sounds. Chest x-ray will reveal cardiomegaly.

The **best initial test** is an EKG, and the **most accurate test** is an echocardiogram. Treatment is NSAIDs and colchicine.

Postcardiac surgery syndrome can be prevented entirely by using colchicine after surgery.

PART 5

Sports Medicine

by Philip J. Koehler III, DO, MS

Upper Extremity: Shoulder, Elbow, Forearm, and Hand

Common Shoulder Pathology				
Pathology	**Presentation**	**Special test**	**Diagnosis**	**Management**
Subacromial impingement syndrome	Pain with abduction, internal rotation, and overhead activities (swimming, throwing). Leads to rotator cuff tears.	Neer Hawkins Painful arc	MRI	Conservative Corticosteroid injection
Rotator cuff tear	Result of trauma fall on outstretched hand (FOOSH) and/or chronic impingement. Most commonly torn is supraspinatus (first 15° of abduction). Causes weakness and pain with abduction and external rotation.	Jobe (empty can) Drop arm	MRI	Surgery for full-thickness tear or failed conservative treatment
Biceps tendinitis and rupture	**Tendinitis:** overuse injury from overhead activities or sports in adults >40 years old with impingement. Associated with other shoulder pathology (labral tear, rotator cuff tear) in elderly. Most common: proximal long head of biceps in bicipital groove. **Rupture:** pain, audible snap, ecchymosis, visible bulge (Popeye sign)	Speed Yergason	Clinical Ultrasound (US) or MRI can help confirm	**Tendinitis:** conservative +/− corticosteroid injection **Rupture:** surgical reattachment in young patients
Adhesive capsulitis (frozen shoulder)	Active and passive range of motion (ROM) restricted >50% in all planes (especially abduction, external rotation). Stiffness exceeds pain. Result of chronic inflammation, fibrosis, and contracture of joint capsule. Risk factors: prior trauma, diabetes mellitus, CVA, hypothyroidism, female, age >40 years.	Limited AROM and PROM	Clinical Imaging can help confirm	Physical therapy Manipulation under anesthesia OMT (Spencer technique)
AC separation	Pain with palpation over AC joint and adduction of arm. Result of massive force on adducted arm, usually a fall onto the tip of the shoulder (football tackle, wrestling throw, ice-hockey check).	Cross-arm adductor	X-ray	**Types 1–2** (no clavicular displacement): conservative + sling **Types 3–6:** surgical open reduction internal fixation (ORIF)

(continued)

Common Shoulder Pathology (*cont'd*)				
Pathology	**Presentation**	**Special Test**	**Diagnosis**	**Management**
DJD of glenohumeral joint	Uncommon; caused by trauma or repetitive use. Pain with abduction and internal rotation.	Limited AROM and PROM	X-ray	Conservative Arthroplasty (replacement)
Labral or SLAP (superior labrum anterior to posterior) tear	Similar symptoms to shoulder instability (pain, locking, clicking). Overuse injury from overhead sports. Associated with biceps tendon rupture. "Dead arm" syndrome—shoulder fatigue, pain, numbness, and/or paresthesias in throwing position or overhead position.	O'Brien Load and shift	MRI	Physical therapy for strengthening Arthroscopic surgery for refractory cases
GH dislocation	**Anterior**: most common (>90%); involves risk of axillary nerve damage. Arm held in abduction with external rotation. Commonly caused by FOOSH. **Posterior**: uncommon (<10%); result of seizure or electrocution. Arm held in adduction with internal rotation.	Observation Apprehension test	X-ray (initial) MRI (**most accurate**)	Reduction followed with a sling Surgery for repeated occurrences
Clavicular fracture	Trauma (FOOSH)	Palpation	X-ray **Angiogram** for vascular injury if neurovascular compromise is suspected (subclavian artery and brachial plexus)	Simple arm sling ORIF for severe displacement

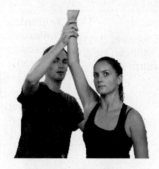

Figure 5.1 Neer Test

Neer test

- Subacromial impingement syndrome
- Place one hand on patient's scapula, other hand on arm
- Internally rotate arm and forcibly flex arm to ear
- Pain = positive test
- Remember "Neer to the ear"

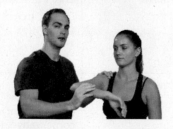

Figure 5.2 Hawkins-Kennedy Test

Hawkins-Kennedy test

- Subacromial impingement syndrome
- Place the patient's arm in 90° of shoulder flexion with the elbow flexed to 90°, and then internally rotate the arm
- Pain = positive test

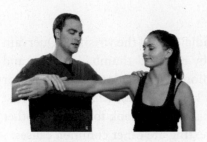

Figure 5.3 Jobe/Empty Can Test

Jobe/empty can test

- Test for rotator cuff tear (supraspinatus)
- Have patient flex arm to 90°, abduct to 45°, and internally rotate with thumb down
- Resisted flexion causes pain = positive test

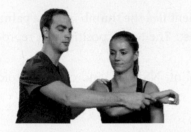

Figure 5.4 Cross Arm/Adductor Test

Cross arm/adductor test

- Acromioclavicular joint separation/tear
- Forward elevation to 90° and active adduction
- Pain = positive test

Epicondylitis

Lateral (tennis elbow):

- The most common cause of elbow pain
- Pain over the distal **lateral epicondyle** that radiates into forearm and increases with repetitive supination or forearm extension; results from microtrauma to the common extensor origin, or extensor carpi radialis brevis (ECRB)
- Often causes weakness in grip strength
- Common in the dominant hand of younger patients (40–55 years old) who perform repetitive motions (carpenters, plumbers, tennis players)

Medial (golfer's elbow, little leaguer's elbow, pitcher's elbow):

- Pain over the **medial epicondyle** that increases with repetitive or excessive forearm valgus stress or pronation motions (golfing, pitching)
- Results from microtrauma to the common flexor tendon

Diagnostic Tests

Diagnose epicondylitis with physical exam:

- Lateral: pain with passive wrist flexion or resisted supination or forearm extension
- Medial: pain with resisted wrist flexion and pronation

Treatment

Treatment is conservative: NSAIDs, rest, and physical therapy, inelastic counterforce sleeve and corticosteroid injection into common tendons (lateral) are effective >90% of patients.

De Quervain Tenosynovitis

This presents as pain and tenderness over radial side of the wrist. De Quervain tenosynovitis is an overuse injury caused by repeated thumb abduction and extension. The pain results from inflammation of the tendons of the extensor pollicis brevis (EPB) and abductor pollicis longus (APL), which are the first compartment of the wrist, in the anatomic snuffbox. Look for a new mother constantly holding her baby. Bowling and texting are other common causes.

Diagnostic Tests and Treatment

- Finkelstein test (**best initial test**): Have patient flex the thumb into the palm, making a fist, then ulnarly deviate the wrist. The test is positive if it reproduces pain.
- Treatment is conservative: thumb spica splint, NSAIDs, and corticosteroid injection.

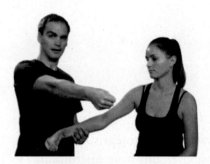

De Quervain tenosynovitis

- Overuse of abductor pollicis longus, extensor pollicis brevis
- Finkelstein test
- Thumb is tucked inside fingers/fist, and wrist is ulnarly deviated
- Pain = positive test

Figure 5.5 Finkelstein Test

Scaphoid Fracture

Scaphoid fracture is also known as fall on outstretched hand (FOOSH) because it is caused by a fall or trauma on an outstretched and dorsiflexed wrist. The scaphoid is the most commonly fractured carpal bone (>70%). This injury involves the risk of avascular necrosis (AVN) of the scaphoid due to unusual blood supply that flows distal to proximal from the radial artery.

Look for pain with palpation over the anatomic snuffbox.

Diagnostic Tests and Treatment

- Plain x-rays (**best initial test**). If fracture is not seen on imaging but is suspected, treat as a fracture: Immobilize the wrist in thumb spica cast for 10–14 days and then repeat x-ray to confirm fracture.
- MRI or CT can make immediate diagnosis but is not the best initial test. CT is best test for patients that are still symptomatic after 4–6 weeks of treatment.
- Treat nondisplaced fracture with thumb spica cast for 6+ weeks.
- Treat displaced fracture (>2 mm) with ORIF.

Lower Extremity: The Hip, Knee, and Foot

Avascular Necrosis of the Femoral Head

This is an insidious onset of hip and groin pain that is worsened by activity (stairs, incline) and weight-bearing but relieved by rest. Avascular necrosis of the femoral head results when the vascular supply to the femoral head is disrupted. Look for a younger patient (<40 years old) with the following risk factors: steroid use, sickle cell disease, alcohol abuse, osteomyelitis, SLE, or previous fracture, dislocation, or surgical fixation. Age and risk factors are main clues to differentiate AVN from OA of the hip.

Diagnostic Tests and Treatment

- MRI (**most sensitive test**)
- X-rays are normal in first few months of pathology
- ESR, CRP, WBC: also normal

Treatment for avascular necrosis of the femoral head is total hip arthroplasty replacement.

Osteoarthritis of the Hip

Look for progressive hip and groin pain that is worse with movement in patients >50 years old. Pain at rest usually correlates to clinically significant x-ray findings. Osteoarthritis of the hip is caused by overuse, trauma, and chronic degeneration of articular cartilage.

Diagnostic Tests

- X-ray
- Physical exam demonstrates limited range of motion and positive FABER/Patrick test

Treatment

Conservative until pain is intolerable, then total hip arthroplasty replacement.

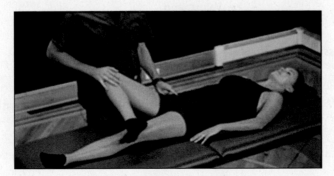

Figure 5.6 FABER/Patrick Test

Knee Injuries

ACL Tear

This is the most common ligament injury of the knee. It is a noncontact but dramatic injury caused by dramatic cutting, deceleration, and hyperextension of the knee (football, soccer, skiing). It can also be caused by valgus stress on a flexed, planted, and rotated knee. More than 50% of patients with an ACL tear have a concurrent meniscal injury. Look for an injury described as starting with an audible pop with anterior knee pain, instability, and effusion.

Diagnostic Tests

- Physical exam demonstrates decreased knee flexion secondary to effusion/ hemarthrosis. Joint line tenderness is common due to secondary pathology (meniscus).

- Anterior drawer: With patient supine and knee flexed to 90 degrees, pull anteriorly on the tibia, if it slides easily in relationship to femur it is a positive test.

- Lachman (**more sensitive**): With patient supine and knee flexed to 30 degrees, pull anteriorly on the tibia; if it slides easily in relationship to the femur it is a positive test.

- MRI is the **best initial test** (80–95% sensitive).

- Arthroscopy is the **most accurate test** (100% sensitive).

Treatment

Most require arthroscopic surgical reconstruction with graft.

Common Knee Pathologies				
Pathology	**Presentation**	**Special test**	**Diagnosis**	**Management**
Ligament tear (ACL, PCL, MCL, or LCL)	**ACL:** noncontact injury, most common, cutting injury **PCL:** hyperflexion, posterior force on a planted leg, rare (car accident dashboard injury) **MCL:** valgus force from a blow on a planted leg (football, soccer) **LCL:** rare, devastating injury, associated with multiple pathology and neurovascular injury	• Anterior and posterior drawer • Lachman • Valgus and varus stress	MRI	• Conservative (especially MCL) • Arthroscopic reconstructive surgery
Meniscus tear	**Joint-line** knee pain and clicking, popping, or locking with movement. Results from cutting maneuvers that cause tibial rotation on a flexed and fixed knee (football, soccer).	• McMurray • Thessaly • Apley grind	MRI	• Conservative • Arthroscopic reconstructive surgery
ITBS	**Lateral** knee pain over Gerdy tubercle where the Iliotibial band (ITB) inserts.	Ober	Clinical	• Conservative • Physical therapy

(continued)

Common Knee Pathologies (*cont'd*)				
Pathology	**Presentation**	**Special test**	**Diagnosis**	**Management**
Patellofemoral syndrome (runner's knee)	**Anterior** knee pain under patella. Caused by overuse, muscular imbalance of quadriceps, and poor biomechanics (bowlegged). Prolonged sitting and excessive activity are exacerbating factors.	Patellar grind test	Clinical	• Conservative • Physical therapy
Patellar tendinitis (jumper's knee)	**Inferior** patellar knee pain. Episodic pain. Commonly occurs in athletes in jumping sports (basketball, volleyball). Overuse injury caused by repetitive overload of quadriceps on patellar tendon.	Pain with palpation over inferior pole of patella	Clinical	• Conservative • Physical therapy
Osteoarthritis of the knee	**Medial > lateral joint-line pain**, age >50 years, obese, limited ROM, crepitus with ROM, small effusion, varus or valgus angulation, pain with weight bearing or activity.	Limited AROM and PROM	X-ray	• Conservative • Arthroplasty (replacement)

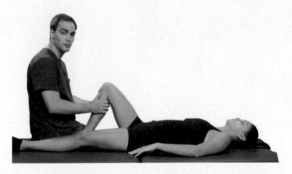

Figure 5.7 Anterior/Posterior Drawer Test

Anterior/posterior drawer test

- Hip flexed 45°, knee flexed to 90°
- Anterior pull on tibia
- Ligament laxity = ACL pathology/tear
- Posterior push on tibia
- Ligament laxity = PCL pathology/tear

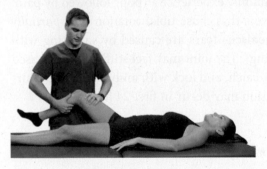

Figure 5.8 Lachman Test

Lachman test

- Hip slightly flexed, knee flexed to 30°
- Anterior pull on tibia
- Ligament laxity = ACL pathology/tear

O'Donoghue Unhappy Triad

This is a triple injury to the ACL, MCL, and medial meniscus.

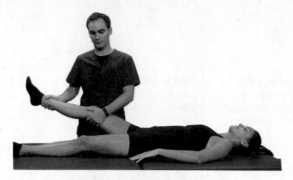

Figure 5.9 Varus Stress Test

Valgus/varus stress tests

- Hip flexed to 30°, knee extended to 180°
- Valgus/lateral force
- Ligament laxity = MCL pathology/tear
- Varus/medial force
- Ligament laxity = LCL pathology/tear

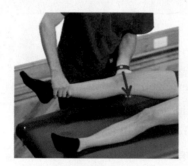

Figure 5.10 Valgus Stress Test

Meniscal Tear

Meniscal tear occurs in younger patients, who commonly experience a "pop" followed by pain. Medial meniscus tears result from cutting maneuvers that cause tibial rotation on a *partially* flexed and fixed knee (football, soccer). Lateral meniscus tears are caused by squatting with *full* flexion of knee and rotation (wrestling, squatting). The joint may feel stiff, with decreased range of motion, especially with flexion. It will pop, catch, and lock with ambulation and stair-climbing. Joint-line tenderness and significant effusion may occur in first 24 hours.

Diagnostic Tests

- Physical exam reveals decreased knee flexion secondary to effusion, joint-line tenderness, and pain or locking with provocative maneuvers.
- McMurray test: With the patient supine and the hip and knee flexed, palpate the joint line of the knee bilaterally. Externally rotate the tibia and apply valgus force while extending the knee to examine the medial meniscus. Internally rotate the tibia and apply varus force while extending the knee to examine the lateral meniscus. Popping, clicking, and pain indicate a positive test. McMurray test is **the most commonly described exam** on standardized tests.
- Thessaly test: Patient stands on the affected limb and rotates the femur on the tibia.
- Apley grind: With patient prone and knee flexed to 90 degrees, the physician places compression through heel while internally and externally rotating tibia to grind the meniscus.
- MRI is the gold standard.

Treatment

- Mild symptoms and patients >40 years old: conservative management rest, activity modification, NSAIDs
- Young patients with >3–4 weeks of symptoms: arthroscopic surgical repair

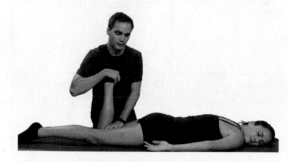

Figure 5.11 Apley Compression Test

Apley compression test

- Patient prone, knee flexed to 90°
- Axial compression down leg into knee
- Pain = positive test (indicates a meniscal tear)

Foot Injury

Common Foot Pathologies			
Pathology	**Presentation**	**Diagnosis**	**Treatment**
Plantar fasciitis	**Heel pain** focal to the rear foot. Pain is greatest with **first steps** in the morning and then improves. Prolonged daily activity often causes a return of the pain at night.	• **Clinical:** point tenderness distal to heel • X-rays are not useful	• Conservative with stretching of plantar fascia • Steroid injection can be useful to refractory cases
Stress fracture	Pain in midfoot (**2nd metatarsal** most common) due to repeated tension. Most commonly caused by dramatic increase in activity (military, athletes). Can occur with poor nutrition – vit D, calcium or **female athlete triad**: low calorie, low bone density, amenorrhea	• **Clinical** • X-rays are normal for 3–6 weeks • **MRI**/CT/bone scans are more sensitive early on	• Conservative with rest and wide, hard-soled footwear • CAM boot if more aggressive for 5th metatarsal
Jones fracture	**5th metatarsal fracture** at junction of metaphysis and diaphysis. Common fracture with ankle sprains and caused when heel is off the ground but forefoot is planted. Risk of delayed healing if untreated.	X-rays	Nondisplaced: 6–8 weeks in cast and non–weight bearing
Morton neuroma	Numbness and burning pain between **3rd and 4th digits**. Caused by an interdigital neuroma. Thought to be a result of mechanical injury but unclear etiology. Happens to both athletes and nonathletes.	• **Clinical** • **Mulder sign** (squeezing metatarsal joints causes pain and crepitus at 3rd/4th digits) • US or MRI to confirm diagnosis	• Conservative, metatarsal support pads or wide, hard-soled footwear (**first-line treatment**) • Injections and surgery for refractory symptoms

(continued)

Common Foot Pathologies (*cont'd*)			
Pathology	**Presentation**	**Diagnosis**	**Treatment**
Tarsal tunnel syndrome	Similar presentation to carpal tunnel syndrome except it occurs on **medial side of the sole of the foot**. Pain, tingling, and burning with activity or at rest. Etiology is entrapment of tibial nerve under flexor retinaculum by tenosynovitis of tibialis posterior, flexor digitorum longus, and flexor hallucis longus. (Mnemonic for order of ligaments and neurovascular bundle at tunnel: Tom, Dick, and A Very Nervous Harry.)	• **EMG** confirms diagnosis • Clinical exam + Tinel sign at the tarsal tunnel	• NSAIDs • Steroid injection • Tunnel release for progressive nerve damage
Hallux valgus (bunion)	Deformity causing pain over the great toe at the **metatarsophalangeal (MTP)** joint. Pain with walking and blisters can occur. Don't confuse with gout, which has similar location but different etiology.	• Clinical • X-ray	Orthotics and surgery

Miscellaneous Orthopedics

Common Bursitis		
Location	**Pathology**	**Presentation and Management**
Posterior knee	Baker cyst, popliteal cyst	Inflammation of synovium causing an outpouching in posterior popliteal space. Asymptomatic bulge that when it ruptures causes pain that can mimic a **DVT** because of increased warmth and edema. **Ultrasound** is best diagnostic test to rule out DVT. Risk factors are OA, RA, meniscal tears, or other articular trauma.
Medial knee	Pes anserine	Pain with palpation just inferior or **distal to the medial joint line of the knee.** Insertion of three muscles (sartorius, gracilis, semitendinosus), which all have different actions and therefore is associated with overuse.
Superior knee	Suprapatellar	This bursa communicates with **joint space of the knee** and becomes inflamed and enlarged with osteoarthritis.
Inferior knee	Prepatellar housemaid's knee	This bursa is superficial to the patella and therefore easily exposed to trauma. **Repetitive kneeling** in professions such as cleaners, carpenters, plumbers, etc., commonly develop this.
Lateral hip	Greater trochanter	**Lateral hip pain** over greater trochanter where gluteus medius inserts. Pain while sleeping on side or with external rotation and resisted abduction. Associated with iliotibial band syndrome (ITBS).
Olecranon	Student's elbow, craftsman's elbow, miner's elbow	Posterior elbow pain. Most commonly occurs from recurrent **gout** exacerbations. However, it can be a result of minor trauma from occupations that cause patients to put pressure on their elbows (student, carpenter, housemaid).

Diagnosis

- Clinical: physical exam revealing swelling and tenderness with palpation over bursa
- Aspiration of the bursa if septic bursitis is suspected (erythema, warmth)

Treatment

- Avoidance behavior and conservative therapy: rest, NSAIDs, ice, and corticosteroid injection
- Antibiotics for 7–10 days in septic bursitis

Atlantoaxial Instability

Atlantoaxial (AA) joint instability is defined as excessive mobility of C1 on C2. This can lead to subluxation and spinal cord injury. Overall, 13% are asymptomatic, 1–2% cause pain, myelopathy, and upper motor neuron signs and can cause behavioral issues. AA is a very common comorbidity of Down syndrome (10–15% of patients) and rheumatoid arthritis. Precaution should be used in patients undergoing intubation.

Diagnose with lateral x-ray films with flexion and extension.

Treat with surgical fusion.

Pediatric Orthopedics

Osgood-Schlatter Disease (Tibial Tuberosity Avulsion – Traction Apophysitis)

Osgood-Schlatter is anterior knee pain, often bilateral (around 25–50% of cases), of **tibial tuberosities** in adolescent children (age 10–11 in girls, 13–14 in boys) who are athletic and undergoing a growth spurt. It is caused by repetitive stress from the quadriceps tendon pulling on the tibial tuberosities during rapid growth spurts. Sports with jumping, running, and kneeling make it worse. Rest improves symptoms.

- Diagnosis is clinical: pain with palpation over tibial tuberosities, and reproduced with resisted knee extension.
- Imaging is not needed, but lateral plain films often show soft tissue swelling and may reveal avulsion fracture; these can be used to rule out more insidious pathology.

Treatment is conservative, and symptoms resolve when bones completely ossify (up to 18 months). Use NSAIDs to relieve pain and patellar strap to distribute force around insertion of patellar tendon.

Nursemaid's Elbow (Radial Head Subluxation)

This condition occurs in children age 1–5 because of traction on forearm, commonly when the child is swung by the arms or yanked by the arm. The radial head slips outside the annular ligament and gets stuck, causing pain and limited ROM.

Diagnosis is clinical: The arm is held still in the pronated position and is mildly tender. There is no erythema or deformity.

Treatment is with physical maneuvers. The physician should effect hyperpronation and/or supination with hyperflexion while continuously applying force over the radial head. Usually both maneuvers are performed, resulting in reduction and instantaneous relief of pain.

PART 6

Ear, Nose, and Throat (ENT)

The Ear

Otitis Media

Otitis media presents with redness, immobility, bulging, and a decreased light reflex of the tympanic membrane. Pain is common. Decreased hearing and fever also occur.

Tympanocentesis for a fluid sample for culture (**most accurate test**) is done if there are recurrences or no response to antibiotics.

Radiologic tests for otitis are always the wrong answer.

> Which of the following is the most sensitive physical finding for otitis media?
>
> a. Redness
> b. Immobility
> c. Bulging
> d. Decreased light reflex
> e. Decreased hearing
>
> Answer: **B.** Immobility is so sensitive a physical finding that a fully mobile tympanic membrane essentially excludes otitis media.

Treatment is amoxicillin (**best initial treatment**). If there is no response or the patient has recently been treated with amoxicillin, use the following:

- Amoxicillin/clavulanate
- Azithromycin, clarithromycin
- Cefuroxime, cefdinir, cefpodoxime, cefprozil
- Levofloxacin, gemifloxacin, moxifloxacin

> Quinolones are relatively contraindicated in children.

Otitis Externa

Otitis externa is a cellulitis of the skin of the external auditory canal, also known as "swimmer's ear." Exposure to water raises the pH of the canal, facilitating bacterial growth. Maceration of the canal with cotton swabs also promotes bacterial growth. There is pain on moving the tragus.

Culture of the yellow-white discharge is not helpful, as all ear canals will grow *Staphylococcus*, *Propionibacterium acnes*, and *Pseudomonas*. Treat with topical neomycin-polymyxin, topical quinolones, or gentamicin. Use hydrocortisone ear drops to decrease inflammation and relieve pain. Removing desquamated skin and cerumen will make it easier to disinfect the ear canal.

> Acetic acid (vinegar) inhibits bacterial growth in the ear canal.

Malignant (Necrotizing) External Otitis

Although the name sounds similar to otitis externa, this infection is actually cranial osteomyelitis in the portion of the skull near the auditory canal, caused by *Pseudomonas*. It is common in poorly controlled diabetics. Severe ear pain is common.

Malignant external otitis can be rapidly fatal as the pseudomonads aggressively invade the base of the skull of the elderly, immunocompromised patient and spread.

The **best initial test** is CT or MRI of the skull base. The **most accurate test** is biopsy.

> Topical antibiotics are useless in malignant external otitis.

Treatment is IV antibiotics that are effective against *Pseudomonas*, such as ceftazidime (or cefepime), quinolones, aztreonam, or the antipseudomonal penicillins (e.g., piperacillin/tazobactam). If the exam question asks you to choose a single agent, the answer is ciprofloxacin.

Mastoiditis

Mastoiditis is an infection of the mastoid air cells that occurs when nearby otitis media spreads. The skin over the mastoid process can become red and the area tender. Inadequate or delayed treatment can result in deafness and meningitis.

The organisms are the same with pneumococcus, *Haemophilus*, and *Moraxella*. CT or MRI is the **best initial test**. If there is no response, the **most accurate test** is a biopsy.

Treat with ceftriaxone or levofloxacin. Surgical debridement is sometimes needed. Recurrent or chronic infection is treated like osteomyelitis. Biopsy and use vancomycin combined with piperacillin/tazobactam.

Cerumen Impaction

Impacted earwax causes hearing loss, earache and ear fullness, tinnitus, and dizziness. Diagnose cerumen impaction with otoscopy. Remove earwax when symptomatic:

- Melt it out with cerumenolytics such as hydrogen peroxide, mineral oil, or liquid docusate.
- Alternative: jet irrigation (high-pressure water)
- Cerumenolytics, irrigation, and manual removal are all equally effective.

Vertigo/Nystagmus

Vertigo is the feeling of the room spinning around you. Any cause of vertigo can produce the jerky eye movements known as nystagmus. Any cause of nystagmus and vertigo can also lead to nausea and vomiting. The distinguishing factor among the causes of vertigo is the presence or absence of hearing loss and tinnitus.

Central Nervous System Causes of Vertigo

CNS causes of vertigo and nystagmus are not associated with hearing loss and tinnitus. It is easy for a stroke to damage speech, but not hearing. Stroke of the posterior circulation of the brain (the vertebral/basilar system) is not associated with hearing loss or tinnitus. Neither is multiple sclerosis. But you need a brain MRI for both. Another cause of vertigo/nystagmus that does not cause hearing problems is phenytoin toxicity.

Peripheral/Inner Ear Causes of Vertigo

Both **labyrinthitis and Meniere disease** cause vertigo and nystagmus in association with hearing loss and tinnitus. Labyrinthitis is acute; Meniere disease is chronic and recurrent. If there is acute hearing loss, glucocorticoids should be used. Meniere is treated with diuretics and carbonic anhydrase inhibitors. If the pain, hearing loss, and vertigo are debilitating and chronic, ablation of the inner ear on the affected side is performed. Meclizine may help.

In addition to hearing loss/tinnitus, patients with **acoustic neuroma/eighth cranial nerve tumor** could have ataxia. A CT or MRI specifically looking at the internal auditory canal localizes the lesion, which must be surgically removed.

In **perilymph fistula**, a history of barotrauma or exposure to explosions is critical to the diagnosis. The leaking hole in the oval window of the inner ear can only be fixed surgically.

In **benign positional vertigo (BPV)** there is no hearing loss or tinnitus or ataxia. This is a transient problem in the vestibular/semicircular canal system of the inner ear. Repositioning the head suddenly can correct the problem. Nearly all resolve in a few hours. There is no effective medical therapy for BPV. The only effective therapy is repositioning maneuvers, such as the Epley maneuver.

The table summarizes types of vertigo and their management.

Vertigo Types and Management					
	Central	**Labyrinthitis**	**Meniere disease**	**BPV**	**Perilymph fistula**
Etiology	• Stroke • MS	Viral	Unknown	Unknown	Barotrauma
Unique feature	• Focal neuro findings • No hearing loss or tinnitus	• Hearing loss, tinnitus • Acute	Same as labyrinthitis, but chronic	• No hearing loss • No tinnitus	History of explosions
Diagnostic test	MRI	None	None	Worsens with head position	Surgical exploration
Treatment	Underlying cause	• Steroids • Meclizine	• Sodium restriction • Diuretics	• Head repositioning • Epley maneuver	Surgical closure of oval window

The Nose and Sinus

Sinusitis

A 34-year-old woman presents with facial pain, discolored nasal discharge, bad taste in her mouth, and fever. On physical examination she has facial tenderness. Which of the following is the most accurate diagnostic test?

a. Sinus biopsy or aspirate
b. CT scan
c. X-ray
d. Culture of the discharge
e. Transillumination

Answer: **A.** In infectious diseases, the radiologic test is never "the most accurate test." Only a biopsy or aspirate can provide a precise microbiological diagnosis. There is a difference between a question that says, "What is the most accurate test?" and one that asks, "What will you do?" CT scan is the most common *wrong answer* to this question. You cannot stain or culture a CT scan.

Diagnostic Testing and Treatment

If the question describes typical symptoms of sinusitis such as face pain, discolored nasal discharge, and fever, answer "Start antibiotics (e.g., amoxicillin) and a decongestant." No radiological testing is needed.

If the question asks "What is the first diagnostic test?" the answer is CT of the sinuses, *not* an x-ray. X-ray does not have enough sensitivity or specificity to be the first test.

Do a biopsy only if infection frequently recurs or if there is no response to different empiric therapies.

▶ **TIP**

Culture of nasal discharge is always the wrong answer for sinusitis.

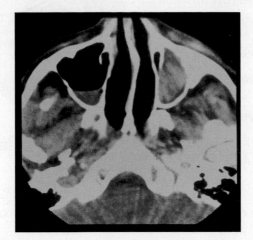

Figure 6.1 Sinusitis CT.
Source: Conrad Fischer, MD.

A 34-year-old woman presents with facial pain, a discolored nasal discharge, bad taste in her mouth, and fever. On physical examination she has facial tenderness. What is the most appropriate next step, action, or management?

a. Linezolid
b. CT scan
c. X-ray
d. Amoxicillin/clavulanic acid and a decongestant
e. Erythromycin and a decongestant

Answer: D. When the diagnosis is as clear as it is here, radiologic testing is unnecessary. Amoxicillin/clavulanic acid is the first-line therapy for both otitis and sinusitis. (If rash from penicillin use cefpodoxime, cefdinir, cefuroxime; if anaphylaxis use doxycycline, levofloxacin, gemifloxacin, or moxifloxacin.) Amoxicillin/clavulanic acid is as effective as newer or more "broad spectrum" agents such as quinolones. Imaging is done if the diagnosis is equivocal. A decongestant is used in all cases to promote sinus drainage. Erythromycin is inadequate because of poorer coverage for *Streptococcus pneumoniae*. Linezolid, although excellent for resistant gram-positive organisms, would not cover *Haemophilus*. Antibiotics are rarely needed, because most cases are viral in etiology. Antibiotics are used with fever and discolored nasal discharge.

Cavernous Sinus Thrombosis

The cavernous sinus is a venous drainage system that receives venous drainage from the face, nose, orbits, and tonsils. The cavernous sinus is adjacent to the sphenoid sinus, allowing sinusitis to thrombose the cavernous venous sinus.

Patients have fever, headache, ptosis, and proptosis. Symptoms arise from damage of cranial nerves III, IV, and VI, which travel through the cavernous sinus. The key to the "most likely diagnosis" question is a history of sinusitis and diplopia with the inability to move the eyes normally on examination.

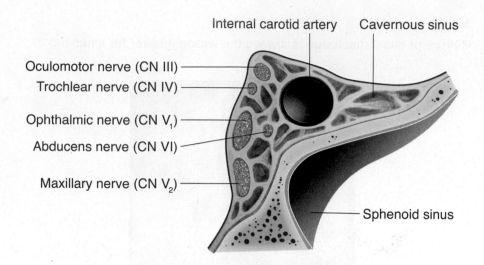

Figure 6.2 Sphenoid Sinus and Cavernous Sinus. © Kaplan

The **best initial test** is CT or MRI with contrast showing the thrombosis. In most patients, lumbar puncture shows CSF with neutrophils. The infectious organisms are *Staphylococcus*, *Streptococcus*, and anaerobes.

Treatment is vancomycin, ceftriaxone, and possibly anaerobic antimicrobials. Ampicillin/sulbactam with vancomycin is a good choice. Steroids decrease inflammation. Anticoagulation is essential.

Tolosa-Hunt Syndrome

This is a granulomatous inflammation of the cavernous sinus with ophthalmoplegia. Look for eye pain and paralysis of the same cranial nerves (III, IV, and VI) that are involved in cavernous sinus thrombosis. Diagnose with MRI. Treat with steroids.

Epistaxis

- 90–95% are anterior, venous bleeds of the Kiesselbach venous plexus.
  - Have patient blow the nose and hold it closed for 5 minutes.
  - More severe cases need vasoconstrictor drops, silver nitrate, sealants, glue, and occasionally nasal packing. Give phenylephrine or oxymetazoline.
- 5% are posterior, arterial bleeds. These are very dangerous and need packing or balloon.
  - After packing, give cephalexin to prevent growth of *Staphylococcus* and toxic shock.
  - Check platelet count if bleeding persists or recurs frequently.

The Throat and Neck

Pharyngitis

Presents with:

- Pain on swallowing
- Enlarged lymph node in the neck
- Exudate in the pharynx
- Fever
- No cough and no hoarseness

When these features are present, the likelihood of streptococcal pharyngitis exceeds 90%.

Diagnostic Tests

The **best initial test** is the "rapid strep test," an office-based test that determines within minutes whether a patient has group A beta hemolytic streptococci.

A negative test is not always sufficiently sensitive to exclude disease. When all the criteria suggesting infection are present, antibiotics are needed until culture is back.

Positive rapid strep test = Positive pharyngeal culture

- Small vesicles or ulcers: HSV or herpangina
- Membranous exudates: diphtheria, Vincent angina, or EBV

Treatment

1. Penicillin or amoxicillin is the **best initial therapy**.
2. Penicillin-allergic patients are treated with cefdinir or cefpodoxime if the reaction is only a rash. If the allergy is anaphylaxis, use clindamycin or a macrolide.

There are many choices of antibiotics for pharyngitis. You cannot be asked to choose between clarithromycin, azithromycin, and erythromycin. Erythromycin is only different in having more adverse effects, such as nausea, vomiting, and diarrhea.

> Streptococcal pharyngitis is treated to prevent rheumatic fever.

Lemierre Syndrome (Septic Jugular Thrombophlebitis)

Lemierre syndrome occurs when an infection of *Fusobacterium necrophorum* (from pharyngitis, peritonsillar abscess, mastoiditis, or parotitis) expands beyond the mouth to infect the neurovascular bundle around the jugular vein; this allows easy spread of bacteria both locally and into the bloodstream. Untreated sepsis causes >90% mortality.

Diagnose with CT of the neck. Treat with ampicillin/sulbactam or piperacillin/tazobactam combined with a beta-lactam/beta-lactamase inhibitor (same anaerobic coverage as metronidazole or clindamycin). Other choices are carbapenems or ceftriaxone with metronidazole.

Ludwig Angina

This is cellulitis of the floor of the mouth. It is caused by the spread of oral flora from dental infection of the mandibular molars into the submandibular and sublingual spaces. Because Ludwig angina causes the tongue to swell, it can compromise the airway, necessitating intubation or tracheostomy.

The **best initial test** is CT of the neck. Treat like Lemierre syndrome with ampicillin/sulbactam or piperacillin/tazobactam (or if anaphylaxis use clindamycin and levofloxacin).

Salivary Gland Disorders

Sialolithiasis

Sialolithiases are stones (calculi) in the ducts draining the salivary glands that cause postprandial pain and local swelling. Recurrent stones lead to strictures and sialadenitis. Treatment:

- Stones can be palpated and removed manually or by incising the distal duct.
- Stones can also be removed with sialoendoscopy, lithotripsy, or surgery.

Sialadenitis

This is an acute bacterial infection of the parotid or submandibular gland, most often caused by *Staphylococcus aureus*. Eating meals causes swelling and increased pain in the erythematous duct. Often pus can be expressed from the duct.

- Diagnose clinically; U/S or CT can help.
- Manage with antibiotics, warm compresses, massage, and sour candy to increase salivary flow.

PART 7

Pediatrics

by Niket Sonpal, MD

Management of the Newborn

Routine Management

Pediatric medicine begins just after the birth with routine management of the newborn, which involves a physical examination, Apgar scoring, eye care, and routine disease prevention and screening.

A 28-year-old G_1P_0 woman delivers a 3.9 kg male infant whose Apgar scores are 9 and 10 at 1 and 5 minutes respectively. The delivery was uncomplicated and both mother and child are in no acute distress. What is the most appropriate next step in management?

a. Intubate the child.
b. Send cord blood for arterial blood gas.
c. Suction the mouth and nose.
d. Place a nasogastric tube.
e. Give prophylactic antibiotics.

Answer: **C.** Once the child is delivered, the mouth and nose are suctioned, followed by clamping and cutting of the umbilical cord. The newborn is then dried, wrapped in clean towels, and placed under a warmer as he has just descended from an environment of 37 C (98.6 F) to approximately 18.3 C (65 F). Gentle rubbing or stimulating the heels of the newborn helps to stimulate crying and breathing. Intubation and ABG analysis of the child are indicated only if the newborn is not breathing or is in respiratory distress. Nasogastric tube placement is indicated when GI decompression is needed. Antibiotics are indicated for sepsis.

Apgar Score

Apgar score delineates a quantifiable measurement for the need and effectiveness of resuscitation. It does not predict mortality.

- **1-minute score** evaluates conditions during labor and delivery
- **5-minute score** evaluates the response to resuscitative efforts

A low Apgar score is not associated with future cerebral palsy.

Criteria of the Apgar Score				
Acronym	**Criterion**	**0 points**	**1 point**	**2 points**
Appearance	Skin color/ complexion	Blue all over	Normal except extremities	Normal all over
Pulse	Pulse rate	<60 bpm or asystole	>60 bpm but <100 bpm	>100 bpm
Grimace	Reflex irritability	No response	Grimace/feeble cry	Sneeze/cough
Activity	Muscle tone	None	Some flexion	Active movement
Respiration	Breathing	Absent	Weak or irregular	Strong

Eye Care

A 3.9 kg female infant whose Apgar scores were 9 and 10 at 1 and 5 minutes after delivery, respectively, is brought in by her parents because her eyes are red. The delivery was without any complications and both mother and child are in no acute distress. What is the most likely diagnosis at 1 day, at 2–7 days, and at >7 days?

a. Chemical irritation
b. *Neisseria gonorrhoeae*
c. *Chlamydia trachomatis*
d. Herpes simplex
e. All of the above

Answer: **E.** To diagnose the cause of conjunctivitis in the newborn, you must consider when the redness and irritation begins.

The most likely cause of conjunctivitis depends on time since delivery:

- **1 day**: chemical irritation
- **2–7 days**: *Neisseria gonorrhoeae*
- **>7 days**: *Chlamydia trachomatis*
- **≥3 weeks**: herpes infection

In the delivery room, all newborns must be given 2 types of antibiotic drops in each eye to prevent ophthalmia neonatorum. This condition can be attributed most commonly to *Neisseria gonorrhoeae* or *Chlamydia trachomatis*. Use erythromycin ointment or oral azithromycin.

A 1-week-old newborn is brought to the ED after a home delivery. His parents state they do not believe in vaccinations and they did not seek any medical attention after delivery. They have noticed bright red blood per rectum from the infant and he is very lethargic. The infant has unequal pupils and his diaper has gross red blood. What is the most likely diagnosis?

a. Cerebrovascular accident
b. Meckel diverticulum
c. Vitamin K–deficient bleeding
d. Crohn disease

Answer: C. As this child received no routine newborn care, it is very likely he is suffering from a vitamin K deficiency. Newborns are at most risk as their immature livers do not utilize vitamin K to develop the appropriate clotting factors. Breast milk typically has very low levels of vitamin K. The child's lethargy is likely from intracranial bleeding, and the bright red blood per rectum is mucosal bleeding. The child's age precludes a diagnosis of CVA, Crohn disease, or a Meckel diverticulum.

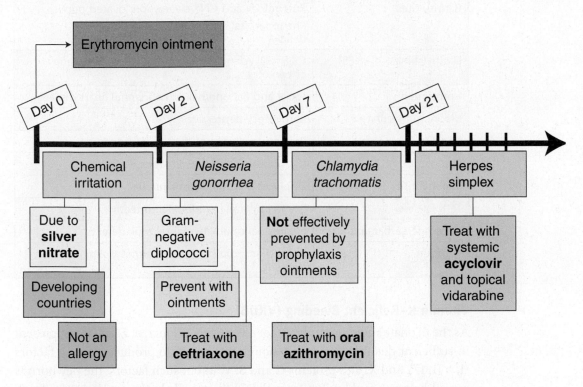

Figure 7.1 Preventive eye care begins in the delivery room with erythromycin ointment.

Retinoblastoma

Retinoblastoma is the most common intraocular malignancy of childhood. It typically presents as leukocoria (white reflex) in a child age <3 years. Rb is a tumor suppressor gene located on chromosome 13. Children with a family history of retinoblastoma should undergo clinical screening and/or genetic testing for the condition.

Diagnosis is made through dilated indirect ophthalmoscopic examination; in retinoblastoma, this shows a chalky, off-white retinal mass with a soft, friable consistency. *Do not biopsy* the mass, as there is risk of seeding. Treat with local and systemic chemotherapy, cryotherapy, laser photocoagulation, and surgical enucleation.

Common Teratogens and Their Effect on the Neonate

Drug	Effect
ACE inhibitors	Craniofacial abnormalities
Anesthetics	Respiratory and CNS depression
Barbiturates	Respiratory and CNS depression, dilated pupils Phenobarbital is associated with vitamin K deficiency.
Diethylstilbestrol (DES)	Clear-cell adenocarcinoma (CCA) of the vagina or cervix
Isotretinoin	Facial and ear anomalies, congenital heart disease
Magnesium sulfate	Respiratory depression
NSAIDs	Premature closure of ductus arteriosus
Phenytoin	Hypoplastic nails, typical facies, IUGR
Sulfonamides	Displaces bilirubin from albumin
Tetracycline	Enamel hypoplasia, discolored teeth
Valproate/carbamazepine	Intellectual disability, neural tube defects
Warfarin	Facial dysmorphism and chondrodysplasia, bone stippling

Vitamin K–Deficient Bleeding (VKDB)

As the neonate's colonic flora has not adequately colonized, *E. coli* is not present in sufficient quantities to make enough vitamin K to produce clotting factors II, VII, IX, and X, and proteins C and S. Without such factors, the newborn is more likely to have bleeding from the GI tract, belly button, and urinary tract.

To prevent VKDB (formerly known as hemorrhagic disease of the newborn), a single intramuscular dose of vitamin K is recommended and has been shown to decrease the incidence of VKDB.

> Anything that decreases mortality is most likely to be tested on the USMLE Step 2 CK.

Screening Tests

All neonates must be screened for these diseases prior to discharge:

- PKU
- Congenital adrenal hyperplasia (CAH)
- Biotinidase
- Beta thalassemia
- Galactosemia
- Hypothyroidism
- Homocystinuria
- Cystic fibrosis

The most commonly tested disorders in newborns:

- **G6PD deficiency**: X-linked recessive disease characterized by hemolytic crises. Treatment involves reducing oxidative stress and specialized diets.

- **Phenylketonuria (PKU)**: autosomal recessive genetic disorder characterized by a deficiency in the enzyme phenylalanine hydroxylase (PAH) that leads to intellectual disability. Treatment is with a special diet low in phenylalanine for at least the first 16 years of the patient's life.

- **Galactosemia**: a rare genetic disorder that precludes normal metabolism of galactose. Treatment is to cut out all lactose-containing products.

- **Congenital adrenal hyperplasia**: any of several autosomal recessive diseases resulting in errors in steroidogenesis. Treatment is to replace mineralocorticoids and glucocorticoid deficiencies and possible genital reconstructive surgery.

- **Congenital hypothyroidism**: compromises brain development. Must have normal thyroid function for normal brain development.

- **Hearing test**: excludes congenital sensory-neural hearing loss. Necessary for early detection to maintain speech patterns and assess the need for cochlear implantation.

- **Cystic fibrosis**: autosomal disorder causing abnormally thick mucus.
  - **Best initial test**: sweat chloride
  - **Most accurate test**: genetic analysis of the CFTR gene
  - Classic findings on the USMLE: combination of an elevated sweat chloride, presence of mutations in CFTR gene, and/or abnormal functioning in at least one organ system

Hepatitis B Vaccination

Every child gets a hepatitis B vaccination, but only those with HBsAg-positive mothers should receive hepatitis B immunoglobulin (HBIG) in addition to the vaccine.

A woman who has hepatitis C from a long history of injection drug use has given birth to a baby girl, who is in postdelivery care. The infant was born via normal spontaneous vaginal delivery. What is the best response to the mother and obstetrics team regarding breastfeeding?

a. Allow the mother to breastfeed.
b. Instruct the mother to give the baby formula only.
c. Breastfeeding is safe if mother is using interferon.
d. Breastfeeding is safe if mother is using velpatasvir and sofosbuvir.
e. Send a breast milk sample for HCV analysis.

Answer: **A**. Allow the mother to breastfeed. There is no documented evidence that breastfeeding spreads hepatitis C or hepatitis B. If the mother's nipples or surrounding areola are cracked and bleeding, she should stop nursing temporarily and switch to the other breast.

Transient Conditions

Transient Polycythemia of the Newborn

Hypoxia during delivery stimulates erythropoietin and causes an increase in circulating red blood cells. The newborn's first breath will increase O_2 and cause a drop in erythropoietin, which in turn will lead to normalization of hemoglobin.

Splenomegaly is a normal finding in newborns.

Transient Tachypnea of the Newborn

Compression of the rib cage by passing through the mother's vaginal canal helps to remove fluid from the lungs. Newborns who are delivered via cesarean birth may have excess fluid in the lungs and therefore be hypoxic. If tachypnea lasts >4 hours, it is considered sepsis and must be evaluated with blood and urine analysis.

Lumbar puncture with CSF analysis and culture is done when the newborn displays neurological signs such as irritability, lethargy, temperature irregularity, and feeding problems.

Transient Hyperbilirubinemia

Over 60% of all newborn infants are jaundiced. This is due to the infant's spleen removing excess red blood cells that carry Hgb F. This excess breakdown of RBCs leads to a physiological release of hemoglobin and in turn a rise in bilirubin.

Delivery-Associated Conditions in the Newborn

Subconjunctival Hemorrhage

Minute hemorrhages may be present in the eyes of the infant due to a rapid rise in intrathoracic pressure as the chest is compressed while passing through the birth canal. No treatment is indicated.

Skull Fractures

There are 3 major types of skull fractures in the newborn:

1. Linear: **most common**

2. Depressed: can cause further cortical damage without surgical intervention

3. Basilar: **most fatal**

Scalp Injuries

Caput succedaneum is a swelling of the soft tissues of the scalp that **does cross** suture lines. Cephalohematoma is a subperiosteal hemorrhage that **does not cross** suture lines. Diagnosis is made clinically, and improvement occurs gradually without treatment over a few weeks to months.

Neonatal Brachial Plexus Palsy

Brachial plexus injuries are secondary to births with traction in the event of shoulder dystocia. Brachial palsy is most commonly seen in macrosomic infants of diabetic mothers and has 2 major forms.

Duchenne-Erb Paralysis: C5–C6

- "Waiter's tip" appearance; secondary to shoulder dystocia
- The infant is unable to abduct the shoulder or externally rotate and supinate the arm.

Diagnosis is made clinically, and physical therapy with immobilization is the best treatment.

Klumpke Paralysis: C7–C8 +/− T1

- "Claw hand" due to a lack of grasp reflex
- Paralyzed hand with Horner syndrome (ptosis, miosis, and anhidrosis)

Diagnosis is made clinically, and immobilization is the best treatment.

Clavicular Fracture

This is the most common newborn fracture as a result of shoulder dystocia. X-ray is the **best diagnostic test**, and the fracture is treated with immobilization, splinting, and physical therapy.

Facial Nerve Palsy

Facial nerve palsy is paralysis of structures innervated by the facial nerve, caused by trauma secondary to forceps use in delivery. During crying, the mouth of an affected infant is drawn over to the unaffected side. Diagnosis is made clinically, and the condition usually resolves gradually over a few weeks to months. If no recovery is seen, however, surgical nerve repair is necessary.

Amniotic Fluid Abnormalities and Associated Manifestations

- In amniotic fluid, 80% is a filtrate of the mother's plasma.
- The baby produces the remaining 20% by swallowing, absorbing, filtering, and urinating.

Polyhydramnios: Too Much Fluid Secondary to Fetus Not Swallowing

Causes are:

- Neurological Werdnig-Hoffman
  - Infant unable to swallow
- GI
  - Intestinal atresias

> Shoulder dystocia occurs when, after delivery of the fetal head, the baby's anterior shoulder gets stuck behind the mother's pubic bone.

Oligohydramnios: Too Little Fluid Because Fetus Cannot Urinate

Causes are:

- Prune belly: lack of abdominal muscles, so unable to bear down and urinate
  - Treatment is with serial Foley catheter placements, but carries high risk of UTI
- Renal agenesis: incompatible with life
  - Associated with Potter syndrome
- Flat facies due to high atmospheric pressure causing compression of the fetus that is normally buffered by the amniotic fluid

Meconium Aspiration Syndrome

Meconium aspiration syndrome (MAS) is seen in a post-term infant born through meconium-stained fluid. Meconium obstructs the airway and causes respiratory distress. The leading three causes of MAS are:

- Physiologic maturational event
- Acute hypoxic event
- Chronic intrauterine hypoxia

The diagnosis of MAS is based on a clinical finding of a meconium-stained infant, respiratory distress, and chest x-ray findings of patchy infiltrates, coarse streaking of both lung fields, and flattening of the diaphragm.

Manage as follows:

- Airway management and ventilatory support with oxygen therapy
- Inhaled nitric oxide
- If the patient worsens, initiate surfactant therapy, which works to break up meconium in the alveoli.
- If the patient still does not improve, the next step in management is extracorporeal membrane oxygenation (ECMO).

Necrotizing Enterocolitis (NEC)

NEC presents in a premature infant with low Apgar scores. The **greatest risk factor** for NEC is premature delivery. It presents with sudden changes in feeding tolerance, abdominal distension, bilious gastric retention vomiting, rectal bleeding, and diarrhea. Physical findings may include abdominal wall erythema, crepitus, and induration. The most common late gastrointestinal complications of NEC are strictures and short bowel syndrome.

The **best initial diagnostic test** is an abdominal x-ray that shows pneumatosis intestinalis, pneumoperitoneum, or hepatobiliary gas.

Manage NEC as follows:

- Stop all feeds.
- Decompress the gut with NG tube.
- Begin antibiotics that cover aerobic and anaerobic intestinal bacteria.
- Surgery is required if intestinal perforation occurs or the patient does not improve with medical therapy.

Abnormal Abdominal Findings

A premature infant born at 28 weeks is in respiratory distress, with grunting, nasal flaring, and the use of accessory muscles. Bowel sounds are heard upon auscultation of the back, and chest x-ray shows air-fluid levels. Which of the following is the most likely diagnosis?

a. Hydrocele
b. Gastroschisis
c. Diaphragmatic hernia
d. Hiatal hernia
e. Omphalocele

Answer: **C.** A hernia in the diaphragm will allow bowel contents to move into the chest and impair ventilation. Hydrocele is a urinary defect and is not seen on x-ray. It cannot be gastroschisis or omphalocele, as those are defined as an extrusion of abdominal contents outside of the body. Hiatal hernia is a benign finding most commonly seen in elderly or obese patients.

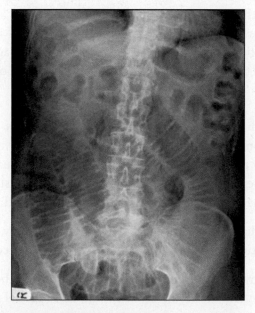

Figure 7.2 Multiple air-fluid levels are seen during obstruction and can be a clue to guide the clinician.
Source: Niket Sonpal, MD.

Diaphragmatic Hernia

Diaphragmatic hernia is a hole in the diaphragm that allows the abdominal contents to move into the thorax.

- Bowel sound in the chest can be heard.
- Air fluid levels are seen on chest x-ray.

Omphalocele

An omphalocele is a defect in which intestines and organs form beyond the abdominal wall with a sac covering. It results from failure of the GI sac to retract at 10–12 weeks' gestation.

Screening is conducted by maternal alpha fetoprotein (AFP) levels and ultrasound. Surgical reintroduction of contents is needed. Omphalocele is highly associated with Edwards syndrome (trisomy 18).

> - Elevated AFP levels indicate both neural tube defects and abdominal wall defects.
> - The most common cause for elevated AFP is incorrect dating.

Umbilical Hernia

With umbilical hernia there is a congenital weakness of the rectus abdominis muscle which allows for protrusion of vessels and bowel. It is highly associated with congenital hypothyroidism. Ninety percent close spontaneously by age 3. After the age of 4, surgical intervention is indicated to prevent bowel strangulation and subsequent necrosis.

Gastroschisis

Gastroschisis is a wall defect lateral to midline with intestines and organs forming beyond the abdominal wall with no sac covering. Multiple intestinal atresias can occur. Treatment calls for immediate surgical intervention with gradual introduction of bowel and silo formation. Overly aggressive surgical reintroduction of the bowel will lead to third spacing and bowel infarction.

> Wilms tumor is the most common abdominal mass in children.

> The combination of **W**ilms tumor, **a**niridia, **g**enitourinary malformations, and intellectual disability (formerly called mental **r**etardation) is referred to as WAGR syndrome. The syndrome results from a deletion on chromosome 11.

Wilms Tumor

With Wilms tumor, a large palpable abdominal mass is felt. It is caused by hemihypertrophy of one kidney due to its increased vascular demands. Aniridia is highly associated with this malignancy and is usually the clinician's most valuable clue. An affected child will show signs of constipation and complain of abdominal pain that is accompanied by nausea and vomiting.

Wilms tumor is diagnosed with abdominal ultrasonography, which is the **best initial** imaging study. Contrast-enhanced CT is the **most accurate test**.

Total nephrectomy with chemotherapy and radiation may be indicated based upon staging. Bilateral kidney involvement indicates partial nephrectomy.

> Neuroblastomas are statistically the most common cancers in infancy and the most common extracranial solid malignancy.

Neuroblastoma

Neuroblastoma is an adrenal medulla tumor similar to a pheochromocytoma but with fewer cardiac manifestations. The percentage of cases presenting with metastases is in the range of 50–60%. Increased vanillyl mandelic acid (VMA) and metanephrines on urine collection are diagnostic.

Growth, Weight, and Vaccinations

What is the best indicator for acute malnutrition?

- Weight/height ratio <5th percentile

What is the best indicator for under- and overweight children?

- BMI

What is the most common cause of failure to thrive?

- Psychosocial deprivation (all age groups)

What is the next step in management of cases of underfeeding?

- Report to Child Protective Services (CPS)

Vaccinations

Vignette presents...	You answer...
Premature infants or low-birth-weight babies	• Do not delay immunizations; immunize at chronological age. • Do not dose-adjust immunizations.
Immunocompromised patients	Do not give live vaccinations.
Concerned parent with sick child in office who is due for vaccination	The following **are not contraindications** to immunization: • A reaction to a previous DPT of temperature <40.5 C (105 F), redness, soreness, and swelling • A mild, acute illness in an otherwise well child • A family history of seizures or sudden infant death syndrome
Report from parent that child has egg allergy	• MMR: Documented egg allergy is not a contraindication. • Yellow fever vaccine: Egg allergy does contraindicate. • Influenza vaccine: Egg allergy is not a contraindication.
Parent's concern about side effects of vaccination	• MMR does not cause autism or inflammatory bowel disease. • Hepatitis B vaccine does not cause demyelinating neurologic disorders. • Meningococcal vaccination is not related to development of Guillain-Barré.

Developmental Achievements

Reflexes

1. Sucking reflex: Baby automatically sucks on a nipplelike object.
2. Grasping reflex
3. Babinski reflex: When outer sole of the foot is stroked, toes extend.
4. Rooting reflex: When cheek is touched, baby turns to that side.
5. Moro reflex: When baby is scared, arms spread symmetrically.
6. Stepping reflex: walking-like maneuvers when toes touch the ground
7. Superman reflex: When baby is held facing the floor, arms go out.

Cardiology

Cyanotic Lesions

A 5-year-old boy is seen for routine examination by his doctor, but his parents have stated that lately he becomes short of breath while playing with his friends and his lips have a bluish cast when he comes back from playing. The boy's teacher also says he finds the boy squatting while playing outside during recess. Which of the following is the most likely diagnosis?

a. Atrial septal defect
b. Patent foramen ovale
c. Hypertrophic obstructive cardiomyopathy
d. Tetralogy of Fallot
e. Restrictive cardiomyopathy

Answer: **D**. The history of exercise intolerance and squatting while playing outside (tet spells) is pathognomonic for tetralogy of Fallot. The other options do not present with tet spells such as squatting during exertion.

Tetralogy of Fallot

Tetralogy of Fallot (TOF) is a condition characterized by:

- Overriding aorta
- Pulmonary stenosis
- Right ventricular hypertrophy
- Ventricular septal defect (VSD)

Its cause is thought to be due to genetic factors and environmental factors. It is associated with chromosome 22 deletions.

▶ TIP

Tetralogy of Fallot is the most common cyanotic heart defect in children.

TOF presents with:

- Cyanosis of the lips and extremities
- Holosystolic murmur best heard at the left lower sternal border
- Squatting after exertive activities
  - Causes an increased preload and increased systemic vascular resistance. This decreases the right-to-left shunting, leading to increased pulmonary blood flow, and increased blood oxygen saturation.

Diagnose with a chest x-ray (**best initial test**) showing:

- Boot-shaped heart
- Decreased pulmonary vascular marking

Surgical intervention is the only definitive therapy.

VSDs are common in **Down** (trisomy 21), **Edwards** (trisomy 18), and **Patau** (trisomy 13).

▶ **TIP**

There are only 3 holosystolic murmurs:

1. Mitral regurgitation
2. Tricuspid regurgitation
3. Ventricular septal defect

> The most common congenital heart defect in Down syndrome is endocardial cushion defect of atrioventricular canal.

Transposition of the Great Vessels

Transposition of the great vessels (TOGV) is characterized by an aorta that originates from the right ventricle and pulmonary artery that comes from the left ventricle. No oxygenation of blood can occur without a patent ductus arteriosus (PDA), atrial septal defect (ASD), or VSD.

Early and severe cyanosis is seen. A single S2 is heard. Chest x-ray will show an "egg on a string."

Treatment is to ensure that the neonate has a PDA. This requires prostaglandin E1 to keep the ductus open. NSAIDs are contraindicated because they will cause closure of the ductus.

Two separate surgeries are necessary; however, each surgery carries a 50% mortality rate. Therefore, only 1 in 4 will survive the surgeries.

> TOF is the most common cyanotic condition in children **after** the neonatal period. TOGV is the most common cyanotic lesion **during** the neonatal period.

Pulses

- Pulsus alternans: sign of left ventricular systolic dysfunction
- Pulsus bigeminus: sign of hypertrophic obstructive cardiomyopathy (HOCM)
- Pulsus bisferiens: in aortic regurgitation
- Pulsus tardus et parvus: aortic stenosis
- Pulsus paradoxus: cardiac tamponade and tension pneumothorax
- Irregularly irregular: atrial fibrillation

Hypoplastic Left Heart Syndrome

This is a syndrome consisting of left ventricular hypoplasia, mitral valve atresia, and aortic valve lesions.

This condition presents as follows:

- Absent pulses with a single S2
- Increased right ventricular impulse
- Gray rather than bluish cyanosis
- Inaudible murmurs
- Hyperdynamic precordium

Best initial test is chest x-ray, which will show a globular-shaped heart with pulmonary edema. Echocardiogram is the **most accurate diagnostic test**.

The only therapies are 3 staged surgeries or a heart transplant.

Truncus Arteriosus

Truncus arteriosus (TA) occurs when a single trunk emerges from both right and left ventricles and gives rise to all major circulations.

Symptoms occur within the first few days of life and are characterized by:

- Severe dyspnea
- Early and frequent respiratory infections

Single S2 is heard as there is only one semilunar valve and a systolic ejection murmur is heard because these valve leaflets are usually abnormal in functionality. Peripheral pulses are bounding.

Testing is chest x-ray, which will show cardiomegaly with increased pulmonary markings.

Treat with prompt surgery. Surgery must be completed early to prevent pulmonary hypertension, the most severe sequela of this condition. Without surgery, pulmonary hypertension will develop within 4 months.

Total Anomalous Pulmonary Venous Return

In total anomalous pulmonary venous return (TAPVR), there is no venous return between pulmonary veins and the left atrium. Oxygenated blood instead returns to the superior vena cava. This congenital condition has 2 forms: with or without obstruction of the venous return. *Obstruction* refers to the angle at which the veins enter the sinus.

TAPVR with and without Obstruction			
	Signs/symptoms	**Diagnostic tests**	**Treatment**
TAPVR with obstruction	Early in life with respiratory distress and severe cyanosis	CXR: pulmonary edema Echocardiography (**definitive**)	Surgery
TAPVR without obstruction	Age 1–2 years with right heart failure and tachypnea	CXR: snowman or figure 8 sign Echocardiogram (**most accurate** diagnostic test)	Surgical intervention

Tricuspid Valve Atresia

Tricuspid valve atresia presents as severe cyanosis in a newborn.

- Caused by lack of communication between the right heart chambers. Results in:
  - Hypoplastic right ventricular and pulmonary outflow tract
  - Underdeveloped pulmonary valve and/or artery

Patients with tricuspid valve atresia must also have an associated congenital PFO, ASD, or VSD, or they would not be alive; this additional abnormality allows for mixing of oxygenated and deoxygenated blood—and hence the infant's survival.

Chest x-ray will show decreased pulmonary flow. EKG will confirm left axis deviation and small or absent R waves in the precordial leads, along with left ventricular hypertrophy.

Treatment is as follows:

- Prostaglandin E1 to keep the PDA open until an aortopulmonary shunt can be performed
- Possible atrial balloon septostomy to enlarge the ASD
- Staged surgical correction

Acyanotic Lesions

A 3-month-old female infant is brought in because her parents say she will not eat anymore. Upon physical examination, a loud pansystolic murmur is observed. The child also appears small for her age, but her records show no maternal or delivery complications. Which of the following is the most likely finding on EKG?

a. Right ventricular hypertrophy
b. Right bundle branch block
c. ST segment elevation
d. QT interval prolongation
e. P wave inversion

Answer: **A.** The key to this case is understanding that a child who was otherwise healthy but presents with a holosystolic murmur and symptoms of failure to thrive most likely has a VSD. Right ventricular hypertrophy occurs from blood shunting from the high pressure left system to the low pressure right system. This could later lead to Eisenmenger syndrome (ES). ES is defined as the process in which a left-to-right shunt caused by a VSD reverses into a right-to-left shunt due to hypertrophy of the right ventricle.

Mitral lesions radiate to the axilla.

Tricuspid and pulmonary lesions radiate to the back.

Aortic lesions radiate to the neck.

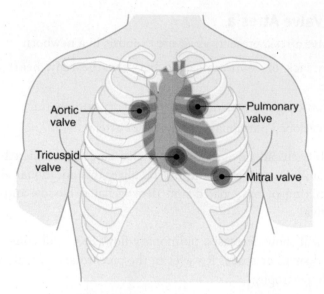

Figure 7.3 VSD, Murmurs, and Auscultation. © Kaplan

Summary of Cyanotic Heart Defects				
	R to L shunt	**PDA dependent**	**VSD**	**Surgery**
Tetralogy of Fallot	X		X	X
TGV	X	X		X
Hypoplastic left heart syndrome	X	X		X
Truncus arteriosus	X		X	X
TAPVR	X			X
Notes: PDA = patent ductus arteriosus; TAPVR = total anomalous pulmonary venous return; TOGV = transposition of the great vessels; VSD = ventricular septal defect.				

Ventricular Septal Defect

VSD is the most common congenital heart lesion. Look for:

- Dyspnea with respiratory distress
- High-pitched holosystolic murmur over lower left sternal border
- Loud pulmonic S2

Diagnostic testing is as follows:

- Chest x-ray shows increased vascular markings.
- Echocardiogram is diagnostic and cardiac catheterization is definitive.

Smaller lesions usually close in the first 1–2 years, while larger or more symptomatic lesions require surgical intervention. Diuretics and digoxin can be used for more conservative treatment. If left untreated, complications can lead to congestive heart failure (CHF), endocarditis, and pulmonary hypertension.

▶ **TIP**

Pansystolic = Holosystolic = Throughout systole

A 17-year-old boy who just flew from Australia and landed in New York presents in the ED with facial drooping, altered mental status, and left side paralysis. He took some diphenhydramine to get through the flight. Physical exam reveals a swollen left calf muscle. Which of the following is the most likely process underlying this patient's condition?

a. Emboli from his carotid artery
b. Emboli from his middle cerebral artery
c. Trauma brain injury
d. Paradoxical emboli from deep leg veins
e. Medication side effect

Answer: **D**. The patient most likely has thrown a clot to his brain. The clot was formed in the setting of venous stasis and was able to travel to his brain via a patent ASD. Without the ASD, this clot would have embolized to the pulmonary circulation. Choices (A) and (B) are incorrect because the patient is too young for such advanced vascular disease; (C) is incorrect because there is no history of trauma; diphenhydramine does not cause emboli, ruling out choice (E).

Atrial Septal Defect

ASD is a hole in the septum between both atria that is twice as common in females as in males.

There are 3 major types of ASD:

1. Primum defect: concomitant mitral valve abnormalities
2. Secundum defect: most common and located in the center of the atrial septum
3. Sinus venosus defect: least common

Patients are usually asymptomatic except for a fixed wide splitting of S2.

The **most definitive test** is cardiac catheterization. However, echocardiography is less invasive and can be just as effective. Chest x-ray (CXR) shows increased vascular markings and cardiomegaly.

The vast majority close spontaneously. Surgery or transcatheter closure is indicated for all symptomatic patients. ASD leads to dysrhythmias and possible paradoxical emboli from DVTs later in life.

Patent Ductus Arteriosus (PDA)

PDA is defined as the failure of spontaneous closure of the ductus. It usually closes when PO_2 rises above 50 mm Hg. Low PO_2 can be caused by pulmonary compromise due to prematurity. Areas of high altitude have an increased occurrence of PDA due to low levels of atmospheric oxygen.

▶ **TIP**

PDA is a normal finding in the first 12 hours of life. **After 24 hours it is considered pathologic.**

The condition presents with:

- "Machinery-like" murmur
- Wide pulse pressure
- Bounding pulses

A high occurrence of CHF and pulmonary hypertension is the most common complication later in the child's life.

Echocardiography is the **best initial test**, while cardiac catheterization is the **most accurate test**. EKG may show LVH secondary to high systemic resistance.

Treatment is to close the PDA unless it is needed to live in concurrent conditions such as TOF. Give ibuprofen (NSAID inhibits prostaglandins). Do surgical ligation if NSAID fails.

> Give **prostaglandins** to **pop** open a PDA.
> Give **NSAIDs** to **inhibit** popping.

Cardiac X-Ray Findings

- Pear-shaped: pericardial effusion
- Boot-shaped heart: tetralogy of Fallot
- Jug handle appearance: primary pulmonary artery hypertension
- "3"-like appearance or rib notching: coarctation of the aorta

---

Coarctation of the Aorta

Coarctation of the aorta is a congenital narrowing of the aorta in the area of ductus arteriosus. It has a frequent association with Turner syndrome.

▶ **TIP**

If the exam question mentions a short girl with webbed neck, shield chest, streak gonads, horseshoe kidneys, or shortened fourth metacarpal, think coarctation of the aorta.

Presentation is as follows:

- Severe CHF and respiratory distress within the first few months of life
- Differential pressures and pulses between the upper and lower extremities
- Reduced pulses in the lower extremities and hypertension in the upper extremities due to narrowing

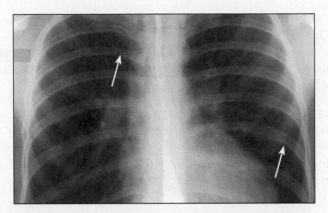

Figure 7.4 Due to increased pressure in the vasculature of the subcostal vessels, the ribs become eroded, leading to the notched appearance seen here. *Source: Niket Sonpal, MD.*

Diagnostic testing:

- Chest x-ray showing rib notching and a "3" sign
- Echocardiogram (**best initial test**)
- MRA (**most accurate test**)
- Echocardiography is the confirmatory test. Cardiac catheterization is the answer if the patient cannot get an MRA.

Primary treatment is surgical resection of the narrowed segment and then balloon dilation if recurrent stenosis occurs.

Long QT Syndrome

A 12-year-old boy is brought in by his mother after she found him unconscious. He quickly woke on the ride to the hospital and was without confusion. The mother states that he did not lose urinary continence and there were no episodes of shaking. He has had hearing loss since birth. An uncle died suddenly from a "heart condition." The boy has blood pressure of 123/75 mm Hg and a pulse rate of 76/min. His mucous membranes are wet, and his blood pressure does not change with standing.

1. What is the most likely diagnosis?

a. Seizure
b. Long QT syndrome
c. Orthostatic hypotension
d. Stroke
e. Vertigo

2. What is the best initial treatment for this patient?

a. Procainamide
b. Verapamil
c. Dronedarone
d. Amiodarone
e. Metoprolol

Answer 1: B. The combination of hearing loss, syncope, normal vital signs and physical exam, and the family history of sudden cardiac death is consistent with long QT syndrome. Seizure is not correct, as the child was not disoriented or postictal after the syncopal episode. Orthostatic BP was normal in the history. Stroke is unlikely in a 12-year-old boy. Vertigo does not cause a loss of consciousness.

Answer 2: E. The best treatment for long QT syndrome is a beta blocker such as metoprolol. Beta blockers may shorten the QT interval by decreasing activation from the left stellate ganglion and reducing cardiac excitation during exertion. If this child has symptoms again while on a beta blocker, then a pacemaker with implantable cardioverter-defibrillator capability may be indicated.

> Sotalol is the only beta blocker that prolongs the QT interval.

Rheumatic Fever

Rheumatic fever is an autoimmune disease resulting from untreated pharyngeal streptococcal infection, caused by cross-reactions between streptococcal antigens and the antigens on joint and heart tissue. Rheumatic heart disease (RHD) is a possible long-term consequence of rheumatic fever. While RHD can involve any heart valve, mitral stenosis is the most common outcome.

The Jones criteria establish the diagnosis of rheumatic fever. A patient is positive for rheumatic fever when either 2 of the major criteria or 1 major criterion plus 2 minor criteria are present, along with evidence of streptococcal infection (i.e., elevated or rising antistreptolysin O titer or DNase).

> Diagnosis is rheumatic fever in the presence of either of the following:
> - 2 major Jones criteria
> - 1 major criterion + 2 minor criteria

Major criteria	Minor criteria
• Migratory polyarthritis	• Fever
• Carditis (myocarditis, pericarditis)	• Arthralgias
• Erythema marginatum	• Elevated ESR/CRP
• Subcutaneous nodules	• Prolonged PR internal
• Chorea	• Heart block on EKG

Treat rheumatic fever with antibiotics to eradicate group A streptococcal bacteria. Patients with mitral valve disease from rheumatic fever should receive:

- Chronic penicillin therapy
  - Reduces recurrence risk of group A strep pharyngitis infection
  - Reduces progression of rheumatic heart disease
- NSAIDs or steroids to control inflammation

Ebstein Anomaly

Ebstein anomaly is a congenital heart defect in which the tricuspid valve is downwardly displaced into the right ventricle. This condition is associated with maternal lithium use in pregnancy. Physical examination will show a holosystolic murmur of tricuspid regurgitation over most of anterior left chest. EKG will show tall P waves and right axis deviation. Echocardiography is the best test to evaluate the anatomy, and cardiovascular MRI is used if the echo is nondiagnostic.

> Patients with Ebstein anomaly may have Wolff-Parkinson-White syndrome (delta wave and short PR interval).

Vascular Ring

Abnormal development of the aortic arch that forms a vascular ring can result in tracheal, bronchial, and/or esophageal compression. Patients with this congenital abnormality will present with biphasic stridor or dysphagia with spitting up after meals from compression. Key facts to look for in the patient history are respiratory symptoms that improve with neck extension and a statement from the parents that their child is a "noisy breather."

There are 2 types of vascular ring:

- Complete: circumferential around trachea and esophagus
- Incomplete: pulmonary artery sling

The diagnostic test of choice is CT or MRI. Patients with symptomatic vascular rings should undergo surgical correction. Asymptomatic, incidentally found rings should be monitored.

> Vascular rings can be seen in genetic or malformation syndromes such as DiGeorge syndrome or Down syndrome.

Gastroenterology

Pathologic Jaundice in the Newborn

Hyperbilirubinemia is considered pathological when:

- It appears on the first day of life.
- Bilirubin rises more than 5 mg/dL/day.
- Bilirubin rises above 19.5 mg/dL in a term child.
- Direct bilirubin rises above 2 mg/dL at any time.
- Hyperbilirubinemia persists after the second week of life.

The **most serious complication** is the deposition of bilirubin in the basal ganglia called kernicterus. Kernicterus presents with hypotonia, seizures, choreoathetosis, and hearing loss.

Diagnostic Testing

If jaundice presents in the first 24 hours, workup includes:

- Total and direct bilirubin
- Blood type of infant and mother: Look for ABO or Rh incompatibility.
- Direct Coombs test
- CBC, reticulocyte count, and blood smear: Assess for hemolysis.
- Urinalysis and urine culture if elevated direct bilirubin: Assess for sepsis.

To diagnose prolonged jaundice (>2 weeks), look at conjugated bilirubin.

	Think of:
Unconjugated bilirubin	• UTI or other infection • Bilirubin conjugation abnormalities (e.g., Gilbert syndrome, Crigler-Najjar syndrome) • Hemolysis • Intrinsic red blood cell membrane or enzyme defects (spherocytosis, elliptocytosis, glucose-6-phosphate dehydrogenase deficiency, pyruvate kinase deficiency)
Conjugated bilirubin	**Cholestasis:** Check liver function tests, ultrasound, and liver biopsy

Treatment

- Phototherapy when bilirubin >10–12 mg/dL (normally decreases by 2 mg/dL every 4–6 hours)
- Exchange transfusion in any infant with suspected bilirubin encephalopathy or failure of phototherapy to reduce total bilirubin and risk of kernicterus

Bilirubin-Induced Neurologic Dysfunction (BIND)

BIND is an umbrella term for the toxic sequelae of indirect bilirubin entering the brain (i.e., acute bilirubin encephalopathy and kernicterus). Unconjugated bilirubin, which is not bound to albumin, can enter the brain and cause cell death by apoptosis and/or necrosis.

Acute Bilirubin Encephalopathy

Acute bilirubin encephalopathy is the acute form of BIND. Symptoms are grouped by severity into phases.

- **Phase 1**: infant is sleepy but arousable and has a high-pitched cry
- **Phase 2**: infant is more lethargic, with a poor sucking reflex and the development of hypertonia, beginning with backward arching of the neck (retrocollis) and trunk (opisthotonos) with stimulation; next step in management is emergent exchange transfusion
- **Phase 3**: infant is apneic, unable to feed, and experiencing fever, seizures, and coma; may result in death due to respiratory failure or intractable seizures

Kernicterus

Kernicterus is the chronic and permanent neurologic sequelae of BIND. It is characterized by:

- Choreoathetoid cerebral palsy
- Significant hearing loss due to auditory neuropathy
- Gaze palsy, especially upward gaze
- Dental enamel dysplasia

Gilbert Syndrome

This is the most common inherited disorder of bilirubin glucuronidation. Gilbert syndrome is characterized by recurrent episodes of jaundice, often triggered in situations of high physical stress (dehydration, fasting, menstruation, overexertion). Patients are typically asymptomatic except for the jaundice.

Gilbert syndrome results from a mutation in the gene that codes for the enzyme uridine diphosphoglucuronic-glucuronosyltransferase 1A1 (UGT1A1), which is responsible for the conjugation of bilirubin with glucuronic acid. No specific therapy is required.

Esophageal Atresia

Upon her first feeding, a 1-day-old child begins to choke and exhales milk bubbles from her nose, then appears to be in significant respiratory distress. Chest x-ray reveals an air bubble in the upper esophagus and no gas pattern in the remainder of the GI tract. A coiled nasogastric tube is also seen. What is the most common complication of this condition?

a. Meningitis
b. Pneumonia
c. Dental caries
d. Dyspepsia
e. Belching

Answer: **B.** The signs described both on physical exam and radiological exam point toward an esophageal atresia with a tracheoesophageal fistula. Aspiration pneumonia is a severe and common complication of this condition as food contents are aspirated via the fistula in the respiratory system. Aspiration leads to abscess formation from anaerobic proliferation. Dental caries cannot form because the child is only 1 day old and therefore does not have teeth. Food cannot reach the stomach, so there is no possibility for either dyspepsia or belching.

In esophageal atresia (EA), the esophagus ends blindly. In nearly 90% of cases, it communicates with the trachea through a fistula known as a tracheoesophageal fistula (TEF).

Presentation

The child will typically exhibit "vomiting with first feeding" or choking/coughing and cyanosis due to the TEF. There will be a history of possible polyhydramnios.

Recurrent aspiration pneumonia occurs when food and secretions travel into lungs via the TEF.

If you see **recurrent aspiration pneumonia**, consider TEF.

Diagnostic Tests

- A gastric air bubble and esophageal air bubble can be seen on chest x-ray (CXR).
- Coiling of the NG tube seen on CXR and an inability to pass it into the stomach are diagnostic.

- CT or esophagram with water-soluble contrast is the **most accurate test**.
- TEF/EA is often part of a constellation of other abnormalities (CHARGE syndrome, VACTERL association). Echocardiography and renal ultrasonography should be performed in all infants in whom TEF has been identified.

Treatment

Treatment of TEF consists of surgical separation of the trachea and esophagus by ligation of the fistula. The most common long-term complications are dysphagia and GERD.

- Antibiotic coverage for anaerobes must also be considered due to high risk of lung abscess formation secondary to aspiration.
- Fluid resuscitation before surgery must be done to prevent dehydration of the infant.

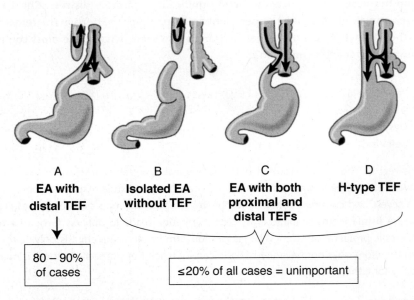

A	B	C	D
EA with distal TEF	**Isolated EA without TEF**	**EA with both proximal and distal TEFs**	**H-type TEF**

80 – 90% of cases

≤20% of all cases = unimportant

Figure 7.5 Esophageal Fistula Types

A 1-month-old child is fed, after which he has vomitus that is forceful, projecting across the nursery. The vomitus is nonbloody and nonbilious. Physical examination reveals a palpable mass in the abdomen. An upper GI series is ordered. Which of the following is the most likely finding on this radiologic exam?

a. String sign
b. Doughnut sign
c. Bird's beak sign
d. Steeple sign
e. Murphy sign

Answer: **A.** Projectile vomiting and palpable abdominal mass are characteristic of pyloric stenosis. String sign is seen on upper GI series (barium is swallowed, and its passage is watched under fluoroscopy). Doughnut sign is seen during intussusceptions. Bird's beak is seen in achalasia, steeple sign is seen during croup, and the Murphy sign is not a radiological sign, but rather a physical exam sign with right upper quadrant tenderness that causes cessation of breathing.

Pyloric Stenosis

A hypertrophic pyloric sphincter prevents proper passage of GI contents from the stomach into the duodenum. The most common cause is idiopathic.

Hypertrophy of the pylorus is not commonly found at birth but rather becomes most pronounced by the first month of life. It can present as late as 6 months after birth.

Look for the following features:

- Succussion splash on auscultation (sound of stomach contents slapping into the pylorus like waves on a beach)
- Nonbilious projectile vomiting (hallmark feature)
  - Due to hypochloremic, hypokalemic metabolic alkalosis
  - Aldosterone release in response to hypovolemia worsens potassium loss by increasing urinary excretion of potassium
- Olive sign is highly associated (i.e., palpable mass the size of an olive in the epigastric region)

The **best initial test** is an abdominal ultrasound that will show a thickened pyloric sphincter.

The **most accurate test** is an upper GI series, which will show 4 signs:

1. String sign: thin column of barium leaking through the tightened muscle
2. Shoulder sign: filling defect in the antrum due to prolapse of muscle inward
3. Mushroom sign: hypertrophic pylorus against the duodenum
4. Railroad track sign: excess mucosa in the pyloric lumen resulting in 2 columns of barium

Treat as follows:

- Replace lost volume with IV fluids
  - Replacement of lost electrolytes, specifically potassium, is crucial to close the anion gap.
- NG tube to decompress the bowel
- Surgical myotomy must follow

> On the USMLE, hypochloremic hypokalemic metabolic alkalosis is almost always caused by vomiting.

Atresias		
Esophageal atresia	**Choanal atresia**	**Duodenal atresia**
Blind esophagus Presents with: • Frothing, cough, cyanosis, and respiratory distress **with feeds** • No respiratory distress **at rest** Initial test: • Chest x-ray Concerns: • Aspiration pneumonia	Buccopharyngeal membrane **Yes** respiratory distress Best initial step: • Pass NG tube Most diagnostic: • CT scan First step in management: • Secure airway!	Failed duodenal canalization **No** respiratory distress Bilious vomiting Initial test: • Abdominal x-ray • Double-bubble Trisomy 21 First step in management: • IV fluids

Choanal Atresia

In choanal atresia, the infant is born with a membrane between the nostrils and pharyngeal space that prevents breathing during feeding. This condition is associated with CHARGE syndrome.

> **CHARGE syndrome is a set of congenital defects seen in conjunction:**
>
> **C:** coloboma of the eye, CNS anomalies
>
> **H:** heart defects
>
> **A:** atresia of the choanae
>
> **R:** retardation of growth and/or development
>
> **G:** genital and/or urinary defects (hypogonadism)
>
> **E:** ear anomalies and/or deafness

A child with this condition will turn blue when feeding and then pink when crying. This recurrent series of events is clinically diagnostic.

Diagnosis is confirmed by CT scan.

The only definitive treatment is surgical intervention to perforate the membrane and reconnect the pharynx to the nostrils.

Hirschsprung Disease

Hirschsprung disease is a congenital lack of innervation of the distal bowel by the Auerbach plexus. This lack causes a constant contracture of muscle tone. There is a frequent association with Down syndrome, and it is more common in boys than in girls (approximately 4:1).

Hirschsprung disease presents in the neonate as follows:

- First meconium passed >48 hours or none passed at all (90% of unaffected infants pass first meconium ≤24 hours)
- Extreme constipation followed by large bowel obstruction
- Extremely tight sphincter on rectal exam; inability to pass flatus also common

Diagnostic testing is as follows:

- Plain x-rays show distended bowel loops with a lack of air in the rectum. Contrast enemas will show retention of barium for >24 hours.
- Manometry will show high pressures in the anal sphincter.
- The mainstay of diagnosis is a full thickness biopsy that reveals a lack of ganglionic cells in the submucosa.

Treatment is surgical repair.

Imperforate Anus

With imperforate anus, the opening to the anus is missing and the rectum ends in a blind pouch with conservation of the sphincter. The cause is unknown, but the condition is highly associated with Down syndrome.

Complete failure to pass meconium is diagnostic. A physical exam will reveal no anus. Surgery is curative.

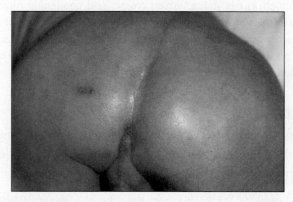

Figure 7.6 Imperforate anus is a clinical diagnosis from extreme constipation and absence of an anal orifice on physical exam. *Source: Niket Sonpal, MD.*

> Imperforate anus is one of the components of VACTERL syndrome:
> **V:** vertebral anomalies
> **A:** anal atresia
> **C:** cardiovascular anomalies
> **T:** tracheoesophageal fistula
> **E:** esophageal atresia
> **R:** renal anomalies
> **L:** limb anomalies

> The most common **wrong answers** for diagnostic testing are barium study and rectal manometry.

A 1-day-old child is given her first feeding, at which time she begins to vomit very dark green fluid. On physical examination, the child has oblique eye fissures with epicanthic skin folds and a single palmar crease. A holosystolic murmur is also heard. Abdominal x-ray reveals a double bubble sign. Which of the following is the most likely diagnosis?

a. Biliary atresia
b. Duodenal atresia
c. Volvulus
d. Intussusception
e. Pyloric stenosis

Answer: **B.** The child's bilious vomiting on the first day of life is the prototypic finding in children with this condition. Furthermore, the description of Down syndrome–like characteristics such as eye shape, simian crease, and congenital murmur also points to duodenal atresia. Volvulus and intussusception would present with symptoms of obstruction such as distension and failure to pass flatus and stool, and do not have vomiting as a presenting symptom. Biliary atresia would not have any bilious vomiting, nor would pyloric stenosis. Pyloric stenosis has a projectile vomitus.

Duodenal Atresia

Duodenal atresia (DA) is due to an absence of apoptosis (programmed cell death) that leads to improper canalization of the lumen of the duodenum. It is associated with an annular pancreas and Down syndrome.

Typical presentation of DA is characterized by the onset of bilious vomiting within 12 hours of birth.

Test as follows:

- Abdominal x-ray: shows classic double bubble sign
- Upper gastrointestinal contrast study with water-soluble contrast (**most accurate test**)

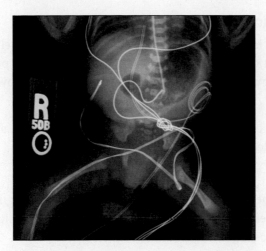

Figure 7.7 X-ray of Duodenal Atresia with Double Bubble Sign.
Source: James C. Pascual, MD.

Treat DA by replacing lost volume with IV fluids, taking special care to replace lost electrolytes. Potassium is often low from vomiting. Use a nasogastric tube to decompress the bowel. Surgical duodenostomy is the most common surgical procedure and **definitive treatment**.

Volvulus

A volvulus is a bowel obstruction in which a loop of bowel has twisted on itself abnormally.

The signs are nonspecific and include vomiting and colicky abdominal pain. On upper GI series, multiple air-fluid levels are visible and a "bird's beak" appearance is typically seen at the site of rotation.

Treatment is emergently needed to avoid life-threatening sepsis from bowel necrosis and perforation.

- **Best initial therapy**: endoscopic decompression
- **Most effective therapy** (if endoscopy fails): surgical decompression

> A 1-year-old child is having his diaper changed when his father notices the stool looks like a purple jelly. He is rushed to the ED, where the father reports that the previous night, the child was very irritable, complained of pain, and had an episode of vomiting. On physical exam the child seems lethargic and a firm sausage-shaped mass is palpated. Which of the following is the most likely diagnosis?
>
> a. Biliary atresia
> b. Duodenal atresia
> c. Volvulus
> d. Intussusception
> e. Pyloric stenosis
>
> **Answer: D.** Intussusception presents with currant jelly stool, sausage-shaped mass, neurologic signs, and abdominal pains. The remaining choices do not fit this description.

> In children, volvulus occurs in the midgut, with the majority being in the ileum.

Intussusception

Intussusception is a condition in which part of the bowel telescopes into another segment of bowel distal to it. It can be caused by a polyp, hard stool, or lymphoma, or can even have a viral origin. Most often, however, there is no clear etiology.

It presents with colicky abdominal pain, bilious vomiting, and currant jelly stool. A right-sided, sausage-shaped mass can be palpated.

Test as follows:

- Ultrasound (**best initial test**) will show a doughnut sign or target sign, which is generated by concentric alternating echogenic (mucosa) and hypoechogenic (submucosa) bands.
- Barium enema (**most accurate test**)
  - Both diagnostic and therapeutic
  - Contraindicated if signs of peritonitis, shock, or perforation

Treat as follows:

- Fluid resuscitation and rebalancing electrolytes (K^+, Ca^{+2}, Mg^{+2}) (**most important initial steps**)
- NG tube decompression of the bowel
- Barium enema; must carefully monitor (approximately 10% of intussusceptions recur within 24 hours)
- Emergent surgical intervention (if barium enema is not curative) to prevent bowel necrosis

> **Currant jelly** is seen with *Klebsiella* pneumonia in the lungs as sputum, or as stool in the setting of intussusception.

A 16-month-old boy is brought in by his mother after she notices bright red blood in his diaper. The mother states the child has not been crying more than usual and has not had any changes in feeding habits. His examination reveals a mass palpated in the left upper quadrant, and his vital signs are stable. Labs show a normal hematocrit. What is the most accurate test for this condition?

a. Colonoscopy
b. Flexible sigmoidoscopy
c. CT scan
d. Meckel scan
e. Repeat hemoglobin

Answer: **D**. When presented with painless bright red blood per rectum in a male child age <2 years, you must consider Meckel diverticulum. A technetium-99m (99mTc) pertechnetate scan, also called a Meckel scan, is the most accurate test for this presentation. Endoscopy is not indicated in this condition, and CT scan has low yield for diagnosis. Rechecking the hemoglobin will not be of any value, as the amount of bleeding is not drastic enough to cause a modest decrease.

Bilious Vomiting			
Condition	**Duodenal atresia**	**Volvulus**	**Intussusception**
Onset	Within the first day of life	Within the first year of life	Within the first year of life
Initial Test	AXR	AXR	Ultrasound "doughnut"
First Step	"Double bubble" Intravenous fluids	Intravenous fluids	Intravenous fluids
Treatment	Surgery	Surgery	Air enema

> Meckel diverticulum is a true congenital diverticulum and involves all layers of the bowel.

Meckel Diverticulum

Meckel diverticulum is the only true congenital diverticulum in which the vitelline duct persists in the small intestinal tract. It can contain ectopic gastric tissue. Meckel diverticulum is the most common congenital anomaly of the gastrointestinal tract.

The classic presentation is with painless rectal bleeding. Massive frank bright red blood per rectum is due to gastric acid secretion by the ectopic tissue causing searing of the nearby small bowel tissue.

The **most accurate test** for Meckel diverticulum is a technetium 99m scan. It is so accurate that it has been dubbed a "Meckel scan." Surgical removal of the diverticulum is the only curative therapy.

> **Meckel Diverticulum Rule of 2s**
> - Affects 2% of population
> - Occurs 2 feet from the ileocecal valve
> - Affects 2 types of ectopic tissue (gastric and pancreatic)
> - Male patients 2 times more affected
> - Patient age <2 years
> - Only 2% of patients symptomatic
> - About 2 inches long

Diarrhea and Gastroenteritis

Acute diarrhea—the acute loss of fluids and electrolytes in the stool due to underlying pathologic process—is the second most common cause of infant death worldwide. Gastroenteritis is the inflammation of the GI tract secondary to microbiologic infiltrate and spread.

> Acute diarrhea is the #2 cause of infant death worldwide.

Presentation

- Inflammatory diarrhea will have fever, abdominal pain, and possibly bloody diarrhea.
- Noninflammatory diarrhea will have vomiting, crampy abdominal pain, and watery diarrhea.

Diagnostic Tests

- Send stool for blood and leukocyte count to detect the presence of invasive toxins.
- Stool cultures with O&P for identifying the causative agent
- PCR for *C. difficile* is the single **most accurate test**.

Treatment

The most important next step is rehydration.

- **Mild** cases: oral fluids
- **Severe** cases: IV fluids

Antidiarrheal compounds such as loperamide are never correct.

Endocrinology

Infants of Diabetic Mothers (IDMs)

A 10.5-pound infant is born to a mother with type 1 diabetes. Upon examination the newborn is shaking, and a holosystolic murmur is heard over the precordium. The baby's right arm is adducted and internally rotated. His lab findings show elevated bilirubin. Which of the following is the most appropriate next step in management?

a. IV insulin
b. Blood sugar level
c. Serum calcium levels
d. Serum TSH
e. CT head and neck

Answer: **B.** Infants of diabetic mothers (IDMs) are born macrosomic, with plethora, and can be very jittery. In utero, these infants usually had dramatically high circulating levels of glucose, but upon delivery, maternal glucose is no longer available. This child is still producing high levels of insulin, and thus his blood sugar levels have dropped. Cardiac anomalies are common, as in this child, who most likely has a VSD. When we think of diabetes, our first thought is insulin treatment. This is the most common *wrong* answer, since it would further exacerbate these newborns' problems.

Findings in IDM include macrosomia; small left colon syndrome; and cardiac, renal, and metabolic abnormalities.

Macrosomia

With macrosomia, all organs are enlarged except for the brain. An increased output from the bone marrow leads to polycythemia and hyperviscosity. Possible shoulder dystocia and brachial plexus palsy can also be in the history.

Small Left Colon Syndrome

A congenitally smaller descending colon leads to distension from constipation. It can be diagnosed by a barium study and treated with smaller and more frequent feeds.

Cardiac Abnormalities

The major cardiac change in IDM is asymmetric septal hypertrophy due to obliteration of the left ventricular chamber, leading to decreased cardiac output. It is diagnosed with echocardiography and treated with beta blockers and IV fluids.

Renal Vein Thrombosis

- Flank mass and possible bruit can be appreciated
- Hematuria and thrombocytopenia

Metabolic Findings and Effects

- Hypoglycemia: seizures
- Hypocalcemia: tetany
- Hypomagnesemia: hypocalcemia and PTH decrease
- Hyperbilirubinemia: icterus and kernicterus

Orthopedics/Rheumatology

A 2-year-old girl who resides in England is brought in for a routine visit. She appears to walk abnormally and falls a great deal when she tries to play with her older brother. The child's delivery was unremarkable. She does not like milk and withdrew from both breastfeeding and cow's milk quite early. Physical exam reveals a very unsteady gait and bowing of the tibia, and x-ray reveals a beading of the ribs and genu varum. What is the most likely diagnosis?

a. Rickets
b. Kartagener syndrome
c. Coarctation of the aorta
d. Traumatic fracture
e. Cerebellar injury

Answer: **A.** Vitamin D–deficient rickets is a disorder caused by a lack of vitamin D and calcium. This child's risk factors include living in a sunless environment and low milk intake. The child displays classic signs including a "rachitic rosary" of the ribs on CXR and bowing of tibia. Kartagener syndrome is characterized by infertility and situs inversus. Coarctation has rib notching on the CXR; traumatic injury would show a clearer break of the tibia; and cerebellar injury would present with ataxia rather than simply an unsteady gait.

Musculoskeletal Diseases				
Disease	**Age**	**Presentation**	**Diagnosis**	**Treatment**
Congenital hip dysplasia	Infants	Usually found on newborn exam screening	Ortolani and Barlow maneuver "Click" or "clunk" in the hip	Pavlik harness
Legg-Calvé-Perthes disease (avascular necrosis of femoral head)	Ages 2–8	Painful limp	X-rays show joint effusions and widening	Rest and NSAIDs Follow with surgery on both hips: If one necroses, eventually so will the other
Slipped capital femoral epiphysis	Adolescence, especially in obese patients	Painful limp Externally rotated leg	X-ray shows widening of joint space	Internal fixation with pinning

Rickets

Rickets is a disorder caused by a lack of vitamin D, calcium, or phosphate. It leads to softening and weakening of the bones, making them more susceptible to fractures. Children 6–24 months are at highest risk because their bones are rapidly growing. There are 3 main etiologies of rickets:

1. Vitamin D-**deficient** rickets caused by a **lack of enough vitamin D** in the child's diet.

2. Vitamin D-**dependent** rickets is the **inability to convert** 25-OH to $1,25(OH)_2$ and therefore the infant is dependent on vitamin D supplementation.

3. X-linked **hypophosphatemic** rickets occurs when an innate kidney defect results in the **inability to retain phosphate**. Without phosphate, adequate bone mineralization cannot take place and bones are weakened.

Child will present with ulnar/radial bowing and a waddling gait due to tibial/femoral bowing.

Diagnostic testing includes:

- Chest x-ray of the costochondral joints shows rachitic rosary-like appearance, with cupping and fraying of the epiphyses
- Bowlegs (characteristic sign)

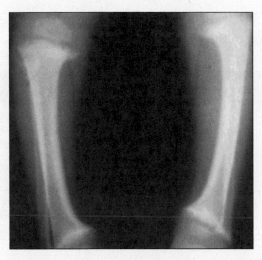

Figure 7.8 Bowlegs are a common physical finding in deficient rickets.
Source: Niket Sonpal, MD.

Treatment is replacement of phosphate, calcium, and vitamin D in the form of ergocalciferol or 1,25(OH)$_2$, calcitriol. Monitor vitamin D with blood testing annually.

Chemical Consequences of Vitamin D Disorders				
Type	**Calcium**	**Phosphate**	**1,25(OH)$_2$ Vit. D**	**25(OH) Vit. D**
Vitamin D-deficient	Normal or decreased	Decreased	Decreased	Decreased
Vitamin D-dependent	Decreased	Normal	Decreased	Normal
X-linked hypophosphatemia	Normal	Decreased	Normal	Normal

Lead Poisoning

Look for a child with a recent loss of appetite, intermittent abdominal pain, vomiting, decreased hours of sleep at night, and withdrawal from school activities. Learning disabilities and behavioral problems are also common in children with lead poisoning.

The **best initial test** is a capillary blood finger-stick for lead level. The **most accurate test** is a serum venous blood level. Intervention is needed if the value is >10 mcg/dL.

The **best initial step** is to remove the child from the offending exposure. Depending upon the degree of lead poisoning, chelation therapy with dimercaprol or succimer may be indicated.

Osteogenesis Imperfecta (OI)

OI is the most likely diagnosis when a young child presents with repeated fractures caused by fragile bones, blue sclerae, and early deafness.

The most **accurate test** for OI is skin biopsy analyzed for collagen synthesis by culturing dermal fibroblasts.

There is no cure for OI. Therapy is aimed at fracture management, increasing bone mass, and correcting of deformities.

Type	X-ray appearance	Most accurate diagnostic test	Therapy
Ewing sarcoma	Onionskin pattern due to lytic lesions causing laminar periosteal elevation	Analysis for a translocation t(11;22) via bone biopsy	Multidrug chemotherapy as well as local disease control with surgery and radiation
Osteogenic sarcoma	Sclerotic destruction causing a "sunburst" appearance	CT scan of the leg	Therapy includes chemotherapy and ablative surgery
Osteoid osteoma	Round central lucency with a sclerotic margin	CT scan or MRI of the affected leg	NSAIDs for pain, because the condition will resolve spontaneously

Juvenile Idiopathic Arthritis

Juvenile idiopathic arthritis (JIA), also known as juvenile rheumatoid arthritis (JRA) or adult Still disease, is difficult to define and there is no known etiology. This does not stop it, however, from appearing on virtually every USMLE exam as either the correct answer or one of the distracters.

Juvenile idiopathic arthritis (JIA) is the most common type of arthritis in children, and "JIA" is an umbrella term for 6 conditions. All 6 are chronic idiopathic synovitis of peripheral joints associated with soft tissue swelling, joint effusion, and elevated markers of inflammation such as ESR and CRP.

Systemic-onset JIA causes inflammation in one or more joints. It is often accompanied by a high-spiking fever lasting ≥2 weeks accompanied by a salmon-pink macular rash that comes and goes. Other possible findings include hepatosplenomegaly, lymphadenopathy, serositis, hepatitis anemia, and lymphadenopathy. Rheumatoid factor and ANA are generally negative in systemic JIA.

Oligoarticular JIA causes arthritis in up to 4 joints—typically the large ones e.g., knees, ankles, elbows. Uveitis is a common extraarticular manifestation. A positive antinuclear antibody (ANA) is highly associated with the greatest risk of developing eye conditions.

The hip is spared in oligoarticular JIA.

- If ANA is positive: do an eye exam every 3 months
- If ANA is negative and patient age >7: do an eye exam every 6 months

Polyarticular JIA causes inflammation in 5 or more joints. It is symmetric in presentation and is common in the hands, neck, and jaw, but large weightbearing joints are also affected. Polyarthritis can be either positive or negative for rheumatoid factor; positive serology is associated with more severe sequelae.

Juvenile psoriatic arthritis is arthritis that usually occurs in combination with psoriasis. The psoriasis may begin many years before any joint symptoms. A positive family history of psoriasis in a first-degree relative is commonly seen, plus dactylitis, pitting of the fingers, or onycholysis.

Enthesitis-related JIA is characterized by tenderness where the bone meets a tendon, ligament, or other connective tissue. Sacroiliac joint tenderness, axial joint involvement, and a family history of IBD are common. Affected children will often test positive for the HLA-B27 gene.

"What Is the Most Likely Diagnosis?"

The **most important feature** of JRA is the presence of high, spiking fever (often >40 C (104 F) in a young person with no clearly identified etiology but is associated with a rash.

Still disease:

- Salmon-colored rash
- Temperature elevation
- Ill-appearing patient
- Lymphadenopathy
- Leukocytosis
- Splenomegaly

Diagnostic testing is as follows:

- No clear diagnostic test
- Anemia, hypoalbuminemia, and leukocytosis (common)
- Normal ANA
- Markedly elevated ferritin (an acute phase reactant that rises with inflammation)

Treatment starts with aspirin or NSAIDs (50% success rate). If there is no response, use steroids. Steroid-resistant cases are treated with TNF drugs.

Marfan Syndrome

Marfan syndrome is an autosomal dominant mutation of the FBN1 gene on chromosome 15. This gene encodes fibrillin protein, which makes up a major part of bones, connective tissue, and blood vessels.

Look for a tall, thin patient with long extremities (arm span exceeds height), arachnodactyly, pectus excavatum, and hypermobile joints.

Diagnosis is made clinically, but genetic testing is the **most accurate test**.

- Aortic root dissection is common in Marfan, so do a transthoracic echocardiogram at the time of diagnosis and again 6 months later to establish whether the aortic root is stable; consider surgical intervention if dilation is seen.
- Annual ophthalmologic evaluation is recommended to screen for ectopia lentis.

Treatment is supportive.

> Aortic dissection is the most common cause of death in Marfan syndrome.

Kawasaki Disease

Kawasaki disease is necrotizing febrile vasculitis of medium-sized vessels that primarily affects the large coronary blood vessels. It occurs in children. Look for a child with >5 days fever and all 5 of the following criteria:

1. Rash

2. Mucositis

3. Edema or erythema of hands and feet

4. Cervical lymphadenopathy

5. Limbus-sparing bilateral conjunctivitis

Other symptoms are elevated WBC and platelets, transaminases, and acute phase reactants, as well as anemia and pyuria.

Treatment is IVIG and aspirin as soon as the diagnosis is made, to prevent the development of coronary artery aneurysm (**most important complication**). IVIG reduces the risk (mechanism of action unknown).

Steroids are of no help in Kawasaki and actually increase aneurysm formation.

Infectious Disease

A 6-month-old boy is brought in by his mother after what she describes as a seizure. He has had a fever of 38 C (100.4 F) for 3 days and has been very irritable. In the ED, he appears unresponsive. Physical examination reveals a markedly delayed capillary refill and blood pressure 80/20 mm Hg. What is the most likely diagnosis?

a. Febrile seizure

b. Absence seizure

c. Dog bite

d. Cocaine withdrawal

e. Epilepsy

Answer: **A.** This child has febrile seizure secondary to sepsis. The key here is to evaluate the child for the underlying cause of the sepsis. Understanding he has had a febrile seizure is only the surface of the case. A full sepsis evaluation must be ordered: CBC with differential blood and urine cultures, urinalysis, chest x-ray, and lumbar puncture (if irritability or lethargy is mentioned = meningitis). Dog bite does not present with seizure. Cocaine withdrawal does not cause seizure.

Neonatal Sepsis

Sepsis	
Most common causes	Pneumonia Meningitis
Most common organisms	Group B strep *E. coli* *S. aureus* *Listeria monocytogenes*
Diagnostic tests	Blood culture Urine culture Chest x-ray
Treatment	Ampicillin and gentamicin

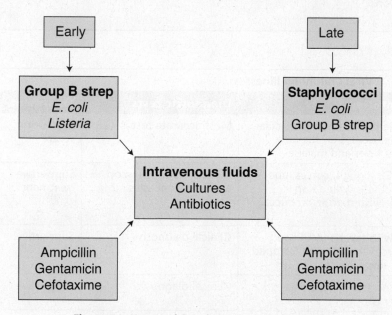

Figure 7.9 Neonatal Sepsis Onset and Treatment

T: toxoplasmosis

O: other infections such as *Syphilis*

R: rubella

C: cytomegalovirus

H: herpes simplex virus

TORCH Infections			
Type	**Presentation**	**Diagnostic tests**	**Treatment**
Toxoplasmosis	Chorioretinitis, hydrocephalus, and multiple ring-enhancing lesions on CT caused by *Toxoplasma gondii*	Best initial test is elevated IgM to toxoplasma; most accurate test is PCR for toxoplasmosis.	Pyrimethamine and sulfadiazine
Syphilis	Rash on the palms and soles, snuffles, frontal bossing, Hutchinson eighth nerve palsy, and saddle nose	Best initial test is VDRL or RPR; most accurate test is FTA ABS or dark field microscopy.	Penicillin
Rubella	PDA, cataracts, deafness, hepatosplenomegaly, thrombocytopenia, blueberry muffin rash, and hyperbilirubinemia	Maternal IgM status along with clinical diagnosis. Each disease manifestation must be individually addressed.	Supportive
CMV	Periventricular calcifications with microencephaly, chorioretinitis, hearing loss, and petechiae	Best initial test is urine or saliva viral titers; most accurate test is urine or saliva PCR for viral DNA.	Ganciclovir with signs of end organ damage
Herpes	Week 1: shock and DIC Week 2: vesicular skin lesions Week 3: encephalitis	Most accurate test is PCR.	Acyclovir

Viral Childhood Illnesses				
Virus	**Etiology**	**Presentation**	**Diagnostic tests**	**Treatment**
Varicella	Varicella zoster virus	Multiple highly pruritic vesicular rash that begins on the face; possible fever and malaise	Most accurate test is PCR	Acyclovir if severe
Rubeola or measles	Paramyxovirus	The 3 C's: cough, coryza, and conjunctivitis with a Koplik spot (grayish macule on buccal surface)	Clinical diagnosis; most accurate is measles IgM antibodies	Supportive treatment
Fifth disease or erythema infectiosum	Parvovirus B19	Starts with fever and URI and progresses to rash with "slapped cheek" appearance	Clinical diagnosis	Supportive
Roseola	Herpesvirus types 6 and 7	Fever and URI progressing to diffuse rash	Clinical diagnosis	Supportive
Mumps	Paramyxovirus	Fever precedes classic parotid gland swelling with possible orchitis.	Clinical diagnosis	Supportive

A 5-year-old girl is noted to be fatigued and lethargic in class. Her schoolteacher observes that she has a beefy, swollen tongue, and the school nurse calls your office because she is febrile. The nurse says the girl's skin feels coarse, like sandpaper, and her tongue looks like a strawberry. Upon examination, you find that the child's rash blanches easily. There is no desquamation of the lips. What is the next step in management?

a. Order blood cultures.
b. Start antibiotics.
c. Start IVIG.
d. Check ESR.
e. Continue observation.

Answer: **B.** Penicillin is the best next step in management. Scarlet fever is an infectious disease caused by *Streptococcus pyogenes* that presents with sore throat, strawberry tongue, and a sandpaper-like rash that blanches easily. The rashes in the inguinal areas and axillary folds of the body are known as Pastia lines. Complications are acute rheumatic fever and glomerulonephritis. IVIG does nothing for scarlet fever. ESR is too nonspecific to be helpful.

Scarlet Fever

Scarlet fever is a diffuse erythematous eruption that is concurrent with pharyngitis. It is caused by erythrogenic toxin made by *Streptococcus pyogenes* and typically lasts 3–6 days.

Symptoms include a classic pentad of (1) fever, (2) pharyngitis, (3) sandpaper rash over trunk and extremities, (4) strawberry tongue, and (5) cervical lymphadenopathy.

Diagnosis of scarlet fever is made clinically; however, it can be correlated with an elevated antistreptolysin O titer, ESR, and CRP.

Treatment is with penicillin, azithromycin, or cephalosporins.

Retropharyngeal Abscess

Retropharyngeal abscess is a deep neck-space infection. Because of its potential for airway compromise and other catastrophic complications, **it can pose an immediate life-threatening emergency**. The most common cause is group A beta-hemolytic streptococci.

Look for a patient with decreased or painful range of motion of the neck or jaw. Some patients may present with a muffled "hot potato" voice and deviated uvula.

CT of the neck can distinguish between an abscess and cellulitis. Incision and drainage of the abscess is the best therapy. The fluid should be collected and sent for culture. While waiting for culture results, administer ampicillin-sulbactam.

Pulmonary Disease

A 2-year-old girl is brought in for a severe cough, fever, and runny nose. The cough sounds like a bark and she is in obvious respiratory distress. Upon physical examination she refuses to lie flat. Neck x-ray shows a steeple sign. What is the most appropriate next step in management?

a. Intubate
b. Racemic epinephrine
c. Empiric antibiotics
d. Acetaminophen
e. CT neck

Answer: **B**. These are the signs of croup, an inflammation that is quite literally choking off the upper airway. The seal-like barking cough with URI-like symptoms gives it away. **This is a medical emergency.** To prevent asphyxiation and probable tracheostomy, administer racemic epinephrine and steroids to decrease swelling. Do not waste time with radiology. There is no medical evidence suggesting that intubation, antibiotics, or antipyretics decrease mortality.

Croup

Croup is an infectious upper airway condition characterized by severe inflammation. It is most commonly caused by parainfluenza virus types 1 and 2. Respiratory syncytial virus (RSV) is the second most common cause.

Croup presents with barking cough, coryza, and inspiratory stridor. The child will have more difficulty breathing when lying down and may show signs of hypoxia such as peripheral cyanosis and accessory muscle use. Chest x-ray will show the classic steeple sign, a narrowing of the air column in the trachea. However, x-ray is rarely done and is always the wrong answer to question "What is the most appropriate next step?"

Diagnosis of croup is made clinically and can be aided by radiology if the symptoms are mild.

Treatment is steroids and nebulized epinephrine for moderate or severe symptoms.

> Hypoxia helps to differentiate croup from epiglottitis.
> - **Croup**: hypoxia on presentation
> - **Epiglottitis**: hypoxia imminent

Foreign Body Aspiration

Foreign body aspiration is most common in children age 1–3 years who present with the sudden onset respiratory distress without a preceding illness. The most common location for the aspirated object to lodge into is the right mainstem bronchus.

The most frequent symptoms are choking and sudden onset of respiratory distress. Physical exam will show focal monophonic wheezing with diminished air movement on the affected side. However, a chest x-ray is the **best initial diagnostic test** because about two-thirds of aspirated objects are radiolucent. Immediate rigid bronchoscopy is both the **most accurate test** and the appropriate treatment.

Epiglottitis

A 4-year-old boy is brought in because of extreme irritability and refusal to eat. He refuses to lean back, speaks in muffled words, looks extremely ill, and is drooling. Chest x-ray shows a thumbprint sign. What is the most appropriate next step in management?

a. Intubate
b. Racemic epinephrine
c. Empiric antibiotics
d. Physical examination
e. CT neck

Answer: **A.** This child presents with signs of epiglottitis, **the truest medical emergency in pediatrics**. He must be intubated at once. Do not waste time with anything else, including a full examination, as his airway may close off any minute. This case mentions a thumbprint sign to aid your studies, but chest x-ray is rarely done with such a convincing presentation. The remaining choices are not indicated until airway management is conducted.

Epiglottitis is a severe, life-threatening swelling of the epiglottis and arytenoids.

Look for a child with a history of vaccination delinquency with:

- Hoarseness
- Fever
- Drooling in the tripod position
- Refusal to lie flat

Physical examination will reveal an extremely hot cherry-red epiglottis.

Diagnosis is made clinically, and x-ray may reveal "thumbprint sign."

To treat:

- Intubate the child in the OR (the preferred setting, in case unsuccessful intubation makes tracheostomy necessary)
- Treat with ceftriaxone and vancomycin

Whooping Cough

Whooping cough is a form of bronchitis caused by *Bordetella pertussis*.

Symptoms include:

- **Catarrhal stage**: severe congestion and rhinorrhea—14 days in duration
- **Paroxysmal stage**: severe coughing episodes with extreme gasp for air (inspiratory whoop) followed by vomiting—14 to 30 days in duration
- **Convalescent stage**: decrease of frequency of coughing—14 days in duration

Diagnosis is made clinically based on whooping inspiration, vomiting, and burst blood vessels in the eyes. Additionally:

- Chest x-ray shows "butterfly pattern"
- PCR of nasal secretions or *Bordetella pertussis* toxin ELISA

Treatment is as follows:

- Azithromycin or clarithromycin (helpful only in catarrhal stage, not in paroxysmal stage)
- Isolation
- Macrolides to all close contacts
- DTaP vaccine to reduce incidence

Upper and Lower Airway Diseases				
Disease	**Etiology**	**Presentation**	**Diagnosis**	**Treatment**
Bronchitis	Various bacteria and viruses causing inflammation of the airways	Productive cough lasting 7–10 days with fever	Clinical	Supportive
Pharyngitis	Inflammation of the pharynx and adjacent structures caused by group A beta hemolytic strep	Cervical adenopathy, petechiae, fever above 40 C (104 F), and other URI symptoms; acute rheumatic fever and glomerulonephritis	Rapid DNase antigen detection test	Oral penicillin for 10 days or macrolides for penicillin allergy
Diphtheria	Membranous inflammation of the pharynx due to bacterial invasion by *Corynebacterium diphtheriae*	Gray highly vascular pseudomembranous plaques on the pharyngeal wall. **Do not scrape.**	Culture of a small portion of superficial membrane	Antitoxin: remember, antibiotics do not work

Seizures

Seizures classically present with subtle repetitive movements, such as chewing, tongue thrusting, apnea, staring, blinking, or desaturations. Tonic-clonic movements are uncommon. The overall goal is to uncover the cause of the seizure and treat it.

Diagnostic Testing

- EEG (may be normal)
- CBC, electrolytes, calcium, magnesium, glucose (hypoglycemia is a common cause of seizures in infants of diabetic mothers)
- Rule out infectious causes
- TORCH infection studies
- Blood and urine cultures
- Lumbar puncture if meningitis is suspected
- Ultrasound of head in preterm neonates to look for intraventricular hemorrhage

Treatment

Correct the underlying cause, including electrolyte abnormalities. For acute seizure, use lorazepam or diazepam (rectally). Treatment for chronic seizures depends on type; with absence seizures, use ethosuximide.

Pediatric Seizure Disorders			
Seizure disorder	**Classic features**	**EEG findings**	**Treatment**
Absence seizures	• Frequent seizures with cessation of motor activity or speech, blank facial expression, and flickering of eyelids • More common in girls, rare in children <4 years, rarely lasts longer than 30 seconds • No aura or postictal state	3 per second spike and generalized wave discharge	• First line: ethosuximide • Alternative: valproic acid
Juvenile myoclonic epilepsy (JME)	• Jerky movement occurring in the morning • Onset around adolescence	Irregular spike-and-wave pattern	First line: valproic acid
Simple febrile seizure	• Generalized tonic-clonic seizure <10 min duration occurring with rapid-onset high fever in a child age 9 months to 5 years • Usually positive family history • No increased risk of epilepsy		• Evaluate for meningitis • Control fever
West syndrome (infantile spasms)	• Infantile spasms during the first year of life • Clusters of mixed flexor/extensor spasms of trunk and extremities persisting for minutes, with brief intervals between spasms • 75% have an underlying CNS disorder (Down syndrome is most common)	Hypsarrhythmia (very high-voltage slow waves, irregularly interspersed with spikes and sharp waves)	First line: ACTH, prednisone, vigabatrin, pyridoxine (vitamin B6)
Partial seizure	• Simple: tonic or clonic movements involving most of the face, neck, and extremities and lasting 10–20 seconds; no postictal period • Complex: includes impaired consciousness	Spike and sharp waves or multifocal spikes	First line: carbamazepine and valproic acid
Generalized seizure	• Aura, LOC, eyes roll back, tonic contraction, apnea then clonic rhythmic contractions alternating with relaxation of all muscle groups • Tongue biting, loss of bladder control • Prominent postictal state	Anterior temporal lobe shows sharp waves or focal spikes	First line: valproic acid

Vitamin Deficiency and Toxicity

Vitamin Deficiencies and Toxicities		
Vitamin	**Findings in deficiency**	**Findings in toxicity**
Vitamin A	• Poor night vision • Hypoparathyroidism	• Pseudotumor cerebri • Hyperparathyroidism
Vitamin B1 (thiamine)	• Beriberi • Wernicke encephalopathy	Water soluble, therefore no toxicity
Vitamin B2 (riboflavin)	• Angular cheilosis • Stomatitis • Glossitis	Water soluble, no toxicity
Vitamin B3 (niacin)	Pellagra (4 D's: diarrhea, dermatitis, dementia, death)	Water soluble, no toxicity
Vitamin B5 (pantothenic acid)	Burning feet syndrome	Water soluble, no toxicity
Vitamin B6 (pyridoxine)	• Peripheral neuropathy • Must be given with INH	Water soluble, no toxicity
Vitamin B9 (folate)	• Megaloblastic anemia • Hypersegmented neutrophils	Water soluble, no toxicity
Vitamin B12 (cyanocobalamin)	• Megaloblastic anemia • Hypersegmented neutrophils • Peripheral neuropathy of the dorsal column tracts	Water soluble, no toxicity
Vitamin C	Scurvy (ecchymosis, bleeding gums, and petechiae)	Water soluble, no toxicity
Vitamin D	Rickets in children	• Hypercalcemia • Polyuria • Polydipsia
Vitamin K	• Increased prothrombin time / INR • Signs and symptoms of mild to severe bleeding • Analogous to warfarin therapy	Toxicity is rare and an upper limit has not been established.

Glycogen Storage Diseases

		Glycogen Storage Diseases			
Type	**Defective/ deficient enzyme**	**Organ(s) affected**	**Clinical manifestation(s)**	**Diagnostic testing**	**Treatment**
I. Von Gierke	Glucose-6-phosphatase	Liver and kidney	• Ketotic hypoglycemia • Hepatomegaly	• Liver biopsy • DNA testing	• Cornstarch • Allopurinol • Granulocyte-colony stimulating factor (G-CSF)
II. Pompe	Lysosomal acid maltase deficiency	All organs	• Hypotonia (floppy baby) • Hypertrophic cardiomyopathy	• Muscle or liver enzyme assay • DNA testing	Enzyme replacement
III. Cori	Debranching enzyme	Muscle and liver	• Hepatomegaly • Hypoglycemia	Muscle or liver biopsy	• High-protein diet • Liver transplant
IV. Andersen	Glycogen branching enzyme deficiency	Liver and spleen	Cirrhosis of the liver and liver failure by age 2	• Liver biopsy • DNA testing	Liver transplant
V. McArdle	Muscle phosphorylase deficiency	Muscle	• Fatigability • Limited physical activity	• Muscle enzyme assay • DNA testing	Sucrose prior to strenuous activity

Child Abuse (Non-Accidental Trauma)

Child abuse may be broadly defined as injury inflicted upon a child by a parent or caretaker. Without intervention, abused children are highly likely to be maltreated again and are at increased risk for death.

Diagnostic testing includes:

- Laboratory studies: PT, PTT, platelets, bleeding time, CBC
- Skeletal survey
- If there are severe injuries (even without neurological signs):
  - Head CT scan ± MRI
  - Ophthalmologic examination
- If there is abdominal trauma:
  - Test urine and stool for blood
  - Liver and pancreatic enzymes
  - Abdominal CT scan
- Urine toxicology screen, especially if the case describes altered mental status

Treatment starts with addressing the medical and/or surgical issues. Then report any child suspected of being abused or neglected to Child Protective Services (CPS). Initial action includes a phone report; in most states, a written report is then required within 48 hours.

The following are indications for hospitalization:

- Medical condition requires it.
- Diagnosis is unclear.
- There is no alternative safe place.

If parents refuse hospitalization or treatment, the physician must get an emergency court order. You must explain to the parent why an inflicted injury is suspected abuse, that you are legally obligated to report it, that you have made a referral to protect the child, and that a CPS worker and law enforcement officer will be involved.

Lysosomal Storage Diseases				
	Deficient/defective enzyme	**Inheritance pattern**	**Accumulated substance**	**Clinical findings**
Tay-Sachs disease	Hexosaminidase A	• Autosomal recessive disease • Chromosome 15q	Ganglioside	• Cherry red macula • Intellectual disability and developmental delay; death by age 2 years • Seizures • Lysosomes with onionskin-whorled membranes
Gaucher disease	β-glucocerebrosidase **(most common of all)**	• Chromosome 1 • Autosomal recessive disease	Glucocerebroside	• Hepatosplenomegaly • Aseptic necrosis of femur • Lytic lesions • Gaucher cells: macrophages that look like crumpled paper due to fibrillary cytoplasm
Krabbe disease	Galactocerebrosidase	Autosomal recessive	Galactocerebroside	• Optic atrophy • Developmental delay
Fabry disease	Alpha-galactosidase A	X-linked recessive	Ceramide trihexoside	Peripheral neuropathy (burning pain) of hands/feet
Niemann-Pick disease	Sphingomyelinase	• Autosomal recessive disease • Chromosome 11p	Sphingomyelin	• Cherry red macula • Neurodegeneration • Hepatosplenomegaly • Foam cells: foamy vacuolated macrophages in the marrow
Metachromatic leukodystrophy	Arylsulfatase A	Autosomal recessive disease	Cerebroside sulfate	Demyelination with ataxia and dementia

PART 8

Obstetrics

by Victoria Hastings, DO, MPH, MS

The most common first symptom of pregnancy in women with regular menstruation is amenorrhea. However, in patients who have irregular menses, amenorrhea may be missed. Other symptoms include breast tenderness, nausea, and vomiting. Pregnant women experience a surge in estrogen, progesterone, and beta-human chorionic gonadotropin (beta-hCG) that leads to these symptoms.

> **Amenorrhea =**
>
> No menses in 3 months if regular
>
> No menses in 6 months if irregular

A 27-year-old woman presents with nausea and vomiting for the past 2 weeks. Symptoms are worse in the morning but can occur at any time during the day. She has a decrease in appetite. Her last menstrual period (LMP) was 6 weeks ago. Physical examination is unremarkable.

Which of the following is the best next step in management?

a. Complete blood count
b. Beta-hCG
c. HIDA scan
d. Comprehensive metabolic panel
e. Urinalysis

Answer: **B.** A pregnancy test should be done first in all symptomatic women of childbearing age. Her LMP occurred 6 weeks ago and the patient is experiencing "morning sickness." Morning sickness is caused by an increase in beta-hCG produced by the placenta. This can occur until the 12th to 14th week of pregnancy. A complete blood count (CBC), comprehensive metabolic panel (CMP), and urinalysis are used to evaluate the severity of dehydration, not the etiology. A HIDA scan is done in patients with suspected cholecystitis.

Definitions

Embryo: fertilization to 8 weeks

Fetus: 8 weeks to birth

Infant: birth to age 1 year

Dating Methods

Nägele rule: LMP – 3 months + 7 days = Estimated day of delivery

Gestational age (GA): number of days/weeks since the last menstrual period

Nägele rule: estimation of the day of delivery by taking the last menstrual period, subtracting 3 months, and adding 7 days. For example, a woman with an LMP of October 1, 2021, will have an estimated delivery date of July 8, 2022.

Trimester Breakdown

First trimester: fertilization until up to 14 weeks

Second trimester: 14 weeks until 28 weeks

Third trimester: 28 weeks until delivery

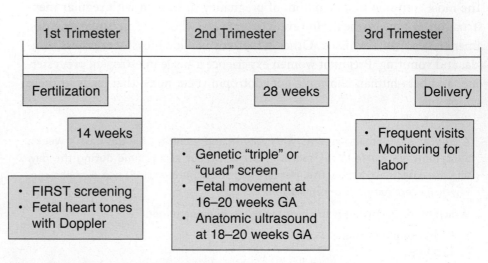

Figure 8.1 Trimester Breakdown. © Kaplan

Term Lengths

Previable: fetus born before 22–25 weeks

- **Before 22 weeks**: no resuscitation
- **23–25 weeks**: discussion of risks and benefits with parents; decision to resuscitate made on case-by-case basis
- **After 25 weeks**: resuscitation always initiated

Preterm: fetus born between 25 weeks and 36 weeks, 6 days

Term:

- **Early term**: fetus born between 37 weeks and 38 weeks, 6 days
- **Full term**: fetus born between 39 weeks and 40 weeks, 6 days
- **Late term**: fetus born between 41 weeks and 41 weeks, 6 days
- **Postterm**: fetus born after 42 weeks

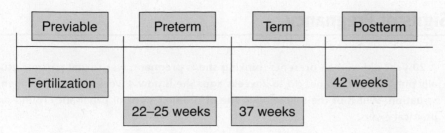

Figure 8.2 Term Length. © Kaplan

Gravidity/Parity

Gravidity is the number of times a patient has been pregnant. **Parity** is what happens to the pregnancy. This is broken down into 4 numbers (using the mnemonic "TPAL"):

1. **Term births**
2. **Preterm births**
3. **Abortions** (both spontaneous and induced)
4. **Living children** (if a patient has a multiple gestation pregnancy, one birth results in 2 living children)

For example, a 35-year-old woman presents to the office for her sixth pregnancy. She has had 2 abortions, 2 children born at term, and a set of twins born preterm. This patient's gravidity and parity are: G6P2124.

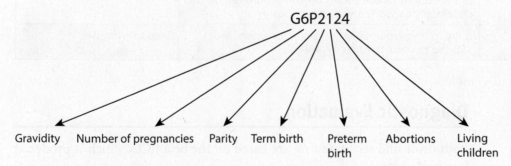

G = Gravidity, or the number of pregnancies (in this example, G = 6).
P = Parity, which is made up of four numbers:

- the number of term births (e.g., 2)
- the number of preterm births (e.g., 1)
- the number of abortions (e.g., 2)
- the number of living children (e.g., 4)

Figure 8.3 Explanation of Gravidity/Parity

▶ **TIP**

Term birth (T); Preterm birth (P); Abortions (A); Living children (L) = TPAL

Signs of Pregnancy

A 20-year-old woman presents thinking she is pregnant. Her sexual partner usually pulls out but did not do so 2 weeks ago. She is now 4 weeks late for her menstruation. Which of the following is one of the first signs of pregnancy found on physical exam?

a. Quickening
b. Goodell sign
c. Ladin sign
d. Linea nigra
e. Chloasma

Answer: **B.** One of the first signs of pregnancy that is seen on physical exam is the Goodell sign, softening of the cervix that is felt first at 4 weeks. Quickening is the first time the mother feels fetal movement.

Signs of Pregnancy		
Sign	**Physical finding**	**Time from conception**
Goodell sign	Softening of the cervix	4 weeks (first trimester)
Ladin sign	Softening of the midline of the uterus	6 weeks (first trimester)
Chadwick sign	Blue discoloration of vagina and cervix	6–8 weeks (first trimester)
Telangiectasias/palmar erythema	Small blood vessels/reddening of the palms	First trimester
Chloasma	The "mask of pregnancy" is a hyperpigmentation of the face most commonly on forehead, nose, and cheeks; it can worsen with sun exposure.	16 weeks (second trimester)
Linea nigra	A line of hyperpigmentation that can extend from xiphoid process to pubic symphysis	Second trimester

Diagnostic Evaluation

Both urine and serum testing are based on the beta-hCG, which is produced by the placenta.

- In the first trimester, beta-hCG is produced rapidly, doubling every 48 hours for the first 4 weeks.
- At 10 weeks of gestation, beta-hCG peaks.
- In the second trimester, levels typically drop.
- In the third trimester, levels increase slowly again to level 20,000–30,000 IU/mL.

Beta-hCG tests are all highly sensitive. **Ultrasound (U/S) is used to confirm an intrauterine pregnancy.** At 5–6 weeks or beta-hCG 1,500 IU/mL, a gestational sac with a yolk sac should be seen on U/S.

> The best initial test when pregnancy is suspected is serum or urine beta-hCG.

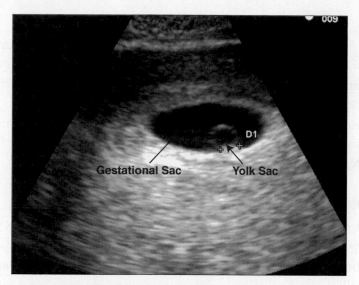

Figure 8.4 Ultrasound of Intrauterine Pregnancy.
Source: X. Compagnion, commons.wikimedia.org.

Physiologic Changes in Pregnancy

There are many physiologic changes in pregnancy; however, only a few are tested on the USMLE.

Cardiology

- Increased blood volume will increase preload.
- Decreased systemic vascular resistance will decrease afterload.
- Cardiac output increases.
- Heart rate increases.

Respiratory

- Elevation of diaphragm from gravid uterus → decreased RV (residual volume)
- Unchanged FEV1/FVC
- Increased tidal volume → increased minute ventilation → decreased pCO_2 → respiratory alkalosis
- No change in respiratory rate

Gastrointestinal

- **Morning sickness:** Nausea and vomiting occur anytime throughout the day and are **caused by an increase in estrogen**, **progesterone**, and hCG made by the placenta.
- Gastroesophageal reflux: Lower esophageal sphincter has decreased tone from the effects of progesterone.
- **Constipation:** Motility in the large intestine is decreased.

Renal

- Kidney volume increases by ≤30% due to increased vascular and interstitial volume.
- Dilation of renal pelvises can occur, resulting from progesterone effect and compression of the ureters by the enlarging uterus.
- Increased plasma volume coupled with decreased peripheral resistance leads to an increase in GFR and a decrease in creatinine concentration.
  - BUN/creatinine decreases

Physiologic

- Excess production of neutrophils in pregnancy can lead to leukocytosis in the absence of infection.
- Gestational thrombocytopenia is common; initiate workup if platelets are <80,000/μL.

Hematology

- **Anemia** from an increase in plasma volume by 50%
- **Hypercoagulable state**
  - No increase in PT, PTT, or INR
  - Increase in fibrinogen
  - Virchow triad elements occur
    - Venous stasis

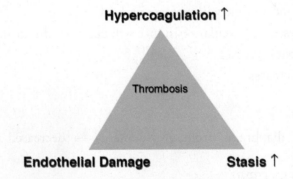

Figure 8.5 Physiologic Changes in Pregnancy. © Kaplan

Prenatal Care

First Trimester

Ideally, women should be taking folic acid 0.4 mg daily *prior to conception*, and folic acid should be prescribed as soon as pregnancy is diagnosed. In the first trimester, patients should be seen every 4–6 weeks. An ultrasound should be done to confirm gestational age. Blood tests, Pap smear, and gonorrhea/chlamydia tests are also performed. Screening tests for fetal aneuploidy should be performed. Maternal beta-hCG, maternal pregnancy-associated plasma protein A (PAPP-A), and nuchal translucency comprise the "combined test," which should be performed at 11–14 weeks.

Cell-free DNA testing can also be done in the first trimester as early as 7 weeks of gestational age. This test is used to detect fetal sex, undertake routine prenatal screening for Rh factor and aneuploidy, and do genetic studies for high-risk patients. Cell-free DNA testing is a noninvasive blood test that evaluates fragmented fetal DNA circulating in the mother's bloodstream.

> Give the flu vaccine at any point during pregnancy. Give the Tdap vaccine after 26 weeks' gestation. Avoid live vaccines during pregnancy.

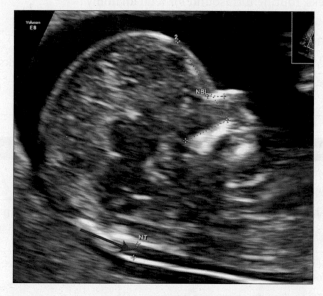

Figure 8.6 A thickened or enlarged nuchal translucency is an indication of Down syndrome. *Source: Dr. Wolfgang Moroder, WikiCommons.*

Second Trimester

Visits in the second trimester are used to screen for genetic and congenital problems. At 15–23 weeks, perform a "triple" or a "quad" screen.

A triple screen includes maternal serum alpha fetoprotein (MSAFP), beta-hCG, and estriol. The quad screen adds inhibin A to the triple screen and increases the sensitivity.

Quad Screen Results with Suspected Trisomies					
Aneuploidy	**Chromo-some**	**AFP**	**Estriol**	**hCG**	**Inhibin A**
Patau syndrome	13	Increased	Unchanged	Unchanged	Unchanged
Edwards syndrome	18	Unchanged	Decreased	Decreased	Unchanged
Down syndrome	21	Decreased	Decreased	Increased	Increased

> Patau → Puberty → chromosome 13
>
> Edwards → Election → chromosome 18
>
> Down → Drinking → chromosome 21

An increase in MSAFP may indicate a dating error, neural tube defect, or abdominal wall defect. A decrease in MSAFP may indicate chromosomal abnormalities. The addition of beta-hCG, estriol, and inhibin A helps increase the sensitivity of the MSAFP test to detect trisomies 13, 18, and 21. The following are also done in the second trimester:

- Auscultation of fetal heart rate
- 16–20 weeks: quickening (feeling fetal movement for the first time)
  - Multiparous women feel the quickening earlier than primiparous women.
- 18–20 weeks: routine ultrasound for fetal anatomy

Third Trimester

In the third trimester, visits are every 2–3 weeks until 36 weeks. **After 36 weeks, there is a visit every week.**

Third Trimester Testing		
Week	**Test**	**Action**
27	Complete blood count Syphillis screen	If hemoglobin <11, replace iron orally
24–28	1-hour glucose challenge test (GCT)	If glucose >130–140 at one hour, perform **oral glucose tolerance test**
36	Cervical cultures for chlamydia and gonorrhea	Treatment if positive
	STD testing if patient was positive during pregnancy or has a risk factor	
	Rectovaginal culture for group B *Streptococcus*	Prophylactic antibiotics during labor

Braxton-Hicks Contractions

Braxton-Hicks contractions occur during the third trimester. They are sporadic and do not cause cervical dilation. If they become regular, the cervix should be checked to rule out preterm labor before 37 weeks. Preterm labor opens the cervix, but Braxton-Hicks contractions do not.

Glucose **challenge** test: fasting or nonfasting ingestion of **50 g** of glucose, and serum glucose check **1 hour** later.

Glucose **tolerance** test: fasting serum glucose, ingestion of **100 g** of glucose, serum glucose checks at **1, 2, and 3 hours**. Elevated glucose during any two of these tests is gestational diabetes.

Diagnostic Genetic Testing

Chorionic Villus Sampling

- Done at 10–13 weeks if genetic aneuploidy screening test is positive
- Obtains fetal karyotype
- Catheter into intrauterine cavity to aspirate chorionic villi from placenta (can be done transabdominally or transvaginally)

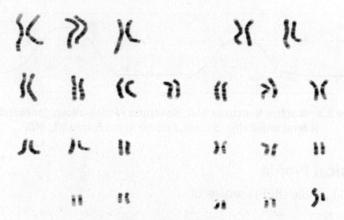

Figure 8.7 Chorionic Villus Sampling.
Source: National Human Genome Research Institute, WikiCommons.

Amniocentesis

- Done at 15–17 weeks if genetic aneuploidy screening test is positive
- Obtains fetal karyotype (advanced maternal age)
- Needle inserted transabdominally into the amniotic sac to withdraw amniotic fluid

Fetal Testing

Nonstress Test (NST)

The NST allows the physician to check for fetal well-being while still in the uterus. A reactive NST is defined as ≥2 accelerations within 30 minutes of fetal heart rate tracing. An acceleration is defined as an abrupt increase of ≥15 bpm above the baseline with onset to peak <30 seconds.

A **reactive** NST reliably indicates adequate fetal oxygenation. If the NST is **nonreactive**, the fetus could be sleeping. Vibroacoustic stimulation is done to wake up the baby.

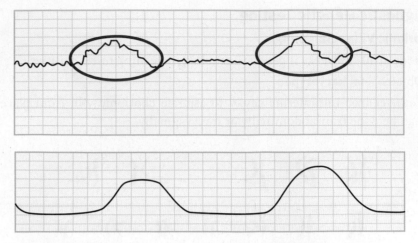

Figure 8.8 Reactive Nonstress Test. Nonstress testing allows for evaluation of fetal well-being in utero. *Source: Jason Franasiak, MD.*

Biophysical Profile

Biophysical profile (BPP) consists of:

- Reactive NST
- Fetal breathing (count episodes of fetal chest expansions; normal is ≥ 1 episode lasting ≥ 30 seconds within a 30-minute time period)
- Fetal movement (count fetal movements; normal is >3 in 30 minutes)
- Fetal muscle tone (≥ 1 episode of flexion and extension of extremity within 30 minutes)
- Amniotic fluid index (maximum vertical pocket ≥ 2 cm)

Each category is worth 2 points; a BPP ≤ 4 may indicate fetal compromise.

Normal Labor

Electronic Fetal Monitoring

When a patient presents in labor, an external tocometer and fetal heart rate monitor are placed on the gravid abdomen to measure the fetal heart rate and uterine contractions.

Fetal Heart Rate

Normal: 110–160 beats per minute

Bradycardia: baseline <110 beats per minute for 10 minutes

Tachycardia: baseline >160 beats per minute for 10 minutes

Accelerations

Normal accelerations are an increase in heart rate of 15 or more beats per minute above the heart rate baseline for longer than 15–20 seconds. If this happens twice in 20 minutes, it is reassuring or normal.

Decelerations			
Type	**Description**	**Decelerations**	**Cause**
Early decelerations	Decrease in heart rate that occurs with contractions (a "mirror image")	Autonomic changes in fetal intracranial pressure and/or cerebral blood flow cause temporary decrease in heart rate.	Head compression
Variable decelerations	Decrease in heart rate and return to baseline with no relationship to contractions	Compression of umbilical cord reduces venous return. Baroreceptor-mediated reflex raises heart rate in response. Further compression occludes umbilical arteries, abruptly raising peripheral resistance and BP. Heart rate reflexively decreases.	Umbilical cord compression
Late decelerations (most serious and dangerous)	Decrease in heart rate after contraction started. No return to baseline until contraction ends	Uterine contraction causes transient hypoxemia, triggering reflexive drop in fetal heart rate. Compression of maternal blood vessels → decreased placental perfusion → reduced oxygen diffusion to fetus → decreased fetal pO_2 → chemoreceptor-mediated reflex drop in heart rate.	Fetal hypoxia

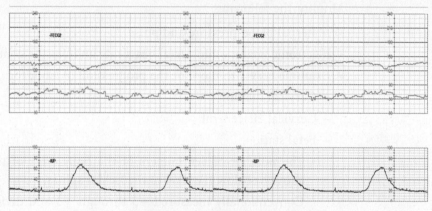

Figure 8.9 Early Decelerations.
Source: Victoria Hastings, DO, MPH

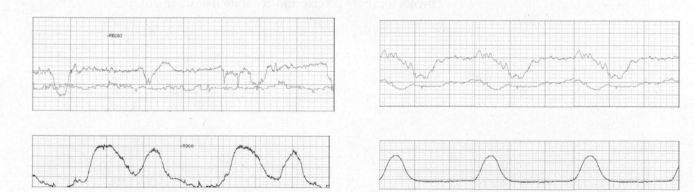

Figure 8.10 Variable Decelerations.
Source: Victoria Hastings, DO, MPH

Figure 8.11 Late Decelerations.
Source: Victoria Hastings, DO, MPH

Physiological Changes Before Labor

- **Lightening**: fetal descent into the pelvic brim
- **Braxton-Hicks contractions**: benign contractions that do not result in cervical dilation; they routinely start to increase in frequency toward the end of the pregnancy
- **Bloody show**: blood-tinged mucus from vagina that is released with cervical effacement

Stages of Labor

- **Stage 1**: onset of labor → full dilation of cervix
  - Latent phase: from onset of labor to 6 cm dilation
  - Active phase: from 6 cm dilation to full dilation
- **Stage 2**: full dilation of cervix → delivery of neonate
- **Stage 3**: delivery of neonate → delivery of placenta

Stage 1

Monitor the following:

- Maternal blood pressure and pulse
- Electronic fetal monitor: fetal heart rate and uterine contractions
- Examine cervix to monitor the progression of labor for:
  - Cervical dilation
  - Cervical effacement
  - Fetal station
    - The number of centimeters of the bony edge of the presenting part above or below the level of the ischial spines.
    - Conventionally measured −3 through +3 and divided the upper and lower parts of the pelvis into thirds. More recently measured in a system of −5 through +5, in which the pelvis is divided based on 1 cm increments for more precise and accurate measurement.

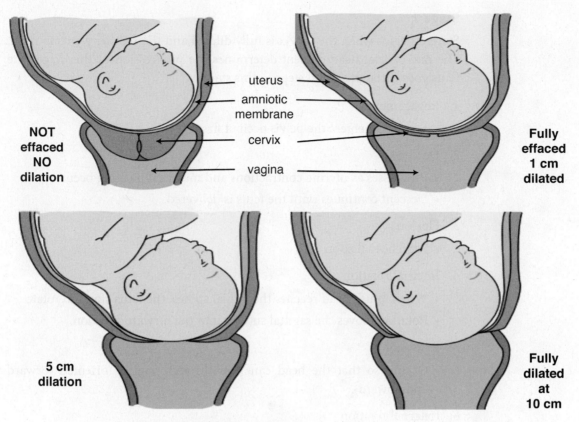

NOT effaced NO dilation

Fully effaced 1 cm dilated

uterus
amniotic membrane
cervix
vagina

5 cm dilation

Fully dilated at 10 cm

Figure 8.12 Labor and Delivery.
Source: Fred the Oyster, commons.wikimedia.org.

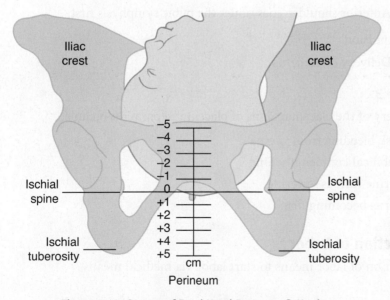

Iliac crest

Iliac crest

Ischial spine

Ischial spine

Ischial tuberosity

Ischial tuberosity

−5
−4
−3
−2
−1
0
+1
+2
+3
+4
+5
cm

Perineum

Figure 8.13 Stages of Fetal Head Descent. © Kaplan

Stage 2

Stage 2 begins when the cervix is fully dilated and the mother wants to push. The rate of fetal head descent determines the progression of this stage. The fetus goes through several steps in this stage:

1. Engagement
   - Fetal head enters the pelvis occiput first.

2. Descent
   - Progresses as uterine contractions and maternal pushing occur.
   - Descent continues until the fetus is delivered.

3. Flexion
   - Fetal head flexion

4. Internal rotation
   - When fetus's head reaches the ischial spines, the fetus starts to rotate.
   - Rotation moves the sagittal sutures into the forward position.

5. Extension
   - Occurs so that the head can pass through vagina (oriented forward and upward).

6. External rotation
   - During fetal head delivery, external rotation occurs, giving the shoulders room to descend.
   - Anterior shoulder goes under the pubic symphysis first.

7. Expulsion
   - Delivery of the fetus

Stage 3

Delivery of the placenta. Signs of placental separation include:
- Fresh bleeding from vagina
- Umbilical cord lengthening
- Uterine fundus lowering
- Uterus becoming firm

Induction of Labor

Induction of labor means to start labor via medical means.

Methods of Induction

- **Prostaglandin E$_2$** is used for cervical ripening.
- **Oxytocin**
  - Exaggerates uterine contractions
  - Normally found in the posterior pituitary (drug is a version of the naturally occurring substance)
- **Amniotomy**
  - Puncture of the amniotic sac via an amnio hook
    - Inspect for a prolapsed umbilical cord before puncturing the amniotic sac.

Early Pregnancy Complications

A 29-year-old woman with a medical history of chlamydia presents with left lower quadrant abdominal pain for 8 hours. She also has some abnormal vaginal bleeding. Her LMP was 6 weeks ago. On physical exam her temperature is 37.2 C (99 F), heart rate 100 bpm, blood pressure 130/80 mm Hg, and respiratory rate 13/min. Which of the following is the most likely diagnosis?

a. Ectopic pregnancy
b. Menstrual cramps
c. Diverticulitis
d. Ovarian torsion
e. Ovarian cyst

Answer: **A.** This is likely an ectopic pregnancy. Diverticulitis causes left lower quadrant abdominal pain and rectal bleeding, not vaginal bleeding. The age range of the patients has almost no overlap between ectopic pregnancy and diverticulitis. Ovarian torsion and ovarian cysts do not cause vaginal bleeding. Menstrual cramps are not associated with an altered menstrual pattern.

Ectopic Pregnancy

Ectopic pregnancy is a pregnancy that implants in an area outside the uterus. This most commonly occurs in the ampulla of the fallopian tube.

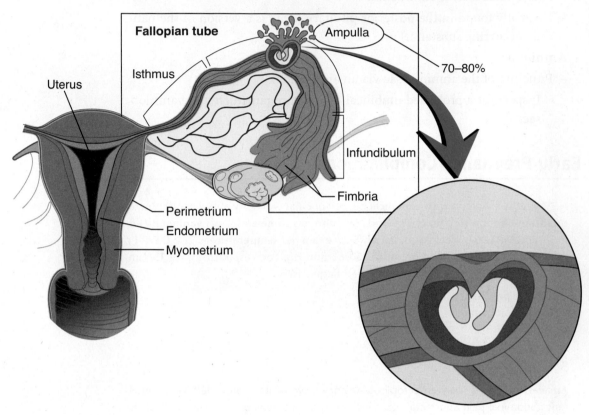

Figure 8.14 Ectopic Pregnancy. © Kaplan

Risk factors include:

- Pelvic inflammatory disease (PID)
- Levonorgestrel intrauterine device (IUD)
- In vitro fertilization (IVF) pregnancy
- Previous ectopic pregnancies (strongest risk factor)

Symptoms include:

- Unilateral lower abdominal or pelvic pain
- Vaginal bleeding
- If ruptured, can be hypotensive with peritoneal irritation

Diagnostic testing includes beta-hCG to confirm the presence of a pregnancy and U/S to locate the site of implantation of the ectopic pregnancy.

Treatment for unstable patients (low BP, high HR) is fluids and immediate surgery.

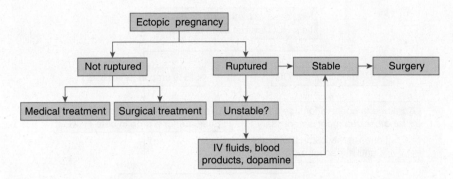

Figure 8.15 Management of Ectopic Pregnancy

Medical treatment should begin with baseline exams such as:

- CBC to monitor for anemia
- Blood type/screen
- Transaminases to detect changes indicating hepatotoxicity that could potentially result from treatment

After these are obtained, manage as follows:

- Consider giving methotrexate, a folate receptor antagonist
- Follow patient's beta-hCG to see if there is a 15% decrease between days 4 and 7
  - If no decrease, a second dose of methotrexate may be given.
  - If still no decrease in beta-hCG after the second dose, proceed with surgery.
    - Surgery is done to try to preserve the fallopian tube by cutting a hole in it (salpingostomy).
    - However, removal of the whole fallopian tube (salpingectomy) may be necessary.
    - Mothers who are Rh negative should receive anti-D Rh immunoglobulin (RhoGAM) so that subsequent pregnancies will not be affected by hemolytic disease.
  - Follow beta-hCG weekly until it reaches zero.

Methotrexate is a folic acid antagonist that is cleared by the kidneys. Exclusion criteria for methotrexate include:

- Immunodeficiency: methotrexate is an immunosuppressive drug
- Noncompliance: patients need to return for evaluation
- Liver disease: hepatotoxicity is a serious side effect of methotrexate; baseline liver disease increases the risk of subsequent toxicity
- Ectopic is 3.5 cm or larger: the larger the ectopic, the greater the risk of treatment failure
- Fetal heartbeat: a pregnancy developed enough to have a heartbeat has an increased risk of failure
- Breastfeeding
- Coexisting viable pregnancy (**heterotopic pregnancy**)

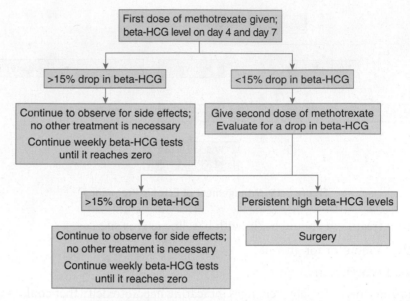

Figure 8.16 Treatment of Ectopic Pregnancy

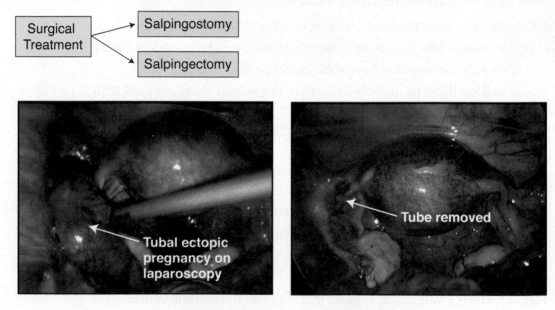

Figure 8.17 Surgical Treatment for Ectopic Pregnancy.
Source: Jason Franasiak, MD.

Abortion

A 20-year-old woman presents to the ED for vaginal bleeding and lower abdominal pain for one day. She is 15 weeks pregnant. Vital signs include temperature 37.2 C (99 F), heart rate 100 bpm, blood pressure 110/75 mm Hg, and respiratory rate 12/min. On pelvic exam, there is blood present in the vault and the cervical os is 3 cm dilated. Ultrasound shows a gestational sac with a yolk sac inside the uterus and a fetal heartbeat is visualized. Which of the following is the most likely diagnosis?

a. Complete abortion
b. Incomplete abortion
c. Inevitable abortion
d. Threatened abortion
e. Septic abortion

Answer: C. An inevitable abortion is characterized by vaginal bleeding with a dilated cervix. Products of conception can be felt or visualized through the internal os. (See "Types of Abortion" algorithm later in this section for details of other answer choices.)

Abortion is defined as a pregnancy that ends <20 weeks' gestation or a fetus <500 grams. Almost 80% of spontaneous abortions occur <12 weeks' gestation.

Chromosomal abnormalities in the fetus account for 60–80% of spontaneous abortions. However, maternal factors that increase risk of abortion include:

- Anatomic abnormalities
- Infections (STDs)
- Immunological factors (antiphospholipid syndrome)
- Endocrinological factors (uncontrolled hyperthyroidism or diabetes)
- Malnutrition
- Trauma
- Rh isoimmunization

Symptoms include cramping abdominal pain and vaginal bleeding. The patient may be stable or unstable, depending on the amount of blood loss.

Diagnostic testing includes:

- CBC to evaluate blood loss and need for transfusion
- Blood type and Rh screen in case blood needs to be transfused, and to evaluate need for anti-D Rh immunoglobulin
- Ultrasound to distinguish between the types of abortion
- Digital exam to determine whether cervical os is open

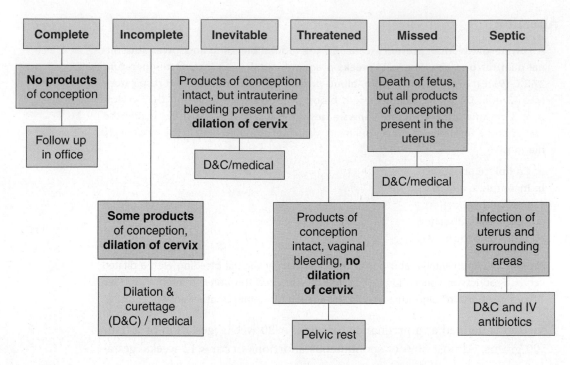

Figure 8.18 Types of Abortion. © Kaplan

Medical treatment can occur via giving medications that induce labor, i.e., misoprostol (a prostaglandin E$_1$ analog). These agents help open the cervix and expulse the fetus.

▶ **TIP**

Mothers who are Rh negative should also receive anti-D Rh immunoglobulin at this time.

Recurrent Fetal Loss

Recurrent fetal loss is defined as 3 consecutive miscarriages that occur before 20 weeks' gestation. There are many reasons for recurrent fetal loss, and often no etiology is identified.

Possible causes of recurrent loss include:

- Genetic factors: maternal/paternal aneuploidy
- Anatomical factors: bicornuate uterus, cervical insufficiency
- Endocrine factors: uncontrolled thyroid, hyperprolactinemia
- Immunological factors: antiphospholipid syndrome, SLE
- Thrombophilia: factor V Leiden mutation, prothrombin mutation

Cervical Insufficiency

Cervical insufficiency is the inability of the cervix to hold a pregnancy in the second trimester in the absence of contractions. Women with at least 2 prior-second-trimester spontaneous births without contractions or abdominal pain are considered to have cervical insufficiency, and they are treated in future pregnancies with a cervical cerclage. Women with no history and findings of short cervix ≤2.5 cm on ultrasound at less than 24 weeks are at risk for cervical insufficiency and are treated with vaginal progesterone.

Multiple Gestations

Symptoms include exponential growth of the uterus; rapid weight gain by mother; and elevated beta-hCG and MSAFP (levels higher than expected for estimated gestational age is the **first clue to multiple gestation**).

Ultrasound is done to visualize the fetuses.

> Fertility drugs increase multiple gestations.

Complications of multiple gestation include the following:

- Spontaneous abortion
- Premature labor and delivery
- Placenta previa
- Anemia

Types of Twins		
Types	**Fertilization**	**Characteristics**
Monozygotic	1 egg and 1 sperm that splits	Identical twins: same gender, same physical characteristics, same blood type, fingerprints differ
Dizygotic	2 eggs and 2 sperm	Fraternal twins: different or same sex; they resemble each other, as any siblings would

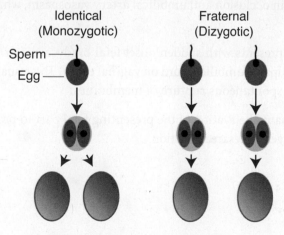

Figure 8.19 Multiple Gestations.
Source: Trlkly, commons.wikimedia.org.

Neonatal Infections

Infections in Pregnancy			
Infection	**Infectious agent**	**Diagnosis**	**Infant complication**
Toxoplasmosis	*Toxoplasma gondii*	Toxoplasmosis IgM and IgG	Chorioretinitis, intracranial calcifications, hydrocephalus
Syphilis	*Treponema pallidum*	VDRL/RPR confirmed with an FTA-ABS	• If acquired early: nonimmune hydrops fetalis, vesicular rash, anemia, thrombocytopenia, hepatosplenomegaly, high perinatal mortality • Late congenital: Hutchinson teeth, saber shins, saddle nose, deafness
Congenital rubella	Single-stranded RNA *Togaviridae*	Rubella IgM and IgG	Sensorineural deafness, cataracts, cardiac issues, intellectual disability, hepatosplenomegaly, thrombocytopenia, "blueberry muffin" rash
Herpes simplex virus	Genital herpes	HSV culture from a vesicle or HSV PCR	High mortality rate, meningoencephalitis, intellectual disability, pneumonia, hepatosplenomegaly, jaundice, petechiae
Congenital CMV	HHV-5	CMV IgM and IgG	IUGR, prematurity, microcephaly, jaundice, petechiae, periventricular calcifications, chorioretinitis
Congenital varicella	HHV-3	Clinical	Zigzag lesions, limb hypoplasia, microcephaly, microphthalmia, chorioretinitis, cataracts
Congenital Zika	Mosquito-borne flavivirus	Zika IgM and PCR	Microcephaly, facial disproportion, hypertonia, seizures, irritability, sensorineural hearing loss

Late Pregnancy Complications

Umbilical Cord Prolapse

Umbilical cord prolapse occurs when the cord extends beyond the presenting part of the fetus and protrudes into the vagina. A prolapsed cord is susceptible to umbilical vein occlusion and umbilical artery vasospasm, which reduce fetal oxygenation.

Cord prolapse presents with sudden onset fetal bradycardia or variable decelerations and palpable umbilical cord on vaginal exam. This usually occurs after amniotomy or spontaneous rupture of membranes.

Treatment is manual elevation of the presenting fetal part to prevent compression, and emergency cesarean section.

A 28-year-old woman in her 28th week of pregnancy presents with severe lower back pain. The pain is cyclical and increasing in intensity. On physical examination the patient seems to be in pain. Her temperature is 37.1 C (98.9 F), HR 104 bpm, BP 135/80 mm Hg, and RR 15/min. On pelvic examination the cervix is 3 cm dilated. Which of the following is the most likely diagnosis?

a. Premature rupture of membranes
b. Preterm labor
c. Cervical incompetence
d. Preterm contractions

Answer: **B.** Preterm labor is diagnosed when there is a combination of contractions with cervical dilation. A premature rupture of membranes patient would have a history of a "gush of fluid" from the vagina. Patients with cervical incompetence do not have a history of contractions, but there is painless dilation of the cervix. Preterm contractions do not lead to cervical dilation.

Preterm Labor

Risk factors include:

- Premature rupture of membranes
- Multiple gestation
- Previous history of preterm labor
- Placental abruption
- Maternal factors
  - Uterine anatomical abnormalities
  - Infections (chorioamnionitis)
  - Preeclampsia
  - Intraabdominal surgery

Symptoms include:

- Contractions (abdominal pain, lower back pain, or pelvic pain)
- Dilation of the cervix
- Occurs between 20 weeks and 36 weeks, 6 days

The fetus should be evaluated for weight, gestational age, and the presenting part (cephalic versus breech).

Circumstances in which preterm labor should *not* be stopped with tocolytics and delivery should occur are:

- Maternal severe hypertension (preeclampsia/eclampsia)
- Maternal cardiac disease
- Maternal cervical dilation of more than 4 cm
- Maternal hemorrhage (abruptio placenta, DIC)
- Fetal death
- Chorioamnionitis

▶**TIP**

When any of these is present, answer "delivery."

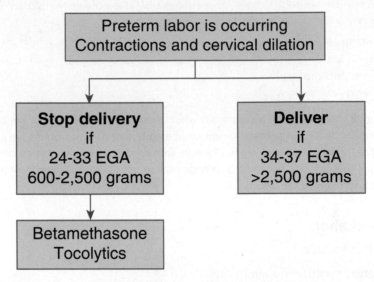

Figure 8.20 Preterm Labor Algorithm

Treatment is as follows:

"Mature the fetus's lungs" means increase surfactant.

- Corticosteroids, e.g., betamethasone, to mature the fetus's lungs. The effects begin within 24 hours, peak at 48 hours, and persist for 7 days. Corticosteroids reduce the risk of respiratory distress syndrome and neonatal mortality.
- A tocolytic should follow the steroids, to allow time for them to work.
  - Tocolytics slow the progression of cervical dilation by decreasing uterine contractions.
  - CCBs are the preferred tocolytic; they prevent calcium influx and inhibit release of intracellular calcium from the sarcoplasmic reticulum. This inhibits phosphorylation of myosin light chain kinase, leading to myometrial relaxation. Side effects include headache, flushing, and dizziness.
- The beta-adrenergic receptor agonist terbutaline also causes myometrial relaxation. It is not used as a tocolytic; however, it can be given to temporarily stop contractions in a laboring patient with a nonreassuring fetal heart tracing. Maternal effects include increase in heart rate leading to palpitations and hypotension.

▶**TIP**

Indomethacin is used as a tocolytic only in patients at <32 weeks' gestation. After birth, it is used to close a patent ductus arteriosus.

Prelabor Rupture of Membranes

Prelabor rupture of membranes (PROM) can happen at any time throughout pregnancy. It becomes the biggest problem when the fetus is preterm or with prolonged rupture of membranes. "Prolonged" means that labor starts >24 hours before delivery.

PROM leads to preterm labor, cord prolapse, placental abruption, and chorioamnionitis.

Symptoms include a history of a gush of fluid from the vagina. Sterile speculum examination should confirm the fluid as amniotic fluid:

- Fluid is present in posterior fornix.
- Fluid turns nitrazine paper blue because the pH is more basic.
- When placed on slide and allowed to air dry, fluid has ferning pattern.
- Amniotic fluid volume (AFI) may be low and aid in diagnosis.

Treatment of PROM depends on the fetus's gestational age and the presence of chorioamnionitis.

- If chorioamnionitis, deliver immediately.
- If no chorioamnionitis and the fetus is at term, wait 6–12 hours for spontaneous delivery; if there is no spontaneous delivery, then induce labor.

Preterm fetuses without chorioamnionitis should be treated with betamethasone (to mature the lungs), ampicillin, and 1 dose of azithromycin (to decrease risk of developing chorioamnionitis while waiting for steroids to begin working). If the patient is penicillin allergic but low-risk for anaphylaxis, use cefazolin and 1 dose of azithromycin. If high-risk for anaphylaxis, use clindamycin and 1 dose of azithromycin.

> Avoid multiple digital exams in patients with PROM to decrease the risk of chorioamnionitis.

Chorioamnionitis or "Triple I"

Intrauterine infection and/or inflammation is referred to as "triple I." Etiology is typically polymicrobial, involving vaginal flora such as *Ureaplasma*, *Mycoplasma*, *Gardnerella vaginalis*, or group B *Streptococcus*.

Risk factors include:

- Prolonged labor
- Prolonged rupture of membranes
- Multiple digital vaginal exams
- Cervical insufficiency
- Invasive testing
- Internal fetal monitoring
- STDs

Symptoms include:

- Maternal fever
- High WBC count
- Maternal and fetal tachycardia
- Uterine tenderness

Treatment of triple I is delivery of the baby and administration of antibiotics. Give ampicillin and gentamicin for a vaginal delivery. If delivery is by C-section, add clindamycin for anaerobic coverage.

Third-Trimester Bleeding

Placenta Previa

A 24-year-old woman in her 32nd week of pregnancy presents to the ED, having woken up this morning in a pool of blood. She has had no contractions or pain. Heart rate is 105 bpm and blood pressure 110/70 mm Hg. Which of the following is the best next step in management?

a. Digital vaginal exam
b. Transabdominal ultrasound
c. Immediate vaginal delivery
d. Immediate cesarean delivery
e. Transvaginal ultrasound

Answer: **B**. Transabdominal ultrasound is done before a digital vaginal exam in all third-trimester bleeding. This patient has painless vaginal bleeding, which may be indicative of placenta previa. If a digital vaginal exam is done, it can result in increased separation of the placenta and the uterus, leading to an increase in bleeding. Delivery is premature at this point. Do an ultrasound to distinguish between cesarean and vaginal delivery modes should it become necessary.

Placenta previa (cause of 20% of prenatal hemorrhages) is an abnormal implantation of the placenta over the internal cervical os. Risk factors include:

- Previous cesarean deliveries
- Previous uterine surgery
- Multiple gestations
- Previous placenta previa

Symptoms include painless vaginal bleeding.

It may be detected on routine U/S before 28 weeks, but usually does not cause bleeding until >28 weeks.

Ultrasound identifies the type of placenta previa.

- Transabdominal U/S is done first.
- Transvaginal U/S (**confirmatory test**) may be done afterward; the transvaginal probe must be held at least 2 cm away from the cervix and is unlikely to induce separation.

Digital vaginal exam is **contraindicated** in placenta previa. It may lead to increased separation between placenta and uterus, resulting in a severe hemorrhage.

- Transvaginal U/S helps monitor placement of the placenta in the uterus during pregnancy.
- The placenta must be more than 2 cm away from the internal cervical os to allow for a vaginal delivery. When the placenta is within 2 cm of the os, a cesarean section is necessary.

Treatment of placenta previa is done when there is large-volume bleeding or a drop in hematocrit.

- Strict pelvic rest, with nothing put into the vagina (intercourse)
- Immediate cesarean delivery only if indicated: unstoppable labor (cervix dilated >4 cm), severe hemorrhage, or fetal distress
  - Prepare for life-threatening bleeding by type and screen of blood, CBC, and prothrombin time.

Preterm fetuses should also be prepared for delivery with betamethasone to mature the fetus's lungs. Should delivery occur, cesarean birth is the mode of choice.

Vasa Previa and Velamentous Cord Insertion

A velamentous umbilical cord occurs when umbilical vessels lack the protective layer of Wharton jelly close to the placental insertion. These vessels are susceptible to compression and rupture. When this tenuous vascular connection overlies the cervical os, vasa previa can result.

Patients present with spontaneous rupture of membranes with heavy vaginal bleeding. Fetal heart rate changes may be present. The bleeding comes from the torn umbilical vessels crossing the os. If untreated, the result is rapid fetal exsanguination and death.

Treatment for all cases of vasa previa is emergency cesarean section.

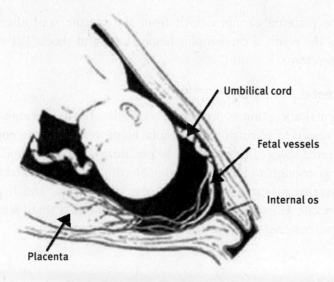

Figure 8.21 Vasa Previa.
Source: Elizabeth August, MD.

Placental Invasion (Accreta, Increta, Percreta)

The placenta may also abnormally adhere to different areas of the uterus (placenta accreta), which is associated with placenta previa. This becomes a problem when the placenta must detach from the uterus after the fetus is born. Often placental invasion cannot be seen on prenatal ultrasound, but it does result in a significant amount of postpartum hemorrhage. Patients are usually asymptomatic unless invasion into the bladder or rectum results in hematuria or rectal bleeding.

- **Placenta accreta**: abnormally adheres to the superficial uterine wall
- **Placenta increta**: attaches to the myometrium
- **Placenta percreta**: invades into uterine serosa, bladder wall, or rectal wall

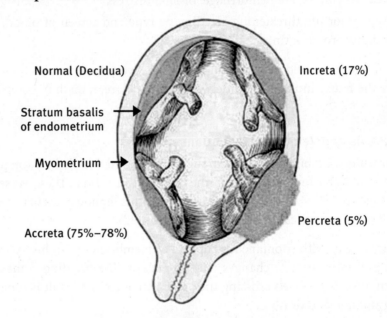

Figure 8.22 Types of Placental Invasion.
Source: Elizabeth August, MD.

If the placenta cannot detach from the uterine wall after delivery of the fetus, the result is catastrophic hemorrhage and shock. Patients often require hysterectomy.

Placental Abruption

Placental abruption is premature separation of the placenta from the uterus. This results in tearing of the placental blood vessels and hemorrhaging into the separated space. This can occur before, during, or after labor. If the separation is large enough and life-threatening bleeding occurs, premature delivery, uterine tetany, disseminated intravascular coagulation, and hypovolemic shock can occur. However, if the degree of separation is small with minor hemorrhage, then there may be no clinical signs or symptoms.

The primary etiology is unknown. However, there are several precipitating factors:

- Maternal hypertension (chronic, preeclampsia, eclampsia)
- Prior placental abruption
- Maternal cocaine use or smoking during pregnancy
- Maternal external trauma

Placental abruption presents with:

- Third-trimester vaginal bleeding
- Severe abdominal pain
- Contractions
- Possible fetal distress

▶ TIP

Placenta previa presents with **painless** vaginal bleeding, while placental abruption presents with **painful** vaginal bleeding.

Types of Placental Abruption		
Type	**Description**	**Complications**
Concealed	Blood is within uterine cavity	Serious complications (occur with larger abruptions) • Disseminated intravascular coagulation • Uterine tetany • Fetal hypoxia • Fetal death • Sheehan syndrome (postpartum hypopituitarism)
External	Blood drains through cervix	

Indications for cesarean delivery are:

- Uncontrollable maternal hemorrhage
- Rapidly expanding concealed hemorrhage
- Fetal distress
- Rapid placental separation

Vaginal deliveries are indicated if:

- Placental separation is limited
- Fetal heart tracing is reassuring
- Separation is extensive and fetus is dead

Uterine Rupture

Uterine rupture is life-threatening to both the mother and the fetus and usually occurs during labor.

> Life-threatening to mother or baby = Immediate delivery

Risk factors include:

- Previous cesarean deliveries (both types): classical (longitudinal along uterus) has higher risk of uterine rupture, or low transverse
- Trauma (most commonly, car accidents)
- Uterine myomectomy
- Uterine overdistention: polyhydramnios, multiple gestations
- Placenta percreta

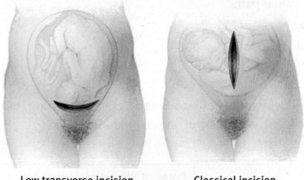

Low transverse incision   Classical incision

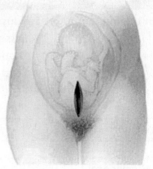

Low vertical incision

Figure 8.23 Types of Cesarean Scars.
Source: Elizabeth August, MD.

Symptoms include:

- Sudden onset of extreme abdominal pain
- Abnormal bump in abdomen
- No uterine contractions
- Loss of fetal station: fetus was moving toward delivery, but is no longer in the canal because it withdrew into the abdomen

Treatment is immediate laparotomy with delivery of the fetus. Cesarean delivery is not done because the baby may not be in the uterus (but floating in the abdomen). Repair of the uterus or hysterectomy will follow. If the patient undergoes a repair of the uterus, all subsequent pregnancies will be delivered via cesarean birth at 36 weeks.

> Uterine rupture requires immediate laparotomy and delivery of the fetus.

Rh Incompatibility

Rh incompatibility occurs when the mother is Rh negative and the baby is Rh positive. This is generally not a problem in the first pregnancy, as the mother has not developed antibodies to the "foreign" Rh-positive blood yet. When the first baby is delivered or fetal RBCs cross the placenta into the mother's bloodstream, she makes antibodies against the Rh-positive blood. When the mother gets pregnant for the second time, her antibodies attack the second Rh-positive baby. This leads to hemolysis of the fetus's RBCs or hemolytic disease of the newborn.

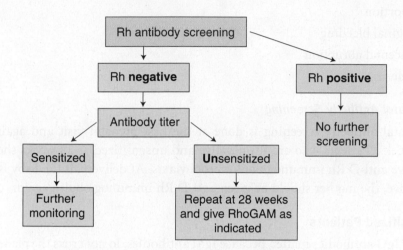

Figure 8.24 Rh Antibody Screening Algorithm. © Kaplan

Hemolytic Disease of Newborn

Hemolytic disease of the newborn results in fetal anemia and extramedullary production of RBCs because the baby's bone marrow is not able to make enough RBCs, so the liver and spleen help. Hemolysis results in increased heme and bilirubin levels in plasma. Bilirubin can be neurotoxic. These effects can lead to erythroblastosis fetalis, characterized by high fetal cardiac output (CHF).

▶ **TIP**

Extramedullary means "outside the bone marrow."

Initial Prenatal Visit

During the initial prenatal visit, an Rh antibody screening test is done. Patients who are Rh negative will have an Rh antibody titer done.

- Rh negative, **no** antibodies: **unsensitized**
- RH negative, **yes** antibodies: **sensitized**

▶ **TIP**

Antibody screen: done to see if mother is Rh− or Rh+

Antibody titer: done to see how many antibodies to Rh+ blood the mother has

Unsensitized Patients

Unsensitized patients do not yet have antibodies to Rh-positive blood. The goal is to keep it that way, so any time that fetal blood cells may cross the placenta, anti-D Rh immunoglobulins (RhoGAM) are given. The following are some scenarios where fetal blood cells may cross into the mother's blood:

- Amniocentesis
- Abortion
- Vaginal bleeding
- Placental abruption
- Delivery

Prenatal Antibody Screening

Prenatal antibody screening is done at the first prenatal visit and again at 28 weeks. Patients who are Rh negative and unsensitized at 28 weeks should receive anti-D Rh immunoglobulin prophylaxis. At delivery, if the baby is Rh positive, the mother should be given anti-D Rh immunoglobulin again.

Sensitized Patients

Only IgG antibodies matter, because IgM antibodies do not cross the placenta. Significant fetal anemia can occur if a critical titer is reached, usually 1:8–1:32. A higher titer level suggests severe fetal anemia, and an amniocentesis should be performed.

> Unsensitized = No anti-Rh antibodies present

Fetal Growth Abnormalities

Intrauterine Growth Restriction

Fetuses with intrauterine growth restriction (IUGR) weigh in the bottom 10% for their gestational age. The terms "symmetric growth" and "asymmetric growth" are no longer used.

Causes include:

- Chromosomal abnormalities
- Neural tube defects
- Infections
- Multiple gestations

- Maternal hypertension or renal disease
  - Maternal malnutrition and maternal substance abuse (**smoking is most preventable cause in United States**)

Ultrasound is done to confirm the gestational age and fetal weight.

Complications include:

- Premature labor
- Stillbirth
- Fetal hypoxia
- Lower IQ
- Seizures
- Intellectual disability

There is no conclusive treatment for IUGR other than prevention. Patients who smoke should quit. Prevent maternal infection with immunizations (but *not* live immunizations).

Macrosomia

Fetuses with an estimated birth weight >4,000 g are considered macrosomic babies. Risk factors include:

- Maternal diabetes or obesity
- Advanced maternal age
- Postterm pregnancy

On physical exam, normally the fundal height should equal the gestational age in weeks (i.e., if the patient is 28 weeks, the fundal height should be 28 cm). In macrosomia, the fundal height will be at least 3 cm greater than the gestational age (i.e., the patient is 28 weeks and the fundal height is 31 cm).

If the fundal height >3 cm greater than the gestational age, do an U/S, which will confirm the estimated gestational weight by:

- Femur length
- Abdominal circumference
- Head circumference
- Biparietal diameter

Complications include shoulder dystocia, birth injuries, low Apgar scores, and hypoglycemia.

Treatment is as follows:

- If lungs are mature **before** the fetus >4,500 g in weight: possible induction of labor

- If fetus >4,500 g in weight (diabetic mother) or >5,000 g in weight (nondiabetic mother): Cesarean delivery

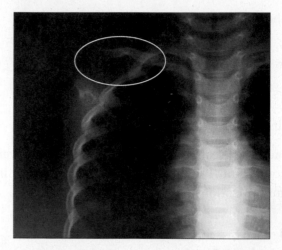

Figure 8.25 Birth Injuries: Clavicle Fracture and Brachial Plexus Injuries.
Source: Nevit Dilman, commons.wikimedia.org.

Medical Complications in Pregnancy

Hyperemesis Gravidarum

This is severe nausea and vomiting in pregnancy that leads to >5% decrease in body weight or weight loss of >6 lb compared with prepregnancy weight. Weight loss may be accompanied by electrolyte changes, including hypokalemia, hypochloremic metabolic alkalosis, hypomagnesemia, and hypocalcemia. Hyperemesis gravidarum usually resolves on its own midway through the pregnancy.

Weight gain recommendations in pregnancy:

BMI	Weight
<18.5 kg/m^2	28–40 lb
18.5–24.9 kg/m^2	25–35 lb
25–29.9 kg/m^2	15–25 lb
≥30 kg/m^2	11–20 lb

The answer to the "**best initial therapy**" question is dietary modification, avoidance of triggers, and nonpharmacological treatments such as acupuncture, ginger, or vitamin B6. In women with severe symptoms, the answer is antihistamines such as doxylamine or diphenhydramine. If the patient does not improve, then the "**best next step in management**" is to give dopamine antagonists such as metoclopramide. The final choice is serotonin antagonist such as ondansetron.

Asymptomatic Bacteriuria

Asymptomatic bacteriuria is typically screened for at 12–16 weeks of gestational age. If a urine specimen sent for culture returns positive, *the patient should receive antibiotic treatment* even if she has no UTI-like symptoms. If left untreated, asymptomatic bacteriuria can result in preterm birth, low birth weight, and perinatal mortality.

The **best empiric treatment** is nitrofurantoin, amoxicillin, or cephalexin. Adjust treatment based on culture results.

Acute Cystitis

Establishing a diagnosis of acute cystitis is the same as in nonpregnant women: The patient is positive for urinary frequency, dysuria, and the presence of WBCs on UA. Begin empiric treatment with nitrofurantoin until the results of sensitivity return. Then tailor the antibiotics to the results.

Acute Pyelonephritis

Symptoms and diagnostic tests are the same as in a nonpregnant woman. However, pregnancy in a patient with acute pyelonephritis warrants hospital admission and IV ceftriaxone. Aztreonam is used in penicillin-allergic patients. After treatment, evaluate urine cultures monthly for recurrent bacteriuria.

> Avoid in pregnant patients:
> - Trimethoprim-sulfamethoxazole in first trimester: Trimethoprim is a folic acid antagonist.
> - Aminoglycosides: associated with ototoxicity
> - Doxycycline and fluoroquinolones: causes yellow discoloration of bones and cartilage

Pulmonary Embolism and DVT in Pregnancy

Pregnancy and the postpartum period are well-known risk factors for thromboembolism. It can manifest as either a deep vein thrombosis (DVT) or pulmonary embolism (PE). The fact that dyspnea is a common symptom among pregnant women—and is physiologic in the majority—makes the diagnosis of pulmonary embolism more difficult. But you must differentiate between the two.

The **best diagnostic test** for PE in pregnancy is a V/Q scan. If the V/Q scan is indeterminate, answer CT pulmonary angiogram.

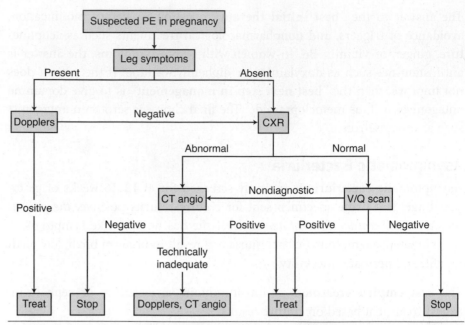

PE: pulmonary embolism; Dopplers: lower extremity Doppler ultrasounds; CXR: chest x-ray; CT angio: computed tomographic pulmonary angiogram; V/Q scan: ventilation-perfusion scan

Figure 8.26 Diagnosis of Suspected Pulmonary Embolism in Pregnancy. © Kaplan

> Warfarin is contraindicated in pregnancy owing to its teratogenic effects: nasal bone hypoplasia, laryngomalacia, congenital heart defects, and growth retardation.

Treatment of PE/DVT is low-molecular-weight (LMW) heparin.

- Stop the LMW heparin 24 hours before delivery, if a set time for delivery is known.
- Resume 12 hours after C-section and 6 hours after vaginal delivery, and continue for 6 weeks postpartum.

Warfarin, direct thrombin inhibitors, and factor Xa inhibitors are contraindicated in pregnancy.

Cervical Cancer during Pregnancy

Cervical cancer is screened via Pap during pregnancy. If the Pap smear is abnormal, treatment is the same as if the patient were not pregnant. Colposcopy with cervical biopsy is needed if there are atypical glandular cells and also if a high-grade squamous intraepithelial lesion is either present or cannot be excluded.

While colposcopy is safe in pregnancy under these indications, endocervical curettage should not be performed. Diagnostic tests are otherwise completed as in nonpregnant patients. If a pregnant patient has invasive disease, she must decide whether to carry the pregnancy to term or terminate; this decision will guide patient management.

PEP/PUPPP

Polymorphic eruption of pregnancy (PEP), also called pruritic urticarial papules and plaques of pregnancy (PUPPP), is a benign, self-limiting pruritic inflammatory disorder that is common in pregnancy. PUPPP presents as erythematous papules within striae that spread outward to form urticarial plaques. It typically occurs in the first pregnancy after 35 weeks or postpartum and usually resolves spontaneously by 15 days postpartum. The face, palms, and soles are spared. All patients with PUPPP have extreme pruritus. Treatment is topical corticosteroids such as clobetasol or betamethasone to decrease the pruritus.

Intrahepatic Cholestasis of Pregnancy

Intrahepatic cholestasis of pregnancy (ICP) is characterized by pruritus in the absence of rash accompanied by an elevated serum bile acid concentration. ICP usually develops during the third trimester and resolves with delivery. Affected women present with moderate to severe pruritus, predominantly on the palms and soles, that is worse at night. Etiology is not well understood; a possibility is high concentrations of estrogen and progesterone oversaturating the hepatic biliary system.

Physical exam shows no primary skin lesions, only excoriations from scratching. Lab results for AST, ALT, GGT, alkaline phosphatase, and bilirubin may be elevated *or* within normal limits. Elevated bile acids, cholic acid, and chenodeoxycholic acid confirm the diagnosis.

ICP carries an increased risk of intrauterine fetal death. Treat with ursodeoxycholic acid and induction of labor at term.

Acute Fatty Liver of Pregnancy (AFLP)

AFLP results from microvesicular fatty infiltration of hepatocytes in the third trimester. The most frequent symptoms are nausea, vomiting, abdominal pain, malaise, anorexia, and jaundice. About half of patients have signs of preeclampsia at some time during the course of illness.

Laboratory findings include:

- LFT (AST, ALT) and bilirubin: elevated
- WBCs: may be elevated
- Platelet counts: occasionally decreased
- Severe cases: high serum ammonia, prolonged prothrombin time, and hypoglycemia from hepatic insufficiency; acute kidney injury and hyperuricemia often occur together

Diagnosis is based on clinical suspicion and laboratory values. Liver biopsy is the gold standard for diagnosis.

Treatment is maternal stabilization (fluids, glucose monitoring, possible transfusion as needed) and prompt delivery.

> The clinical similarities between AFLP and HELLP syndrome (hemolysis, elevated liver enzymes, low platelets) make it difficult to distinguish between them. Signs of **hepatic insufficiency (hypoglycemia, encephalopathy) and abnormalities in coagulation profile** point toward a diagnosis of AFLP.

A 29-year-old woman G2P1 in her 30th week of pregnancy presents for a routine prenatal visit. She has no real complaints except that her wedding ring is getting too tight. On physical exam her blood pressure is 150/100 mm Hg, heart rate 92/min, respiratory rate 12/min, and temperature 37.2 C (99 F). Urine dipstick done in the office reveals 1+ protein. Which of the following is the most likely diagnosis?

a. Chronic hypertension
b. Gestational hypertension
c. HELLP syndrome
d. Preeclampsia
e. Eclampsia

Answer: **D.** Preeclampsia is characterized by hypertension, edema, and protein-uria. Eclampsia is preeclampsia with seizures. HELLP syndrome is a complication of preeclampsia with elevated liver enzymes and low platelets. Chronic hypertension is increased blood pressure that was present before the patient became pregnant. Gestational hypertension begins during pregnancy but has no edema or proteinuria.

Hypertension

Chronic Hypertension

Chronic hypertension is hypertension defined as a BP >140/90 mm Hg before the patient became pregnant or before 20 weeks of gestation. It may lead to preeclampsia. Treat the patient with methyldopa, labetalol, or nifedipine.

Gestational Hypertension

Gestational hypertension is defined as a BP >140/90 mm Hg that starts after 20 weeks' gestation. There is no proteinuria and no edema.

> ACE inhibitors and ARBs cause fetal malformations. Do not use them in pregnancy.

The patient is treated only during pregnancy with methyldopa, labetalol, or nifedipine.

Preeclampsia

> The only definitive treatment in preeclampsia is delivery.

Risk factors for preeclampsia include chronic hypertension, renal disease, and history of preeclampsia in a prior pregnancy. Patients with risk factors can be placed on aspirin therapy early in the pregnancy to reduce their risk.

Presentation of Types of Preeclampsia		
	Preeclampsia without severe features	**Preeclampsia with severe features**
Hypertension	>140/90	>160/110
Proteinuria	Dipstick 1+ to 2+; 24-hour urine >300 mg	Not necessary for diagnosis once severe features present
Mental status changes	No	Yes
Vision changes	No	Yes
Right upper quadrant pain	No	Yes
Severe headache	No	Yes

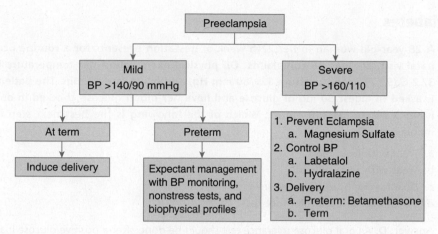

Figure 8.27 Preeclampsia Algorithm

> **Etiology of pain in preeclampsia:**
>
> Impaired liver function → Swelling of Glisson capsule → RUQ pain

Eclampsia

Eclampsia is defined as a tonic-clonic seizure occurring in a patient with a history of preeclampsia.

To treat eclampsia, first stabilize the mother, then deliver the baby. Seizure control should be done with magnesium sulfate and blood pressure control with hydralazine.

> Eclampsia = preeclampsia + seizures

HELLP Syndrome

Patients have:

HELLP = **h**emolysis; **e**levated **l**iver enzymes; **l**ow **p**latelets

Treatment is the same as for eclampsia.

The table differentiates hypertensive disorders in pregnancy.

Disorder	BP (mm Hg)	Proteinuria?	Warning signs?	Other features
Chronic hypertension (Dx <20 weeks)	≥140/90 but ≤160/110	No	No	
Gestational hypertension (Dx >20 weeks)	≥140/90 but ≤160/110	No	No	
Preeclampsia without severe features	≥140/90 but ≤160/110	Yes	No	
Severe gestational hypertension	≥160/110	No	No	
Preeclampsia with severe features (1)	≥140/90	Yes	Yes	
Preeclampsia with severe features (2)	≥160/110	Yes	No	
Eclampsia	Elevated			Seizures with no alternative organic cause
HELLP syndrome				Hemolytic anemia, elevated LFTs, low platelets

Diabetes

A 28-year-old woman in her 27th week of gestation presents for a routine pre-natal visit. She has no complaints. On physical examination her temperature is 37.2 C (99 F), blood pressure 120/80 mm Hg, and heart rate 87/min. The patient is asked to ingest 50 mg of glucose and have her blood glucose checked in one hour; it returns as 190 mg/dL. Which of the following is the best next step in management?

a. Treat with insulin.
b. Treat with sulfonylurea.
c. Do a fasting blood glucose level.
d. Do an oral glucose tolerance test.

Answer: **D.** An oral glucose tolerance test should be done after a positive glucose load test (described in the question). Fasting blood glucose is not used to diagnose gesta-tional diabetes. Treatment with insulin is premature without a diagnosis of gestational diabetes. Sulfonylurea has been used, but it does not have better pregnancy outcomes than insulin.

Pregestational Diabetes

Pregestational diabetes means that a woman had diabetes before she became pregnant. She can be a type 1 or a type 2 diabetic.

Complications

- Increased maternal risk of:
  - Preeclampsia
  - Spontaneous abortion
  - Infection
  - Postpartum hemorrhage
- Increased fetal risk of:
  - Congenital anomalies (heart and neural tube)
  - Macrosomia (possible complications include shoulder dystocia, in which fetus's shoulder gets stuck under the symphysis pubis during delivery)

Evaluation

These tests should be done in addition to the usual prenatal tests:

- EKG
- 24-hour urine for baseline renal function
  - Creatinine clearance
  - Protein
- HbA1c
- Ophthalmological exam for baseline eye function and assessing the condi-tion of the retina

Gestational Diabetes

Complications

- Preterm birth
- Fetal macrosomia
- Birth injuries from fetal macrosomia
- Neonatal hypoglycemia: There is an increase in fetal insulin, secondary to living in a hyperglycemic environment. When the fetus leaves the hyperglycemic environment, the excess insulin causes the glucose to drop.
- Mothers with gestational diabetes are 4–10 times more likely to develop type 2 diabetes later in life.

Evaluation

Gestational diabetes is routinely screened for between 24 and 28 weeks of gestational age. Human placental lactogen (hPL), recently renamed human somatomammotropin, is a hormone produced by the placenta that peaks at this time and decreases maternal insulin sensitivity owing to its similar biochemical properties. A glucose load test is done first. It consists of nonfasting ingestion of 50 g of glucose, with a measurement of serum glucose one hour later. If the serum glucose is above 130–140 mg/dL, then a glucose tolerance test is done. The glucose tolerance test consists of the ingestion of 100 g of glucose after a fast and fasting blood glucose is taken. Glucose has been then measured 3 times (at 1, 2, and 3 hours). If 2 of the 4 measurements are abnormal, the test is positive for gestational diabetes.

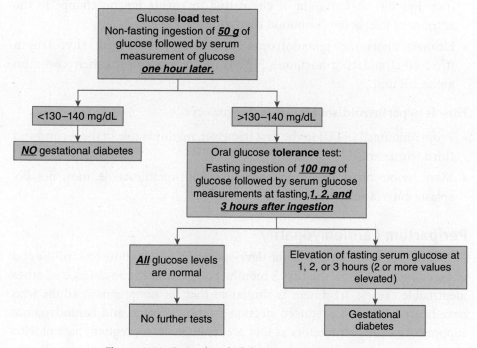

Figure 8.28 Gestational Diabetes Testing Algorithm

Treatment for gestational diabetes starts with diabetic diet and exercise (walking). If that fails to control blood sugars (fasting >90 mg/dL and 2 hour postprandial >120mg/dL), medication is indicated, with insulin the gold standard. For patients who refuse insulin, glyburide and metformin are safe alternatives.

▶ **TIP**

Do *not* tell pregnant patients to lose weight. It is the most common wrong answer.

Thyroid Disease

When it comes to thyroid disease in pregnancy, there are a few key things to know.

What crosses the placenta?

- TRH
- Immunoglobulins against TSH receptor

What does not cross the placenta?

- TSH
- T4

What physiologic changes in pregnancy affect thyroid disease?

- There is an increase in serum thyroxine-binding globulin (TBG), which increases the total amount of circulating thyroxine but no change in the amount of free, active, unbound thyroxine.
- Human chorionic gonadotropin (hCG) stimulates the thyrotropin (thyroid-stimulating hormone [TSH]) receptor owing to their common alpha subunit.

How is hyperthyroidism treated in pregnancy?

- Propylthiouracil (PTU) in the first trimester, methimazole in the second and third trimesters
- More serious birth defects are associated with methimazole, most notably aplasia cutis (a scalp defect).

Peripartum Cardiomyopathy

Peripartum cardiomyopathy is the development of heart failure toward the end of pregnancy or within the first 5 months postpartum in the absence of other identifiable causes. Treatment is similar to that for nonpregnant adults who have heart failure with reduced ejection fraction: oxygen and hemodynamic support. Avoid ACE inhibitors as they are teratogenic. A pregnant patient with peripartum cardiomyopathy should deliver the fetus, as heart failure will only worsen under the ongoing hemodynamic changes of pregnancy.

Hemoglobinopathies

Pregnant women with thalassemia or sickle cell disease should be referred to a genetic counselor regarding risks of transmission to offspring. They should also receive folic acid and iron supplementation. Their risk of requiring a blood transfusion remains high.

Labor and Delivery Complications

A 22-year-old nullipara in her 39th week of pregnancy presents with intense abdominal pain that is intermittent. She states that she felt a gush of fluid from her vagina almost 3 hours ago. On physical exam her cervix is 3 cm dilated and 50% effaced, and the fetus's head is felt at the –2 station. For the next 3 hours she continues to progress so that her cervix is 8 cm dilated, 60% effaced, and fetal head is felt at –1 station. Six hours after presentation, her cervix is 8 cm dilated and 60% effaced, and fetal head is felt at 0 station. Which of the following is the most likely diagnosis?

a. Prolonged latent stage
b. Protracted cervical dilation
c. Arrest of descent
d. Arrest of cervical dilation

Answer: **D.** Arrest of cervical dilation is when there is no dilation of the cervix for >2 hours. Patients who are >6 cm dilated are considered to be in active stage 1 labor. Patients with prolonged latent stage take more than 20 hours (in primipara) to reach 6 cm of dilation. Protracted cervical dilation occurs when the primipara's cervix does not dilate more than 1.2 cm in 1 hour. It is dilating slowly, but still dilating. Arrest of descent is when the fetal head does not move down into the canal.

Prolonged Latent Stage

Prolonged latent stage occurs when the latent phase lasts >20 hours for primipara and >14 hours for multipara.

Causes include sedation, unfavorable cervix, and uterine dysfunction with irregular or weak contractions.

Treatment is rest and hydration. Most will convert to spontaneous delivery in 6–12 hours.

Protracted Cervical Dilation

Protraction occurs when there is slow dilation during the active phase of stage 1 labor, <1.2 cm per hour in nulliparous patients, and <1.5 cm per hour in multiparous patients.

The etiology is the 3 Ps:

- **Power**: strength and frequency of uterine contractions
- **Passenger**: size and position of fetus
- **Passage**: if passenger is larger than pelvis = cephalopelvic disproportion

Treatment of cephalopelvic disproportion is cesarean delivery. If the uterine contractions are weak, oxytocin may be given.

Malpresentation

A 25-year-old woman in her 35th week of gestation presents for a routine prenatal checkup. She has no complaints. On physical examination her temperature is 36.6 C (98 F), blood pressure 130/90 mm Hg, heart rate 87/min, and respiratory rate 12/min. Her abdomen is gravid. On palpation of the abdomen, a hard circular surface is felt in the proximal part of the uterus. Which of the following is the next step in management?

a. External cephalic version
b. Ultrasound
c. CT scan
d. X-ray

Answer: **B**. This patient is showing signs of a possible breech presentation on physical exam (the hard circular surface is the fetal head). Breech presentation should be confirmed via ultrasound before therapeutic measures such as external cephalic version are implemented. X-ray and CT scan are avoided during pregnancy secondary to the radiation exposure.

Presentation includes:

- Lower half of fetus (pelvis and legs) is the presenting part.
  - The presenting part is the part of the fetal body that is closest to the vaginal canal and will be engaged when labor starts. Normally it is the head (cephalic presentation); however, in malpresentation, it can be a foot or a buttock.
- Can be felt on physical exam
  - Leopold maneuvers are a set of 4 maneuvers that estimate the fetal weight and the presenting part of the fetus.
  - Vaginal exam: With malpresentation, you feel a soft mass instead of the normal hard surface of skull.

Ultrasound is needed to visualize the fetus and confirm the diagnosis.

Types of Breech Presentation	
Type	**Description**
Frank breech	Fetus's hips are flexed with extended knees bilaterally
Complete breech	Fetus's hips and knees are flexed bilaterally
Footling breech	Fetus's feet are first: one leg (single footling) or both legs (double footling)

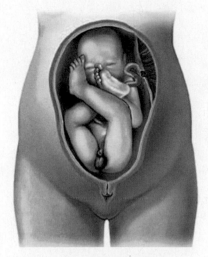

Figure 8.29 Frank Breech.
Source: Elizabeth August, MD.

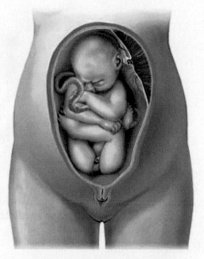

Figure 8.30 Complete Breech.
Source: Elizabeth August, MD.

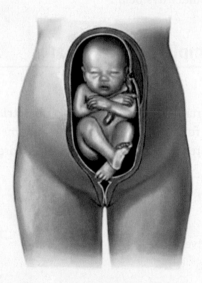

Figure 8.31 Footling Breech (Incomplete Breech).
Source: Elizabeth August, MD.

With external cephalic version, the caregiver maneuvers the fetus into a cephalic presentation (head down) through the abdominal wall. You should not perform this maneuver until after 37 weeks' gestation. The fetus can maneuver itself into a cephalic presentation (head first) before 37 weeks.

Shoulder Dystocia

Shoulder dystocia occurs when the fetus's head has been delivered but the anterior shoulder is stuck behind the mother's pubic symphysis.

> Any factor that indicates that a fetus is too big or the pelvis is too small is a risk factor for shoulder dystocia.

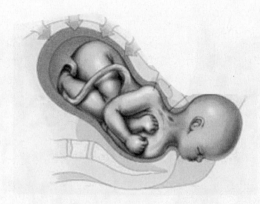

Figure 8.32 Shoulder Dystocia.
Source: Elizabeth August, MD.

Risk factors include:

- Maternal diabetes and obesity cause fetal macrosomia.
- Postterm pregnancy allows the baby more time to grow.
- History of prior shoulder dystocia

Postpartum Complications

Uterine Inversion

Uterine inversion is a rare complication and an **obstetrical emergency**. Inversion occurs when the fundus collapses into the endometrial cavity and turns inside out. It is often related to excessive umbilical cord traction and fundal pressure during Stage 3 of labor.

Risk factors include:

- Macrosomia
- Rapid labor and delivery
- Short umbilical cord
- Uterine abnormalities
- Placenta accreta

Symptoms include vaginal bleeding, lower abdominal pain, and a smooth round mass protruding from the cervix and vagina.

Diagnosis is based on clinical presentation.

Treatment is to return the uterus back to its correct position.

- **Stop all uterotonic drugs.** You need to have the uterus relaxed to return it to its proper position.
- **Manually reposition the uterus.** If uterine repositioning is not possible with manual maneuvers alone, try a uterine relaxing agent such as nitroglycerine, terbutaline, or magnesium sulfate.

If all else fails, perform laparotomy to reposition the uterus.

Lactational Mastitis

Lactational mastitis is inflammation of the breast with fever, myalgia, pain, and erythema. It can be either infectious or noninfectious. Although it usually occurs during the first 6 weeks postpartum, it can occur at any time during the period of breastfeeding. Diagnosis is based on clinical presentation.

Treat with dicloxacillin or cephalexin, anti-inflammatory medications, and cold compresses. Breastfeeding should be continued.

Postpartum Blues and Depression

Postpartum blues is a transient condition that starts 2–3 days after delivery and resolves in 2 weeks. It appears to be related to a change in hormones. The condition is characterized by sadness, tearfulness, anxiety, insomnia, and decreased concentration.

Risk factors for postpartum blues:

- Family history of depression
- Depression symptoms during pregnancy
- History of PMS/PMDD
- Stress surrounding child care

Treatment is not needed, as postpartum blues is self-limiting. It may, however, progress to postpartum depression.

Risk factors for postpartum depression:

- Depression in the past
- History of abuse
- Young age
- Unplanned pregnancy
- Stressful life events, such as lack of social or financial support
- No partner or intimate partner violence
- Gestational diabetes
- Not breastfeeding
- Miscarriage/stillbirth

Symptoms include:

- Anxiety and panic attacks
- Irritability and anger
- Feeling inadequate or overwhelmed with taking care of the baby
- Feelings of failure as a mother
- Fear of hurting self or baby

> Postpartum psychosis is postpartum depression plus delusions, hallucinations, and disorganized thoughts and behavior.

Many of the symptoms of postpartum depression overlap with the effects of being a new mom—such as fatigue, trouble sleeping, and low libido—so it can often be hard to distinguish between the two. Although postpartum depression is common, women are often reluctant to ask for help.

Diagnosis and treatment for depression in a postpartum patient are the same as for the general population.

Hemorrhage

Postpartum hemorrhage is defined by blood loss ≥1,000 mL or bleeding with signs and symptoms of hypovolemia within 24 hours of delivery. **Early** postpartum bleeding occurs within 24 hours of delivery, while **late** postpartum bleeding occurs 24 hours to 12 weeks later.

> *a* = without
>
> *tony* = contractions

Normally, postpartum, the uterine contractions compress the blood vessels to stop blood loss. In uterine atony, this does not occur. Uterine atony accounts for 80% of postpartum hemorrhage. Other causes include laceration, retained parts, and coagulopathy.

Risk factors for atony include:

> Sheehan syndrome after postpartum hemorrhage presents as inability to breastfeed.

- Anesthesia
- Uterine overdistention (such as in twins and polyhydramnios)
- Prolonged labor
- Retained placenta (can occur with placenta accreta)
- Coagulopathy

Treatment starts with a bimanual examination of the uterus. Assure that there is no rupture of the uterus and there is no retained placenta.

If the examination is unremarkable, bimanual compression and massage should be done. This will control most cases of postpartum bleeding. If the bimanual massage does not control the postpartum bleeding, administer oxytocin to make the uterus contract, constricting the blood vessels and decreasing the blood flow.

Breastfeeding

Benefits
- Enhanced infant gastrointestinal function
- Decreased risk of infant infection
- Increased rate of maternal recovery
- Decreased maternal and neonatal stress
- Higher rate of maternal weight loss postpartum

- Decreased risk of maternal breast, ovarian, and endometrial cancer
- Decreased risk of maternal cardiovascular disease and type II diabetes mellitus

Contraindications

Maternal

- HIV/HTLV-1
- Active tuberculosis
- Active herpes virus breast lesions
- Maternal use of drugs of abuse
- Cytotoxic medications (methotrexate, cyclosporine)

Neonatal

- Galactosemia

PART 9

Gynecology

by Victoria Hastings, DO, MPH, MS

Normal Menstrual Cycle

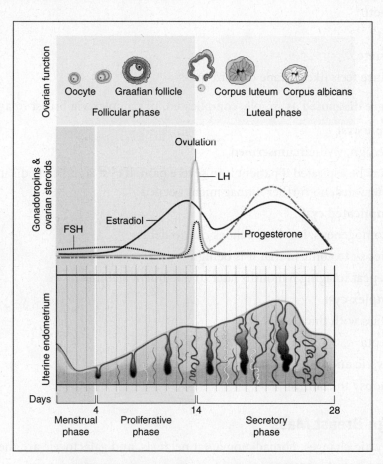

Figure 9.1 Normal Menstrual Cycle. © Kaplan

The normal menstrual cycle begins on the first day of menstruation and continues until menstruation begins again. At the end of menses during the follicular phase, increasing levels of estradiol initially suppress LH and FSH as part of a negative feedback system. Eventually, the level of estradiol increases to the point that it stimulates production of both follicle-stimulating hormone (FSH) and luteinizing hormone (LH), which are released into circulation. This "LH surge" leads to ovulation, and progesterone levels increase to support and stabilize the endometrial lining. If a pregnancy does not occur, progesterone levels will fall and menstruation will occur.

Mittelschmerz is the diagnosis in women who report mild unilateral pelvic pain that occurs monthly at the time of ovulation.

Breast Lesions

Breast Cyst

A breast cyst presents as a painful or painless mass in the breast that can arise suddenly or enlarge acutely. It may be related to the menstrual cycle. On physical exam, cysts will be:

- Smooth
- Firm
- Discrete
- Texture feels like a grape or hard mass

Cysts are diagnosed as simple, complicated, or complex via breast imaging.

- **Simple cyst**
  - Benign, well-circumscribed
  - May be aspirated if patient is in severe pain; if cyst completely disappears afterward, no further management needed
- **Complicated cyst**
  - Homogenous; low level echoes due to debris
  - Biopsy to confirm that it is benign
  - Repeat imaging 6 months later to document stability
- **Complex cyst**
  - Mass with thick walls
  - Septa
  - Cystic and solid components
  - Biopsy to confirm

Benign Breast Mass

Fibrocystic changes, fibroadenoma, fat necrosis, and galactocele are the most common breast masses.

Benign Breast Lesions				
Disease	**Etiology**	**Physical findings**	**Diagnosis**	**Management**
Fibrocystic changes	Cyclical breast pain: increases with approach of menses, returns to baseline once menstruation starts	• Nodular tissue bilaterally • Diffuse tenderness • Mass not discrete or well defined	Physical exam	Observation
Fibroadenoma	• Benign solid tumors with glandular and fibrous tissue • 20% bilateral • May increase in size with pregnancy and decrease with menopause	Well-defined mobile mass	• Ultrasound • Definitive diagnosis with core needle biopsy	• Observation with repeat ultrasound 3–6 months • Excise if increases in size to rule out malignancy
Fat necrosis	Results from breast trauma or surgery	• Clinically detected hard lump • May be confused with malignancy	Mammogram	Observation (self-limiting)
Intraductal papilloma	Papillary cells growing into cyst lumen	Bloody nipple discharge	Core needle biopsy	Surgical excision to rule out hidden cancer
Mastitis	Prolonged engorgement in breastfeeding women or inflammation in non-breastfeeding women	Painful, swollen, erythematous breast(s)	Cultures	Cover for *S. aureus*: dicloxacillin or cephalexin
Breast abscess	Localized collection of pus in breast tissue	Fluctuant, tender, palpable mass with fever and malaise		• Needle aspiration, surgical drainage, and antibiotics (dicloxacillin or cephalexin) • If MRSA suspected: TMP-SMX or clindamycin

Breast Cancer

A 52-year-old woman with a medical history of hypertension presents for a routine physical exam. She states that she is feeling well, although tired at times. Her colonoscopy, mammogram, and Pap smear done at age 50 were normal. Blood pressure today is 135/80 mm Hg, RR 12, temperature 36.9 C (98.5 F), and BMI 29. Physical exam is within normal limits. Which of the following screening tests is indicated at this time?

a. Colonoscopy

b. DEXA scan

c. Mammogram

d. Pap smear

e. Hepatitis B screen

Answer: **C.** Screening mammogram is recommended every other year for women age 50–74. Colonoscopy is done every 10 years in the general population; repeat colonoscopy is done every 3–5 years if there is a polyp present. Osteoporosis screening with a DEXA scan starts at age 65. Pap smear is done every 3 years if cytology alone is done or every 5 years if done in conjunction with HPV testing. Hepatitis B screening is not conducted routinely unless the patient is at high risk; however, a onetime screen for hepatitis C is done in patients born 1945–1965.

Breast Cancer Screening

According to the United States Preventive Services Task Force (USPSTF), breast cancer screening should be conducted every 2 years in the general population, starting at age 50 and ending at age 74. Mammogram is the best screening test for breast cancer, and it has been proven to decrease mortality. In patients with a family history of breast cancer, start screening at age 40.

BRCA Screening

BRCA gene screening and genetic counseling are recommended for patients with:

- A family member with ovarian, fallopian tube, primary peritoneal cancer
- Two family members with breast cancer age <50
- Two or more primary breast cancers
- A personal history of triple-negative breast cancer diagnosed age <60
- A male family member with breast cancer
- Breast, prostate, or pancreatic cancer diagnosed at any age in 2 relatives
- A personal history of breast cancer age <50

A 55-year-old woman presents to the office for a breast mass that she felt. The mass is painless and mobile, and it has been present for the past week. Mammogram done last year was negative. Vital signs are stable. Physical exam is significant for a 3 cm × 3 cm, round, firm mass that is mobile and nontender, located on the right breast at the 4 o'clock position. No nipple discharge or skin changes are noted, and no axillary lymph nodes are palpated. What is the next step in management?

a. Biopsy
b. Mammogram
c. Breast ultrasound
d. Breast MRI
e. No further treatment

Answer: **B.** Diagnostic mammogram is done as the first-line test in women with a palpable breast mass, regardless of when the last mammogram was done. Even in a woman under the age of 30, *a mammogram should be performed first*. Breast ultrasound is done first only if the woman is breastfeeding or pregnant. Breast MRI is not a screening test. Biopsy is never the first step in the workup.

Malignant and Premalignant Breast Lesions				
Disease	**Etiology**	**Physical findings**	**Diagnosis**	**Management**
Paget disease of the breast	Migration of neoplastic ductal epithelial cells to nipple	Scaly, vesicular, ulcerated lesion +/− bloody nipple discharge	• Bilateral mammogram • Wedge or punch biopsy • Underlying breast cancer in 85% of cases	• Simple mastectomy • Breast conservation surgery in select cases
Phyllodes tumor	Papillary projections of epithelial-lined stroma with varying degrees of hyperplasia and atypia	Smooth mobile rapidly growing breast mass or abnormal radiographic findings	• Ultrasound • Core needle biopsy	Excision
Lobular carcinoma in situ (LCIS)	Atypical proliferation within terminal duct lobules	Usually an incidental finding diagnosed on breast biopsy performed for another reason	Core biopsy	Surgical excision
Ductal carcinoma in situ (DCIS)	Proliferation of neoplastic epithelial cells within mammary ducts without stromal invasion	Suspicious microcalcifications on mammography	Core biopsy	Lumpectomy with radiation therapy OR mastectomy
Lobular carcinoma	Invasion of neoplastic cells into mammary stroma and adipose in a single-file pattern	Hard, immovable, single dominant lesion with irregular borders	• Mammogram • Core biopsy	Surgery +/− radiation therapy +/− chemotherapy
Ductal carcinoma	Nests of tumor cells within glandular tissue			

Amenorrhea

Amenorrhea is the absence of menstruation. It can be primary or secondary.

Primary Amenorrhea

Primary amenorrhea is the absence of menstruation by the age of 15 years in a female who has normal secondary sexual characteristics. If a girl has not developed secondary sexual characteristics (i.e., breasts) by age 13, begin a workup for primary amenorrhea. Causes include:

- Gonadal dysgenesis (Turner syndrome)
- Müllerian agenesis
- Delay of puberty
- Polycystic ovary syndrome (PCOS)
- Hypopituitarism

This is not an exhaustive list. Also remember that secondary amenorrhea can present as primary amenorrhea, so always rule out pregnancy.

Diagnostic Tests

Initial testing for primary amenorrhea includes:

- β-HCG
- TSH
- Prolactin
- FSH
- Pelvic ultrasound (to assess for presence of a uterus)

Treatment depends on the cause of the amenorrhea.

Secondary Amenorrhea

Secondary amenorrhea is the absence of menses for >3 months in a female who menstruates regularly or absence of menses for 6 months in a female who menstruates irregularly. Causes include:

- Pregnancy (**most common**)
- Hypothalamic amenorrhea
- Hyperprolactinemia
- Primary ovarian insufficiency
- Polycystic ovarian syndrome
- Thyroid abnormalities

Diagnostic Tests

Best initial test is β-HCG—this is done first.

The workup for secondary amenorrhea is *very high yield* for Step 2. The algorithm for workup is provided.

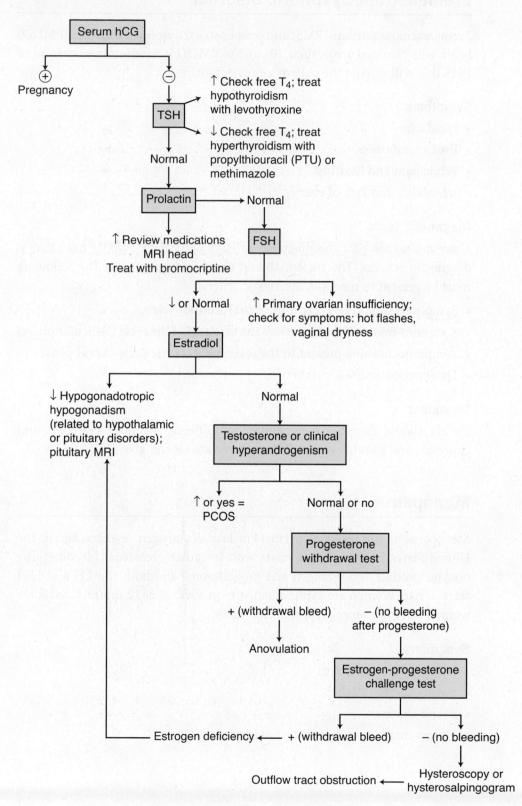

Figure 9.2 Workup for Amenorrhea Algorithm

Premenstrual Syndrome and Premenstrual Dysphoric Disorder

Premenstrual syndrome (PMS) and premenstrual dysphoric disorder (PMDD) begin when women are in their 20s to 30s. PMDD is a more severe version of PMS that will disrupt the patient's daily activities.

Symptoms

- Headache
- Breast tenderness
- Pelvic pain and bloating
- Irritability and lack of energy

Diagnostic Tests

There are no tests for the diagnosis of PMS or PMDD; PMDD has DSM-V diagnostic criteria. The patient should chart her symptoms. The following must be present to meet the diagnostic criteria:

- Symptoms should be present for 2 consecutive cycles
- Symptom-free period of 1 week in the first part of the cycle (follicular phase)
- Symptoms must be present in the second half of the cycle (luteal phase)
- Dysfunction in life

Treatment

Patient should decrease consumption of caffeine, alcohol, cigarettes, and chocolate and should exercise. If symptoms are severe, give SSRIs.

Menopause

Menopause is the result of permanent loss of estrogen (average age in the United States is 51 years). It starts with irregular menstrual bleeding. The oocytes produce less estrogen and progesterone, and both the LH and FSH start to rise. Women are symptomatic for an average of 12 months, but some women can experience symptoms for years.

Symptoms

- Menstrual irregularity
- Sweats and hot flashes
- Mood changes
- Dyspareunia (pain during sexual intercourse)

Physical Exam Findings

- Atrophic vaginitis
- Decrease in breast size
- Vaginal and cervical atrophy

| ↓ estrogen = osteoporosis |

Diagnostic Tests/Treatment

The diagnosis is based on clinical presentation. If the diagnosis is unclear, an increased FSH level is diagnostic. Hormone replacement therapy (HRT) is indicated for short-term symptomatic relief as well as the prevention of osteoporosis. SSRIs can be used to treat symptoms of depression and some are also effective for vasomotor symptoms.

Vaginal atrophy and dyspareunia can be treated with topical estrogen cream.

Dyspareunia can also be treated with prasterone, a dehydroepiandrosterone (DHEA) analogue with weak androgenic and weak estrogenic activity. May be preferred if it is beneficial to have weaker estrogen exposure.

| HRT is associated with endometrial hyperplasia and can lead to endometrial carcinoma. For this reason, HRT use is limited to **5 years**. |

Contraindications

- Estrogen-dependent carcinoma (breast or endometrial cancer)
- History of pulmonary embolism or DVT

Contraception

Barrier Methods

Barrier methods include male condoms, female condoms, and vaginal diaphragms. Male condoms protect against sexually transmitted infections. Barrier methods are not very effective for pregnancy prevention.

Oral Contraceptive Pills (OCPs)

OCPs are most commonly a combination pill of both estrogen and progesterone. The pill is taken for 21 days and a placebo is taken for 7 days. During the 7 days of the placebo pills, the patient will experience menstruation. OCPs reduce the risk of ovarian carcinoma, endometrial carcinoma, and ectopic pregnancy. They cause a slight increase in the risk of thromboembolism. OCPs are contraindicated in women with a history of migraine with aura or hypertension and smokers age >35.

Vaginal Ring

A flexible vaginal ring that releases both estrogen and progesterone is inserted into the vagina for 3 weeks. Hormones are released on a constant basis. When the ring is removed, withdrawal bleeding will occur. The vaginal ring has similar side effects and efficacy to OCPs.

Transdermal Patch

A transdermal patch with a combination of estrogen and progesterone is placed on the skin for 7 days. Each week the previous patch is removed and a new patch is placed. Three weeks of patches are followed by a patch-free week, during which the patient will experience withdrawal bleeding. Patches should not be placed on the breast. The side effects and efficacy are the same as OCPs.

Intramuscular Injection

Depot medroxyprogesterone acetate is a progesterone-only intramuscular injection that is effective contraception for 3 months. Adverse effects include weight gain, acne, and unpredictable vaginal spotting.

Intrauterine Device

There are 2 types of intrauterine devices (IUDs), a copper device and a levonorgestrel device. The copper IUD impairs sperm migration and viability, impairs implantation, and works for ≤10 years. The levonorgestrel device (containing progesterone) thickens cervical mucus, which impairs implantation, and works for 3–5 years, depending on the dose. A urine pregnancy test must be performed prior to insertion, and patients should be offered testing for gonorrhea and chlamydia.

> When in doubt, answer IUD.
> - First-line contraceptive option offered to all women
> - Copper IUD: first-line for emergency contraception

Sterilization

Surgical sterilization can be done on both men and women. Sterilization via tubal ligation and vasectomy is permanent and can be reversed only by surgery, which is not always successful.

Tubal Ligation

Tubal ligation is a surgical procedure that women may choose to undergo for permanent contraception. The risk of pregnancy is very low, but if it occurs, there is an increased incidence of ectopic pregnancy.

Vasectomy

Vasectomy is a surgical procedure in which ligation of the vas deferens is performed.

Emergency Contraception

Method	Mechanism	Timing
Copper IUD	Prevents fertilization via effect of copper ions on sperm function, prevents endometrial receptivity	Up to 5 days
Ulipristal or mifepristone	Progesterone receptor modulator; delays/inhibits ovulation	Up to 5 days
Levonorgestrel	Progesterone receptor agonist; delays/inhibits ovulation	Up to 3 days
Estrogen + progesterone	Delays/inhibits ovulation (but more side effects)	Up to 5 days

Vulva and Vagina

Labial Fusion

Labial fusion occurs when excess androgens are present either from extraneous androgen administration or increased androgen production. 21-B hydroxylase deficiency is the **most common cause**.

Treatment is reconstructive surgery.

Epithelial Abnormalities			
Abnormality	**Age group affected**	**Description**	**Treatment**
Lichen sclerosus	Any age can be affected; however, if postmenopausal, there is an increased risk of cancer.	White, thin skin extending from labia to perianal area	Topical steroids
Squamous cell hyperplasia	Any age; patients who have had chronic vulvar pruritus	Patients with chronic irritation develop hyperkeratosis (raised white lesion).	Sitz baths or lubricants (relieve the pruritus)
Lichen planus	30s–60s	Violet, flat papules	Topical steroids

Bartholin Gland Cyst

Bartholin glands are located on the lateral sides of the vulva. They secrete mucus and can become obstructed, leading to a cyst or abscess which causes pain, tenderness, and dyspareunia. Physical exam shows edema and inflammation of the area with a deep fluctuant mass.

Treatment is drainage with a simple incision and drainage (I&D). Culture the fluid for an STD such as *Neisseria gonorrhoeae* or *Chlamydia trachomatis*. For recurrent cysts, consider marsupialization, a form of I&D in which the cyst is opened and the cyst walls are sutured to the vaginal mucosa.

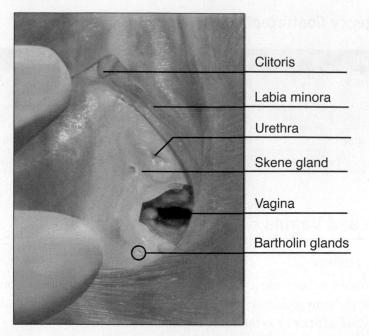

Clitoris

Labia minora

Urethra

Skene gland

Vagina

Bartholin glands

Figure 9.3 Bartholin Gland Cyst.
Source: Nicholasolan, commons.wikimedia.org

Lichen Sclerosus

Lichen sclerosus (LS) is a benign chronic condition of the vulvar epithelium that causes pruritus and pain. It tends to occur in both prepubertal and postmenopausal women. LS presents with white atrophic papules that coalesce into plaques. Treat with topical steroids.

Vaginitis

A 19-year-old woman presents for vaginal pruritus and discharge for 1 week. She states that the discharge is green and profuse. She has had multiple sexual partners in the past 2 months. Her last menstrual period was 2 weeks ago. On wet mount, the vaginal discharge has motile flagellates present. Which of the following is the most likely diagnosis?

a. Chlamydia
b. Bacterial vaginosis
c. Neisseria gonorrhoeae
d. Candidiasis
e. Trichomonas vaginalis

Answer: **E.** Trichomonas presents with a profuse, green, frothy discharge. Neisseria is a bacterial infection that is identified by culture. Chlamydia is diagnosed by serology DNA probe. Candidiasis is associated with white, cheesy vaginal discharge. Bacterial vaginosis is associated with vaginal discharge and a fishy odor, without pruritus.

Risk factors for vaginitis include any factor that will increase the pH of the vagina, such as:

- Antibiotic use (*Lactobacillus* normally keeps vaginal pH <4.5)
- Diabetes
- Overgrowth of normal flora

Symptoms include itching, pain, abnormal odor, and discharge.

Types of Vaginitis			
Disease	Bacterial vaginosis	Candidiasis	Trichomonas (the most common nonviral STD)
Pathogen	*Gardnerella*	*Candida albicans*	*Trichomonas vaginalis*
Symptom	Vaginal discharge with fishy odor; gray white	White, clumpy vaginal discharge	Profuse, green, frothy vaginal discharge
Diagnostic test	Saline wet mount shows **clue cells**, which are epithelial cells covered with bacteria. **Figure 9.4** Clue Cells. *Source: Per Grinsted, commons.wikimedia.org.*	KOH shows **pseudohyphae.** **Figure 9.5** Pseudohyphae. *Source: Nephron, commons.wikimedia.org.*	Most accurate test is NAAT. Saline wet mount shows **motile flagellates.** **Figure 9.6** Trichomonas. *Source: Alex Brollo, commons.wikimedia.org.*
Treatment	Metronidazole or clindamycin	Miconazole or clotrimazole, fluconazole, or nystatin	Treat both patient and partner with metronidazole.

▶ **TIP**

If trichomonas is diagnosed, both partners need to be treated.

Chancroid

A chancroid is a genital ulcer caused by the gram-negative rod *Haemophilus ducreyi*. The ulcer is painful, with an erythematous base, and may be accompanied by lymphadenopathy. Treat with azithromycin, ceftriaxone, or ciprofloxacin.

Syphilis

Syphilis is a sexually transmitted disease caused by the spirochete *Treponema pallidum*. Primary syphilis presents with a painless chancre and lymphadenopathy. If left untreated, secondary syphilis can develop, which presents with diffuse, symmetric macular or papular rash involving the trunk, extremities, palms, and soles. Late syphilis can develop years after initial infection with gummas (granulomas within skin and bones), cardiac abnormalities, or CNS abnormalities such as tabes dorsalis.

Malignant Disorders

Paget Disease of the Vulva

Paget disease is an intraepithelial neoplasia that most commonly occurs in postmenopausal Caucasian women. Paget presents with vulvar soreness and pruritus appearing as a red lesion with a superficial white coating. A biopsy is needed for a definitive diagnosis. Treatment for a bilateral lesion is a radical vulvectomy. If there is a unilateral lesion, a modified vulvectomy can be done.

Squamous Cell Carcinoma

Squamous cell carcinoma is the most common type of vulvar cancer. It presents with pruritus, bloody vaginal discharge, and postmenopausal bleeding. The physical exam can range from a small ulcerated lesion to a large cauliflower-like lesion. A biopsy is essential for diagnosis. Staging is done while the patient is in surgery.

Treatment for unilateral lesions without lymph node involvement is a modified radical vulvectomy. Treatment for bilateral involvement is radical vulvectomy. Lymph nodes that are involved must undergo lymphadenectomy.

Cervical Abnormalities

Cervicitis

Acute cervicitis, or inflammation of the uterine cervix, is usually caused by infection, although a specific microbe is not identified in the majority of cases. Gonorrhea and chlamydia are sexually transmitted infections that cause cervicitis. Chronic cervicitis is usually noninfectious.

Women may present with mucopurulent vaginal discharge, dyspareunia, or postcoital bleeding. However, most cases of gonorrhea and chlamydia infection are asymptomatic.

Treat chlamydia empirically with azithromycin or doxycycline. If gonorrhea is also suspected, add a single dose of ceftriaxone.

> When gonorrhea is diagnosed, the patient should also be treated for chlamydia.

Lymphogranuloma venereum (LGV) is a genital ulcer disease caused by the L1, L2, and L3 serovars of *Chlamydia trachomatis*. Primary infection is characterized by small genital ulcers or mucosal inflammatory reaction. Buboes are unilateral painful inguinal lymph nodes that develop with initial infection. Genital elephantiasis is a late feature of disease.

Treat with doxycycline.

Pelvic Inflammatory Disease

Pelvic inflammatory disease is defined as acute infection of the upper genital tract including the uterus, fallopian tubes, and/or ovaries. The majority of cases are caused by sexually transmitted pathogens, most commonly *Neisseria gonorrhea* and *Chlamydia trachomatis*.

Clinical findings include pelvic or lower abdominal pain, cervical motion tenderness with chandelier sign on exam, and signs of infection. Long-term sequelae of PID may include infertility, ectopic pregnancy, and chronic pelvic pain.

> **Chandelier sign** occurs when pelvic exam elicits pain, causing the patient to reach up toward the ceiling for relief.

Treatment is as follows:

- Outpatient: ceftriaxone + azithromycin or doxycycline
- Inpatient: cefoxitin or cefotetan + doxycycline
  - Indications for inpatient include pregnancy, failure of outpatient therapy or nonadherence, inability to tolerate oral medication (nausea, vomiting), severe clinical symptoms, or presence of tubo-ovarian abscess (TOA)
  - For penicillin-allergy, use gentamicin and clindamycin

Tubo-Ovarian Abscess (TOA)

TOA is regarded as a complication of PID. It classically presents with cervical motion tenderness, acute lower abdominal pain, fever, and chills. Suspect a ruptured TOA if the patient also has hypotension, tachycardia, tachypnea, and acute peritoneal signs (abdominal tenderness, rebound, rigidity, guarding).

> **TOAs** are usually polymicrobial and often contain a mixture of aerobic, facultative, and anaerobic bacteria.

Workup includes CBC and culture for gonorrhea/chlamydia. Best initial imaging is a transvaginal ultrasound showing a complex, multilocular mass. CT scan is preferred if bowel pathology must also be excluded; findings will reveal a thick-walled, rim-enhancing adnexal mass.

Treatment is inpatient IV antibiotics: cefoxitin and doxycycline (or in penicillin-allergic patients: clindamycin and gentamicin). **Ruptured TOA is a surgical emergency.** If there is no improvement with antibiotics alone in 48–72 hours or when abscess is large (>9 cm), do image-guided percutaneous drainage.

Fitz-Hugh and Curtis Syndrome

This is a perihepatitis arising from inflammation of the liver capsule and peritoneal surfaces of the anterior right upper quadrant in a patient with acute PID. Suspect Fitz-Hugh and Curtis syndrome in patients with RUQ pain that is referred to the right shoulder and worse with inspiration. LFTs are usually normal or slightly elevated.

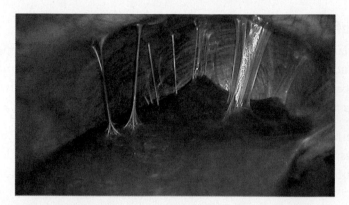

Figure 9.7 Perihepatic adhesions with violin-string appearance.
Source: Hic et nunc, commons.wikimedia.org.

On laparoscopy, perihepatitis is visualized by fibrinous exudates ("violin-string" adhesions), which spare the liver parenchyma.

Cervical Cancer Screening

> **HPV types and associations:**
> - Cervical cancer: 16 and 18
> - Condyloma acuminata (genital warts): 6 and 11

In asymptomatic, immunocompetent women, cervical cancer screening with Pap smear starts at age 21, regardless of sexual activity.

- If age <30, screen with Pap alone every 3 years
- If age >30, screen with Pap alone every 3 years or Pap + HPV co-testing every 5 years, for as long as both tests are negative

Abnormal Cervical Cancer Screening

Patients with abnormal screening tests should have prompt follow-up. If risk of HPV is high, do a colposcopy.

Management of abnormal Pap results differs based on the results:

- Atypical glandular cells present: colposcopy with endometrial sampling
- Atypical endometrial cells: endometrial and endocervical sampling

> Cervical cancer screening has historically been confusing and also changes quite rapidly.

Manage abnormal HPV with negative Pap in patients age >30 with either HPV DNA typing for 16 and 18 now or repeat co-testing in 1 year.

Cervical Cancer Screening and Management			
	Age 21–25	**Age 25–30**	**Age 30–65**
Routine screening	Cytology every 3 years	Cytology every 3 years	• Cytology every 3 years *OR* • Cytology and HPV testing every 5 years *OR* • HPV testing alone every 5 years*
ASCUS	Repeat cytology in 1 year	Order HPV: • **HPV+**, colposcopy and ECC • **HPV−**, repeat Pap in 3 years	Order HPV: • **HPV+**, colposcopy and ECC • **HPV−**, repeat Pap in 3 years
LSIL	Repeat cytology in 1 year	Colposcopy and ECC	Order HPV: • **HPV+**, colposcopy and ECC • **HPV−**, repeat Pap in 1 year
HSIL	Colposcopy and ECC required regardless of age		
Abbreviations: ASCUS = atypical squamous cells of undetermined significance; ECC = endocervical curettage (ECC); LSIL = low-grade squamous intraepithelial lesion; HSIL = high-grade squamous intraepithelial lesion.			

*United States Preventive Task Force recommendation as of 9/13/2017.

HPV Prevention

HPV vaccination is administered to both male and females, starting at age 11, with the goal of eradicating HPV and preventing cervical cancer before it starts. Both males and females can get the vaccine until age 45.

Abnormal Uterine Bleeding

Abnormal uterine bleeding (AUB) is menstrual bleeding of abnormal quantity, duration, or schedule. The classification system for categorizing the wide range of AUB etiologies is referred to by the acronym PALM-COEIN.

P: Polyp

A: Adenomyosis

L: Leiomyoma

M: Malignancy/hyperplasia

C: Coagulopathy

O: Ovulatory dysfunction

E: Endometrial

I: Iatrogenic (anticoagulants, OCPs, IUD) or infection/inflammation

N: Not yet classified

> Postcoital bleeding is cervical cancer until proven otherwise.

Diagnostic Tests

- CBC to see if hemoglobin and hematocrit have dropped
- PT/PTT to evaluate for coagulation disorder
- Pelvic ultrasound to visualize any anatomical abnormality

When is an endometrial biopsy indicated?

- *Any* postmenopausal bleeding
- AUB in women >45 years old
- In women <45 years old with BMI ≥30, chronic unopposed estrogen exposure, failed medical management of AUB, or high risk of endometrial cancer
- Atypical glandular cells on Pap smear

Ovulatory Dysfunction

In an ovulatory cycle, the ovary produces estrogen, but no corpus luteum is formed. Without the corpus luteum, progesterone is not produced. This prevents the usual withdrawal bleeding. The continuously high estrogen continues to stimulate growth of the endometrium. Bleeding occurs only once the endometrium outgrows the blood supply.

Diagnostic testing should rule out systemic reasons for anovulation, such as hypothyroid and hyperprolactinemia. Transvaginal U/S will help show whether structural causes are responsible for AUB.

Treatment is as follows:

- Long-acting reversible contraception (LARC) (**best initial therapy** for patients with anovulatory bleeding after other etiologies have been ruled out); the levonorgestrel IUD is preferred but OCPs are an alternative
- D&C for acute hemorrhage, to stop the bleeding

AUB is regarded as severe if patients are anemic, bleeding is uncontrolled with medical management, or patients report a compromised lifestyle. Treat with endometrial ablation or hysterectomy.

Postmenopausal Bleeding

Postmenopausal bleeding is vaginal bleeding in a woman who has already gone through menopause. It is considered endometrial cancer until proven otherwise. Endometrial biopsy is the best initial step for postmenopausal bleeding.

Postmenopausal bleeding itself is usually self-limited. The main objective is to rule out cancer!

Uterine Abnormalities

Structural causes of AUB include endometrial polyps, adenomyosis, and leiomyoma.

> Any patient age >45 with abnormal bleeding should undergo endometrial biopsy to rule out endometrial carcinoma.

> For postmenopausal bleeding, endometrial biopsy is the **best initial test**.

Endometrial Polyp

An endometrial polyp is a hyperplastic overgrowth of endometrial glands and stroma that projects from the endometrial surface. It originates from endometrial tissue.

Endometrial polyp may be visualized on transvaginal U/S or operative hysteroscopy. Polypectomy is performed to confirm the diagnosis histologically, but 95% of cases are benign.

Adenomyosis

Adenomyosis is the invasion of endometrial glands into the myometrium, and it commonly occurs in women age 35–50. Risk factors are endometriosis and uterine fibroids. Symptoms include dysmenorrhea and menorrhagia.

Adenomyosis is a clinical diagnosis. On physical examination the uterus is large, globular, and boggy.

MRI is the **most accurate test**. Treatment is hysterectomy (the only definitive treatment and the only way to definitively diagnose adenomyosis).

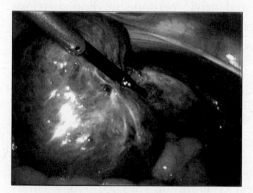

Figure 9.8 Adenomyosis.
Source: Hic et nunc, commons.wikimedia.org

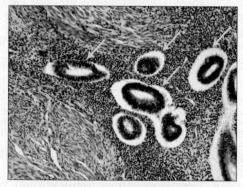

Figure 9.9 Histopathological Image of Uterine Adenomyosis. *Source: Hic et nunc, commons.wikimedia.org*

Leiomyoma

Leiomyomata, or uterine fibroids, are benign monoclonal tumors that stem from the smooth muscle cells of the myometrium. They can occur under the serosa, within the myometrial wall, or within the endometrial cavity. They are common in obese and African American women.

Symptoms include heavy, irregular menstrual bleeding with pelvic pain and pressure. These tumors are hormonally sensitive—growing in pregnancy and shrinking with menopause.

Bimanual exam will reveal an enlarged, mobile, and irregular nontender uterus. Diagnostic testing starts with transvaginal U/S. Note that submucosal myoma cannot be visualized on transvaginal U/S, so use saline infusion sonography or hysteroscopy.

Treatment ranges from hormonal contraceptives (including levonorgestrel IUD) to myomectomy to hysterectomy once childbearing is complete.

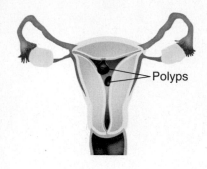

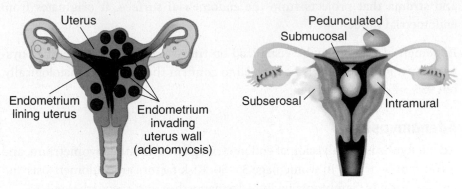

Figures 9.10, 9.11, 9.12 Structural Sources of Abnormal Uterine Bleeding: Polyp (left), Adenomyosis (center), Leiomyoma (right). © Kaplan

Endometriosis

Endometriosis is the implantation of endometrial tissue outside of the endometrial cavity. Although the endometrial tissue can implant anywhere, the most common sites are the ovary and pelvic peritoneum. Endometriosis occurs in women of reproductive age and is more common if a first-degree relative (mother or sister) has endometriosis.

Endometriosis presents with:

- Cyclical pelvic pain that starts 1–2 weeks before menstruation, peaks 1–2 days before menstruation, and ends with menstruation
- Abnormal bleeding (**common**)
- Physical exam finding of nodular uterus and adnexal mass

Diagnosis can be made only by direct visualization via laparoscopy. Direct visualization of the endometrial implants looks like rusty or dark brown lesions. On the ovary, a cluster of lesions called an endometrioma looks like a "chocolate cyst."

Treatment is NSAIDs, hormonal contraceptives, gonadotropin-releasing hormone (GnRH) agonists, and/or aromatase inhibitors, depending on patient preference, side effects, and treatment efficacy. (There are no data proving that one treatment is superior to another.)

- For moderate to severe symptoms, use danazol or leuprolide acetate to decrease FSH and LH.
  - Danazol is an androgen derivative; side effects include acne, oily skin, weight gain, and hirsutism.
  - Leuprolide acetate is a GnRH agonist, and when given continuously it suppresses estrogen; side effects include hot flashes and decreased bone density.

> Dysmenorrhea and dyspareunia are common in endometriosis.

- For severe symptoms or infertility, surgery can remove all the endometrial implants and adhesions and restore pelvic anatomy. For patients who have completed childbearing, consider total abdominal hysterectomy or bilateral salpingo-oophorectomy.

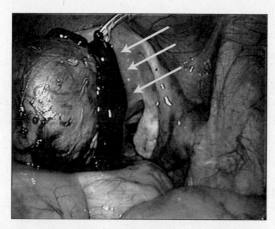

Figure 9.13 Severe endometriosis may require surgery.
Source: Hic et nunc, commons.wikimedia.org

Endometrial Hyperplasia/Carcinoma

Endometrial hyperplasia and carcinoma often coexist. The majority of the cases occur secondary to chronic exposure of the endometrium to unopposed estrogen. They present with abnormal uterine bleeding or postmenopausal bleeding.

> **Adipose tissue has aromatase,** which converts androgens to estrogens and is responsible for increased risk of endometrial hyperplasia in obese women. For the same reason, obese women are less likely to experience menopausal symptoms.

Endometrial hyperplasia is classified into 2 categories:

- **Hyperplasia without atypia** (benign): proliferative endometrium with dilated and contorted glands
- **Atypical hyperplasia** (endometrial intraepithelial neoplasm): epithelial crowding with increased gland to stroma ratio and cells appearing distinct from normal endometrial cells

Risk Factors

- Obese, postmenopausal woman
- PCOS
- Tamoxifen therapy
- Early menarche
- Late menopause
- Lynch syndrome

Treatment is surveillance, progestin therapy, or hysterectomy. Benign endometrial hyperplasia without atypia has a low risk of progression to endometrial carcinoma (<5%). Atypical hyperplasia, however, has a high risk, so hysterectomy is the treatment of choice.

Ovarian Abnormalities

Polycystic Ovary Syndrome

Diagnosis of polycystic ovary syndrome is made when 2 of the following 3 conditions are present:

- Amenorrhea or irregular menses
- Signs of hirsutism
- Polycystic ovaries on U/S

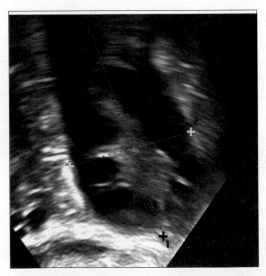

Figure 9.14 Polycystic Ovary Showing "String of Pearls" Appearance as Seen on Sonography. *Source: Schomyny, commons.wikimedia.org.*

Diagnostic testing is as follows:

- Pelvic U/S may show bilaterally enlarged ovaries with multiple cysts
- Free testosterone will be elevated secondary to the high androgens
- High androgens and obesity lead to an increase in estrogen formation outside the ovary; this stimulates LH secretion and inhibits FSH secretion, where the LH:FSH ratio >3:1.

Treatment begins with weight loss, which will decrease the insulin resistance. Additionally:

- For patients who **do not wish to conceive**: OCPs to control the amount of estrogen and progestin in the body (this both controls the androgen level and prevents endometrial hyperplasia)
- For patients who **wish to conceive**: clomiphene or letrozole and metformin

Ovarian Torsion

Ovarian torsion occurs when the ovary rotates around the infundibulopelvic ligament, compromising its own blood supply. Suspect ovarian torsion in women of reproductive age who have sudden onset of severe unilateral pelvic pain and an ovarian cyst or mass, often accompanied by nausea and vomiting. Transvaginal ultrasound may reveal decreased or absent blood flow to the affected ovary. Treatment is emergency laparoscopy or laparotomy.

Ovarian Cancer

Among gynecological cancers, ovarian cancer is one of the leading causes of death. Presentation is acute or subacute.

- **Acute presentation**, such as pleural effusion or bowel obstruction, indicates late disease and poor prognosis.
- **Subacute presentation**, such as abdominal pain or an adnexal mass, can occur early or late in the disease.

Symptoms include bloating/feeling full quickly; urinary urgency and frequency; pelvic pain; and abdominal pain. Because subacute presentation involves many nonspecific symptoms, it is often not diagnosed until late in the disease.

Diagnostic testing is by pelvic ultrasound or CT of the pelvis. A biopsy must be performed to confirm the diagnosis.

There is no screening test for the general population. Family history of ovarian cancer is an indication to do BRCA gene screening.

Gestational Trophoblastic Disease

Gestational trophoblastic disease (GTD) is a group of diseases that originate from placental tissue and have the ability to invade the uterus and metastasize. Hydatidiform molar pregnancy is a premalignant disease that is characterized as partial or complete.

Characteristics of GTD		
Feature	**Partial mole**	**Complete mole**
Fetal parts	Present	Absent
Karyotype	69 XXX or 69 XXY	46 XX or 46 XY
Villous edema	Mild	Severe
Risk of persistent disease	1–5%	15–20%

If the question describes a patient who sounds like she has preeclampsia but is <20 weeks' gestation, molar pregnancy is the most likely diagnosis. Sonographically, molar pregnancies have a classic "snowstorm appearance." Treatment is uterine evacuation.

Other Female Reproductive Tract Disorders

Müllerian Anomalies

The uterus and upper portion of vagina are embryologically formed from the paramesonephric ducts. Normally, these migrate to the midline and fuse, and then the septum is resorbed.

Müllerian agenesis occurs when there are no paramesonephric structures; patients have normal ovaries and external female secondary sex characteristics, but the vagina ends in a blind pouch and there is no uterus.

Bicornuate uterus results from a partial failure of the paramesonephric ducts to fuse.

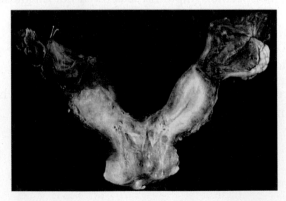

Figure 9.15 Bicornuate Uterus. *Source: Ed Uthman, commons.wikimedia.org*

Septate uterus results from a failure of the midline septum to resorb after fusion of the paramesonephric ducts.

Imperforate Hymen

The hymenal membrane is composed of fibrous connective tissue attached to the vaginal wall. Incomplete degeneration of the hymen results in an imperforate hymen. Patients will present with primary amenorrhea and cyclical pelvic pain. Treatment is surgical.

Female Sexual Arousal Disorder

Significantly reduced arousal or interest in sexual activity characterizes this condition (previously known as hypoactive sexual desire disorder and female sexual arousal disorder). Treatment includes psychotherapy.

Genitopelvic Pain/Penetration Disorder

This condition (previously known as vaginismus and dyspareunia) involves persistent or recurrent difficulty and pain with vaginal penetration, or intense fear in anticipation of vaginal pain prior to penetration. Treatment includes psychotherapy and pelvic floor physical therapy.

Asherman Syndrome

Aggressively performed dilation and curettage can result in Asherman syndrome. When the endometrial lining is scraped down below the basalis layer, scar tissue forms and the patient develops secondary amenorrhea and infertility.

Pelvic Organ Prolapse

Prolapse occurs when pelvic organs herniate beyond the vaginal walls. Patients may present with sensations of a bulge or vaginal pressure, or with associated urinary, defecatory, or sexual dysfunction. Initial treatment is conservative and includes pessary and pelvic floor therapies.

PART 10

Radiology

Plain X-Rays

Chest X-Ray

Chest x-ray is the best initial radiologic test for all forms of pulmonary complaints such as:

- Cough
- Shortness of breath (dyspnea)
- Chest pain, particularly when pleuritic or changing with respirations
- Sputum and hemoptysis

Chest x-ray is also the best initial radiologic test for any abnormality on physical examination of the lungs, i.e., rales/rhonchi; wheezing; dullness to percussion; chest wall tenderness; tracheal deviation; possible superior vena cava syndrome (jugulovenous distention, plethora of the face, venous distention of the chest wall).

- **Posterior/anterior (PA) film** (standard of care for chest x-ray); the patient must be able to stand up

  - If a pleural effusion is found on a PA film, use **decubitus film** to evaluate; after patient lies down, effusion is confirmed if fluid in the chest is freely mobile and forms a layer on the side of the x-ray

  - If an infiltrate is found on a PA film, use **lateral chest x-ray** to identify the precise location; **best initial test for an effusion**, since it can detect as little as 50–75 mL of fluid (as opposed to a PA chest x-ray, which requires 200–300 mL of fluid to become abnormal)

- **Anterior/posterior (AP) film** (standard of care for chest x-ray in ICU) for the unstable patient who cannot stand up; often done bedside with portable equipment

- **Apical lordotic film** is almost never the right answer. Lordotic x-ray of the chest is done with the patient leaning backward to take ribs out of the way in order to examine the upper lobes.

> - PA film showing widening of the mediastinum is the best test of a dissection of the thoracic aorta.
> - Decubitus x-ray is the best test to distinguish an effusion from an infiltrate caused by pneumonia.

> Lordotic film was originally the best initial test for TB, which has an increased predilection for the apices of the lung. However, today, chest CT scan is preferred.

Abdominal X-Ray

Abdominal x-ray has very few indications. The best indication for its use is small bowel obstruction or ileus, where it will show multiple air-fluid levels in the small bowel. However, note the following:

- Abdominal x-ray is not accurate for stones of the kidney, and will miss at least 20% of cases.
- Abdominal x-ray is not accurate for finding air under the diaphragm because it does not always visualize the top of the diaphragm, especially in a tall person.

> Abdominal x-ray is good only for an ileus.

▶ TIP

For perforation of the bowel, get an upright chest x-ray, not an abdominal x-ray.

Bone X-Ray

X-ray of the bone is the **best initial test** for osteomyelitis. You will see elevation of the periosteum. Long-standing bone infection gives destroyed bone with periosteal new bone formation. Although it will take at least 2 weeks for the bone x-ray to become abnormal with osteomyelitis, you should still do this study first. You will only obtain an MRI of the bone or a nuclear bone scan if the x-ray does not show osteomyelitis.

Skull X-Ray

There is no first-class indication for skull x-ray. It is **never the best initial or most accurate test**. On the USMLE exam, it is rarely the correct answer.

- A normal skull x-ray does not exclude intracranial hemorrhage.
- An abnormal skull x-ray does not mean there is a hemorrhage.

Computed Tomography (CT Scan)

Head CT

Non-contrast head CT is the best initial test for:

- Severe head trauma, especially with loss of consciousness or altered mental status
- Stroke
- Any form of intracranial bleeding including subarachnoid hemorrhage

CT scan **with contrast**:

- Cancer and infection will enhance with contrast. You cannot distinguish between neoplastic disease and an abscess by CT scan or MRI, but the head CT with contrast is the best initial test for any form of intracranial mass lesion.

- Do not order contrast with severe renal failure.
- Hydrate with saline with mild renal insufficiency.
- Stop metformin prior to using contrast.

Abdominal CT

Choose abdominal CT to visualize the pancreas. It should be performed with both IV and oral contrast. Oral contrast is indispensable for outlining abdominal structures that are pressed against each other and difficult to visualize. Abdominal CT is also good for:

- Retroperitoneal structures: Organs such as the pancreas are difficult to visualize with sonography. In sonography, the transducer is placed against the anterior abdominal wall. This makes it difficult to visualize structures that are further away from the anterior abdominal wall.
- Appendicitis and other intraabdominal infections
- Kidney stones (**most accurate test**)
- Diverticulitis (**most accurate test**)
- Nephrolithiasis (**most accurate test**) but *contrast is not needed*
- Masses within abdominal organs such as the liver and spleen

Chest CT

When is chest CT the answer?

- Hilar nodes such as sarcoidosis
- Mass lesions such as cancer
- Cavities
- Interstitial lung disease: Chest CT adds considerable definition to the chest x-ray. Chest x-ray shows only interstitial infiltrates, while CT shows much more detail in evaluating parenchymal lung disease.
- Pulmonary emboli: The spiral CT or CT angiogram has supplanted the V/Q scan in confirming pulmonary emboli.

CT is neither the "best initial" nor "most accurate" test of bone.

MRI

MRI is the most accurate test for all CNS diseases with the exception of looking for hemorrhage. The indication for the use of contrast with MRI is the same as with CT scan. Contrast detects cancer and infectious mass lesions.

When is MRI the answer?

- Demyelinating diseases such as multiple sclerosis
- Posterior fossa lesion in the cerebellum
- Brainstem
- Pituitary lesions
- Facial structures such as the orbits and sinuses
- Bone lesions, particularly osteomyelitis. MRI is the best visualization of bone, although it cannot determine a precise microbiologic etiology.
- Spinal cord and vertebral lesions

▶ TIP

With cancer and infection, the radiologic test is never the most accurate test; biopsy is.

Ultrasound (Sonography)

When is ultrasound the answer?

- Gallbladder disease, including the ducts for stones and obstruction
- Renal disease, although CT is more sensitive for nephrolithiasis
- Gynecologic organs: uterus, ovaries, adnexa
- Prostate evaluation (transrectal approach)

Endoscopic Ultrasound

Endoscopic ultrasound (EUS) is the most accurate method of assessing:

- Pancreatic lesions, particularly in the head
- Pancreatic and biliary ductal disease
- Gastrinoma localization (Zollinger-Ellison syndrome)

With EUS, a sonographic device is placed at the end of the scope and placed into the duodenum to allow outstanding visualization of hard-to-reach intra-abdominal structures.

Nuclear Scans

- **HIDA (hepatobiliary) scan**: only functional test of the biliary system that allows detection of cholecystitis
- **Bone scan**: equal in sensitivity to the MRI in detecting osteomyelitis, but far less specific than the MRI; use as a sensitive test to detect occult metastases from cancer
- **Gallium scan**: fever of unknown origin; gallium follows iron metabolism and is transported on transferrin. Gallium increases in uptake with infection and in some cancers because of increased iron deposition.
- **Indium scan**: fever of unknown origin; superior in assessing the abdomen, which can be obscured in gallium scan. Indium is a tagged WBC scan: to detect infection, the patient's WBCs are tagged with indium, then reinjected to see where they localize.
- **Ventilation/perfusion (V/Q) scan**: A normal V/Q scan essentially excludes a pulmonary embolus. Low-probability scans still have a clot in 15% of cases and high-probability scans do not have a clot in 15% of cases. V/Q is no longer the standard of care in detecting pulmonary emboli. It has been replaced by the spiral CT (CT angiogram) in the confirmation of pulmonary emboli. The only time a V/Q scan is more accurate than a CT angiogram is in diagnosing chronic thromboembolic disease.
- **Multiple-gated acquisition scan (MUGA)** or nuclear ventriculography is the most accurate method to measure ejection fraction.

PART 11

Ophthalmology

Conjunctivitis

Comparison of Viral and Bacterial Conjunctivitis	
Viral conjunctivitis	**Bacterial conjunctivitis**
Bilateral	Unilateral
Watery discharge	Purulent, thick discharge
Easily transmissible	Poorly transmissible
Normal vision	Normal vision
Itchy	Not itchy
Preauricular adenopathy	No adenopathy
No specific therapy	Topical antibiotics

▶ **TIP**

The "must know" subjects in ophthalmology are:

- The red eye (emergencies)
- Diabetic retinopathy
- Artery and vein occlusion
- Retinal detachment

The Red Eye (Ophthalmologic Emergencies)

Etiologies of the Red Eye				
	Conjunctivitis	**Uveitis**	**Glaucoma**	**Abrasion**
Presentation	Itchy eyes, discharge	Autoimmune diseases	Pain	Trauma
Eye findings	Normal pupils	Photophobia	Fixed midpoint pupil	Feels like sand in eyes
Most accurate test	Clinical diagnosis	Slit lamp examination	Tonometry	Fluorescein stain
Best initial therapy	Topical antibiotics	Topical steroids	Acetazolamide, mannitol, pilocarpine, timolol, apraclonidine	Patch not clearly beneficial, antibiotics

Glaucoma

Chronic Glaucoma

Chronic glaucoma is most often asymptomatic and is diagnosed by routine screening. Confirmation is with tonometry indicating extremely elevated intraocular pressure.

Treatment is medication to decrease the production of aqueous humor or to increase its drainage.

- Prostaglandin analogues: latanoprost, travoprost, bimatoprost
- Topical beta blockers: timolol, carteolol, metipranolol, betaxolol, or levobunolol
- Topical carbonic anhydrase inhibitors: dorzolamide, brinzolamide
- Alpha-2 agonists: apraclonidine
- Pilocarpine

> Uveitis involves the iris, ciliary body, and choroid.

If no response with medical therapy, consider laser trabeculoplasty.

Acute Angle-Closure Glaucoma

Look for the sudden onset of an extremely painful, red eye that is hard to palpation. Walking into a dark room can precipitate pain because of pupillary dilation. The cornea is described as "steamy" and the pupil does not react to light because it is stuck. The cup-to-disc ratio is greater than the normal 0.3.

Diagnosis is confirmed with tonometry.

Treatment is:

- IV acetazolamide
- IV mannitol to act as an osmotic draw of fluid out of the eye
- Pilocarpine, beta blockers, and apraclonidine to constrict the pupil and enhance drainage; beta blockers also decrease production of aqueous humor
- Laser iridotomy

Herpes Keratitis

Keratitis is an infection of the cornea. The eye may be very red, swollen, and painful. Do not use steroids. Fluorescein staining of the eye helps confirm the dendritic pattern seen on examination. Steroids markedly increase the production of the virus.

Treatment is oral acyclovir, famciclovir, or valacyclovir. Topical antiherpetic treatment is trifluridine and idoxuridine.

> **Beware of steroid use for herpes keratitis.** Steroids make the condition worse.

Cataracts

There is no medical therapy for cataracts. Surgically remove the lens and replace with a new intraocular lens. The new lens may automatically have a bifocal capability. Early cataracts are diagnosed with an ophthalmoscope or slit lamp exam. Advanced cataracts are visible on examination.

Diabetic Retinopathy

Annual screening exams should detect retinopathy before serious visual loss has occurred. Nonproliferative or "background" retinopathy is managed by controlling glucose level. The **most accurate test** is fluorescein angiography. Proliferative retinopathy is treated with vascular endothelial growth factor (VEGF) inhibitors. These are injected into the patient's eyes to control neovascularization. Laser photocoagulation is used in those who cannot come for VEGF injections.

Vitrectomy may be necessary to remove a vitreous hemorrhage obstructing vision.

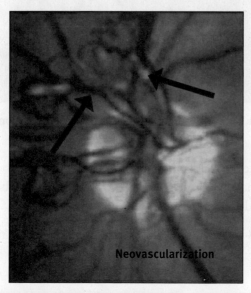

Figure 11.1 New blood vessel formation obscures vision.
Source: Conrad Fischer, MD

Retinal Artery and Vein Occlusion

Both conditions present with the sudden onset of monocular visual loss. You cannot make the diagnosis without retinal examination.

There is no conclusive treatment for either condition.

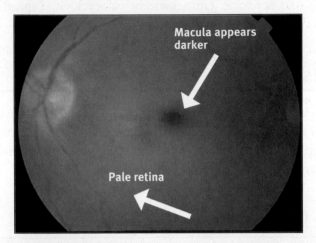

Figure 11.2 Retinal artery occlusion presents with sudden loss of vision and a pale retina and dark macula. *Source: Conrad Fischer, MD*

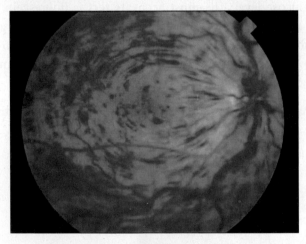

Figure 11.3 Retinal vein occlusion leads to extravasation of blood into the retina. *Source: Conrad Fischer, MD*

> The macula is described as "cherry red" in artery occlusion because the rest of the retina is pale.

Treatment of artery occlusion is attempted with thrombolytics and 100% oxygen, ocular massage, acetazolamide, or anterior chamber paracentesis to decrease intraocular pressure.

Try VEGF inhibitors such as ranibizumab for vein occlusion.

Retinal Detachment

Risks include trauma to the eye, extreme myopia that changes the shape of the eye, and diabetic retinopathy. Anything that pulls on the retina can detach it.

Detachment presents with the sudden onset of painless, unilateral loss of vision that is described as "a curtain coming down."

Reattachment is attempted with a number of mechanical methods such as surgery, laser, cryotherapy, and the injection of an expansile gas that pushes the retina back up against the globe of the eye.

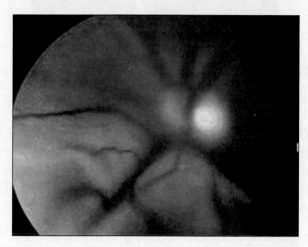

Figure 11.4 Sudden, painless loss of vision is described as "like a curtain coming down." *Source: Conrad Fischer, MD*

Macular Degeneration

Macular degeneration is now the **most common cause of blindness in older persons** in the United States. The cause is unknown. There is an atrophic (dry) type and a neovascular (wet) type.

Visual loss in macular degeneration:

- Far more common in older patients
- Bilateral
- Normal external appearance of the eye
- Loss of central vision

Neovascular disease is more rapid and more severe. New vessels grow between the retina and the underlying Bruch membrane. The neovascular, or wet, type causes 90% of permanent blindness from macular degeneration.

> Atrophic macular degeneration has no proven effective therapy.

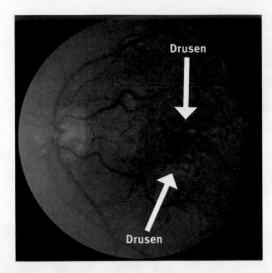

Figure 11.5 Macular degeneration can be diagnosed only by visualization of the retina. This image reveals lesions that are characteristic of dry macular degeneration (drusen). *Source: Conrad Fischer, MD*

The **best initial therapy** for neovascular disease is laser photocoagulation or a VEGF inhibitor such as ranibizumab, bevacizumab, or aflibercept. They are injected directly into the vitreous chamber every 4–8 weeks. Over 90% of patients will experience a halt of progression, and one-third of patients will have improvement in vision.

The majority of macular degeneration (80%) is dry, or atrophic. Dry macular degeneration cannot be reversed with treatment.

PART 12

Psychiatry

Contributing author Niket Sonpal, MD

Childhood Disorders

Intellectual Disability

Intellectual disability is more common in boys than girls, with the highest incidence in school-age children. Causes include fetal alcohol syndrome (**most common**) and genetic causes (Down syndrome and fragile X syndrome most common).

Risk factors include inborn errors of metabolism, intrauterine infection, exposure to toxins and heavy metals, poor prenatal care, physical trauma, and social deprivation.

To identify the level of intellectual disability, both intellectual functioning (cognitive abilities) and social adaptive functioning (ability to do daily activities) must be exhibited.

Treatment is as follows:

- Genetic counseling, prenatal care, and safe environments for expectant mothers
- Special education to improve the level of functioning
- Behavioral therapy to help reduce negative behaviors

Autism Spectrum Disorders

Autism spectrum disorders (ASDs) are characterized by difficulty in social interactions, behavior, and language that impair daily functioning. ASDs tend to be diagnosed in children <3 years. This diagnosis has replaced autism, Rett syndrome, and Asperger disorder.

Children with ASDs have ongoing deficits in social communication and social interaction across various areas. The deficits include lack of social connection, poor eye contact, and problems with language, relationships, and understanding others. Other features include stereotyped or repetitive movements, inflexibility, and unusual interest in sensory aspects of the environment.

> ASDs are associated with prenatal or perinatal infections such as rubella or CMV.

ASDs are associated with a higher incidence of abnormal EEGs, seizures, and abnormal brain morphology. By adulthood, 25% of patients develop seizures.

The goal of treatment is to improve the patient's ability to develop relationships, attend school, and achieve independent living.

- Behavioral modification to help with language and the ability to connect with others
- Antipsychotic medication (e.g., risperidone or aripiprazole) to help with aggression

Early behavioral interventions improve outcomes.

A 2-year-old boy is taken to the pediatrician by his parents. His problems started at 18 months of age, when he did not speak much. He does not have much attachment to his parents and seems aggressive toward other children. What is the most likely diagnosis?

a. Deafness
b. Schizophrenia, childhood onset
c. Child abuse
d. Autism spectrum disorder
e. Learning deficit

Answer: **D.** Autism spectrum disorder is seen more frequently in boys and usually starts by age 3. Children with autism tend to have problems with language and aggression, lack separation anxiety, and are withdrawn. If parents report that a child does not respond when his name is called, first evaluate the child for hearing impairment. Child abuse should also be considered and ruled out.

Attention Deficit Hyperactivity Disorder

Attention deficit hyperactivity disorder (ADHD) is characterized by inattention, short attention span, or hyperactivity that is severe enough to interfere with daily functioning.

ADHD is associated with lower levels of dopamine.

- Symptoms must be present >6 months, usually age <7.
- Symptoms must be present in ≥2 areas, such as home and school.
  - At home, children interrupt others, fidget in chairs, and run or climb excessively; are unable to engage in leisure activities; and talk excessively.
  - At school, children are unable to pay attention, make careless mistakes in schoolwork, do not follow through with instructions, have difficulties organizing tasks, and are easily distracted.

Symptoms may persist into adulthood.

Treatment is as follows.

- **First-line**: methylphenidate and dextroamphetamine to reduce inattention and hyperactivity
  - Affect the noradrenergic and dopaminergic pathways of attention
  - Side effects include insomnia, decreased appetite, GI disturbances, increased anxiety, and headache.
- **Second-line**
  - Atomoxetine (a norepinephrine reuptake inhibitor) has fewer side effects and less risk of abuse.
  - Clonidine and guanfacine (alpha-2 agonists) are used if ADHD presents with Tourette syndrome and tics.

The first symptom to disappear after treatment is hyperactivity.

Disruptive Behavioral and Mood Disorders			
Disorder	**Epidemiology**	**Features**	**Treatment**
Oppositional defiant disorder	Usually noted by age 8; seen more in boys than girls before puberty, but equal incidence after puberty	Often argue with others, lose temper, easily annoyed by others, and blame others for their mistakes. Tend to have problems with authority figures and justify their behavior as response to others' actions. These behaviors manifest during interactions with others that do not include siblings.	Teach parents appropriate child management skills and how to lessen the oppositional behavior. Psychotherapy for the child.
Conduct disorder	Seen more frequently in boys and in children whose parents have antisocial personality disorder and alcohol dependence. Diagnosis is given only to those age <18.	Persistent **rule-breaking** behavior: aggression toward others (bullying, cruelty to animals, fighting, using weapons), destroying property (vandalism, setting fires), stealing items or lying to obtain goods from others, violating rules (truancy, running away from home, breaking curfew).	Behavioral intervention using rewards for prosocial and nonaggressive behavior. If aggressive, antipsychotic medications may be used.
Disruptive mood dysregulation disorder (DMDD)	Seen more frequently in boys age 6–10 years. Should not be diagnosed age <6 or >18. Children with DMDD usually do not develop bipolar disorder in adulthood; they are more likely to develop depression or anxiety.	**Chronic, severe, persistent irritability with temper outbursts** and angry, irritable, or sad mood between the outbursts. These occur almost every day, are noticeable by others, and are out of proportion to the situation. The outbursts are inconsistent with developmental issues. Symptoms occur year-round; there is no period lasting ≥3 consecutive months without all symptoms. The symptoms are severe enough to **interfere with home, school, or peers.**	Treatment is individualized to the needs of the particular child and family. It may include individual therapy as well as work with the child's family and/or school. It may also include the use of medication to address specific symptoms.

You are asked to evaluate a 9-year-old boy who is having problems at home and school. His teachers report frequent temper tantrums in which he becomes physically aggressive toward his peers (biting and kicking). These usually occur after minor incidents, such as another child cutting in front of him in the cafeteria line. These outbursts have been occurring almost daily since age 8 and have worsened since school started 4 months ago, resulting in several weeks of disciplinary suspension. His parents report the same problems at home (e.g., attacking his older brother when told he could not play outside). His general mood is irritable and angry, though his family noticed a slight improvement in his behavior during the summer months. What is the most likely diagnosis?

a. Intermittent explosive disorder
b. Adjustment disorder with disturbances of conduct
c. Disruptive mood dysregulation disorder
d. Bipolar disorder
e. Oppositional defiant disorder

Answer: **C.** Disruptive mood dysregulation disorder. Children with intermittent explosive disorder are not aggressive on such a continuous basis; they have extended periods of good behavior. There is no mention of a stressor, ruling out diagnosis of adjustment disorder. There is no evidence of mood swings, ruling out diagnosis of bipolar disorder. Children with oppositional defiant disorder mostly have problems with authority figures, not their peers.

Tourette Disorder

Tourette disorder is characterized by the onset of multiple tics for >1 year, and is seen age <18 (often by age 7). Boys > girls.

Tourette is associated with ADHD and OCD.

- The motor tics often involve the muscles of the face and neck, such as head shaking and blinking.
- The vocal tics include grunting, coughing, and throat clearing.

Treatment is dopamine antagonists, such as the antipsychotic medications haloperidol, pimozide, and risperidone. Medications such as clonidine, an alpha-2 agonist, can also be used.

Mood Disorders

Major Depressive Disorder

Major depressive disorder presents with ≥5 of the following symptoms, observable for ≥2 weeks, that represent a change from the previous level of functioning:

- Symptoms always include depressed mood or anhedonia (absence of pleasure). A patient may present with both.
- Additional symptoms include depressed mood for most of the day, weight changes, sleep changes, psychomotor disturbances, fatigue, poor concentration, and thoughts of death and worthlessness.

About 60% of those with major depressive disorder have suicidal ideation at some point.

Major depressive disorder is associated with decreased norepinephrine, serotonin, dopamine, and REM latency, plus increased REM.

To diagnose, first rule out any medical causes (the most common of which is hypothyroidism). The most common neurological associations are Parkinson disease and neurocognitive disorders. Rule out bipolar disorder presenting in the depressed phase (bipolar depression).

Treatment:

- **First-line** treatment: SSRI such as fluoxetine, paroxetine, sertraline, citalopram, or escitalopram (highly effective, have relatively few side effects, and are less toxic in overdose than other antidepressants)
  - After 4–6 weeks, if some improvement is noted but not full response, increase the dose of the SSRI. If no effect is noted, switch to another SSRI.
  - **Do not take SSRIs with MAO inhibitors**, as they will cause a dramatic increase in serotonin.
  - TCAs can be used, but their lethal potential precludes routine use.
- **Second-line** treatment: SNRI such as venlafaxine, duloxetine, or desvenlafaxine (side effects include hypertension and sweating)
- Psychotherapy such as cognitive therapy to teach patients to identify negative thoughts and develop tools for positive thinking

Treatment that combines medication with psychotherapy is superior to either treatment alone.

> Intranasal ketamine can be used in refractory depression but is contraindicated in uncontrolled hypertension.

Exceptions to SSRI Use	
Variety of depression	**Specific alternative to SSRIs**
Patient with depression and neuropathic pain	Use duloxetine, since it is approved for both depression and neuropathy.
Patient with depression who is fearful of weight gain or sexual side effects or is a smoker trying to quit	Use bupropion, since it has fewer sexual side effects and less weight gain than SSRIs. May also be used as adjunct or replacement treatment for SSRI-induced sexual side effects. Bupropion has been approved for smoking cessation. Bupropion lowers seizure threshold.

A 45-year-old woman is seen with complaints of depressed mood, lack of pleasure, sleep disturbance, decreased appetite and weight, low energy, and problems with concentration. The symptoms started when she was fired from her job about 4 weeks ago, and since then, she has been unable to function. Which of the following is the most indicated treatment at this time?

a. Alprazolam
b. Paroxetine
c. Bupropion
d. Venlafaxine
e. Trazodone
f. Electroconvulsive therapy

Answer: **B.** The patient has major depression, and the first-line treatment is an SSRI. All other answer choices, except alprazolam and electroconvulsive therapy, would be useful but are not first-line due to their side effects. Alprazolam is a benzodiazepine and acts as an anxiolytic, not an antidepressant. Electroconvulsive therapy might be useful for severe, persistent depression associated with psychotic features.

A 55-year-old presents with complaints of depressed mood for over 2 months, low energy, decreased appetite, inability to concentrate, and poor sleep. He states that his sleep problems and inability to focus in the morning are impairing his work. Which of the following is the most indicated treatment at this time?

a. Imipramine
b. Venlafaxine
c. Bupropion
d. Zolpidem
e. Mirtazapine

Answer: **E.** Although any antidepressant can be used, mirtazapine is preferable in this patient for both its antidepressant and sedative effects. Imipramine would have too many side effects and is not a first-line agent. Venlafaxine might be considered if the patient had depression alone; since insomnia is a major concern, mirtazapine is the better option. Bupropion tends to cause problems with sleep, so is not indicated. Zolpidem would help this patient sleep but would not treat his depression.

Bipolar Disorder

Bipolar type I disorder is a mood disorder where the patient experiences manic symptoms that cause significant distress in the level of functioning for ≥1 week. Manic symptoms include elevated mood, increased self-esteem, distractibility, pressured speech, decreased need for sleep, an increase in goal-directed activity, racing thoughts, and excessive involvement in pleasurable activities.

Bipolar type 1 typically starts with depression and increased energy, despite lack of sleep.

Diagnosis starts by making sure the condition is not secondary to drug use, such as cocaine or amphetamine use. Obtain a good history and urine drug screen.

> Bipolar disorder is regarded as the illness with the greatest genetic linkage.

> Bipolar disorder is associated with increased levels of norepinephrine and serotonin.

Classification is done with mania and hypomania; the difference between mania and hypomania has to do with the severity of symptoms, level of functioning, and duration.

- **Manic symptoms** last >1 week, affect functioning, and are severe enough to warrant hospitalization.
- **Hypomanic symptoms** last <1 week, do not severely affect functioning, and are not severe enough to warrant hospitalization.

Rapid-cycling bipolar disorder is defined by ≥4 mood episodes in a 12-month period.

Types of Bipolar Disorders	
Bipolar disorder type I	Mania and depression
Bipolar disorder type II	Hypomania and depression

A 21-year-old college student is taken to the ED after acting bizarrely in class. She is talking fast and giggling, and reports that she has not slept for over 4 days. She appears to be paying little attention to her surroundings. Her roommate reports that she has been drinking alcohol excessively over the last few days and has had many sexual contacts with unknown men. What is the most likely diagnosis?

a. Alcohol-induced mood disorder
b. Bipolar disorder type I
c. Bipolar disorder type II
d. Major depression with psychosis
e. Cyclothymia

Answer: **B**. The patient is exhibiting mania, as shown by her pressured speech, decreased sleep, increased libido, and inappropriate behavior. The symptoms are severe enough that her level of functioning is affected. Bipolar disorder occurs more frequently in young individuals.

Treatment begins by identifying whether you are treating acute mania or bipolar depression.

- If **acute mania**, use lithium, valproic acid, and atypical antipsychotics as first-line treatments. If there are severe symptoms, use atypical antipsychotics with a shorter onset of action.
- If **bipolar depression**, use lithium, quetiapine, lurasidone, or lamotrigine. Lurasidone can be used in pregnancy if the benefits outweigh the risk. As with other atypical antipsychotics, fetuses exposed to lurasidone in the third trimester have an increased risk of extrapyramidal symptoms.
- If kidneys are compromised, do not use lithium.
- Avoid divalproex in women of child-bearing age.

Use of an SSRI during bipolar depression risks inducing mania.

▶ **TIP**

Lithium is the first-line treatment for bipolar disorders.

A 33-year-old man is taken to the ED by the police after neighbors complain about his behavior. His family informed the doctor that he has been diagnosed with bipolar disorder and was recently started on lithium. While in the ED, he becomes combative and punches a nurse on the mouth. What is the next step in management?

a. Obtain lithium level
b. Admit to psychiatric unit
c. Refer to psychiatry
d. Add valproic acid
e. Olanzapine

Answer: **E.** The patient is exhibiting mania. Lithium level does not need to be verified given that the symptoms are acute. He apparently has been noncompliant with medications and obtaining a level is not the correct answer. He needs to be medicated, and antipsychotics are considered first-line treatment for bipolar patients presenting with acute mania. Admitting an agitated patient to the psychiatric unit is not as important as administering adequate treatment. "Refer to psychiatry" is never the correct answer on Step 2 CK.

Persistent Depressive Disorder

Persistent depressive disorder is characterized by the presence of depressed mood that lasts most of the day and is present almost continuously. Symptoms must be present for >2 years (1 year in children or adolescents). Treatment is with antidepressant medications and psychotherapy.

Symptoms of persistent depressive disorder are not severe enough for hospitalization.

Cyclothymic Disorder

Cyclothymia is characterized by the presence of hypomanic episodes and mild depression. Symptoms must be present for >2 years. Treatment is lithium, valproic acid or antipsychotic medication, and psychotherapy.

Major Depressive Disorder with Atypical Features

Atypical depression is characterized by reverse vegetative changes such as increased sleep, increased weight, and increased appetite, and interpersonal rejection sensitivity that results in significant social or occupational impairment. The patient's mood tends to be worse in the evening. Patients may complain of extremities feeling "heavy." Treatment is with SSRIs (fluoxetine, sertraline, paroxetine, citalopram, or escitalopram) or MAOIs (phenelzine, isocarboxazid, or tranylcypromine).

▶ **TIP**

MAOIs are the correct answer on USMLE Step 2 CK for the treatment of atypical depression.

Major Depressive Disorder with Seasonal Pattern

This disorder is characterized by seasonal changes in mood during fall and winter. Symptoms include weight gain, increased sleep, and lethargy.

Treatment is phototherapy and bupropion or SSRIs. In phototherapy, patients sit 12–18 inches from a source of 10,000 lux of white fluorescent light without UV wavelengths for 30 min each morning. The eyes should be kept open, but it is not necessary to stare at the light.

> Major depressive disorder with seasonal pattern is thought to be related to abnormal **melatonin** metabolism.

Peripartum Disorders (Formerly Postpartum Disorders)				
Disorder	**Onset**	**Symptoms**	**Mother's feelings toward baby**	**Treatment**
Postpartum blues or "baby blues"	Immediately after birth up to 2 weeks	Sadness, mood lability, tearfulness	No negative feelings	Supportive, usually self-limited
Depressive disorder with peripartum onset	Within 1–3 months after birth	Depressed mood, weight changes, sleep disturbances, and excessive anxiety	May have negative feelings toward baby	Antidepressant medications
• Bipolar disorder with peripartum onset • Brief psychotic disorder with peripartum onset	During pregnancy up to 4 weeks after birth	Depression, mania, hallucinations, delusions, and thoughts of harm	May have thoughts of harming baby	Antipsychotic medication, lithium, and possibly hospital admission

Bereavement (Grief)

Normal bereavement typically begins after the death of a loved one and includes feelings of sadness, worrying about the deceased, irritability, sleep difficulties, poor concentration, and tearfulness. It typically lasts <6 months to 1 year but can go on longer.

Treatment is generally limited to supportive psychotherapy. Pharmacotherapy is the wrong answer.

> **Brexanolone** is a synthetic neuroactive steroid indicated for the treatment of postpartum depression that modulates the GABA-A receptor.

Diagnosis of major depression (greater severity than bereavement):

- Thoughts of death
- Morbid preoccupation with **worthlessness**
- Marked psychomotor retardation
- Psychosis
- Prolonged functional impairment
- **Symptoms last >2 weeks** and adversely affect functioning

A 65-year-old man is brought to the office by his daughter, who is concerned that he has been hopeless and helpless since his wife died 3 months ago. He has had isolative behavior and lack of appetite and expresses feelings of worthlessness. He has lost over 30 pounds. He does not seem interested in getting better and believes he should have died with his wife. What is the most likely diagnosis?

a. Bereavement
b. Persistent depressive disorder
c. Major depressive disorder
d. Adjustment disorder
e. Bipolar disorder

Answer: **C.** Although it has been less than 6 months since his wife died, his symptoms are severe enough to warrant a diagnosis of major depression. He has no interest in things, has lost weight, feels hopeless and helpless, and believes he should have died as well. He needs to be treated with antidepressants, and you must ensure that he is not suicidal since he is at high risk.

Treatment

Medications, Electroconvulsive Therapy, and Side Effects	
Type of medication	**Adverse effects**
Tricyclic antidepressants (amitriptyline, nortriptyline, imipramine)	Hypo/hypertension, dry mouth, constipation, confusion, arrhythmias, sexual side effects, weight gain, GI disturbances
Monoamine oxidase inhibitors (phenelzine, isocarboxazid, tranylcypromine)	Monitor diet, given that food rich in tyramine will produce hypertension. Safe foods include white wine and processed cheese. Unsafe foods include red wine, aged cheese, and chocolate.
Serotonin selective reuptake inhibitors (fluoxetine, paroxetine, sertraline, citalopram, escitalopram, fluvoxamine)	Headaches, weight changes, sexual side effects, GI disturbances
Serotonin norepinephrine reuptake inhibitors (venlafaxine, duloxetine, desvenlafaxine)	Hypertension, blurry vision, weight changes, sexual side effects, GI disturbances
Others (bupropion, mirtazapine, trazodone)	Bupropion has **increased risk for seizures**, trazodone has increased risk for **priapism**, and mirtazapine has increased risk for weight gain and sedation.
Lithium	Tremors, weight gain, GI disturbance, **nephrotoxic**, teratogenic, **leukocytosis**, diabetes insipidus. Lithium has a narrow therapeutic index. Blood levels should be monitored. Severe toxicity gives confusion, ataxia, lethargy, and abnormal reflexes.
Valproic acid	Tremors, weight gain, GI disturbances, alopecia, teratogenic, **hepatotoxic**. Must monitor levels; toxicity causes hyponatremia, coma, or death.
Lamotrigine	Stevens-Johnson syndrome
Electroconvulsive therapy (ECT)	Headaches, transient memory loss

What is the single most effective treatment for depression?

a. Electroconvulsive therapy
b. Fluoxetine
c. Venlafaxine
d. Imipramine
e. Phenelzine

Answer: **A.** Although electroconvulsive therapy is usually used for suicidal patients or those who do not respond to treatment, it is considered the best treatment for depression. It can also be used as an adjunctive treatment for psychosis. All others are equally efficacious, but the SSRIs are used more frequently due to side-effect profiles.

> ECT is safe in all terms of pregnancy.

Serotonin Syndrome

Serotonin syndrome is a potentially life-threatening disorder occurring as a result of therapeutic drug use of SSRIs, often with inadvertent interactions between drugs, overdose, or recreational use of drugs that are serotonergic in origin.

> Drugs that can precipitate serotonin syndrome:
> - Meperidine
> - Lithium
> - Linezolid
> - Metoclopramide

Common symptoms include:

- **Cognitive effects**: agitation, confusion, hallucinations, hypomania
- **Autonomic effects**: sweating, hyperthermia, tachycardia, nausea, diarrhea, shivering
- **Somatic effects**: tremors, myoclonus

Treatment is as follows:

- Stop SSRI medication.
- Symptomatic treatment of fever, diarrhea, hypertension
- Cyproheptadine (serotonin antagonist)

Psychotic Disorders

Before making a psychiatric diagnosis, always rule out organic causes first. Also rule out substance use as a cause of symptoms.

Focus on 2 elements of diagnostic criteria: **duration** of symptoms and **severity** of symptoms.

Classification of Psychotic Disorders			
Disorder	**Duration of symptoms**	**Symptoms**	**Treatment**
Brief psychotic disorder	>1 day but <1 month	Delusions, hallucinations, disorganized speech, grossly disorganized or catatonic behavior	Antipsychotic medication
Schizophreniform disorders	>1 month but <6 months	Delusions, hallucinations, disorganized speech, grossly disorganized or catatonic behavior, and negative symptoms (flat affect, poor grooming, social withdrawal)	Antipsychotic medication
Schizophrenia	>6 months	**Delusions, hallucinations, or disorganized speech**; grossly disorganized or catatonic behavior; and negative symptoms. Severely affects level of functioning.	Antipsychotic medication

> Visual hallucinations suggest an organic cause. Get an MRI to rule out a mass.

▶ TIP

Be careful with duration of symptoms; it is the only thing that distinguishes brief psychosis, schizophreniform, and schizophrenia. If no time is mentioned, always choose schizophrenia as the correct answer to the "What is the most likely diagnosis?" question.

Schizophrenia

Schizophrenia impairs judgment, behavior, and the ability to interpret reality. Symptoms must be present ≥6 months and must affect functioning.

> **Positive** symptoms: **dopamine** receptors
>
> **Negative** symptoms: **muscarinic** receptors

To diagnose, first do a urine drug screen to rule out cocaine or amphetamine use. Symptoms must persist >6 months, with ≥2 of the following:

- Delusions
- Hallucinations
- Disorganized speech
- Negative symptoms
- Disorganized or catatonic behavior

At least one symptom must be delusions, hallucinations, or disorganized speech.

Key imaging findings include:

- CT: later and third ventricular enlargement, decreased cortical volume
- PET scan: hypoactive frontal lobes, hyperactivity in basal ganglion

Treatment

- Hospitalize patients who are acutely psychotic.
- Ensure patient safety and use an atypical antipsychotic as a first-line agent, e.g., risperidone, olanzapine, quetiapine, ziprasidone, aripiprazole, paliperidone, asenapine, iloperidone, or lurasidone.
- In any emergency situation where intramuscular medication is needed, consider the use of short-acting medications such as olanzapine or ziprasidone; haloperidol is still used, but has more side effects, so if given the choice, pick the atypical.
- If the question involves a patient who is noncompliant with medication, consider a long-acting antipsychotic medication such as risperidone or paliperidone as first-line treatment. Haloperidol and fluphenazine are still used but have more side effects.
- Clozapine (**most effective medication for treatment-resistant psychosis**) is used only when patients have no response to 2 trials of typical or atypical antipsychotics; **never used first-line**

Overall prognosis in schizophrenia is divided into thirds:

- 1/3 lead normal lives
- 1/3 are symptomatic but functional
- 1/3 have frequent or long-term hospitalization

A good prognosis of schizophrenia is indicated by late onset, rapid course, positive symptoms, absence of family history, and lack of structural brain abnormalities.

▶TIP

For the USMLE exam, you must know the side-effect profiles of the atypical antipsychotics. As a rule:

- *–pines* (olanzapine, quetiapine, asenapine, clozapine) cause increased risk of weight gain, metabolic syndrome, diabetes
- *–dones* (risperidone, lurasidone, ziprasidone, iloperidone) cause increased risk of movement disorders, cardiac conduction problems

> Quetiapine = quiet (lowest incidence of EPS)
>
> Ziprasidone **zips** through QT.

Pimavanserin is the only FDA-approved drug for treatment of psychosis in Parkinson disease.

Adverse Effects of Atypical Antipsychotic Medications	
Antipsychotic medication	**Specific adverse effects**
Olanzapine	Greater incidence of **diabetes** and **weight gain**; avoid in diabetic and obese patients
Risperidone	Greater incidence of **movement disorders**
Quetiapine	**Lower incidence of movement disorders**; appropriate for use in patients with existing movement disorders
Ziprasidone	Increased risk of **prolongation of QT interval**; avoid in patients with conduction defects
Clozapine	High risk of **agranulocytosis**; need to **monitor CBC** on regular basis; cardiomyopathy
Aripiprazole	Compulsive behavior (gambling)
Lurasidone	Safer for use in pregnant patients

A 22-year-old woman was recently diagnosed with schizophrenia. She is 30 pounds overweight and suffers from type 2 diabetes. She is concerned about her medications and asks for your advice. Which of the following is most indicated?

a. Aripiprazole
b. Olanzapine
c. Quetiapine
d. Clozapine
e. Risperidone

Answer: **A.** Aripiprazole and ziprasidone are the least likely to cause weight gain, diabetes, and metabolic syndrome. Olanzapine and clozapine have the highest risk of metabolic abnormalities. Quetiapine and risperidone have medium risk.

Management of Adverse Effects of Antipsychotic Medications			
Disorder	**Onset of symptoms**	**Symptoms**	**Treatment**
Acute dystonia	Hours to days	Muscle spasms, such as torticollis, laryngeal spasms, oculogyric crisis	Benztropine, trihexyphenidyl, diphenhydramine
Akathisia	Weeks	Generalized restlessness, pacing, rocking, inability to relax	Reduce dose, beta blockers, switch to atypical medication, benzodiazepine
Tardive dyskinesia	Rare before 6 months	Abnormal involuntary movements of head, limb, and trunk. Perioral movements are the most common.	Switch to atypical antipsychotic. Clozapine has least risk. Also used: valbenazine, tetrabenazine, deutetrabenazine
Neuroleptic malignant syndrome	Not time limited	Muscular rigidity, fever, autonomic changes, agitation, and obtundation	Dantrolene or bromocriptine

A 23-year-old man recently diagnosed with schizophrenia has recently been started on haloperidol. Within a few hours, he develops muscle stiffness, and his eyes roll upward and he cannot move them down. What is the most likely diagnosis?

a. Tardive dyskinesia
b. Neuroleptic malignant syndrome
c. Akathisia
d. Serotonin syndrome
e. Acute dystonia

Answer: **E.** Acute dystonia develops within hours of the use of medications. This side effect is typical for haloperidol. The treatment of choice is benztropine or diphenhydramine, which can be given with the haloperidol or after should side effects occur.

Schizoaffective Disorder

Schizoaffective disorder is an uninterrupted period of mood symptoms that meet criteria for major depressive disorder or bipolar disorder in addition to psychotic symptoms.

- A major mood episode must be present for a majority of the total duration of the disorder.
- Psychotic symptoms (≥ 2 of criteria A) must be present for ≥ 1 month and must be present while the patient has no mood symptoms for ≥ 2 weeks.
- Contrast this with a mood disorder with psychotic features, where the psychosis and mood symptoms are present at the same time.
- Functional impairment is also seen, but negative symptoms are not as commonly seen in schizoaffective disorder as they are in schizophrenia.

Treatment begins with a determination about whether hospitalization is indicated. An antidepressant and/or a mood stabilizer is used to control mood symptoms, and an antipsychotic is used for psychotic symptoms.

Delusional Disorder

Delusional disorder is characterized by the prominence of non-bizarre delusions for >1 month and no impairment in level of functioning (e.g., the patient may believe the country is about to be invaded but still obeys the law, goes to work, and pays bills). Hallucinations, if present, are not prominent and are related to the delusional theme. Treatment is with atypical antipsychotic agents as first-line therapy. You may also consider psychotherapy to help promote reality testing.

- With **delusional disorder,** there are **nonbizarre delusions** (false but plausible).
- With **schizophrenia,** there are **bizarre delusions** (false and implausible).

Anxiety Disorders

Panic Disorder

Panic attack is the experience of intense anxiety along with feelings of dread and doom. This is accompanied by ≥4 symptoms of autonomic hyperactivity, such as diaphoresis, trembling, chest pain, fear of dying, chills, palpitations, shortness of breath, nausea, dizziness, dissociative symptoms, and paresthesias. These sensations typically last <30 minutes and may be accompanied by agoraphobia, defined as the fear of places where escape is felt to be difficult.

Panic disorder is defined by recurrent panic attacks and:

- 1 month of persistent worry or fear of having another panic attack and/or
- Significant maladaptive behavior in order to avoid the possibility of another attack

Panic disorder is typically seen in women, can occur at any time, and usually has no specific stressor. It is important to ensure that thyroid disease, hypoglycemia, and cardiac disease have been ruled out.

Treatment

- SSRIs (typically fluoxetine, paroxetine, and sertraline) are indicated for this disorder.
- Along with SSRIs, patients may benefit from benzodiazepines (such as alprazolam, clonazepam, or lorazepam). Begin with both, then taper and discontinue the benzodiazepine given the potential for abuse.
- Behavioral and individual therapy are also helpful *in conjunction with* medication (not as the sole treatment).

> In women, anxiety disorders are the most common psychiatric disorder. In men, anxiety symptoms are most commonly substance-induced.

Which is considered to be the first-line treatment for panic disorder?

a. Alprazolam
b. Buspirone
c. Sertraline
d. Imipramine
e. Fluvoxamine

Answer: **C.** SSRIs are first-line treatment for panic disorder. If the question is *panic attack*, then alprazolam is the correct answer. If a single panic attack is the diagnosis, a benzodiazepine is the treatment.

►TIP

When determining the most likely diagnosis in cases involving panic symptoms, distinguish between direct presentation and patient history.

- If the patient is **presenting with autonomic hyperactivity**, then panic **attack** is the most likely diagnosis and benzodiazepines are the correct treatment.
- If the patient is **telling the doctor a story** about the panic attacks, the diagnosis is most likely panic **disorder** and the treatment of choice is an SSRI.

Phobias

A phobia is the fear of an object or situation and the need to avoid it. Phobias may be learned and involve 2 main types.

The most common phobia is **public speaking**.

Two Types of Phobias	
Type of phobia	**Characteristic of the phobia**
Specific phobia	Fear of an object, such as animals, heights, or cars
Social phobia	Fear of a situation, such as public restrooms, eating in public, or public speaking. These involve situations where something potentially embarrassing may happen.

Diagnosis usually can be made by obtaining a good history where patients indicate anxiety symptoms in specific situations or when in contact with feared objects. The symptoms must last over 6 months and must be persistent and disabling.

Treatment

- **Behavioral modification** techniques such as systematic desensitization, in which the patient while relaxed is exposed, often only in imagination, to progressively more frightening aspects of the feared objects.
- Patients are also taught **relaxation techniques** such as breathing or guided imagery.

Beta blockers such as atenolol or propranolol are used only for performance anxiety such as stage fright. They are given 30–60 minutes before the performance.

A 40-year-old man is referred to a psychiatrist by his physician because he is "too shy." He has trouble going to parties, feels anxious about getting close to others, and stays at home in fear that others would laugh at him. When confronted by others, he develops severe anxiety as well as hyperventilation and increased sweating. Which is the most likely diagnosis?

a. Panic disorder
b. Social anxiety
c. Generalized anxiety disorder
d. Specific phobia
e. Acute stress disorder

Answer: **B.** Social anxiety is characterized by fear of embarrassment in social situations. Patients have problems going out in fear that others will laugh at them.

Obsessive Compulsive Disorder

Obsessive compulsive disorder (OCD) is a disorder where patients typically experience obsessions alone, or in combination with compulsions (**more common**), that often affect level of functioning.

- **Obsessions:** thoughts that are intrusive, senseless, and distressing to the patient, thus increasing anxiety. These include fear of contamination.
- **Compulsions:** rituals, e.g., counting and checking, that are performed to neutralize obsessive thoughts. These are time consuming and tend to lower anxiety.

Features of OCD include increased frontal lobe metabolism and increased size of caudate nucleus.

OCD is seen more frequently in young patients. There is an equal incidence in men and women. OCD can coexist with Tourette disorder.

Treatment is SSRIs; fluoxetine, paroxetine, sertraline, citalopram, and fluvoxamine are the usual first-line agents. The primary behavioral therapy used is exposure and response prevention.

> In obsessive-compulsive personality disorder (**OCPD**), there are no obsessions or compulsions, unlike **OCD**. Further distinctions:
> - OCD = ego-dystonic
> - OCPD = ego-syntonic

▶ TIP

On the USMLE exam, if all the answer choices offered as pharmacotherapy for OCD are TCAs, choose clomipramine.

Hoarding Disorder

Individuals with hoarding disorder have problems discarding their possessions, leading to persistent accumulations of possessions such that the home is overwhelmed by clutter. The hoarding affects the individual's level of functioning and impairs her ability to maintain a safe environment.

Treatment is SSRIs, combined with behavioral modification or psychotherapy.

Body Dysmorphic Disorder

Individuals with body dysmorphic disorder believe that some body part is abnormal, defective, or misshapen, although others do not see these perceived defects. These beliefs significantly impair the patient's level of functioning. Patients spend excessive time checking their appearance in the mirror and seeking reassurance.

Treatment is SSRIs, combined with individual psychotherapy.

Posttraumatic Stress Disorder and Acute Stress Disorder

In both posttraumatic stress disorder (PTSD) and acute stress disorder, individuals have been exposed to a stressor to which they react with fear and helplessness. Patients continually relive the event and avoid anything that reminds them of the event. These stressors are usually overwhelming and involve such events as war, rape, hurricanes, or earthquakes. The symptoms adversely affect the patient's level of functioning. Other symptoms include increased startle response, hypervigilance, sleep disturbances, anger outbursts, and concentration difficulties.

Posttraumatic Stress Disorder versus Acute Stress Disorder	
Disorder	**Duration of symptoms**
Posttraumatic stress disorder	Symptoms last >**1 month.**
Acute stress disorder	Symptoms last >**2 days** and ≤**1 month.** They occur within 1 month of the traumatic event.

Diagnosis is made, first, by determining the time period when the traumatic events occurred in relationship to the symptoms. Depression and substance abuse must be ruled out, because both worsen the prognosis.

Treatment:

- First-line treatment includes paroxetine and sertraline. Prazosin is used to reduce the incidence of nightmares.
- Relaxation techniques and hypnosis
- Psychotherapy after traumatic events to develop coping techniques and acceptance of the event

Generalized Anxiety Disorder

This is a disorder in which patients experience excessive anxiety and worry about most things, lasting >6 months. Typically, the anxiety is out of proportion to the event. This is accompanied by fatigue, concentration difficulties, sleep problems, muscle tension, and restlessness. Patients are usually women, and they report feeling anxious as long as they can remember.

Treatment

- SSRIs such as fluoxetine, paroxetine, sertraline, or citalopram are indicated in this disorder.
- Venlafaxine and buspirone are also effective.
- Psychotherapy and behavioral therapy are beneficial as well.

Therapy + medication is more effective than either treatment alone.

A 35-year-old woman reports palpitations, dizziness, and increased sweating for ≥8 months. She has visited numerous physicians, and none have been helpful. Her husband is concerned because she cannot relax and worries about everything. She worries about her parents' health, even though they are healthy. She worries about her finances, although her husband assures her they are financially secure. What is the most likely diagnosis?

a. Generalized anxiety disorder
b. Phobias
c. Panic disorder
d. Adjustment disorder
e. Social anxiety

Answer: **A.** The main feature of generalized anxiety disorder is the chronic worrying about things that do not merit concern. It is also accompanied by other symptoms of anxiety, as well as sleep and concentration problems.

Antianxiety Medications and Their Adverse Effects	
Antianxiety medication	**Adverse effects**
Benzodiazepines (diazepam, lorazepam, clonazepam, alprazolam, oxazepam, chlordiazepoxide, temazepam, flurazepam)	Sedation, confusion, memory deficits, respiratory depression, and increased addiction potential
Buspirone	Headaches, nausea, dizziness

Antianxiety Medications and Their Specific Indications	
Antianxiety medication	**Specific indications**
Lorazepam	Used frequently in emergency situations because it can be given intramuscularly
Clonazepam	May be used if addiction is a concern given its longer half-life
Chlordiazepoxide, oxazepam, lorazepam	Used frequently in treatment of alcohol withdrawal. Lorazepam and oxazepam are the drugs of choice in patients with liver problems.
Alprazolam	Used frequently in panic attack and panic disorder
Flurazepam, temazepam, triazolam	Approved as hypnotics (rarely used)

> Overdose of benzodiazepine or barbiturate can be fatal.

Flumazenil is a benzodiazepine antagonist that can be used to treat benzodiazepine overdose. It is used only in an acute overdose when it is certain that there is no chronic dependence. If flumazenil is used in a patient with chronic dependence, it can precipitate acute withdrawal symptoms such as seizures or delirium tremens.

Substance-Related Disorders

Some basic definitions:

- **Intoxication:** reversible experience with a substance that leads to psychological or physiological changes
- **Withdrawal:** cessation or reduction of a substance leading to psychological or physiological changes
- **Use:** maladaptive pattern of use of substances which leads to engaging in hazardous situations, legal problems, inability to fulfill obligations, and continued use despite adverse consequences and cravings

▶ **TIP**

Focus on substances with potentially life-threatening potential in withdrawal or overdose.

Presentation and Treatment of Intoxication and Withdrawal				
Substance	**Signs and symptoms of intoxication**	**Treatment of intoxication**	**Signs and symptoms of withdrawal**	**Treatment of withdrawal**
Alcohol	Talkative, sullen, gregarious, moody, disinhibited	Mechanical ventilation if severe	Tremors, hallucinations, seizures, delirium tremens	Benzodiazepines, thiamine, multivitamins, folic acid
Amphetamines and cocaine (synthetic forms: bath salts)	Euphoria, hypervigilance, autonomic hyperactivity, weight loss, pupillary dilatation, perceptual disturbances	Antipsychotics and/or benzodiazepines and/or antihypertensives	Anxiety, tremulousness, headache, increased appetite, depression, risk of suicide	Bupropion and/or bromocriptine
Cannabis (synthetic forms: K2 and spice)	Impaired motor coordination, slowed sense of time, social withdrawal, increased appetite, conjunctival injection	Consider use of antipsychotics if patient is psychotic	Irritability, anger, anxiety, sleep problems, restlessness, appetite problems	Symptomatic
Hallucinogens	Ideas of reference, perceptual disturbances, possible increase in psychosis, impaired judgment, tremors, incoordination, dissociative symptoms	Antipsychotics and/or benzodiazepines and/or talking down	None	None
Inhalants	Belligerence, apathy, aggression, impaired judgment, stupor, or coma	Antipsychotics	None	None
Opiates (synthetic form: desomorphine, a.k.a. krokodil)	Apathy, dysphoria, pupillary constriction, drowsiness, slurred speech, coma, or death	Naloxone	Fever, chills, lacrimation, abdominal cramps, muscle spasms, diarrhea	Clonidine, methadone, or buprenorphine

(continued)

Presentation and Treatment of Intoxication and Withdrawal (cont'd)				
Substance	**Signs and symptoms of intoxication**	**Treatment of intoxication**	**Signs and symptoms of withdrawal**	**Treatment of withdrawal**
Phencyclidine (PCP)	Belligerence, psychomotor agitation, violence, nystagmus, hypertension, seizures	Antipsychotics and/or benzodiazepines and/or talking down	None	None
Anabolic steroids	Irritability, aggression, mania, psychosis	Antipsychotics	Depression, headaches, anxiety, increased concern over body's physical state	SSRIs

The most commonly abused and most commonly tested drug is **alcohol**.

If you suspect someone is an alcoholic, do the **CAGE** test. Two positive responses to the four questions are considered positive and indicate that further assessment is warranted.

C: Have you ever tried to **cut down** on your drinking?

A: Have you ever gotten **annoyed** by others who have criticized your drinking?

G: Have you ever felt **guilty** about your drinking?

E: Have you ever used alcohol as an **eye-opener**?

Treatment

- **Detoxification**: usually 5–10 days, mostly in hospital settings to assure safe detoxification
- **Rehabilitation**: usually ≥28 days, emphasizing relapse prevention techniques
- Alcoholics Anonymous: **most effective**
- Narcotics Anonymous
- Pharmacologic treatments: often include disulfiram (acetaldehyde dehydrogenase inhibitor), naltrexone (opioid receptor antagonist), and acamprosate

Somatic Symptoms and Related Disorders, Factitious Disorder, and Malingering

Somatic Symptom Disorder

Somatic symptom disorder is characterized by the presence of one or more somatic symptoms that are distressing and cause impairment in functioning. The patient has excessive thoughts, feelings, or behaviors related to the somatic symptom that are manifested by disproportionate and persistent thoughts about the seriousness of the symptoms, intense anxiety about the symptoms, and excessive time devoted to the symptoms or health concerns.

A patient must be symptomatic >6 months to be diagnosed with somatic symptom disorder. The disorder is seen more frequently in young women and usually has some psychological component of which the patient is unaware. Psychotherapy is the treatment of choice given the psychological source of the symptoms.

Other Somatic Symptom Disorders	
Type	**Definition/Diagnostic criteria**
Illness anxiety disorder	Patients believe that they have some **specific disease despite constant reassurance.**
Conversion (functional neurological disorder)	Typically affects **voluntary motor or sensory functions** that are indicative of a medical condition: • At least 1 voluntary motor or sensory symptom • Clinical exam shows **incompatibility** between symptoms and recognized medical conditions, and patients show less than expected concern about their neurologic symptoms

A 35-year-old married woman with 3 children was taken to the doctor's office after daily complaints of dizziness, nausea, and headaches for the last 6 months. She is intensely bothered by her symptoms to the point that she now stays home and avoids both going to work and caring for her children. She has been tried on numerous medications, but none has proven to be beneficial. A neurological examination finds some abnormalities. Which of the following would be most indicated in this patient?

a. Lorazepam
b. Sertraline
c. Individual psychotherapy
d. Lithium
e. Risperidone

Answer: **C.** This patient has somatic symptom disorder, which is treated with individual psychotherapy given that psychological issues are the cause of her symptoms. She should have one primary caretaker and not be sent to specialists. Lorazepam, a benzodiazepine, treats anxiety disorder. SSRIs such as sertraline treat fibromyalgia and depression. Lithium treats bipolar disorder. Risperidone is for psychosis.

Factitious Disorder

In factitious disorder, an individual falsifies symptoms in order to get attention and emotional support in the patient role. This can be either a psychological or physical illness. Psychological symptoms include hallucinations, delusions, depression, and bizarre behavior. Physical symptoms include abdominal pain, fever, nausea, vomiting, or hematomas. At times, these individuals may inflict life-threatening injuries on themselves in order to get attention. This behavior may be compulsive at times.

> Factitious disorder is motivated **unconsciously.**
>
> Malingering is motivated **consciously.**

There are 2 principal diagnoses:

- When a caretaker fakes signs and symptoms in another person (usually a child or elderly dependent) in order to assume the sick role, the diagnosis is **factitious disorder imposed on others**.
- When signs and symptoms are faked in oneself, the diagnosis is **factitious disorder imposed on self**.

Diagnosis

Typically, patients with this disorder are women who may have a history of being employed in healthcare. Men more often have physical symptoms. The patient's ultimate goal is to gain admission to the hospital. You must always exclude any medical disorder with similar symptoms.

Treatment

No specific therapy has been proven to be effective in these patients. When a child is involved in factitious disorder imposed on others, child protective services should be contacted to ensure the child's safety.

Malingering

Malingering is characterized by the conscious production of signs and symptoms for a secondary gain, such as avoiding work, evading criminal prosecution, or achieving financial gain. Malingering is not a mental illness.

Malingering is typically diagnosed when there is a discrepancy between the patient's complaints and the actual physical or laboratory findings.

Adjustment Disorder

Adjustment disorder is characterized by a maladaptive reaction to an identifiable stressor, such as loss of job, divorce, or failure in school. The symptoms usually occur within 3 months of the stressor and must remit within 6 months of removal of the stressor. The symptoms include anxiety, depression, or disturbances of conduct. They are severe enough to cause impairment in functioning.

Psychotherapy is the treatment of choice. Both individual and group therapy have been used effectively.

Personality Disorders

This is a group of disorders characterized by personality patterns that are pervasive, inflexible, and maladaptive. Personality disorders are ego-syntonic, lifelong, and difficult to treat.

Factitious disorder cannot be diagnosed without first confirming that a legitimate medical illness is not present.

A lack of cooperation from patients is characteristic of malingering.

Personality disorders are ego-syntonic, meaning that patients are not distressed by them.

Types of Personality Disorder	
Type	**Definition/Diagnostic criteria**
Paranoid	**Suspicious, mistrustful**, secretive, isolated, and questioning of the loyalty of family and friends
Schizoid	Choice of **solitary activities**, lack of close friends, **emotional coldness**, no desire for or enjoyment of close relationships
Schizotypal	Ideas of reference, **magical thinking**, odd thinking, eccentric behavior, increased social anxiety, **brief psychotic episodes**
Histrionic	**Must be the center of attention**, inappropriate sexual behavior, self-dramatization, use physical appearance to draw attention to self
Antisocial	**Failure to conform to social rules**, deceitful, devoid of remorse, impulsive, **aggressive toward others**, irresponsible, must be age >18
Borderline	Unstable relationships, impulsive, recurrent suicidal behaviors, **chronic feelings of emptiness**, **inappropriate anger**, dissociative symptoms when severely stressed, brief psychotic episodes
Narcissistic	**Grandiose sense of self**, belief that they are uniquely special, lack empathy, sense of entitlement, require excessive admiration
Avoidant	**Unwilling to get involved with people**, views self as socially inept, reluctant to take risks, **feelings of inadequacy**
Dependent	Difficulty making day-to-day decisions, **unable to assume responsibility**, unable to express disagreement, fear of being alone, seeks relationship as source of care
Obsessive compulsive personality disorder (OCPD)	**Preoccupied with details**, orderly, perfectionistic, excessively devoted to work; no obsessions or compulsions seen, in contrast to obsessive-compulsive disorder (OCD)

Schizoid patients lack desire for close friendships. Avoidant patients desire intimacy but avoid it.

Patients with borderline personality disorder display self-injurious behavior and are at increased risk for **suicide**.

Treatment

- Individual psychotherapy
- Medications if mood or anxiety symptoms are present

Which of the following personality disorders has been associated with positive psychotic symptoms?

a. Borderline
b. Histrionic
c. Schizoid
d. Paranoid
e. Antisocial

Answer: **A.** Borderline and schizotypal personality disorders may have short-lived psychotic episodes that are brief and usually occur after stressful situations.

Eating Disorders

Anorexia Nervosa

Anorexia is characterized by failure to maintain a normal body weight, fear of and preoccupation with gaining weight, and body image disturbance. There is an unrealistic self-evaluation as overweight. These patients tend to deny their emaciated condition. They show great concern with appearance and frequently examine and weigh themselves. They typically lose weight by maintaining strict caloric control, excessive exercise, purging, and fasting, with laxative and diuretic abuse. Amenorrhea is often present but not required for diagnosis.

Diagnosis

> Patients with a **maternal history** of anorexia are 50% more likely to develop anorexia.

Anorexia is seen more frequently in teenage girls age 14–18. There is evidence of severe weight loss. Hypotension, bradycardia, lanugo hair, and edema may be present. EKG changes such as rhythm disorders occur as a result of potassium deficiency. Arrhythmia is the most common cause of death.

Treatment

- Hospitalization to prevent dehydration, starvation, electrolyte imbalances, and death
- Psychotherapy
- Behavioral therapy
- SSRIs have been used to promote weight gain.

Bulimia Nervosa

Bulimia is characterized by frequent binge eating, as evidenced by eating large amounts of food in a discrete amount of time, as well as a lack of control of overeating episodes. This is accompanied by a compensatory behavior to prevent weight gain in the form of purging, misuse of laxatives and diuretics, fasting, and excessive exercise. The patient's self-evaluation is unduly influenced by body shape and weight.

Diagnosis

Bulimia is seen more frequently in women and occurs later in adolescence than anorexia nervosa. Most of these women are of normal weight but do have a history of obesity.

Treatment

- Does not require hospitalization unless severe electrolyte abnormality is present
- Psychotherapy
- SSRIs

Binge Eating Disorder

The essential feature of binge eating disorder is recurrent episodes of binge eating that occur ≥3 times per week for >3 months. Patients are overweight, and they usually lack a sense of control over their eating habits. The binge eating episodes are associated with eating faster than usual, eating until feeling uncomfortably full, eating large amounts of food in the absence of hunger, eating alone, and feeling disgusted with oneself after the eating episode.

Treatment

- Topiramate has been proven efficacious for binge eating disorder. SSRIs may have limited benefits.
- Lisdexamfetamine dimesylate is FDA-approved for the treatment of binge eating disorder.
- Psychotherapy is indicated, including cognitive behavioral therapy, interpersonal psychotherapy, and dialectic behavioral therapy.

Sleep Disorders

Narcolepsy

Characterized by excessive daytime sleepiness and abnormalities of REM sleep, narcolepsy most frequently begins in young adulthood. Sleep studies are usually indicated in the diagnosis.

No therapy has been found to be curative. The patient is managed with forced naps during the day. Modafinil is a medication used to maintain alertness. Therapy can also include methylphenidate and dextroamphetamine. Gamma-hydroxybutyrate (GHB) may be given at bedtime to induce symptoms of narcolepsy and contain them at night.

> Nightmares: REM sleep
>
> Sleep terrors, somnambulism (sleepwalking): stages 3 and 4

> Loss of **hypocretin** results in inability to regulate sleep.

Psychiatric and Physical Symptoms of Narcolepsy (Sleep Disorder)	
Specific feature of narcolepsy	**Characteristics of sleep disorders**
Sleep attacks	Episodes of **irresistible sleepiness** and feeling **refreshed upon awakening**
Cataplexy	**Sudden loss of muscle tone**: considered pathognomonic and may be precipitated by loud noise or emotions
Hypnagogic and hypnopompic hallucinations	**Hallucinations** that occur as the patient is **going to sleep and waking up**
Sleep paralysis	**Patient awake but unable to move**; this typically occurs upon awakening

Insomnia

> There is a 30% decrease in **GABA** in insomnia.

Insomnia is a disorder characterized by the inability to initiate or maintain sleep. Insomnia may be due to anxiety and depression. It is severe enough to adversely affect level of functioning. It is typically seen in women who complain of feeling tired or have increased appetite and yawning.

Treatment consists of sleep hygiene techniques such as going to bed and waking up at the same time, avoiding caffeinated beverages, and avoiding daytime naps. Behavioral modification techniques include using the bed only for sleeping and not for reading, watching TV, or eating. Medical therapy consists of zolpidem, eszopiclone, zaleplon, or ramelteon.

Human Sexuality

Terminology of Human Sexuality	
Sexual characteristic	**Definition**
Sexual identity	Based on a person's secondary sexual characteristics
Gender identity	Based on a person's sense of maleness or femaleness, established by the age of 3
Gender role	Based on external patterns of behavior that reflect inner sense of gender identity
Sexual orientation	Based on person's romantic or sexual attraction

Sexual Dysfunction

> Erectile disorder:
> - Most often **psychological** in etiology
> - 50% more likely in **smokers**

Types of Sexual Dysfunction		
Disorder	**Definition**	**Treatment**
Erectile disorder	Persistent or recurrent inability to attain or maintain an erection until completion of the sexual act	Rule out medical causes or medication, psychotherapy, couples sexual therapy, PDE5 medications
Premature ejaculation	Ejaculation before penetration or just after penetration, usually due to anxiety	Psychotherapy, behavioral modification techniques (stop and go, squeeze), SSRI medication
Genitopelvic pain disorder (formerly dyspareunia)	Pain associated with sexual intercourse, not diagnosed if due to medical condition	Psychotherapy
Penetration disorder (formerly vaginismus)	Involuntary constriction of the outer third of the vagina preventing penile insertion	Psychotherapy, dilator therapy

Paraphilic Disorders (Formerly Paraphilias)

Paraphilias are a group of disorders that are recurrent, sexually arousing, and seen more frequently in men. They usually focus on humiliation, nonconsenting partners, or use of nonliving objects. Must occur for >6 months and both cause distress and adversely affect level of functioning. Do not diagnose if done in experimentation.

Pedophilia is the most common paraphilia.

Types of Paraphilias	
Type of paraphilia	**Definition**
Exhibitionism	Recurrent urge to expose oneself to strangers
Fetishism	Recurrent use of nonliving objects to achieve sexual pleasure
Pedophilia	Recurrent urges or arousal toward prepubescent children
Masochism	Recurrent urge or behavior involving the act of humiliation
Sadism	Recurrent urge or behavior involving acts in which physical or psychological suffering of victim is exciting
Transvestic fetishism	Recurrent urge or behavior involving cross dressing for sexual gratification; usually found in heterosexual males
Frotteurism	Rubbing, usually one's pelvis or erect penis, against a nonconsenting person for sexual gratification

Treatment

- Individual psychotherapy
- Behavioral modification techniques such as aversive conditioning
- Antiandrogens or SSRIs to reduce sexual drive

Gender Dysphoria

This is a condition characterized by the persistent discomfort and sense of inappropriateness regarding the patient's assigned sex.

Gender dysphoria will manifest by wearing the opposite gender's clothes, using toys typically associated with the opposite sex, playing with opposite-sex children when young, and feeling unhappy about one's own sexual assignment. Older individuals with gender dysphoria may take hormones to deepen the voice, if female, or soften the voice, if male. Women may bind their breasts and men may hide their penis and testicles. Gender dysphoria is seen more frequently in young men.

Treatment

Treatment is either psychotherapy or steps to support the individual's preferred gender through hormone therapy, gender expression and role, or surgery.

Suicide

Suicide (especially violent suicide) is associated with a decreased level of serotonin. Patients with a psychiatric history are at 34 times greater risk of committing suicide. Protective factors include connection to family, pregnancy, responsibility for children, and religious affiliation.

Firearms are the most common method used by *both* men and women to commit suicide. Therefore, be sure to ask about access to guns. Pills/poison is the most common method for women to use to attempt suicide.

> **Native Americans** are the ethnic group with the highest suicide rate.

Presentation

- Recent suicide attempt
- Complaints of suicidal thoughts
- Demonstration of suicidal behaviors (e.g., buying weapons, giving away possessions, or writing a will)

Risk Factors

> Ask about ideation, intent, and plan.

- Men
- Older adults
- Social isolation
- Presence of psychiatric illness or substance use
- Chronic pain or chronic medical illness
- Perceived hopelessness
- Previous attempts—the **#1 risk factor**

Treatment

- Hospitalize patient
- Take all threats seriously
- Treat comorbid disorders (e.g., mood disorder, psychosis)

PART 13

Emergency Medicine

Toxicology/Poisoning/Overdose

Initial Management of Poisoning

A 32-year-old woman with a history of depression comes to the ED 30 minutes after taking a bottle of pills in an attempt to commit suicide. Blood pressure is 118/70 mm Hg, pulse 90/min, and respirations are normal at 14/min. She refuses to tell you what she took. What is the most appropriate next step in management?

a. Induce emesis with ipecac
b. Gastric lavage
c. Psychiatric consultation
d. Serum chemistry
e. Urine toxicology screen
f. Cathartics/laxatives
g. Whole bowel irrigation
h. Naloxone
i. Flumazenil

Answer: B. When ingestion is extremely recent, it is possible that the substance can be removed from the body prior to its absorption. Gastric emptying has very limited value because there is not much time between the ingestion and passage of the pills beyond the pyloric sphincter from where they cannot be removed. Pills, on an empty stomach, can leave in as little as 30–60 minutes. Gastric lavage can be attempted ≤2 hours after ingestion, but it will remove only 50% of pills at 1 hour and 15% at 2 hours. After 2 hours, it is useless. Although serum chemistry and urine toxicology screen should be done, they are not helpful this soon after ingestion. Ipecac for the induction of vomiting is wrong when a patient is already in the emergency department. Inducing vomiting needs 15–20 minutes to work, and only delays the administration of antidotes such as N-acetylcysteine, which can be given orally.

Gastrointestinal Emptying

Gastric lavage may occasionally be useful in the first hour of ingestion. It is dangerous in:

- Altered mental status: may cause aspiration
- Caustic ingestion: causes burning of the esophagus and oropharynx

---

- Gastric lavage is rarely done: It removes 50% of pills at 1 hour, and removes 15% of pills at 2 hours.
- Ipecac is always a wrong answer in the ED.
- Cathartic agents such as sorbitol are always a wrong answer.

Ipecac

Although ipecac has been used as a home remedy in those with accidental overdose or pill ingestion prior to coming to the hospital, there is no benefit in using ipecac in the hospital. Ipecac needs 15–20 minutes to work and delays the administration of antidotes.

Cathartics

Cathartic agents such as sorbitol are always a wrong answer. Speeding up GI transit time does not eliminate the ingestion without absorption.

Forced Diuresis

Giving fluids and diuretics to accelerate urinary excretion is always a wrong answer. More patients are harmed with pulmonary edema with this method than are helped.

Whole Bowel Irrigation

Placing a gastric tube and flushing out the GI tract with polyethylene glycol-electrolyte solution (GoLYTELY) is almost always wrong. Indications for this method are very narrow and limited to massive iron ingestion, lithium, and swallowing drug-filled packets (e.g., smuggling).

Gastric emptying of any kind is **always the wrong answer** with:

- **Caustics** (acids and alkali)
- **Altered mental status**
- **Acetaminophen overdose**

► **TIP**

When the answer is not clear and the cause of overdose is asked, say:

- Acetaminophen
- Aspirin

They are, by far, the most common cause of death by overdose.

► **TIP**

What to do is often unclear. What is useless or dangerous (ipecac, forced diuresis, cathartics) is very clear.

> A woman comes to the ED one hour after taking a bottle of pills. Blood pressure is 118/70 mm Hg, pulse 90/min, and respirations 14/min. She is confused, disoriented, and lethargic. What is the most appropriate next step in management?
>
> a. Flumazenil
> b. Gastric lavage
> c. Psychiatric consultation
> d. Naloxone and dextrose
> e. Intubation
>
> Answer: **D.** The best initial management of altered mental status of unclear etiology is an opiate antagonist and glucose. Opiate ingestion and diabetes are extremely common. Naloxone and glucose work instantaneously and have no adverse effects. If they do not work, perform intubation to protect the airway, possibly followed by gastric lavage. Intubation should not be done first. Naloxone is faster and emergency intubation is associated with aspiration, trauma to teeth, and the possibility of intubating the esophagus. Flumazenil reverses benzodiazepines but can cause seizures from instant withdrawal.

► **TIP**

Psychiatric consultation is indicated when the overdose is from a suicide attempt but is a wrong answer on USMLE Step 2 CK when specific antidotes and diagnostic tests are needed. You do not need a consultant to tell you to give naloxone and dextrose.

- **Opiate** overdose is **fatal.** Give naloxone immediately.
- **Benzodiazepine** overdose by itself is **not fatal** and acute withdrawal causes seizures. *Do not give* flumazenil.

Charcoal

Charcoal is benign and should be given to anyone with a pill overdose. Charcoal may not be effective for every overdose, but it is not dangerous in anyone. Charcoal can also remove toxic substances even after they have been absorbed. Blood levels of toxins drop faster in those given repeated doses of charcoal. Charcoal is superior to lavage and ipecac.

► **TIP**

When you don't know what to do in toxicology, give charcoal.

Acetaminophen

Legal drugs kill more people in the United States than illegal drugs because they are less expensive and more available. Acetaminophen ingestion causes toxicity at >8–10 grams and fatality at >12–15 grams.

Alcoholism decreases the amount of acetaminophen needed to cause toxicity.

The Four Most Common Acetaminophen Overdose Questions

1. If a clearly toxic amount of acetaminophen has been ingested (more than 8–10 grams), the answer is N-acetylcysteine.

2. If the overdose was >24 hours ago, there is no therapy.

3. If the amount of ingestion is unclear, get a drug level.

4. Charcoal does not make N-acetylcysteine ineffective. Charcoal is not contraindicated with N-acetylcysteine.

Aspirin Overdose

The most common question is "What is the most likely diagnosis?" Look for:

- Tinnitus and hyperventilation
- Respiratory alkalosis progressing to metabolic acidosis
- Renal toxicity and altered mental status
- Increased anion gap

Aspirin causes diffuse, multisystem toxicity. It causes ARDS. It interferes with prothrombin production and raises the prothrombin time (PT). The metabolic acidosis is from lactate. Aspirin interferes with oxidative phosphorylation and results in anaerobic glucose metabolism, which produces lactate.

Tinnitus, respiratory alkalosis, and metabolic acidosis are the key to diagnosing aspirin overdose.

Treatment is alkalinizing the urine, which increases the rate of aspirin excretion.

► **TIP**

Know the blood gas in aspirin overdose.

Which of the following is most likely to be found in aspirin overdose? (Normal values: pH 7.40 pCO_2 40 HCO_3^- 24)

a. pH 7.55 pCO_2 50 HCO_3^- 24
b. pH 7.25 pCO_2 62 HCO_3 38
c. pH 7.46 pCO_2 22 HCO_3 16
d. pH 7.35 pCO_2 32 HCO_3 20

Answer: **C.** The blood gas shows a respiratory alkalosis with a low pCO_2 and a metabolic acidosis with decreased bicarbonate. Because the pH is alkalotic, we know that the respiratory alkalosis is not simply compensation for a metabolic acidosis. If it were respiratory compensation, the pH would be <7.4 as in choice (D). Choice (D) is a primary metabolic acidosis with respiratory alkalosis as compensation as would occur in sepsis, DKA, or uremia. Choice (B) shows an increased pCO_2 and an elevated bicarbonate. This represents a primary respiratory acidosis with bicarbonate retention at the kidney as compensation. This is characteristic of COPD.

A patient with depression presents with altered mental status from ingesting multiple toxic substances. You know for certain that he took some lorazepam today, for the first time. There is no response to naloxone or dextrose. The patient is given flumazenil and immediately seizes. What is the most likely cause of the seizure?

a. Cocaine withdrawal
b. Opiate withdrawal
c. Tricyclic antidepressants
d. SSRIs
e. Aspirin

Answer: **C.** Although flumazenil can cause seizures from reversing chronic benzodiazepine dependence, this case quite specifically states the benzodiazepine ingestion was today only. Benzodiazepines, however, can prevent seizures from tricyclic toxicity. When you reverse the benzodiazepines, you remove the suppression of the tricyclic toxicity. Opiate withdrawal does not cause seizures. Cocaine toxicity causes seizures, not withdrawal. Coingestion of tricyclics and benzodiazepines is very common.

What is the best initial test for the patient previously described?

a. Urine toxicology
b. Electroencephalogram
c. EKG
d. Head CT
e. Potassium level

Answer: **C.** Tricyclic antidepressant toxicity is rapidly detectable on EKG. The EKG will show widening of the QRS complex.

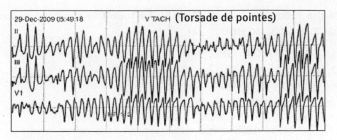

Figure 13.1 Tricyclic antidepressant toxicity prolongs the QT until torsade develops, causing amplitude to undulate as if it were "twisting around a point." *Source: Pablo Lam, MD, and Eduardo Andre, MD*

Tricyclic Antidepressants

Tricyclic antidepressant (TCA) toxicity can cause seizures and arrhythmia leading to death. A wide QRS will tell who is about to have an arrhythmia.

TCA toxicity causes signs of anticholinergic effects, i.e., dry mouth, constipation, and urinary retention. None of these effects causes death.

Treatment of TCA overdose is sodium bicarbonate. Bicarbonate will protect the heart against arrhythmia.

The bicarbonate does not increase urinary excretion of TCAs in the way it does for aspirin.

Caustics

> Steroids do not prevent injury from caustics.

Caustic ingestion of acids and alkalis (e.g., drain cleaner) causes mechanical damage to the oropharynx, esophagus, and stomach including perforation. Do not give alkali to reverse acids, or give acids to reverse alkali. This would cause the release of heat from an exothermic reaction and would only make it worse. Flush out the caustics. Use water in high volumes. Endoscopy is performed to assess the degree of damage.

Carbon Monoxide Poisoning

> The left ventricle cannot distinguish between anemia, carboxyhemoglobin, and a stenosis of the coronary arteries.

Carbon monoxide (CO) poisoning is the most common cause of death in fires (60% of deaths on the first day after a fire). Also look for a history of:

- Gas heaters or wood-burning stoves
- Automobile exhaust, particularly in an enclosed environment

CO binds oxygen to hemoglobin so tightly that carboxyhemoglobin will not release oxygen to tissues. Carboxyhemoglobin acts functionally like anemia. There is no functional difference between the absence of blood and carboxyhemoglobin; 60% carboxyhemoglobin acts like the loss of 60% of blood. CO poisoning presents with dyspnea, lightheadedness, confusion, seizures, and ultimately death from a myocardial infarction.

Which of the following blood gas results would you find in carbon monoxide poisoning?

a. pH 7.55 pCO_2 50 HCO_3^- 24
b. pH 7.25 pCO_2 62 HCO_3 38
c. pH 7.46 pCO_2 22 HCO_3 16
d. pH 7.35 pCO_2 26 HCO_3 18

Answer: D. Carbon monoxide poisoning prevents oxygen release to tissues, so lactic acidosis develops.

> Carbon monoxide poisoning gives a normal pO_2 because oxygen does not detach from hemoglobin.

Diagnostic Tests/Treatment

Since routine oximetry will be falsely normal, the most accurate test is a level of carboxyhemoglobin. You should expect to find a low bicarbonate and low pH (metabolic acidosis) when carbon monoxide levels are very high.

The best initial therapy is to remove the patient from exposure and give 100% oxygen, which detaches carbon monoxide from hemoglobin and shortens the half-life of carboxyhemoglobin. Severe disease is treated with hyperbaric oxygen. Hyperbaric oxygen shortens the half-life of carboxyhemoglobin even more than 100% oxygen. "Severe" symptoms are defined as:

- CNS symptoms
- Cardiac symptoms
- Metabolic acidosis

Whenever any of these are in the question, the answer is hyperbaric oxygen.

Methemoglobinemia

Methemoglobin is oxidized hemoglobin that is locked into the ferric state. Oxidized hemoglobin is brown and will not carry oxygen. Methemoglobinemia occurs from an idiosyncratic reaction of hemoglobin to certain drugs such as:

- Benzocaine and other anesthetics
- Nitrites and nitroglycerin
- Dapsone

The effects of methemoglobinemia are similar to carboxyhemoglobin. Oxygen is not delivered to tissues. In methemoglobinemia, hemoglobin will never pick up the oxygen. With carboxyhemoglobin, the oxygen is picked up, but will not release it to tissues. Severe symptoms appear when blood levels rise above 40%–50%. There is no functional difference for end organs such as the brain and heart. The symptoms are the same and include:

- Dyspnea and cyanosis
- Headache, confusion, and seizures
- Metabolic acidosis

> **Carbon monoxide:** Blood is abnormally **red**.
> **Methemoglobinemia:** Blood is abnormally **brown**.

Diagnostic testing includes methemoglobin level (**most accurate test**). Both methemoglobinemia and carboxyhemoglobin can give a normal pO2 on blood gas. At the same time, there is no delivery of oxygen to tissues.

Treatment is 100% oxygen (**best initial therapy**) and methylene blue (**most effective therapy**), which decreases the half-life of methemoglobin.

▶ **TIP**

Cyanosis + normal pO_2 = methemoglobinemia

Organophosphate (Insecticide) Poisoning and Nerve Gas

> Acetylcholine causes constriction of bronchi and an increase in bronchial secretions.

> Nerve gas and organophosphates are absorbed through the skin.

Organophosphates and nerve gas are identical in their effects. Nerve gas is faster and more severe. It causes a massive increase in the level of acetylcholine by inhibiting its metabolism. Patients present with:

- Salivation
- Lacrimation
- Polyuria
- Diarrhea
- Bronchospasm, bronchorrhea, and respiratory arrest if severe

A 56-year-old military commander has been attacked with nerve gas. She presents with salivation, lacrimation, urination, defecation, and shortness of breath. Her pupils are constricted. What is the first step in management?

a. Atropine
b. Decontaminate (wash) the patient
c. Remove the patient's clothing
d. Pralidoxime
e. No therapy is effective

Answer: **A.** Atropine blocks the effects of acetylcholine that is already increased in the body. Atropine dries up respiratory secretion. Although removing clothes and washing the patient to prevent further absorption is good, this will do nothing for symptoms that are already occurring. Pralidoxime is the specific antidote for organophosphates. Pralidoxime reactivates acetylcholinesterase. It does not work as instantaneously as atropine.

Digoxin Toxicity

> Hypokalemia → digoxin toxicity
>
> Digoxin toxicity → hyperkalemia

Hypokalemia predisposes to digoxin toxicity because potassium and digoxin compete for binding at the same site on the sodium/potassium ATPase. When less potassium is bound, more digoxin is bound.

Symptoms include:

- GI disturbance (**most common**), i.e., nausea/vomiting and abdominal pain
- Hyperkalemia
- Inhibition of the sodium/potassium ATPase
- Confusion
- Visual disturbance such as yellow halos around objects
- Rhythm disturbance (bradycardia, atrial tachycardia, AV block, ventricular ectopy, and arrhythmias such as atrial fibrillation with a slow rate)

Diagnostic testing includes:

The most accurate test is a digoxin level. The best initial tests are a potassium level and an EKG. The EKG will show a downsloping of the ST segment in all leads. Atrial tachycardia with variable AV block is the most common digoxin toxic arrhythmia.

Treatment is control of the potassium and digoxin-specific antibodies, which will rapidly remove digoxin from circulation.

> Digoxin can produce **any** arrhythmia.

> The strongest indications for digoxin-binding antibodies are CNS and cardiac involvement.

Lead Poisoning

Lead is diffusely toxic throughout many organs in the body. Patients present with:

- Abdominal pain (lead colic)
- Renal tubule toxicity (ATN)
- Anemia (sideroblastic)
- Peripheral neuropathies such as wrist drop
- CNS abnormalities such as memory loss and confusion

The most accurate test is a lead level. Lead interferes with hemoglobin production. This gives anemia. There is an increased level of free erythrocyte protoporphyrin.

▶ TIP

The **most accurate test** for sideroblastic anemia is a Prussian blue stain. This detects increased iron built up in red blood cell mitochondria.

Treatment

Chelating agents remove lead from the body. Succimer is the only oral form of lead chelator. Ethylenediaminetetraacetic acid (EDTA) and dimercaprol (BAL) are parenteral agents that bind and remove lead from the body.

Mercury Poisoning

Orally ingested mercury causes neurological problems. Inhaled mercury vapor produces lung toxicity that presents as interstitial fibrosis. Neurological problems present with patients who are nervous, jittery, twitchy, and sometimes hallucinatory.

There is no therapy to reverse the pulmonary toxicity. Chelating agents can remove mercury from the body. Chelating agents such as dimercaprol and succimer are effective in removing mercury from the body and decreasing neurological toxicity. This can prevent progression of pulmonary disease but cannot reverse fibrosis.

Toxic Alcohols: Methanol and Ethylene Glycol

Both methanol and ethylene glycol produce intoxication and metabolic acidosis with an increased anion gap. Both give an osmolar gap and are treated with fomepizole and dialysis.

Differences between Methanol and Ethylene Glycol		
	Methanol	**Ethylene glycol**
Source	Wood alcohol, cleaning solutions, paint thinner	Antifreeze
Toxic metabolite	Formic acid/formaldehyde	Oxalic acid/oxalate
Presentation	Ocular toxicity	Renal toxicity
Initial diagnostic abnormality	Retinal inflammation	Hypocalcemia, envelope-shaped oxalate crystals in urine

Osmolar Gap

The osmolar gap is the difference between the **measured** serum osmolality and the **calculated** osmolality.

$$\text{Serum osmolality} = 2 \text{ times the sodium} + \text{BUN}/2.8 + \text{glucose}/18$$

If you calculate the serum osmolality to be 300, but on measurement you find the osmolality to be 350, it is possible that a toxic alcohol such as methanol or ethylene glycol is accounting for the extra osmoles. Ordinary alcohol (ethanol) also increases the osmolar gap.

Treatment is fomepizole (**best initial therapy**), which inhibits alcohol dehydrogenase and prevents the production of the toxic metabolite. Fomepizole does not remove the substance from the body. Only dialysis (**most effective therapy**) will effectively remove methanol and ethylene glycol from the body.

Snake Bites

The most common injury from snake bites is the local wound. Although 1/3 of bites are not deep enough to deliver venom to the bloodstream, they do deposit venom into the tissues. Proteases and lipases in the venom damage tissue locally.

Death from snake bites is from:

- **Hemolytic toxin**: hemolysis, DIC, damage to the endothelial lining of tissues
- **Neurotoxin**: respiratory paralysis, ptosis, dysphagia, diplopia

Treatment of Snake Bites	
Ineffective or dangerous treatment	**Beneficial therapy**
Tourniquets blocking arterial flow	Pressure
Ice	Immobilization decreases movement of venom
Incision and suction, especially by mouth	Antivenin

Spider Bites

All spider bites present with a sudden, sharp pain that the patient may describe as "I stepped on a nail" or "A piece of glass was in my shoe."

Types of Spider Bites		
	Black widow	**Brown recluse**
Presentation	Abdominal pain, muscle pain	Local skin necrosis, bullae, and blebs
Lab test abnormalities	Hypocalcemia	None
Treatment	Calcium, antivenin	Debridement

Dog, Cat, and Human Bites

Management of dog, cat, and human bites is essentially identical. They are managed with:

- Amoxicillin/clavulanate
- Tetanus vaccination booster if more than 5 years since last injection (Tdap)

Dog and Cats: *Pasteurella multocida*

Humans: *Eikenella corrodens*

> **Human bites** are **more damaging** than dog and cat bites.

> **Rabies vaccine only if:**
> - Animal has **altered mental status**/bizarre behavior.
> - Attack was unprovoked, by a **stray dog** that cannot be observed or diagnosed.

Cannabinoid Hyperemesis Syndrome

The question will describe a patient with recurrent episodes of nausea, vomiting, and crampy abdominal pain. Besides the history of marijuana or cannabinoid use, look for improvement in symptoms with a hot shower or bath.

Treatment is antiemetics (such as ondansetron) or benzodiazepines (such as lorazepam).

> Hot shower "better" = cannabinoid

Head Trauma

Any head trauma resulting in sufficient injury to cause altered mental status or LOC is managed first with a head CT. It does not matter how minor the trauma is if it results in LOC.

Head CT without contrast is the **best initial test to detect blood**. Head CT with contrast detects mass lesions, e.g., cancer and abscess, but not blood.

- **Concussion**: no focal neurological abnormalities. CT will be normal.
- **Contusion**: occasionally (rarely) has focal findings. CT will show ecchymoses (blood mixed in with brain parenchyma).
- **Subdural and epidural hematoma**: usually associated with more severe trauma than a concussion. Impossible to distinguish without a head CT, even though epidural hematoma is more frequently associated with skull fracture.
  - Patients with subdural and epidural hematoma often have lucid intervals, a period of normal consciousness in between two LOCs.
  - The patient wakes up after the initial LOC, but loses consciousness a second time due to the accumulation of blood—several minutes or hours after the initial loss.

▶**TIP**

LOC means do a CT.

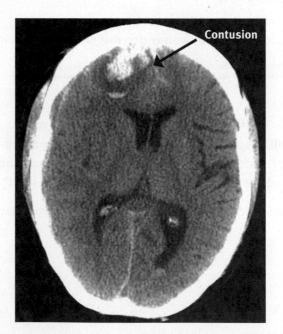

Figure 13.2 Blood Mixed in with Brain but Not Collected in a Way That Allows Drainage. *Source: Saba Ansari, MD*

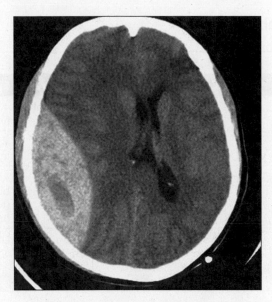

Figure 13.3 Lenticular Hemorrhage from
Higher Pressure Artery. *Source: Saba Ansari, MD*

Treatment is as follows:

- **Concussion**: no specific treatment
  - Those with concussion are safe to go home. Hospitalization is not necessary.
  - Observe at home for altered mental status.
  - Wait at least 24 hours before returning to sports.
- **Contusion**: no specific treatment for vast majority; rarely, surgical debridement needed
- **Subdural and epidural hematoma**: treatment based on size and signs of compression of the brain, i.e., small ones are left alone, and large ones are managed with intubation and hyperventilation, mannitol, and drainage.
  - Hyperventilation works by decreasing pCO_2. Normally, cerebral circulation constricts when the pCO_2 is low. A small decrease in volume results in a large decrease in pressure.
  - Mannitol, an osmotic diuretic, decreases intravascular volume, which decreases intracranial pressure (limited benefit only).

Large Intracranial Hemorrhage

- Compression of ventricles or sulci
- Herniation with abnormal breathing and unilateral dilation of the pupil
- Worsening mental status or focal findings

> Hyperventilation **briefly** slows herniation and is **a bridge to surgery.**

Types of Cerebral Injury

Severe Head Trauma			
Concussion	**Contusion**	**Subdural**	**Epidural**
No focal finding	Rarely focal	+/− focal findings	+/− focal findings
No lucid interval	No lucid interval	+/− lucid interval	+/− lucid interval
Normal CT	Ecchymoses	Venous, crescent	Arterial, biconvex (lens-shaped) hematoma
No specific treatment; observe at home for lucid interval or new focal findings	No specific treatment; observe in hospital	Drain large ones	Drain large ones

A 25-year-old man sustains head trauma in a car accident. A large epidural hematoma is found. Immediately after intubation and mannitol, surgical evacuation is successfully performed. Which of the following will most likely benefit the patient?

a. Repeated doses of mannitol
b. Continued hyperventilation
c. Proton pump inhibitor (PPI)
d. Nimodipine
e. Dexamethasone

Answer: **C.** A PPI is given to prevent stress ulcers. The only clear indications for stress ulcer prophylaxis are head trauma, burns, endotracheal intubation, and coagulopathy (platelets <50,000 or INR >1.5) with respiratory failure. Hyperventilation has very short-term efficacy and is probably ineffective after 24 hours. Nimodipine prevents stroke after subarachnoid hemorrhage. Dexamethasone, a potent glucocorticoid, is ineffective for intracranial hemorrhage.

> Steroids do not benefit intracranial bleeding. They decrease edema around mass lesions.

Burns

For those caught in a fire, the **best initial therapy** is 100% oxygen to treat smoke inhalation and carbon monoxide poisoning.

- **If airway burn is present**: intubate if there is stridor, hoarseness, wheezing, or burns inside the nasopharynx or mouth.
- **If airway burn is not present**: replace fluid, based on the percentage of body surface area (BSA) burned. Fluid volume loss is a leading cause of death from burns.
  - Ringer lactate (if not one of the choices on the USMLE exam, choose normal saline): 1/2 in first 8 hours, 1/4 in second 8 hours, and 1/4 in third 8 hours

– Give 4 mL for each percentage of BSA burned (including second and third degree burns) for each kilogram of body weight

- Head: 9% BSA
- Arms: 9% BSA each
- Legs: 18% BSA each
- Chest or abdomen: 9% BSA each
- Back: 18% BSA
- Hands: 1% BSA each (patchy burns that are not continuous make the percentage of BSA burned hard to assess; use the width of patient's hand to estimate)

What is the most common cause of death several days to weeks after a burn?

a. Infection
b. Renal failure
c. Cardiomyopathy
d. Lung injury
e. Malnutrition

Answer: A. Because of loss of skin, there is a massive loss of body fluids and albumin. Fluid loss, if fatal, will occur immediately. After several days, the loss of the protective barrier of the skin leads to infection with *Staphylococcus*. Rhabdomyolysis causes renal failure, especially combined with volume depletion decreasing renal perfusion (this is not the most common cause of death). Lung injury is an immediate cause of death.

> - Fluid replacement: (4 mL) × (%BSA burned) × weight in kg
> - On the USMLE exam, give the largest amount of Ringer lactate or normal saline listed as an answer choice. It is probably the correct answer.

> Prophylactic topical antibiotics (e.g., silver sulfadiazine) are routinely used, not IV antibiotics.

Thermoregulatory Disorders

Heat Disorders

	Heat cramps/exhaustion	Heatstroke	Neuroleptic malignant syndrome	Malignant hyperthermia
Risk	Exertion; high outside temperatures	Exertion; high outside temperatures	Antipsychotic medications	Anesthetics administered systemically
Body temp	Normal	Elevated	Elevated	Elevated
CPK and potassium level	Normal	Elevated	Elevated	Elevated
Treatment	Oral fluids and electrolytes	IV fluids; evaporation	Dantrolene or dopamine agonists: bromocriptine, cabergoline	Dantrolene

Hypothermia

Look for an intoxicated person with a low body temperature. Unintoxicated people do not fall asleep outside in cold temperatures. The most common cause of death from hypothermia is cardiac arrhythmia. The best initial step is EKG.

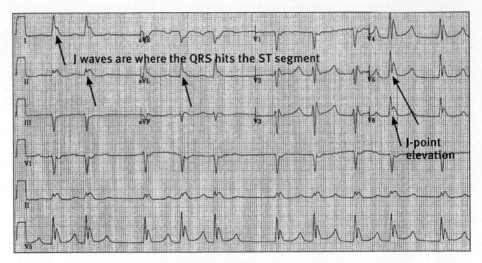

Figure 13.4 Hypothermia results in marked elevation of the J point.
This is not ST elevation or right bundle branch block. All of these abnormalities are
normalized with rewarming. *Source: Juan Hernandez, MD, and Eduardo Andre, MD*

Drowning

Manage with airway and administer positive pressure ventilation.

- Steroids and antibiotics *are not* beneficial.
- **Salt** water drowning: acts like **CHF** with wet, heavy lungs
- **Fresh** water drowning: causes **hemolysis** from absorption of hypotonic fluid into the vasculature

▶ **TIP**

Wrong answers for drowning include:

- Steroids
- Antibiotics

High Altitude Pulmonary Edema (HAPE)

> HAPE is pulmonary edema with normal ejection fraction.

Patients don't start to become short of breath until they go above 2,500 meters (8,200 feet). Slow ascent and training make HAPE unlikely under 5,000 meters. Acclimatization to altitude happens more quickly with the use of acetazolamide.

There is no specific diagnostic test. The clinical diagnosis is based on the presence of ≥2 of the following symptoms and ≥2 of the following signs:

HAPE symptoms	HAPE signs
• Dyspnea	• Crackles or wheezing
• Cough	• Cyanosis
• Weakness	• Tachypnea
• Chest tightness	• Tachycardia

Treat with oxygen, rapid descent, and steroids or nifedipine or sildenafil.

Jellyfish Stings

Patients may not see the tentacle, but they experience pain. Presentation of symptoms can be delayed by several hours. Look for inflamed red skin with burning pain. Equivocal cases are confirmed by microscopy from a sample of wounded tissue showing nematocysts.

Treat by removing nematocysts. Wash the wound with seawater to prevent nematocysts from firing. Scrape off the stingers using a piece of hard plastic, such as a credit card.

After tentacle removal, use hot water on the wound, which inactivates the toxin. Acetic acid (vinegar) may help prevent toxin release from the nematocyst of these tentacles. Topical steroids and antihistamines relieve symptoms.

Cardiac Rhythm Disorders

In any patient with potential cardiac arrest, the first step is to make sure the patient is truly unresponsive—not just sleeping or having a syncopal episode. Rescue breaths on someone who is breathing will be counterproductive, and chest compressions on someone with a pulse will be dangerous.

Once you have confirmed the person is unresponsive, call for help: 911 will alert Emergency Medical Services (EMS).

Next steps are:

1. Check pulse and start chest compressions if pulseless.
2. Open the airway: head tilt, chin lift, jaw thrust
3. Give rescue breaths if not breathing.

When is "precordial thump" the answer?

- Never.

Pulselessness

The sudden loss of a pulse can be caused by:

- Asystole
- Ventricular fibrillation (VF)
- Ventricular tachycardia (VT)
- Pulseless electrical activity (PEA)

The **best initial management** of all forms of pulselessness is CPR.

> CPR does not restart the heart; it just keeps the patient alive until cardioversion can be performed.

Asystole

Besides CPR, treatment for asystole is epinephrine, which constricts blood vessels in tissues such as the skin. This shunts blood into critical central areas like the heart and brain.

Vasopressin is not correct.

Ventricular Fibrillation

The **best initial therapy** for ventricular fibrillation (VF) is immediate, unsynchronized cardioversion, followed by the resumption of CPR if that is not effective. Unsynchronized cardioversion is synonymous with defibrillation.

Generally, all electrical cardioversions should be synchronized to the cardiac cycle, **except VF and pulseless VT**. (In VF, there is no organized electrical activity to synchronize with.)

> Amiodarone is superior to lidocaine for VF.

> Only VF and ventricular tachycardia (VT) without a pulse get unsynchronized cardioversion.

- After another attempt at defibrillation, the most appropriate next step is epinephrine, followed by another electrical shock. Medications do not restart the heart; they make the next attempt at defibrillation more likely to succeed.
- Amiodarone (preferred) or lidocaine is given next to try to get subsequent shocks to be more successful. Magnesium is given with ventricular arrhythmia without waiting for a level.
- Manage with shock, drug, shock, drug, shock, drug, and CPR at all times in between the shocks.

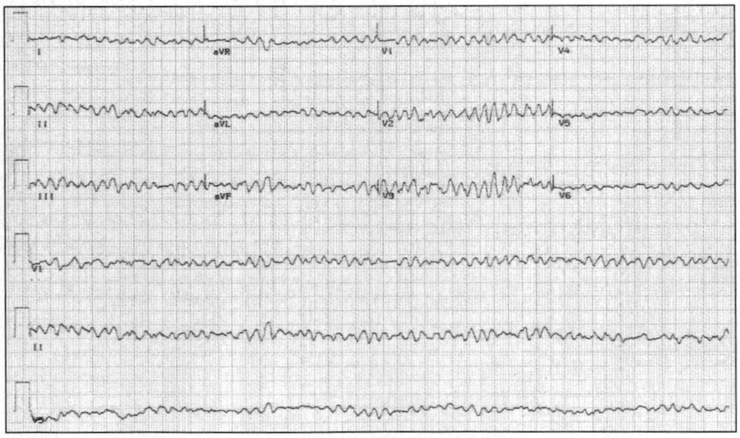

Figure 13.5 Ventricular Fibrillation with No Organized Electrical Activity.
Source: Abhay Vakil, MD

▶ **TIP**

Bretylium is always a wrong answer.

Ventricular Tachycardia

VT is a wide complex tachycardia with a regular rate. Treatment is entirely based on the hemodynamic status.

- Pulseless VT: same management as VF
- Hemodynamically stable VT: medications such as amiodarone, then lidocaine, then procainamide; if all medical therapy fails, then cardioversion
- Hemodynamically unstable VT: electrical cardioversion several times, followed by medication such as amiodarone, lidocaine, or procainamide

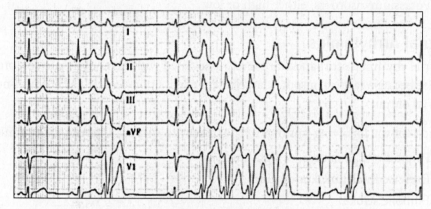

Figure 13.6 Short Run of Nonsustained Ventricular Tachycardia.
Source: Abhay Vakil, MD

Hemodynamic instability is defined as:

- Chest pain
- Dyspnea/CHF
- Hypotension
- Confusion

These qualities of instability are the same for all rhythm disturbances.

We synchronize the delivery of electricity in the cardioversion of VT to prevent worsening of the arrhythmia into ventricular fibrillation or asystole.

▶**TIP**

Direct intracardiac medication administration is always a wrong answer.

Pulseless Electrical Activity

Pulseless electrical activity (PEA) means that the heart is electrically normal but there is no motor contraction. In other causes of PEA, the heart may still be contracting but without blood inside there will be no meaningful cardiac output.

To diagnose PEA, look for a normal EKG and no pulse. Treatment is correction of the underlying cause, i.e., knowing the etiology is identical to knowing the treatment. Causes include:

- Tamponade
- Tension pneumothorax
- Hypovolemia and hypoglycemia
- Massive pulmonary embolus (PE)
- Hypoxia, hypothermia, metabolic acidosis
- Potassium disorders, either high or low

Atrial Arrhythmias

Atrial rhythm disturbances are rarely associated with hemodynamic compromise because cardiac output is largely dependent upon ventricular output—not atrial output.

Look for the following findings in the history to suggest an atrial arrhythmia:

- Palpitations, dizziness, or lightheadedness
- Exercise intolerance or dyspnea
- Embolic stroke

▶ TIP

An irregularly irregular rhythm suggests A-fib as the "most likely diagnosis," even before an EKG is done. **A-fib is the most common arrhythmia in the United States.**

Atrial Fibrillation and Atrial Flutter

A-fib and flutter are caused by anatomic abnormalities of the atria from hypertension or valvular heart disease. They have nearly identical management. The major points of difference are:

- **Flutter**: regular rhythm
- **Fibrillation**: irregular rhythm
- Flutter usually goes back into sinus rhythm or deteriorates into fibrillation.

The anatomic cardiac defects dilating the atrium in A-fib do not go away with cardioversion; that is why the vast majority revert. Many patients with acute A-fib from alcohol, caffeine, cocaine, or transient ischemia will simply convert back to sinus rhythm on their own. Hence, acute disease normalizes spontaneously; don't force it. Chronic disease reverts into the arrhythmia. Don't force it either.

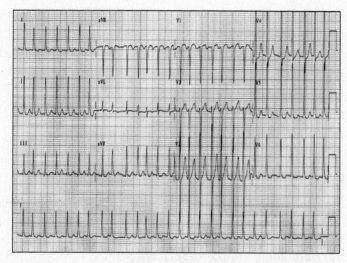

Figure 13.7 Atrial Fibrillation with an Irregularly Irregular Rhythm.
Source: Abhay Vakil, MD

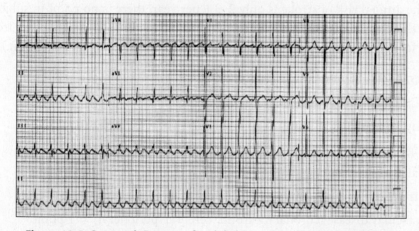

Figure 13.8 Sawtooth Pattern of Atrial Flutter. *Source: Abhay Vakil, MD*

Treatment

Rate control and anticoagulation are the standard of care for A-fib.

- **Hemodynamically unstable atrial arrhythmia** is managed with synchronized cardioversion. Synchronization prevents electricity from being delivered during the refractory period (ST-T wave). Synchronization helps prevent deterioration into VT or VF. Hemodynamic instability is defined as it is for VT: hypotension, confusion, CHF, and chest pain.

- **Chronic A-fib** (lasting >2 days): It takes several days for a clot to form. Routine cardioversion is not indicated. The majority of those who are converted into sinus rhythm will not stay in sinus.

  - Shocking the patient into sinus rhythm does not correct a dilated left atrium. Over 90% will revert to fibrillation even with the use of antiarrhythmic medication.

Unstable, acute disease does not need anticoagulation before cardioversion.

> - Rate control drugs do not convert the patient into sinus rhythm.
> - No matter how much you might think it better to shock every patient into sinus, it just does not work in the long run.

> **Heparin** is **not necessary** before starting a patient on warfarin for A-fib.

> Normally the atrium contributes 10–15% to cardiac output. In a diseased heart, this rises to 30–50%.

> Compared with warfarin, NOACs have better efficacy and fewer adverse effects.

- The best initial therapy for fibrillation and flutter is rate control with BBs, CCBs, or digoxin. Once the rate <100/minute, give dabigatran, rivaroxaban, edoxaban, or apixaban (NOAC). Warfarin is used with metal valves or mitral stenosis. Slow the rate. Then, anticoagulate.
- Dabigatran, rivaroxaban, apixaban, edoxaban, warfarin
  - Without anticoagulation, there will be ~6 embolic strokes per year for every 100 patients with A-fib (6% a year).
  - When INR is maintained at 2–3, the rate is 2–3% a year.
  - NOACs prevent stroke and need no INR monitoring.

The CCBs used to control heart rate with atrial arrhythmias are diltiazem and verapamil. These reliably block the AV node. The other CCBs control BP.

"Lone" Atrial Fibrillation: CHADS-VASc Score ≤1

Patients with a low risk of stroke can have their strokes safely prevented using aspirin alone, without warfarin, dabigatran, or rivaroxaban as an anticoagulant. If the annual risk of stroke is only 2–3% per year, there is no point in subjecting these patients to the 1% a year risk of major bleeding. (*Major bleeding* from warfarin is defined as intracranial hemorrhage or requiring a transfusion.)

CHADS-VASc Score

C: CHF or cardiomyopathy = 1 point

H: hypertension = 1 point

A: age >75 = 2 points

D: diabetes = 1 point

S: stroke or TIA = 2 points

V: vascular disease (coronary, carotid, cerebral, peripheral) = 1 point

A: age 65–74 = 1 point

Sc: sex category (female) = 1 point

When CHADS-VASc score is ≤1, use aspirin.

When CHADS-VASc score is ≥2, use a NOAC or warfarin. Warfarin causes more bleeding than NOACs. NOACs prevent more strokes than warfarin.

Agents to Reverse Anticoagulation

- Adexanet alfa reverses rivaroxaban, apixaban, and edoxaban.
- Idarucizumab reverses dabigatran.
- Prothrombin complex concentrate (PCC) reverses warfarin.

Supraventricular Tachycardia

Supraventricular tachycardia (SVT) presents with palpitations in a patient who is usually hemodynamically stable (based on reentry around the AV node). The **best initial therapy** is:

1. Vagal maneuvers (e.g., carotid massage, Valsalva, dive reflex, ice immersion)

2. If no response to vagal maneuvers, give adenosine

3. If no response to adenosine, give BBs (metoprolol), CCBs (diltiazem), or digoxin

Radiofrequency catheter ablation is curable in many cases.

> Vagal maneuvers both slow and convert SVT. They do not convert A-fib.

▶ TIP

Adenosine is used only therapeutically for SVT.

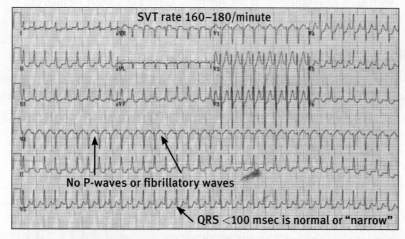

Figure 13.9 Supraventricular tachycardia (SVT) is a narrow complex tachycardia without P waves, fibrillatory waves, or flutter waves. *Source: Abhay Vakil, MD*

Wolff-Parkinson-White Syndrome

Wolff-Parkinson-White syndrome (WPW) is an anatomic abnormality in the cardiac conduction pathway. You answer the "most likely diagnosis" question by looking for:

- SVT alternating with ventricular tachycardia
- SVT that gets worse after diltiazem or digoxin
- Observing the delta wave on the EKG

Cardiac electrophysiology (EP) studies are the **most accurate test**.

Treatment is as follows:

- **Acute disease**: procainamide or amiodarone for both atrial and ventricular rhythm disturbances; use only if an arrhythmia accompanies the WPW
- **Chronic disease**: radiofrequency catheter ablation (curative for WPW), where a heated catheter tip ablates/eliminates the abnormal conduction tract around the AV node (EP studies reveal the location of the anatomic defect)

Digoxin and CCBs are dangerous in WPW. They block the normal AV node and force conduction into the abnormal pathway.

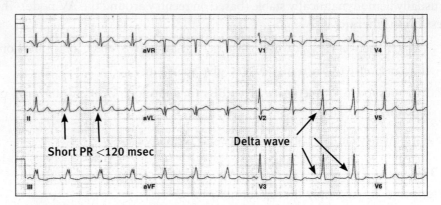

Figure 13.10 Wolff-Parkinson-White syndrome, a preexcitation syndrome with early depolarization of the ventricle, results in a short PR interval.
Source: Juan Marcos Velasquez, MD

Multifocal Atrial Tachycardia

Multifocal atrial tachycardia (MAT) is associated with chronic lung disease such as COPD. Treat the underlying lung disease. Treat MAT as you would A-fib, but avoid beta blockers because of the lung disease.

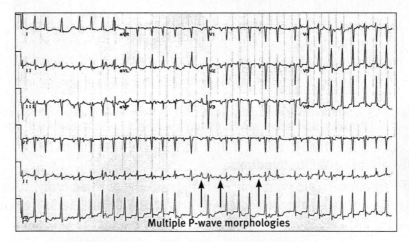

Figure 13.11 MAT has at least 3 P-wave morphologies and is associated with COPD. *Source: Abhay Vakil, MD*

Bradycardia and AV Block

A woman comes to the office for routine evaluation. She is found to have a pulse 40/min and an otherwise completely normal history and physical examination. What is the most appropriate next step in management?

a. Atropine

b. Pacemaker

c. EKG

d. Electrophysiology studies

e. Epinephrine

f. Isoproterenol

g. Nothing; reassurance

Answer: **C.** Bradycardia is common. A normal heart rate is 60–100 bpm, but some people just normally have a heart rate <60 bpm. Bradycardia can also be the initial presentation of third-degree or "complete" heart block. EKG is mandatory to distinguish the cause of bradycardia. The most common wrong answer is "do nothing." If you confirm that this is an asymptomatic sinus bradycardia, then the answer is "reassurance" or "do nothing." Atropine is the answer for an acutely symptomatic patient with signs of hypoperfusion. Pacemaker is used for all patients with third-degree AV block. Epinephrine is dangerous, especially since ischemia is such a common cause of bradycardia. Isoproterenol is an old, rarely used nonspecific beta agonist that speeds up the heart rate but increases ischemia.

▶ **TIP**

Isoproterenol is never the right answer to anything.

Sinus Bradycardia

If asymptomatic, no treatment is needed—no matter how low the heart rate. If symptomatic, atropine is the **best initial therapy**, and a pacemaker is the **most effective therapy**.

First-Degree AV block

Treatment is the same as for sinus bradycardia.

Second-Degree AV block

- **Mobitz I**, or Wenckebach block, is a progressively lengthening PR interval that results in a "dropped" beat. It is most often a sign of normal aging of the conduction system. If asymptomatic, no treatment is needed.
- **Mobitz II** second-degree AV block is far more pathologic than Mobitz I. Mobitz II just drops a beat without the progressive lengthening of the PR interval. Mobitz II progresses, or deteriorates into third-degree AV block. Treat it like third-degree AV block. Treatment for all cases of Mobitz II block is a pacemaker, even if asymptomatic.

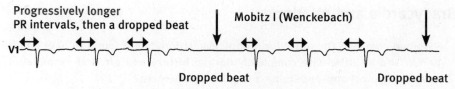

Figure 13.12 Mobitz I (Wenckebach) block is a benign sign of the aging of the conduction system. *Source: Abhay Vakil, MD*

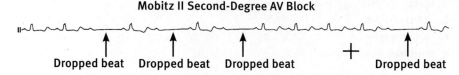

Figure 13.13 Mobitz II Block. *Source: Abhay Vakil, MD*

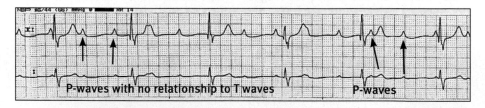

Figure 13.14 Third-Degree or Complete Heart Block. The P-waves and T-waves have no fixed relationship to each other. *Source: Nishith Patel, MD*

Arrhythmia Bonus Questions

A 58-year-old woman is admitted to the hospital with an acute myocardial infarction. On hospital day 2, she develops sustained ventricular tachycardia even though she is on aspirin, heparin, lisinopril, and metoprolol. What is the most appropriate next step in management?

a. Increase the dose of metoprolol
b. Add diltiazem
c. Angiography for angioplasty or bypass
d. Implantable defibrillator
e. EP studies

Answer: **C.** The most common cause of death in the 72 hours surrounding an acute myocardial infarction is a ventricular arrhythmia. Manage arrhythmias from ischemia by correcting the ischemia. Don't put in an implantable defibrillator for an arrhythmia you can prevent or fix by eliminating the cause.

Which of the following tests would you do for this patient to determine a risk of recurrence?

a. EP studies
b. Echocardiography
c. MUGA scan (nuclear ventriculography)
d. Ventilation/perfusion scan
e. Tilt-table testing

Answer: **B.** Left ventricular function is the most important correlate of the risk of recurrence. Although nuclear ventriculography is more accurate, you would never do this test first or before you had done an echocardiogram. Tilt-table testing assesses orthostasis and autonomic instability. Tilt-table testing is done to evaluate syncope of unclear etiology, particularly when there are signs of postural instability. EP studies are used when you are not certain of the diagnosis. EP studies are done if there are short runs or ventricular tachycardia or unexplained syncope and you want to see if you can induce sustained ventricular tachycardia. If the echo shows a normal ejection fraction, her risk of recurrence of ventricular arrhythmia is small.

A 73-year-old man has his third syncopal episode in the last 6 months. An EKG done in the field shows ventricular tachycardia. Stress test is normal. What is the most appropriate next step in management?

a. Metoprolol
b. Diltiazem
c. Angiography
d. Implantable defibrillator
e. EP studies

Answer: **D.** There is no point in doing an EP study when the EKG shows a clear etiology of the syncope. We already know he has an unprovoked ventricular rhythm disorder. Metoprolol is not sufficient when syncope or sudden death has occurred. Calcium channel blockers like diltiazem are useless in preventing or treating ventricular tachycardia. The stress test is normal and there is no chest pain, so there is no point in doing angiography. An implantable defibrillator will prevent the next episode of sudden death or syncope.

A 46-year-old man has intermittent episodes of palpitations, lightheadedness, and near-syncope. His EKG is normal. The echo shows an ejection fraction of 42%. Holter monitor shows several runs of wide complex tachycardia lasting 5–10 seconds. Which of the following will most benefit him?

a. Pacemaker placement
b. Digoxin
c. Warfarin
d. EP studies
e. Swan-Ganz catheter

Answer: **D.** EP studies are useful in detecting a source of ventricular arrhythmia. If you can readily induce sustained ventricular tachycardia, this person would benefit from an implantable defibrillator. He may have episodes of sustained ventricular tachycardia causing his symptoms that have not been detected by the Holter monitor. Digoxin is useless for ventricular arrhythmias. Swan-Ganz is a right heart catheter that assesses intracardiac pressure and cardiac output.

PART 14

Ethics

Every human being of adult years and sound mind has the right to determine what shall be done with his own body; and a surgeon who performs an operation without his patient's consent commits an assault, for which he is liable in damages...except in cases of emergency where the patient is unconscious and where it is necessary to operate before consent can be obtained.

Justice Benjamin Cardozo, *Schloendorff v. Society of New York Hospital*, 211 NY 125, 105 NE 92 (1914)

This landmark decision states in one sentence the fundamental premise which underlies half the ethics questions on Step 2 CK of USMLE:

1. Autonomy
2. Adult
3. Capacity to understand

Autonomy

Patients have the sole right to determine what treatments they shall and shall not accept. Autonomy, ethically, is more important than beneficence. Beneficence, trying to do good for others, is generally a good thing—but trying to help someone is not as important as following her wishes.

> Patients have the right to refuse treatments that are good for them if they do not want them.

> A man has an ugly house that you offer to paint for free in his favorite color. Everyone on the neighborhood council agrees that the house is ugly and that what you are offering is clearly superior to what he has. The man would have no financial or other obligation in exchange. He understands everything you are offering, including the clear benefit to him. The man still refuses. What do you do?
>
> a. Honor the man's wishes: no paint job.
> b. Paint his house against his will.
> c. Ask the neighborhood council to consent to the paint job.
> d. Get a psychiatric evaluation on the man.
> e. Get a court order to allow the paint job.
> f. Ask his family for consent to the paint job.
> g. Wait until he is out of town, then paint his house.

Answer: **A.** This seemingly silly example will allow you to answer the majority of questions. Cost and benefit and the common good are not as important as the autonomy individuals have to just do what they want with their own property. A community board is like an ethics committee. You cannot wait until a person loses consciousness or is sedated to then perform the test or treatment.

A man comes to the ED after a car accident caused his spleen to rupture. At present, he is still fully conscious. He understands that he will die without splenectomy, and that he will live if he has the splenectomy. He refuses the repair and refuses blood transfusion. His whole family is present, including his brother, who is the healthcare proxy. The family and the proxy—both the agent (the person) and the document completed only a few weeks ago—clearly state, "Everything possible should be done, including surgery." What do you do?

a. Honor his current wishes: no surgery.
b. Wait until he loses consciousness, then perform the surgery.
c. Request a psychiatric consultation.
d. Refer to the ethics committee.
e. Request an emergency court order.
f. Follow what is written in the documented health-care proxy.
g. See if there is consensus from the family.

Answer: **A.** You must follow the last known wishes of the patient, even if they are verbal, and even if they contradict the written proxy. You cannot wait until his consciousness is lost, then go against his wishes. The family cannot go against his clearly stated wishes, even if the whole family is in agreement. The proxy cannot go against his wishes. There is no need for a psychiatric consultation if it is clear that the patient has the capacity to understand the problem and the consequences of refusing treatment. A court order or ethics committee cannot contradict an adult with capacity to understand. If a patient writes one thing and 10 minutes later changes his mind, you go with whatever the last clear wishes are.

Advance Directives

Advance directives tell the caregivers the parameters of care that the patient wanted. The agent is the person designated by the patient to carry out the patient's wishes. This term is sometimes used interchangeably with healthcare proxy. The healthcare proxy is the written document outlining the parameters of care. The major problem with the proxy is that the details of care are often not clear. It is not helpful to just say, "No heroic measures." In order to be useful, the document must specifically state, "No intubation, no CPR, no chemotherapy, no dialysis." The proxy can also specifically state wishes about fluid and nutrition. If the proxy says, "No nasogastric tube, no artificial feeding," then it is useful.

The healthcare proxy takes effect only when the patient has lost the capacity to make decisions.

Order of Decision Making

1. **A patient with capacity supersedes all else.**
2. **Healthcare proxy that includes an agent (person) to carry out wishes**

3. **Living will**: The living will is a document outlining a patient's wishes. A document clearly stating, "I never want dialysis" is more valid than a family member or friend saying, "From what I know about him, he would not want dialysis," or "He told me he never wants dialysis." **Advance directives are a matter of documentation**. A written living will that makes concrete statements such as "I never want blood transfusion or chemotherapy" is valid.

4. **Persons clearly familiar with the patient's wishes.** The problem with this is one of documentation. If the patient loses capacity, it is difficult for a friend to document that she knew the patient's wishes better than the family. If the case clearly states that a friend knows and can prove that she knew the patient's wishes, then this is the plan of care that is followed.

5. **Family.** In general, the order of decision making starts with a spouse. If there is no spouse, then it goes to adult children, then parents, then siblings. Unlike life, USMLE Step 2 CK must provide clear circumstances in order to know what to do. If the family is split, then the answer is an ethics committee or court order.

Ethics Committee

The ethics committee is important when a patient has lost capacity to make decisions and the advance directive is missing or unclear. The ethics committee is also important on issues of medical futility. This is when the patient or healthcare proxy is asking for tests and treatments that may have no benefit.

Court Order

The court order is important when the patient has no capacity to understand and the family is in disagreement. It is like a house being left equally to four children who cannot agree what to do with it. Examples of when court order is the right answer:

- A patient has no capacity and no proxy; his family is split about whether to continue care.
- Caregivers want to withdraw care and the ethics committee cannot reach a conclusion.

Psychiatric Evaluation of the Patient

A psychiatric consult is important when it is **not clear** if the patient has capacity to understand. If the question clearly states that the patient has capacity to understand, a psychiatric evaluation is not necessary. If the patient is clearly delirious or psychotic, psychiatric evaluation is not necessary.

Minors

Minors do not have decision-making capacity. They cannot consent to or refuse medical treatments. Only the parents or legal guardian can consent and refuse. Exceptions are contraception, prenatal care, substance abuse treatment, and sexually transmitted diseases (STDs) including HIV/AIDS.

Abortion

The states are split on parental notification laws. Some require it, and some don't. Your answer will be something like "Tell the minor patient to notify her parents."

Brain Death

Brain death is considered death in our legal system. If the patient is brain dead, you do not need consent to stop therapy such as mechanical ventilation or antibiotics. Court order and ethics committee are not correct answers.

▶ **TIP**

USMLE Step 2 CK will want you to discuss, educate, explain, and confer before everything else.

Consent

Only an adult can consent to procedures, and each procedure needs individual consent. Consent is implied in an emergency. The person doing the procedure must obtain consent. Adverse effects of a procedure must be explained to make the consent valid and the consequences of refusing a procedure must be explained to make the consent valid. Pregnant women can refuse procedures and treatments for their unborn children. Telephone consent is valid.

A patient signs consent for an ovarian biopsy on the left side. At surgery, you find cancer of the right side. What do you do?

- Wake the patient up and obtain consent to remove the ovary on the right side.

A patient needs a colonoscopy. The gastroenterologist asks you to obtain consent for the procedure. What do you do?

- Do not agree to obtain the patient's consent. The gastroenterologist who will perform the procedure needs to obtain consent.

For consent to be valid, the person who performs the procedure must obtain the consent. Consider: Do you know all the complications of the procedure and the alternatives? If you do not explain the possibility of perforation because you are unfamiliar with it, the consent is not valid. Do you know that sigmoidoscopy or barium enema are alternatives? If the patient's colon perforates and you did not explain alternate procedures, the consent is not valid.

Do Not Resuscitate Orders

Do not resuscitate (DNR) orders refer only to withholding cardiopulmonary resuscitation. They do not refer to withholding any other form of therapy.

A patient with capacity consents to DNR before losing consciousness. She needs a surgical procedure, but the surgeon refuses because the patient is DNR. What do you do?

- Perform the surgery. DNR does not mean withholding antibiotics, chemotherapy, or surgery. DNR means only that, if the patient dies, you will not attempt resuscitation.

Physician-Assisted Suicide

Physician-assisted suicide is always a wrong answer. This includes states in which it is legal to do so. Ethical requirements for physicians supersede legality. Physician-assisted suicide is administered by the patient, but this is still unethical for the physician.

Euthanasia

Euthanasia is the physician administering treatment intended to end or shorten the life of the patient. It is always wrong.

Terminal Sedation and Law of Double Effect

It is acceptable to administer pain medication even if there is the possibility of the treatment shortening the patient's life. For example, it is acceptable to give pain medications to a person with COPD who has metastatic cancer even if the only way to relieve pain is to give enough opiates that breathing may be impaired, causing the patient to die earlier.

The question is one of intent: If the medications are given with the intent to relieve pain, and as an adverse effect they shorten life, it is ethical. If the primary intent is to shorten life, it is unethical.

Futile Care

A physician is not obligated to render care that is futile even if the family or patient wants it. If a patient is brain dead and the family insists that you continue mechanical ventilation, you are under no obligation to do so. You are under no obligation to perform tests and treatments you consider worthless.

> Physician ethics come before legal requirements. You cannot do something unethical even if it is legal at the moment.

Organ and Tissue Donation

Payment for organ donation is unacceptable; however, payment for renewable tissues such as sperm and eggs is acceptable.

Consent for Organ Donation

Only the organ donor network should ask for consent for the organs. It is an ethical conflict of interest for the physician to ask for consent for organ donation. The organ donor network also has fewer refusals than the physician. Organ donor cards give an indication of the patient's wishes, but the family can refuse organ donation even if the patient has an organ donor card.

Confidentiality

> Confidentiality is important, but not as important as protecting others from harm.

The patient's right to confidentiality **can be broken** when there is danger to others. Examples of ethically acceptable circumstances in which confidentiality can be broken are STDs, HIV/AIDS, airborne communicable diseases such as tuberculosis, and court orders demanding information.

The patient's right to confidentiality **cannot be broken** for employers, coworkers, government agencies, or family and friends.

> A patient with HIV/AIDS has repeatedly refused to disclose his HIV status to his sexual partner. The partner accompanies the patient to the office visits and is in the waiting room. The patient insists you not tell the partner. What do you do?
>
> a. Honor the patient's wishes.
> b. Obtain a court order.
> c. Consult the ethics committee.
> d. Notify the partner.
>
> Answer: **D.** You have the right either to notify the partner or to disclose the patient's HIV status to the health department so that they can notify the partner. Maintaining the confidentiality of the patient is not as important as protecting the health of the partner.

> HIV-positive healthcare workers do **not** have to disclose their status to their patients or their employers.

A woman comes to your office with valid identification from a government agency that works in law enforcement. She requests a copy of your patient's medical records. What do you do?

- Refuse unless she also presents a valid court-issued warrant or subpoena.

You are to provide health-related protected records to government agencies, including those from law enforcement, only if they have a valid warrant or subpoena from the courts. To do otherwise would be a violation of the constitutional protection against illegal search and seizure of property. This would also constitute a violation of HIPAA, which is designed to protect health information.

Doctor/Patient Relationship

A physician is not obligated to accept everyone as a patient. The physician has the right to end the doctor/patient relationship but must give the patient sufficient time to obtain another caregiver. Small gifts from patients are acceptable as long as they are not tied to a specific treatment request. Romantic or sexual contact between patients and their current physicians is never acceptable.

Gifts from Industry

Unlike a small gift from a patient, gifts from industry such as drug companies are never acceptable. Even small items from industry such as pens, penlights, pads, and cups are unacceptable. Meals in direct association with educational activities are not considered gifts.

Doctor and Society

Elder Abuse

You can report elder abuse against the consent of the patient. This is based on the concept that abused older adults may be too weak, fragile, or vulnerable to protect themselves or remove themselves from an environment of potential harm. Elder abuse is treated ethically like child abuse.

Domestic Violence and Spousal Abuse

Unlike child abuse, domestic abuse **cannot be reported** against the patient's wishes. You can report and intervene only with the consent of the patient.

Impaired Drivers (Seizure Disorders and Driving)

This is one of the least clear areas nationally, and the states have no uniformity of laws. You must answer "suggest that the patient find another means of transportation." Wrong answers would be:

- Confiscating car keys and reporting to law enforcement
- Hospitalizing the patient
- Refusing to let the patient get in her car

Execution of Prisoners

It is never ethical for a physician to participate in executions at any level. You cannot ethically formulate a lethal injection or even do so much as pronounce a prisoner dead. Even if state law makes execution legal, you as a physician are not to participate at any level.

Torture

Physicians are **never** to participate in the torture of prisoners or detainees. Even if the question states that you are in the military, your ethical obligation as a physician supersedes your obligation to the military. This would include:

- Refusing orders from military superiors to participate in torture
- Keeping the torture "safe" so that it is not fatal or damaging

The ethics questions on torture are easy to answer because your answer is "no" to any level of involvement, even if you are a military physician in a legal war zone whose role is simply to protect the patient against permanent harm.

> Torture is the ethical equivalent of child abuse. Your participation is never acceptable; you are obligated only to report it.

PART 15

Biostatistics and Epidemiology

Sensitivity and Specificity

Sensitivity and specificity are qualities of diagnostic tests. The sensitivity and specificity of a test does not change based on the prevalence or rate of a disease in a community.

Sensitivity

Sensitivity is the likelihood that a test will detect all the people with the disease.

- A sensitive test means all the people with a disease should test positive.
- A sensitive test means a negative result excludes that disease in a population.
- In a perfectly sensitive test, there will be no false negatives.
- With a sensitive test, a negative result rules a disease out.
- Sensitive: If you have the disease, will you have a positive test?
- Sensitivity $= \dfrac{TP}{TP + FN}$

Specificity

Specificity is the likelihood that people without a disease are correctly identified as disease-negative.

- A specific test means that those with no disease will have a negative test.
- A specific test means that all the people with a positive test will have the disease.
- A positive specific test means a person really has the disease.
- In a perfectly specific test, there will be no false positives.
- With a specific test, a positive result rules a disease in.
- Specific: If you DON'T have the disease, will you have a negative test?
- Specificity $= \dfrac{TN}{TN + FP}$

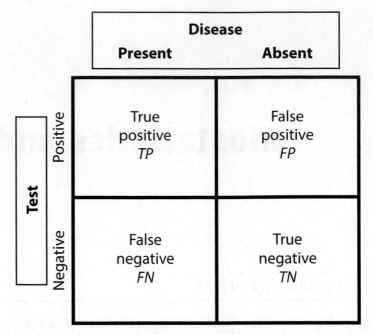

Figure 15.1 Sensitivity and Specificity. © Kaplan

Negative and Positive Predictive Values

Negative predictive value (NPV) and positive predictive value (PPV) vary based on the prevalence of a disease in a community or population. NPV and PPV start with the test.

- **NPV**: If you have a negative test, what is the likelihood you really DON'T have the disease?
- **PPV**: If you have a positive test, what is the likelihood you really DO have the disease?
- **Sensitivity**: If you have the disease, what is the likelihood you will have a positive test?
- **Specificity**: If you DON'T have the disease, what is the likelihood you will have a negative test?

The greater the prevalence of a disease, the greater the PPV. The lesser the prevalence of a disease, the greater the NPV.

Absolute and Relative Risk Reduction

Absolute risk reduction (ARR) is the percentage decrease in the risk of death or disease from a treatment compared with 100% of the people in a population.

For example, for every 100 angioplasty procedures performed, one person has major bleeding leading to death. The rate, or attributable risk (AR), of fatal complications of angioplasty is 1%, or 0.01. This means that for every 100 people we treat, we harm one person. The AR is thus 1%, or 0.01. The number needed to harm (NNH) is $\dfrac{1}{AR}$ or $\dfrac{1}{0.01} = 100$.

Relative risk reduction (RRR) always seems to be a much larger number. RRR can be used to exaggerate the effectiveness of medications. For example, in patients without heart disease with high LDL levels, the use of statin medications may reduce mortality. Going from 3% mortality to 2% mortality is a reduction of 33%. And thus the benefit of statin medications in those without coronary disease or diabetes can be exaggerated by saying "Statins result in a 33% reduction in mortality." Yes, there is a 33% RRR in mortality, but only 1% ARR. On the other hand, the risk of serious liver toxicity is 3% at the least. So, the number needed to harm someone from a statin is 33. The number needed to treat is 100.

Standard Deviation (SD)

- Critical concept for understanding sets of data
- A must-know fact for Step 2 CK
- One SD above the mean indicates that your score is better than 84% of test takers.

The SD for Step 2 is 18 points. You would have to score a 258 (mean of 240 + 18) to be better than 84% of test takers.

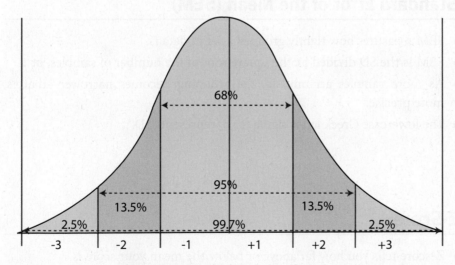

Figure 15.2 Standard Deviation. © Kaplan

When data is normally distributed:

- 1 SD = 68% of scores
- 2 SD = 95% of scores
- 3 SD = 99.7% of scores

Following is a graphical representation of the effect of SD on grouping of data around the mean. The tallest line on the graph shows the smallest SD. This is because the data clusters around the center point, as dictated by the central limit theorem: When you collect more data, it tends to collect around the center of the graph.

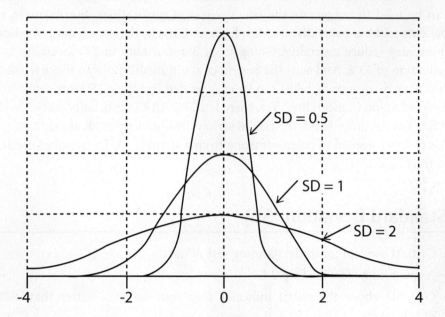

Figure 15.3 Effect of SD on the Mean. © Kaplan

Standard Error of the Mean (SEM)

- SEM measures how tightly grouped a set of data is.
- SEM is the SD divided by the square root of the number of samples, or *n*.
- As more samples accumulate, the grouping becomes narrower—that is, more precise.
- The lowercase Greek letter sigma, or σ, represents SD.

$$\sigma_x = \frac{\sigma}{\sqrt{n}}$$

Z-Score

- Z-score tells you how far above or below the mean your score is.
- One SD above the mean is a Z-score of 1.0; one SD below the mean is also a Z-score of −1.
- Two SDs above the mean is a Z-score of 2.0.

Confidence Intervals

- Confidence intervals (CIs) assess the precision of a collection of data.
- CI records whether data points are centralized around the mean, or scattered.
- More scatter means less precision.
- When the CI crosses 1, it means that the results are not significant: They are not precise enough to be useful. (For instance, if the CI is 0.5 to 1.5, the study has no validity.)

The 95% CI that is used is basically 2 times SEM. SEM is equal to SD divided by the square root of *n*, or the number of measurements. In order to double the precision of the test, you must increase the sample size by *4 times*. This is because you are dividing by a square root.

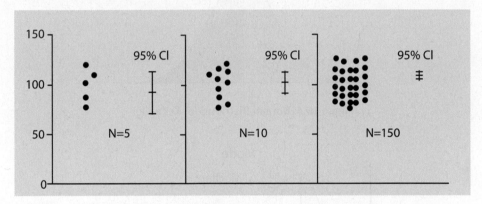

Figure 15.4 Confidence Intervals. © Kaplan

Descriptive Statistics

Mode

- The most frequently appearing measurement in a set of data points
- Example: In 1, 2, 3, 4, 8, 8, 8, 20, 100, the **mode** is 8 because it is the most frequent measurement.

Mean

- The average of all the data points in a data collection
- Example: In 1, 2, 3, 4, 8, 8, 8, 20, 100, the **mean**, or average, is 17.
- Take the sum of the data collection (154) and divide it by the number of data points (9) to calculate the mean (17).

Median

- The data point halfway between the highest and lowest in the collection of measurements
- In the data set above, the **median** is 8 (which is the 5th of 9 data points—exactly in the middle).
- Corrects for outliers in data sets

In a normal distribution of data points, the mean (average), mode (most frequent measurement), and median (data point in the middle) are the same.

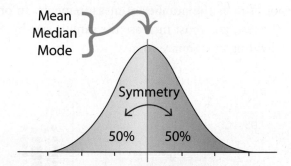

Figure 15.5 Normal Distribution. © Kaplan

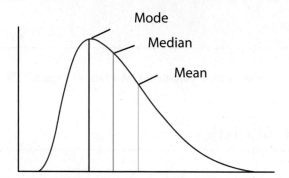

Figure 15.6 Right-Skewed Distribution. © Kaplan

Epidemiology Terms

Incidence

- The rate at which new diseases occur
- Measured in new numbers of cases per unit of time
- Medical therapies that lower mortality *do not change the incidence* of the disease.

Prevalence

- The number of total cases of a disease in a population
- A reduction in mortality *increases the prevalence.*

Precision, Accuracy, and Reliability

Precision

- Measurements are immune from randomness.
- Data points cluster around one point.
- The opposite of scattered or spread out

Accuracy

- The combination of sensitivity and specificity
- Equivalent to validity; if something is true, it is accurate.
- "Gold standard" refers to the most accurate test.

Reliability

- Reproducibility: If you repeat the measurements, they will come out the same again and again.
- The opposite of drift
- Not necessarily accurate: You can also have something come out reliably wrong.

Assessing Data for More Than One group

Correlation Coefficient (r)

- Gives a numerical value to the level of connection or correlation between two variables or two groups.
- In a very strong correlation: value is $+1$
- In a very strong *inverse* correlation: value is -1
- No correlation: value is 0

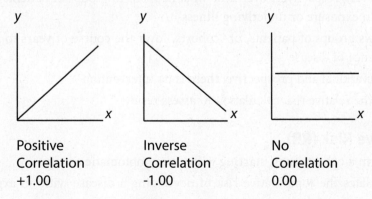

Figure 15.7 Correlation Coefficient Variation. © Kaplan

T-Test (T-Score) and Analysis of Variance (ANOVA)

- Two measures that assess groups of data from different data sets
- T-test is used when there are 2 groups of data to assess.
- ANOVA is used when there are 3 or more groups of data to assess.
- Both t-test and ANOVA can assess more irregular data (data sets that are not in a normal or bell-shaped, Gaussian distribution).
- Also used when only a sample of measurements is known, and not all the values in an entire population
- T-test answers the question: "Are the means between these groups different?"

Chi-Square Test

- Compares multiple groups for statistical difference
- Used when data is in discrete categories
- Answers the question: "Are these groups related (or not)?"

Study Design and Analysis of Results

Randomized Controlled Trial (RCT)

- Most accurate type of study
- Samples are sorted into different arms of the study by a computer or a randomly generated list of assignments.
- Avoids selection bias
- Prospective trial
- If clear harm or clear benefit is evident before the end, the study is stopped by an independent data monitoring group.

Cohort Study

- Observes prospectively over time what happens to groups of patients with a certain exposure or underlying illness
- Follows groups of patients, or "cohorts," over the course of years to record incidence of disease
- Observational and prospective; there is no intervention
- Uses the relative risk calculation to assess results

Relative Risk (RR)

- Used in a cohort study, starting with an asymptomatic group
- Calculates the comparative risk of developing a disease with an exposure versus without the exposure

Case Control Study

- Retrospectively views data looking for the odds of a previous exposure on the development of a rare disease manifestation
- Starts with people who have a disease and looks backward at other groups that are otherwise matched, to assess for risks of exposure
- Subject to recall bias

Odds Ratio

- Assesses case control studies
- Starts with those who have a disease and looks for the chance of past exposure

Types of Bias

Selection Bias

- Uses less-ill patients for the drug end of the trial and sicker patients for the placebo side
- Makes the drug look more successful

Berkson Bias

- Uses hospitalized patients instead of selecting from the general population
- Solved by random selection

Hawthorne Effect

- Study subjects know they are being watched for the effect of a drug or intervention.
- Solved by a placebo control and blinding both the investigator and the participants

Lead-Time Bias

- Confuses early detection with increased survival based on treatment
- Can make screening look like a benefit based on early detection of minor disease

Type I and Type II Error

Type I error is a false positive result. It is when a drug or test is said to make a difference when it really doesn't. The other name for type I error is **alpha error**.

Type I error means:

- Rejecting the null hypothesis when it really is true.
- Saying the new drug works when it really doesn't.
- Saying there is a statistically significant difference in the data when there really isn't.

Type II error is a false negative result. The drug or test is great, but the report says it isn't. The other name for type II error is **beta error**.

Type II error means:

- Saying the drug does not work, when it really does.
- Incorrectly concluding that the drug is ineffective.

PART 16

Patient Safety

by Niket Sonpal, MD

Medical Errors

Medical errors are unintended acts or omissions with the potential to harm patients. The most commonly tested point regarding medical errors on the USMLE is the physician's responsibility to inform the patient: Patients should be made aware of all medical errors regardless of whether there was an adverse outcome. Regular reporting of errors strengthens the patient's ability to make informed decisions, promotes trust, and reduces stress for the patient.

Preventing Falls in the Elderly

A fall in an elderly person is far more deadly than an MI. The only clearly proven treatment is strength training and exercise.

- Screen for visual problems and removing objects in the home.
- Prescribe exercise such as walking, yoga, tai chi, dance, or weight training.

Breaking Bad News

Breaking bad news is a difficult but essential physician responsibility. Deliver bad news with the SPIKES protocol, a practical approach that follows 6 sequential steps:

Step 1: **S**ETTING up the interview. Arrange an appropriate environment, with privacy and without interruptions.

Step 2: Assess the patient's **P**ERCEPTION. Find out how much the patient knows and gauge how far her understanding is from the truth you have to tell.

Step 3: Obtain the patient's **I**NVITATION. Before you proceed, find out how much the patient wants to know.

Step 4: Give **KNOWLEDGE** and information to patient. Respond to his needs for clarification, but follow your agenda of points to impart.

Step 5: Address the patient's **EMOTIONS** with empathic responses. Respond to the patient's feelings; do not argue.

Step 6: **STRATEGY** and **SUMMARY**. Demonstrate an understanding of the patient's concerns, and offer possible plans for the future.

Health Care–Associated Infections

Catheter-Associated Urinary Tract Infections (CAUTI)

CAUTI is the **most common** type of health care-associated infection and the leading cause of nosocomial bacteremia. The diagnosis of CAUTI is made when a patient has catheter-related bacteriuria combined with fever, suprapubic tenderness, costovertebral angle tenderness, and evidence of a systemic inflammatory response syndrome.

> Prophylactic antibiotics have no role in the prevention of CAUTI.

The **most accurate test** is UA with WBCs and urine culture. Treatment involves prompt removal of the catheter and antibiotics.

How is CAUTI prevented?

- Early removal of the catheter has been shown to reduce the risk of CAUTI.

How should a patient's long-term indwelling bladder catheterization be managed?

- Do intermittent catheterization.

Central Line-Associated Bloodstream Infection (CLABSI)

All catheters can introduce bacteria into the bloodstream. If a patient with a central line develops signs of infection, blood cultures are taken from a peripheral vein. If the cultures yield the same organisms, the central line should be removed and antibiotics should be started.

> **Most common CLABSI bugs:**
>
> *S. aureus*, coagulase-negative *staphylococci* or *Candida* species

When should I start antibiotics?

- Start antibiotics immediately after blood cultures are obtained and change the antibiotic as needed based on organismal sensitivities.

Pressure-Induced Skin Injuries

Pressure-induced skin injuries (or "bedsores") are localized areas of damage to the skin and underlying tissue, usually over a bony prominence. They arise as a result of chronic immobility. The table outlines how the severity of pressure-induced skin injuries is staged.

Stage	Description
1	• Skin intact • Nonblanchable redness remains >1 hour after pressure is relieved
2	• Blister or other break in the dermis • Partial-thickness loss of dermis • With or without infection
3	• Full-thickness tissue loss • Subcutaneous fat may be visible; destruction extends into muscle • With or without infection • Undermining and tunneling may be present
4	• Full-thickness skin loss • Involvement of bone, tendon, or joint • With or without infection • Undermining and tunneling often present
Unstageable	• Full-thickness tissue loss • Base of the ulcer covered by slough and/or eschar in the wound bed

The goal regarding pressure-induced skin injuries is prevention:

- Chronically immobile patients should be repositioned at least every 2 hours to relieve pressure on tissues.

- Nutritional intake should be optimized to promote wound healing.

- If necrotic tissue is seen, the next step in management should be wound debridement.

Complementary and Alternative Medicine

The USMLE wants you to know the most commonly taken herbal and nutritional supplements and their adverse effects. Be prepared to answer these favorite questions on Step 2 CK:

How do you know if a patient is taking a specific supplement?

- On each visit, the physician should review and reconcile with the patient all current medications (including prescription, OTC, and supplements) and should document them all in the medical record.

Should the patient take a specific supplement?

- The patient should discuss the risks and benefits of taking any supplement with the physician in an office-based setting.

Common Herbal and Nutritional Supplements				
Name	**Intended purpose**	**Adverse effects**	**Drug interactions**	**Effectiveness**
St. John's wort	Treatment of depression	Insomnia, anxiety, and vivid dreams	• Do not use with antidepressants • Induces CYP3A4	Inconsistent evidence for efficacy
Saw palmetto	Treatment of BPH	Nausea	Bleeding with antiplatelet and anticoagulants	No more effective than placebo
Red yeast rice	Treatment of hyperlipidemia	Abnormal liver function tests and myalgias	• Induces CYP3A4 • Do not take with statins or fibrates	Does not appear to be effective
Milk thistle	Reduction of liver inflammation	Nausea and dyspepsia	Interacts with medications metabolized by CYP2C9 and CYP3A4	Does not appear to be effective
Ginseng	Immune system enhancement	Hypertension, diarrhea, and pruritus	Interacts with MAOIs and warfarin	Inconsistent evidence for efficacy
Ginkgo biloba	Improved cognition	Increased risk of bleeding	INH, NNRTI, and warfarin	Inconsistent evidence for efficacy
Echinacea	Treatment of URI	Unpleasant taste and GERD	None	Does not appear to be effective
Cranberry	Prevention of UTI	None	None	Does not appear to be effective
Black cohosh	Treatment of post-menopausal symptoms	Headache	None	Does not appear to be more effective than placebo

Index